Atlas of the Diabetic Foot

Atlas of the Diabetic Foot

Third Edition

Ioanna Eleftheriadou MD
Postdoctoral fellow in Internal Medicine and Diabetes, First Department of Propaedeutic Internal Medicine, National and Kapodistrian University of Athens, Medical School, Laiko General Hospital, Athens, Greece

Alexandros Kokkinos MD
Associate Professor in Internal Medicine, First Department of Propaedeutic Internal Medicine, National and Kapodistrian University of Athens, Medical School, Laiko General Hospital, Athens, Greece

Stavros Liatis MD
Consultant in Internal Medicine and Diabetology, First Department of Propaedeutic Internal Medicine, National and Kapodistrian University of Athens, Medical School, Laiko General Hospital, Athens, Greece

Konstantinos Makrilakis MD, MPH, PhD
Associate Professor in Internal Medicine, First Department of Propaedeutic Internal Medicine, National and Kapodistrian University of Athens, Medical School Laiko General Hospital, Athens, Greece

Nicholas Tentolouris MD
Professor in Internal Medicine, First Department of Propaedeutic Internal Medicine, National and Kapodistrian University of Athens, Medical School, Laiko General Hospital, Athens, Greece

Anastasios Tentolouris MD
Clinical and Research Fellow, First Department of Propaedeutic Internal Medicine, National and Kapodistrian University of Athens, Medical School, Laiko General Hospital, Athens, Greece

Panagiotis Tsapogas MD
Consultant in Internal Medicine and Diabetes Center for Diabetes and Metabolism, Henry Dunant Hospital Center, Athens, Greece

WILEY Blackwell

This edition first published 2019 © 2019 by John Wiley & Sons Ltd

Edition History [2e, 2010]

Registered Office(s)
John Wiley & Sons, Inc., 111 River Street, Hoboken, NJ 07030, USA
John Wiley & Sons Ltd, The Atrium, Southern Gate, Chichester, West Sussex, PO19 8SQ, UK

Editorial Office
9600 Garsington Road, Oxford, OX4 2DQ, UK

For details of our global editorial offices, customer services, and more information about Wiley products visit us at www.wiley.com.

Wiley also publishes its books in a variety of electronic formats and by print-on-demand. Some content that appears in standard print versions of this book may not be available in other formats.

Library of Congress Cataloging-in-Publication Data

Names: Eleftheriadou, Ioanna.
Title: Atlas of the diabetic foot / by Ioanna Eleftheriadou [and 6 others].
Description: Third edition. | Hoboken, NJ, USA : Wiley-Blackwell, 2018. |
Preceded by Atlas of the diabetic foot / Nicholas Katsilambros ... [et al.].
2nd ed. 2010. | Includes bibliographical references and index. |
Identifiers: LCCN 2018045739 (print) | LCCN 2018046128 (ebook) |
ISBN 9781119255284 (Adobe PDF) | ISBN 9781119255307 (ePub) | ISBN 9781119255239 (hardback)
Subjects: | MESH: Diabetic Foot | Atlases
Classification: LCC RC951 (ebook) | LCC RC951 (print) | NLM WK 17 | DDC 616.4/62–dc23
LC record available at https://lccn.loc.gov/2018045739

Cover Design: Wiley
Cover Images: © ChooChin/Shutterstock, © memorisz/Shutterstock, © Srisakorn/iStock.com, © MIRIAM MASLO/Getty Images

Set in 10/12pt Warnock by SPi Global, Pondicherry, India

10 9 8 7 6 5 4 3 2 1

Contents

Preface to the Third Edition

With this third edition, Nicholas Katsilambros has passed the responsibility for the continuation of this work to the present editors. We accepted the challenge with enthusiasm, subject to his willingness to continue as authors.

Despite advances in medicine, diabetic foot problems continue to be a major concern of every society in the world, even those with the best healthcare systems. As in the previous editions, the purpose of this publication is to offer the knowledge of understanding the basic mechanisms that lead to the appearance of ulcers, preventing and treating of diabetic foot problems by healthcare professionals aiming at reduction of amputations. For this purpose, in addition to theoretical knowledge, we describe actual cases of patients with various foot problems, the diagnostic approach, differential diagnosis, and treatment. The initial chapters describe epidemiology, pathophysiology, and classification of diabetic foot ulcers. Importance is given to the diagnosis of the main risk factors for the diabetic foot, namely diabetic neuropathy, peripheral arterial disease, and to the anatomic deformities of the lower extremities. One chapter is devoted to Charcot foot (neuro-osteoarthropathy) and one chapter to infections. In the following chapters we describe methods of prevention and ulcer healing. In addition, developments in technology help to learn better and to acquire medical skills. In this edition we include five videos demonstrating the methods of examination for diabetic neuropathy and peripheral arterial disease and methods of callus removal and debridement as well as offloading, including the way total contact cast is constructed.

We trust that the new edition of this book will make a real contribution to the understanding of the diabetic foot problems and will help colleagues to better address them.

On behalf of the authors

2018 *N. Tentolouris*

Preface to the Second Edition

It is no exaggeration to state that the new (second) edition of this book resulted from the marked success of the first edition. It must also be noted that the problems of the diabetic foot continue to be a major and very serious concern of every society in the world, even those with the best healthcare systems.

This new edition has been enriched with a relatively large number of representative pictures as well as new information. This work has been achieved through the enormous efforts of my colleagues, co-authors of the book, as well as through the technical help of the publisher.

On behalf of the authors

2010 *N. Katsilambros*

Preface to the First Edition

Diabetes mellitus is a common disease all over the world and its frequency is steadily increasing. The availability of a wide variety of treatment options results in improvement or even normalization of hyperglycemia as well as of the accompanying metabolic disorders. However, people with diabetes continue to suffer from the complications of the disease.

Diabetic foot-related problems occur frequently and may have serious consequences. Amputations at different anatomical levels are the most serious of them.

The present *Atlas* represents a systematic description of the many different foot lesions, which are often seen in diabetic patients. Each figure corresponds to a case treated in our Diabetes Centre in the Athens University Medical School. Our patients are evaluated and treated in collaboration with the Orthopedic Department as well as with other specialists depending upon individual needs. A short text, which follows each illustration, describes the history of the patient, the physical signs observed, the approach of treatment, and is followed by a short comment.

It is hoped that this *Atlas* will be of assistance, as a reference guide and a teaching instrument, not only to diabetologists and surgeons, but also to all doctors involved in the treatment of diabetic patients. This book might help them not only to recognize and to treat the diabetic foot lesions, but also to prevent them.

On behalf of the authors
N. Katsilambros

Acknowledgements

The writers of this *Atlas* express their thanks and gratitude to plastic surgeon Othon Papadopoulos, Professor Emeritus at the University of Athens, for his help with certain cases in his area of specialty. They also thank radiologist Dr. Constantine Revenas at the Laiko General Hospital in Athens for his help in the field of ultrasonography; Dr. Stamatia Georga, specialist in nuclear medicine at the Papageorgiou Hospital in Thessaloniki; radiologist Dr. Constantine Lymperopoulos at the George Gennimatas General Hospital of Athens for his help with the magnetic resonance imaging studies; Dr. Chara Loupa, specialist in Internal Medicine, Diabetes and Infectious Diseases at Amalia Fleming General Hospital, and radiologist Dr. Rania Efthimiadou of the Ygeia Hospital in Athens. We also thank Constantine Mazis, podiatrist at the Laiko General Hospital, and Maureen Bates, podiatrist at the King's College Hospital, UK who kindly helped with or provided the videos for this edition. We also thank Dr. Constantine Kyriakopoulos for his help in editing the videos.

The authors are grateful to the following colleagues for providing photographs: Professor Emeritus Christos Liapis of the University of Athens; Professor Emeritus Elias Bastounis of the University of Athens; Dr. Olympia Tzaida, pathologist at the Metaxa Cancer Hospital in Piraeus; and late Dr. Dimitris Voyatzoglou of the Amalia Fleming Hospital in Athens.

They also express their gratitude to nurse Georgia Markou, the soul of the outpatient Diabetic Foot Clinic, for her precious duty in maintaining proper functioning of the clinic and the patients' records. Many thanks are expressed to Katerina and Eleni Kapsimani for their precious help in providing shoes, insoles and plantar pressure measurement equipment for photographing.

Thanks must also go to the numerous doctors who have assisted the outpatient diabetic foot clinic, either as specialists in infectious diseases or orthopedics, or as scholars in the field of diabetes and the diabetic foot, as well as to the patients of the Diabetic Foot Clinic of the Laiko General Hospital in Athens, whose contribution was the most significant of all.

About the Companion Website

This book is accompanied by a companion website:

www.wiley.com/go/tentolouris/atlas_diabetic_foot

The website includes:

- Videos
- Downloadable images

1
Introduction

N. Tentolouris

First Department of Propaedeutic Internal Medicine, National and Kapodistrian University of Athens, Medical School, Laiko General Hospital, Athens, Greece

1.1 Definition

Diabetic foot is defined as the presence of infection, ulceration and/or destruction of deep tissues associated with neurologic abnormalities and various degrees of peripheral arterial disease (PAD) in the lower limb in patients with diabetes.

1.2 Epidemiology

The prevalence of foot ulceration in the general diabetic population is 4–10%, being lower (1.5–3.5%) in young and higher (5–10%) in older patients. The annual incidence of foot ulceration ranges from less than 1 to 3.6% among people with type 1 or type 2 diabetes. It is estimated that about 5% of patients with diabetes have a history of foot ulceration, whereas the lifetime risk for this complication today is between 19 and 34%. A selection of epidemiologic data on diabetic foot problems from large studies are summarized in Table 1.1. In a community-based study in the northwestern United Kingdom, the prevalence of active foot ulcers identified at screening among persons with diabetes was 1.7%, and the annual incidence was 2.2%. Higher annual incidence rates have been reported in specific populations: 6.0% among Medicare beneficiaries with diabetes, 5.0% among U.S. veterans with diabetes, and 6.3% in the global population of persons with diabetes.

There are ethnic differences in the prevalence of foot problems. Foot ulcers are more common in Caucasians than in Asian patients of the Indian subcontinent. This difference may be related to physical factors (a lower prevalence of limited joint mobility and lower plantar pressures in Asians) and to better foot care in certain religious groups such as Muslims. The risk for foot ulcers is higher in black, Native American and Hispanic American individuals in comparison to white Americans.

It is thought that foot ulcers are more common on the plantar aspect of the feet. However, clinic-based data from 10 European countries participating in the European Study Group on Diabetes and the Lower Extremity (EURODIALE) project showed that 48% of the ulcers affect the plantar aspect of the feet, while 58% are in non-plantar areas. Similar findings have been reported by other authors.

The majority (60–80%) of foot ulcers will heal, 10–15% will remain active, and 5–24% will end up in amputation within a period of 6–18 months after first evaluation. Based on outcome data in specialized tertiary centers, approximately 77% of diabetic foot ulcers heal within one year. Unfortunately, even after the resolution of a foot ulcer, recurrence is common. It was estimated that roughly 40% of patients have a recurrence within one year after ulcer healing, almost 60% within three years, and 65% within five years. Interestingly, 3.5–13% of patients die with active ulcers, probably because the prevalence of co-morbidities such as coronary artery disease and nephropathy is high in patients with foot ulcers especially among those with neuro-ischemic ulcers. The risk of death at 10 years for a patient with diabetes who has had a foot ulcer is twice as high as the risk for a patient who has not had a foot ulcer. Neuropathic wounds are more likely to heal over a period of 20 weeks if they are smaller, of small duration and superficial. Neuro-ischemic ulcers take longer to heal and are more likely to lead to amputation. The patient's vascular status is the strongest predictor of healing rate and outcome.

The major adverse outcome of foot ulceration is amputation. Despite efforts at national levels, the rates of non-traumatic lower extremity amputation in people with diabetes remain 10–20-fold higher than in those without

Atlas of the Diabetic Foot, Third Edition. Ioanna Eleftheriadou, Alexandros Kokkinos, Stavros Liatis, Konstantinos Makrilakis, Nicholas Tentolouris, Anastasios Tentolouris, and Panagiotis Tsapogas.

Companion website: www.wiley.com/go/tentolouris/atlas_diabetic_foot

Table 1.1 Epidemiological data on the diabetic foot.

Reference	Country	Population- or clinic-based	Prevalence (%)		Incidence	
			Foot ulcers	Amputation	Foot ulcers	Amputation
Borssen et al. (1990)	Sweden	Population	0.75	–	–	–
McLeod et al. (1991)	UK	Clinic	2.6	2.1	–	–
Walters et al. 1992	UK	Population	7.4	-	–	–
Moss et al. (1992)	USA	Population	–	3.6	10.1[a]	2.1[a]
Bouter et al. (1993)	The Netherlands	Population	–	–	0.8[b]	0.4
Siitonen et al. (1993)	Finland	Population			–	0.5
Pendsey et al. (1994)	India	Clinic	3.6	–	–	–
Kumar et al. (1994)	UK	Population	1.4	–	–	–
Humphrey et al. (1996)	Nauru	Population	–	–	–	0.76
Abbott et al. (2002)	UK	Population	1.7	1.3	2.2	–
Mueller et al. (2002)	The Netherlands	Population	–	–	2.1	0.6
Centers for Disease Control and Prevention (2003)	USA	Population	11.8	–	–	–
Lavery et al. (2003)	USA	Population	–	–	6.8	0.6
Manes et al. (2002)	Balkan region	Clinic	7.6	–	–	–

[a] Incidence over four years. Data from the Balkan region include Albania, Bulgaria, Greece, Romania, Serbia and the Former Republic of Macedonia.
[b] Include annual incidence of foot ulcers in patients hospitalized for foot problems.

diabetes. Approximately 40–70% of all non-traumatic amputations of the lower limbs are performed on patients with diabetes. Many studies have documented the fact that foot ulcers precede approximately 85% of all amputations performed in patients with diabetes.

In addition, amputations in patients with diabetes are performed at a younger age. The risk for ulceration and amputation increases with both age and the duration of diabetes. According to one report, the prevalence of amputation in diabetic patients was 1.6% for the age range 18–44 years, 3.4% for ages 45–64 and 3.6% in patients over 65 years. The age-adjusted amputation rate for persons with diabetes (5.5 per 1000 persons) was 28 times that of those without diabetes (0.2 per 1000 persons) in 1997, increasing by 26% from 1990.

Regardless of diabetes status, these rates were higher for men than women and higher for Native Americans and non-Hispanic black individuals than Hispanic or non-Hispanic white patients. Lower amputation rates have been reported for South Asians and for African-Caribbean men. The higher prevalence of amputation may be due to aging of the diabetic population, the increasing prevalence of diabetes and better reporting. As the size of the diabetic population increases, more disease-related complications, and consequently more amputations, are expected in the future unless effective interventions aimed at preventing amputations are undertaken.

The efforts of some countries to reduce amputation rates are encouraging. An examination of recent time-trend national data from The Netherlands and Finland showed reductions in amputation rate of 40% between 1995 and 2000 and of 41% between 1984 and 2000, respectively. Data from Leverkusen, Germany, also showed a reduction in both the major and minor amputation rate in patients with diabetes by 37% between the years 1990 and 2005.

There is evidence that the decline in amputation rates is due to a better quality of foot care, including the provision of podiatrists, multidisciplinary foot teams and surgical interventions for lower extremity arterial disease. Clinic- and community-based studies have demonstrated that strategies aiming at patient education, identification of the foot at risk, implementation of preventive measures (proper footwear, podiatrist services) and multidisciplinary management can reduce the rate of amputation in patients with diabetes by almost 50%.

The most common cause of amputation in diabetes is ischemia and infection; critical limb ischemia or non-healing foot ulcer is the cause of amputation in 50–70% and infection in 30–50% of patients with diabetes.

1.3 Economic Aspects

Foot ulceration and amputation affect largely patients' quality of life and place an economical burden on both the patient and the healthcare system. Therefore, prevention of foot ulceration, and consequently amputation, is a major priority of healthcare providers.

Considering the costs related to patients with foot ulcers, studies usually report on direct costs related to hospital (hotel) charges, antibiotics, diagnostic and therapeutic procedures, dressings and off-loading devices. In addition to the direct costs, there are indirect costs, which are more difficult to estimate and are related to value lost in terms of income from work, early retirement and the cost of rehabilitation.

Quality of life is another important issue in patients with foot ulcers that cannot be measured in economic terms. Foot ulceration affects a patient's ability to perform simple daily tasks and leisure activities. Patients with foot ulcers or amputation suffer more often from depression and have a poorer quality of life than those without foot problems.

The EURODIALE study showed that the average cost per patient with a foot wound, including the direct and indirect costs and irrespective of payers and reimbursement systems, was approximately €10 000 in 2005. It should be mentioned that estimates of the indirect costs in this study were based only on the value of lost income from work. The average direct cost of healing of an ulcer in Sweden in 1990 was US$8,950, which is €6,7384 according to 2017 prices. The average direct cost per ulcer episode reported by an American group based on data from 2000 and 2001 was US$13,179 (approximately €10,950) in patients with adequate vascular status, and almost double that (US$23,372 or €19,373) in individuals with inadequate vascular status. Data also for the period 2007–2014 in the United States reported that diabetic foot ulcers represent a substantial cost burden among Medicare beneficiaries with diabetes, suggesting a 1-year cost of US$9–13 billion (approximately €7.6–11 billion), in addition to the costs associated with diabetes itself.

An analysis of the costs related to foot ulcers and the outcome from the EURODIALE project is presented in Table 1.2 and Figure 1.1. It is apparent from these data that the more severe the ulcer, the higher the cost, and that the cost related to major amputations or non-healing ulcers is the highest. Considering the direct costs per ulcer in Europe, almost 40% arise because of hotel cost

Table 1.2 Direct and indirect costs per patient with foot ulcers of various severities.

	No infection or PAD	With infection, no PAD	No infection, with PAD	With both infection and PAD	Not classified	Total
A. Direct costs						
Hospitalization (hotel cost)	808 (18)	3703 (40)	4333 (45)	6787 (40)	4599 (40)	3892 (39)
Amputations	198 (4)	499 (5)	594 (6)	2411 (14)	687 (6)	889 (9)
Revascularization	44 (1)	62 (1)	685 (7)	1309 (8)	1213 (11)	554 (5)
Other interventions/surgery	550 (12)	992 (11)	897 (9)	1553 (9)	937 (8)	986 (10)
Diagnostic procedures	74 (2)	111 (1)	190 (2)	260 (2)	225 (2)	160 (2)
Antibiotics	847 (19)	1146 (12)	1147 (12)	1846 (11)	764 (7)	1197 (12)
Off-loading and orthopedic appliances	435 (10)	448 (5)	447 (5)	503 (5)	445 (4)	457 (5)
Topical treatment	368 (8)	446 (5)	679 (7)	1057 (6)	1029 (9)	658 (7)
Consultations and Outpatient visits	448 (10)	707 (8)	549 (6)	687 (74)	1221 (11)	653 (6)
Total direct costs	**3771**	**8113**	**9622**	**16 414**	**11 120**	**9446**
B. Indirect costs	**743 (16)**	**1160 (13)**	**229 (2)**	**421 (3)**	**335 (3)**	**645 (6)**
C. Total direct and indirect costs	**4514 (100)**	**9273 (100)**	**9851 (100)**	**16 853 (100)**	**11 455 (100)**	**10 091 (100)**

Source: Modified from Prompers et al. (2008), with permission.
The direct and indirect costs per patient are shown in Euros (% of total) according to 2005 prices and have been weighted by purchasing power standards. Indirect costs refer to the costs for patients who were employed and had been on sickness leave because of the foot ulcer. Indirect costs were calculated by multiplying the number of weeks a patient had been on sickness leave by the average income per week of the general population in the country of residence.
PAD, peripheral arterial disease.

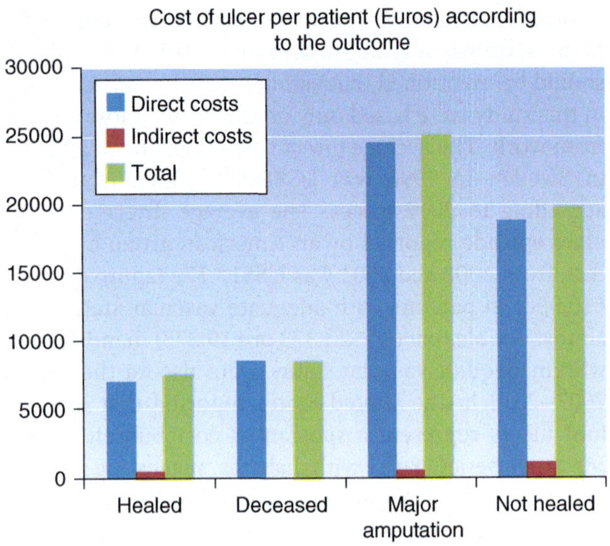

Figure 1.1 Costs of ulcer per patient (Euros) according to outcome in 10 European countries. *Source:* Reproduced from Prompers et al. (2008), with permission.

from hospitalization, followed by antibiotic use, amputations, surgical interventions and off-loading and orthopedic appliances. Most of the excess costs in individuals with peripheral vascular disease (PAD) and infection were related to a higher rate of hospitalization and higher costs of antibiotics, amputations, revascularization and other surgery. Based on the data for Europe for 2017, which showed a prevalence of diabetes of 58 million people and an ulcer incidence among diabetic patients of 2% per year, the costs associated with the treatment of diabetic foot ulcers may be as high as €11.6 billion per year.

1.4 Etiopathogenesis of Foot Problems

The major risk factors for foot ulceration are a loss of protective sensation due to neuropathy, PAD and trauma. Diabetic neuropathy or PAD alone does not cause foot ulceration; it is the combination of these factors with trauma that leads to foot problems. Trauma and loss of protective sensation or PAD are the major contributors to foot ulceration, and diabetic neuropathy is the common denominator in almost 90% of diabetic foot ulcers. Trauma initially causes minor injuries, which are not perceived by the patient with a loss of protective sensation. As the patient continues his or her activities, a small injury enlarges and may be complicated by infection.

Data on the prevalence and incidence of PAD vary considerably in population-based studies depending on the method used for the assessment. PAD is 2–8 times more common in patients with diabetes in comparison to the general population, with a prevalence of 10–20% and an annual incidence of 6–13.5 per 1000 patients with diabetes. In addition, it starts at an earlier age and progresses more rapidly, is usually more severe in extent, and affects the segments between the knee and ankle more commonly in comparison to patients without diabetes.

It is also in itself an independent factor for increased mortality due to associated cardiovascular disease. Whereas before 1980 neuropathic ulcers were more commonly seen in diabetic foot clinics, nowadays ulcers of mixed etiology (neuro-ischemic) predominate, particularly in older patients. PAD is a major contributory factor for foot ulceration and a major predictor of outcome. Even a minor injury, especially if complicated by infection, increases the demand for blood supply and may eventually result in ulceration and amputation.

A diagnosis of PAD can be easily made by a history, clinical examination and determination of the ankle–brachial pressure index (ABI), as discussed in detail in Chapter 7. Smoking cessation, tight blood pressure control, use of antiplatelets, and management of dyslipidemia can reduce the risk for PAD in diabetes. Prospective data have not, however, shown any benefit of tight diabetes control in the prevention of PAD.

Neuropathies are common in diabetes, affect different parts of the nervous system and may present with diverse clinical manifestations. Most common among neuropathies are chronic sensorimotor distal symmetric polyneuropathy and peripheral autonomic neuropathy. Peripheral sensorimotor neuropathy is defined – according to the International Consensus Group on Neuropathy – as "the presence of symptoms and/or signs of peripheral nerve dysfunction in people with diabetes, after exclusion of other causes."

The average prevalence of peripheral sensorimotor neuropathy in diabetes is about 30%, irrespective of gender or type of diabetes. Diabetic neuropathy shows a positive association with both age and duration of diabetes and is very common (a prevalence of up to 60%) in older patients with type 2 diabetes. It should be emphasized that the prevalence of symptomatic neuropathy (burning sensation, pins and needles or allodynia, shooting, sharp and stabbing pain or muscle cramps in the legs) is less common (20–30%) among patients with neuropathy; thus, most of the patients with neuropathy are asymptomatic. Often, the first sign of peripheral neuropathy is a neuropathic ulcer. Other patients have neuropathic pain and on examination are found to have a severe loss of sensation. This combination is described as "painful–painless feet," and these patients are at increased risk for foot ulceration.

Peripheral neuropathy, beyond a loss of protective sensation, leads to small muscle wasting, foot deformities and gait disturbances, all of which are associated with increased plantar pressures and callus formation.

Peripheral autonomic neuropathy affects the distal parts of the lower limbs and leads to reduced sweating, dry skin, fissures and callus formation. Cross-sectional data show that reduced sweating and dryness of the skin of the feet is associated with an increased risk for foot ulceration. With opening of the arteriovenous shunts in the skin, in the absence of severe PAD, the feet may be warm with distended dorsal veins. The warm, insensitive and dry foot is at risk for ulceration partly because the patient has a false sense of security, as most patients perceive vascular disease as the main cause of foot problems.

Trauma, either internal (from calluses, ingrown nails and foot deformities) or external (from ill-fitting shoes and insoles, burns and foreign bodies), is a sufficient cause for skin breakdown. The pathways to foot ulceration are depicted in Figure 1.2. All patients with diabetes should be examined at least annually for peripheral neuropathy, so that those at risk for ulceration can be identified. A diagnosis of peripheral neuropathy should be based on the history and clinical examination and can be made easily in a few minutes at the bedside or on an outpatient basis (see Chapter 2).

1.5 Other Risk Factors of Foot Ulceration

Beyond neuropathy and PAD, a history of previous foot ulceration or amputation, foot deformities, calluses, neuro-osteoarthropathy (Charcot arthropathy) and high plantar pressures have been associated with an increased risk for foot ulceration. Limited joint mobility may result in high plantar pressures. Several, but not all, studies have shown that foot ulcers are more common in male patients. In addition, poor vision, diabetic nephropathy and especially dialysis, and social factors including low social position, poor access to healthcare services, poor education and living alone have all been associated with foot ulceration. Cigarette smoking is also considered a risk factor for foot ulceration because it is associated strongly with both PAD and neuropathy. Another important factor for foot ulceration is poor compliance of the patient with medical instructions and neglectful behavior. Edema may impair the blood supply to the foot, particularly in patients with PAD.

The risk factors for foot ulceration are summarized in Box 1.1.

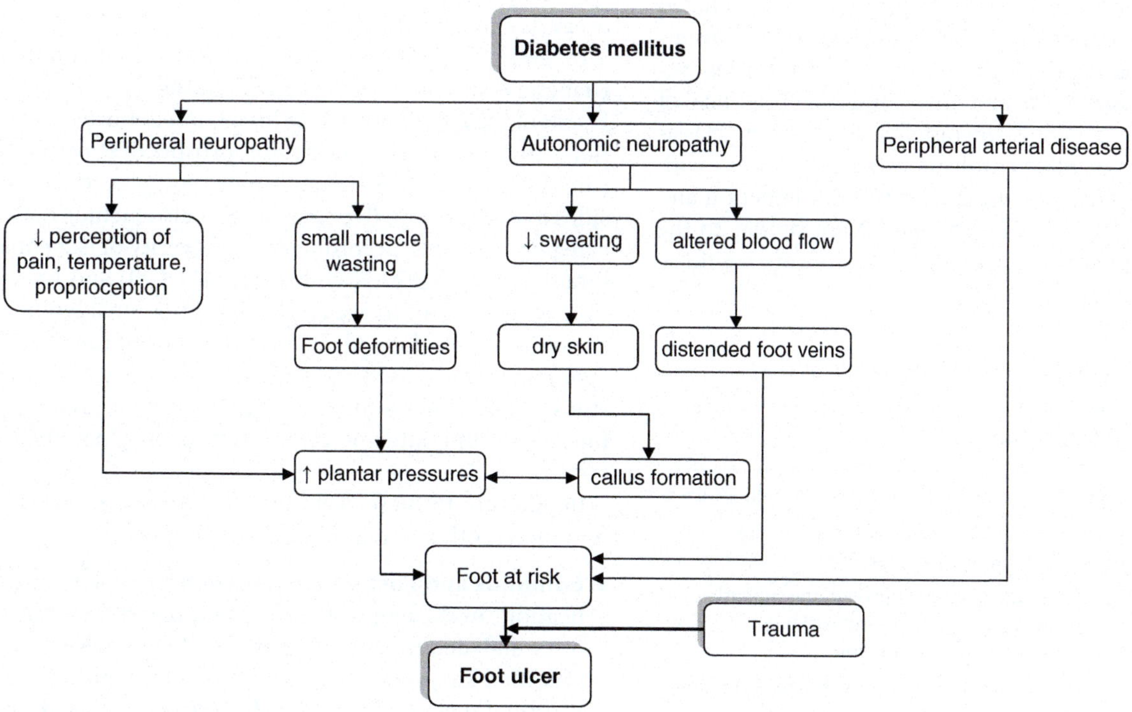

Figure 1.2 The pathways to foot ulceration. *Source:* Modified from Boulton (2000), with permission.

Box 1.1 Risk Factors for Foot Ulcers

- Previous amputation
- Past foot ulcer
- Peripheral neuropathy
- Foot deformity
- Peripheral arterial disease
- Visual impairment
- Diabetic nephropathy (especially patients on dialysis)
- Poor glycemic control
- Cigarette smoking

1.6 Classification of Foot Problems

Classically, diabetic foot ulcers are neuropathic in the presence of neuropathy but no ischemia, ischemic if they are due to ischemia in the absence of neuropathy, and of mixed etiology (neuro-ischemic) if neuropathy and ischemia coexist. However, this is a rather crude classification for the initial evaluation. Many efforts have been made, for both clinical and research purposes, to categorize foot ulcers according to extension, size and depth, location, presence of infection and ischemia.

The **Meggitt-Wagner classification** is the best known and validated system for foot ulcers and is described in Table 1.3. The advantages and disadvantages of this classification system are described in Box 1.2.

The **University of Texas classification system for diabetic foot wounds** has been proposed and validated by the University of Texas (Table 1.4). This system evaluates both the depth of the ulcer – as in the Meggitt-Wagner classification system – and the presence of infection and ischemia. Uncomplicated ulcers are classified as stage A, infected ulcers as stage B, ulcers with ischemia as stage C and ulcers with both infection and ischemia as stage D. Grades 1 and 2 are similar to the Meggitt-Wagner classification. Grade 3 ulcers are those penetrating to bone or joint.

Table 1.3 Meggitt-Wagner classification of foot ulcers.

Grade	Description of the ulcer
Grade 0	Pre- or post-ulcerative lesion completely epithelialized
Grade 1	Superficial, full-thickness ulcer limited to the dermis, not extending to the subcutis
Grade 2	Ulcer of the skin extending through the subcutis with exposed tendon or bone and without osteomyelitis or abscess formation
Grade 3	Deep ulcers with osteomyelitis or abscess formation
Grade 4	Localized gangrene of the toes or the forefoot
Grade 5	Foot with extensive gangrene

Box 1.2 Advantages and Disadvantages of the Meggitt-Wagner Classification System

Advantages

- It is simple in use and has been validated in many studies
- Higher grades are directly related to increased risk for lower limb amputation
- It provides a guide to plan treatment
- It is considered the gold standard against which other systems should be validated

Disadvantages

- Although the presence of infection and ischemia are related to poor outcome, ischemia is not taken into account in patients with grades 1–3 and infection in grades 1, 2 and 4
- The location and size of the ulcer are not evaluated
- Neuropathy status is not evaluated

This system has been evaluated prospectively, showing that the greater the grade and stage of an ulcer, the greater the risk for non-healing and amputation. Thus, the healing rate of foot ulcers was 90% for stage A, 89% for stage B, 69% for stage C and only 36% for stage D. The advantages and disadvantages of the University of Texas system are shown in Box 1.3. The system can be used in every day clinical practice.

In 2003, the International Working Group on the Diabetic Foot proposed the **PEDIS system** (P, perfusion; E, extent/size; D, depth/tissue loss; I, infection; S, sensation) to classify foot ulcers for prospective research (Box 1.4). The PEDIS system is more complex and classifies foot ulcers into five categories. It also includes subcategories (grades) according to the severity of ischemia (grades 1–3), depth/tissue loss (grades 1–3) and infection (grades 1–4), as well as taking into consideration the dimensions of the ulcer. Modifications of the PEDIS system have been used and evaluated prospectively. One study showed that a modified PEDIS system predicted foot ulcers and outcome better than the original PEDIS system.

In addition to these classification systems of diabetic foot ulcers, other systems have been proposed:

- **Edmonds and Foster** have proposed a simpler classification. According to their system, based on clinical tests and determination of the ABI, foot ulcers are classified into neuropathic and neuro-ischemic.
- Brodsky suggested the **depth–ischemia classification**, which is a modification of the Wagner-Meggitt classification. According to this system, ulcers are

Table 1.4 The University of Texas classification system for diabetic foot wounds.

Grade					
Stage		0	1	2	3
	A	Pre- or post-ulcerative lesion completely epithelialized	Superficial wound not involving tendon, capsule or bone	Wound penetrating to tendon or capsule	Wound penetrating to bone or joint
	B	With infection	With infection	With infection	With infection
	C	With ischemia	With ischemia	With ischemia	With ischemia
	D	With infection and ischemia	With infection and ischemia	With infection and ischemia	With infection and ischemia

Box 1.3 Advantages and Disadvantages of the University of Texas Classification System for Diabetic Foot Wounds

Advantages

- It is simple in use and more descriptive
- It has been evaluated and has shown greater association with the outcome of an ulcer, healing or amputation, compared with the Meggitt-Wagner classification
- Cases with infection and/or ischemia are classified
- It provides a guide to plan treatment

Disadvantages

- The location and size of the ulcer are not evaluated
- Neuropathy status is not evaluated

classified as grade 0–3 (like the Meggitt-Wagner classification) and also into four subgroups (A, not ischemic; B, ischemic without gangrene; C, partial gangrene of the foot; D, complete foot gangrene).

- Macfarlane and Jeffcoate proposed the **S(AD)SAD classification** for diabetic foot ulcers. According to this system, ulcers are classified based on Size (Area and Depth), presence of Sepsis, Arteriopathy and Denervation.
- A hybrid of the S(AD)SAD and the University of Texas system, the **SINBAD system** (S, site; I, ischemia; N, neuropathy; BA, bacterial infection; D, depth) has been introduced and evaluated in the UK, Germany and Pakistan. Each abnormality is scored (maximum value 9, minimum 6), and there is an excellent correlation between the total score for the ulcer and the outcome and time to healing.

Box 1.4 The PEDIS System

Perfusion

Grade 1: No symptoms or signs of PAD in the affected foot in combination with:

- palpable foot arteries *or*
- ABI 0.9–1.1 *or*
- TBI > 0.6 *or*
- tcO_2 > 60 mmHg

Grade 2: Symptoms or signs of PAD, but not of CLI:

- presence of intermittent claudication *or*
- ABI <0.9 but with ankle pressure > 50 mmHg *or*
- TBI <0.6 but with systolic toe blood pressure > 30 mmHg *or*
- $TcPO_2$ 30–60 mmHg *or*
- other abnormalities of non-invasive testing, compatible with PAD but not with CLI

Grade 3: CLI, as defined by:

- systolic ankle blood pressure < 50 mmHg *or*
- systolic toe blood pressure < 30 mmHg *or*
- $TcPO_2$ < 30 mmHg

Extent/Size

Wound size (in square centimeters determined by multiplying the largest diameter by the second largest diameter), preferably after debridement

Depth/Tissue Loss

Grade 1: Superficial full-thickness ulcer, not penetrating any structure deeper than the dermis

Grade 2: Deep ulcer, penetrating below the dermis to subcutaneous structures, involving fascia, muscle or tendon

Grade 3: All subcutaneous layers of the foot involved, including bone and/or joint (exposed bone, probing bone)

Infection

Grade 1: No symptoms or signs of infection

Grade 2: Infection involving the skin and the subcutaneous tissue only (without involvement of deeper tissues and without systemic signs, as described below). At least two of the following items are present:

- local swelling or induration
- erythema >0.5–2 cm around the ulcer
- local tenderness or pain
- local warmth
- purulent discharge (thick, opaque to white or sanguineous secretion)

Other causes of inflammatory response of the skin should be excluded (trauma, gout, acute Charcot neuro-arthropathy, fracture, thrombosis, venous stasis)

Grade 3: Erythema >2 cm plus one of the items described above (swelling, tenderness, warmth, discharge) or infection involving structures deeper than skin and subcutaneous tissue such as abscess, osteomyelitis, septic arthritis or fasciitis. No systemic inflammatory response signs, as described below

Grade 4: Any foot infection with the following signs of a systemic inflammatory response syndrome. This response is manifested by two or more of the following conditions:

- temperature > 38 or < 36 °C
- heart rate > 90 beats minutes^{-1}
- respiratory rate > 20 breaths minutes^{-1}
- $PaCo_2$ < 32 mmHg
- white blood cell count > 12 000 or < 4000 mm^{-3}
- greater than 10% immature (band) forms

Sensation

Grade 1: No loss of protective sensation on the affected foot detected, described as the presence of the sensory modalities described below

Grade 2: Loss of protective sensation defined as the absence of perception of the one of the following tests in the affected foot:

- Absent pressure sensation, determined with a 10 g monofilament, on two out of three sites on the plantar surface of the foot, as described by the International Working Group on the Diabetic Foot
- Absent vibration sensation (determined with a 128 Hz tuning fork) or vibration perception threshold >25 V (using semi-quantitative techniques), both tested on the hallux

ABI, ankle–brachial index; CLI, critical limb ischemia; $PaCo_2$, arterial partial pressure of carbon dioxide; PAD, peripheral arterial disease; TBI; toe–brachial index; $TcPo_2$, transcutaneous oxygen pressure

Any valid classification system of foot ulcers should facilitate appropriate treatment, help in monitoring the progress of healing and serve as a communication code across specialties in standardized terms. Despite its disadvantages, the University of Texas classification system offers many advantages over the Meggitt-Wagner system for clinical use, while the PEDIS system may offer advantages for research purposes. In addition, the inclusion of other parameters such as the location of the ulcer, foot deformities and other factors in a classification system, which may be related to the outcome of an ulcer, makes it more complex and cumbersome.

References

Abbott, C.A., Carrington, A.L., Ashe, H. et al. (2002). The North-West Diabetes Foot Care Study: incidence of, and risk factors for, new diabetic foot ulceration in a community-based patient cohort. *Diabet. Med.* 19: 377–384.

Borssén, B., Bergenheim, T., and Lithner, F. (1990). The epidemiology of foot lesions in diabetic patients aged 15-50 years. *Diabet. Med.* 7: 438–444.

Bouter, K.P., Storm, A.J., de Groot, R.R. et al. (1993). The diabetic foot in Dutch hospitals: epidemi-ological features and clinical outcome. *Eur. J. Med.* 2: 215–218.

Boulton, A.J.M. (2000). The pathway to ulceration: aetiopathogenesis. In: *The Foot in Diabetes*, vol. 4 (ed. A.J.M. Boulton and G. Rayman), 51–67. Chichester: Wiley.

Centers for Disease Control and Prevention (CDC) (2003). History of foot ulcer among persons with diabetes--United States, 2000-2002. *MMWR Morb. Mortal. Wkly Rep.* 52: 1098–1102.

Humphrey, A.R., Dowse, G.K., Thoma, K., and Zimmet, P.Z. (1996). Diabetes and nontraumatic lower extremity amputations. Incidence, risk factors, and prevention--a 12-year follow-up study in Nauru. *Diabetes Care* 19: 710–714.

Kumar, S., Ashe, H.A., Parnell, L.N. et al. (1994). The prevalence of foot ulceration and its correlates in type 2 diabetic patients: a population-based study. *Diabet. Med.* 11: 480–484.

Lavery, L.A., Armstrong, D.G., Wunderlich, R.P. et al. (2003). Diabetic foot syndrome: evaluating the prevalence and incidence of foot pathology in Mexican Americans and non-Hispanic whites from a diabetes disease management cohort. *Diabetes Care* 26: 1435–1458.

Macleod, A.F., Williams, D.R., Sonksen, P.H., and Boulton, A.J. (1991). Risk factors for foot ulcers in diabetic patients attending a hospital clinic. *Diabetologia* 34 (Suppl): A39.

Manes, C., Papazoglou, N., Sassidou, E. et al. (2002). Prevalence of diabetic neuropathy and foot ulceration: a population-based study. *Wounds* 14: 11–15.

Moss, S.E., Klein, R., and Klein, B.E. (1992). The prevalence and incidence of lower extremity amputation in a diabetic population. *Arch. Intern. Med.* 152: 610–616.

Muller, I.S., DeGraw, W.J., van Gerwen, W.H. et al. (2002). Foot ulceration and lower limb amputation in type 2 diabetic patients in Dutch primary care. *Diabetes Care* 25: 570–574.

Pendsey, S. (1994). Epidemiological aspects of the diabetic foot. *Int. J. Diabetes Developing Countries* 2: 37–38.

Prompers, L., Huijberts, M., Schaper, N. et al. (2008). Resource utilization and costs associated with the treatment of diabetic foot ulcers. Prospective data from the Eurodiale study. *Diabetologia* 51: 1826–1834.

Siitonen, O.I., Niskanen, L.K., Laakso, M. et al. (1993). Lower-extremity amputations in diabetic and nondiabetic pa-tients. A population-based study in eastern Finland. *Diabetes Care* 16: 16–20.

Walters, D.P., Gatling, W., Mullee, M.A., and Hill, R.D. (1992). The distribution and severity of diabetic foot disease: a community study with comparison to a non-diabetic group. *Diabet. Med.* 9: 354–358.

Further Reading

van Acker, K., Léger, P., Hartemann, A. et al. (2014). Burden of diabetic foot disorders, guidelines for management and disparities in implementation in Europe: a systematic literature review. *Diabetes Metab. Res. Rev.* 30: 635–645.

American Diabetes Association (1999). Consensus Development Conference on Diabetic Foot Wound Care: 7–8 April 1999, Boston, Massachusetts. American Diabetes Association. *Diabetes Care* 22: 1354–1360.

American Diabetes Association (2018). Microvascular complications and foot care: standards of medical care in diabetes-2018. *Diabetes Care* 41 (Suppl 1): S105–S118.

Apelqvist, J., Larsson, J., and Agardh, C.D. (1993). Long-term prognosis for diabetic patients with foot ulcers. *J. Intern. Med.* 233: 485–491.

Armstrong, D.G., Boulton, A.J.M., and Bus, S.A. (2017). Diabetic foot ulcers and their recurrence. *N. Engl. J. Med.* 376: 2367–2375.

Armstrong, D.G., Lavery, L.A., and Harkless, L.B. (1998). Validation of a diabetic wound classification system. *Diabetes Care* 21: 855–859.

Bakker, K., Apelqvist, J., Lipsky, B.A. et al. (2016). The 2015 IWGDF guidance documents on prevention and management of foot problems in diabetes: development of an evidence-based global consensus. *Diabetes Metab. Res. Rev.* 32 (Suppl 1): 2–6.

Boulton, A.J. (2008). The diabetic foot: grand overview, epidemiology and pathogenesis. *Diabetes Metab. Res. Rev.* 24 (Suppl. 1): S3–S6.

Boulton, A.J., Vileikyte, L., Ragnarson-Tennvall, G., and Apelqvist, J. The global burden of diabetic foot disease. *Lancet* 366: 1719–1724.

Boulton, A.J., Vinik, A.L., Arezzo, J.C. et al. (2005). Diabetic neuropathies: a statement by the American Diabetes Association. *Diabetes Care* 28: 956–962.

Brodsky, J.W. (2001). The diabetic foot. In: *Levin and O'Neal's The Diabetic Foot*, 6e (ed. J.H. Bowker and M.A. Pfeifer), 273–282. St Louis: Mosby.

Dormandy, J.A. and Rutherford, R.B. (2000). Management of peripheral arterial disease (PAD). TransAtlantic Inter-Society Consensus (TASC). *Eur. J. Vasc. Endovasc. Surg.* 19 (Suppl. A): S1–S250.

Doupis, J., Grigoropoulou, P., Voulgari, C. et al. (2008). High rates of comorbid conditions in patients with type 2 diabetes and foot ulcers. *Wounds* 20: 132–138.

Edmonds, M.E., Blundell, M.P., Morris, M.E. et al. (1986). Improved survival of the diabetic foot: the role of a specialized foot clinic. *Q. J. Med.* 60: 763–771.

Ince, P., Abbas, Z.G., Lutale, J.K. et al. (2008). Use of the SINBAD classification system and score in comparing outcome of foot ulcer management on three continents. *Diabetes Care* 31: 964–967.

Lavery, L.A., Armstrong, D.G., and Harkless, L.B. (1996). Classification of diabetic foot wounds. *J. Foot. Ankle. Surg.* 35: 528–531.

Lavery, L.A., Peters, E.J., Williams, J.R. et al. (2008). International Working Group on the Diabetic Foot. Reevaluating the way we classify the diabetic foot: restructuring the diabetic foot risk classification system of the International Working Group on the Diabetic Foot. *Diabetes Care* 31: 154–156.

LeMaster, J.W. and Reiber, G.E. (2006). Epidemiology and economic impact of foot ulcers. In: *The Foot in Diabetes*, 4e (ed. A.J.M. Boulton, P.R. Cavanagh and G. Rayman), 1–16. Chichester: Wiley.

Macfarlane, R.F. and Jeffcoate, W.J. (1999). Classification of foot ulcers: the S(SAD)SAD system. *Diabetic Foot* 2: 123–131.

Oyibo, S.O., Jude, E.B., Tarawneh, I. et al. (2001). A comparison of two diabetic foot ulcer classification systems: the Wagner and the University of Texas wound classification systems. *Diabetes Care* 24: 84–88.

Pecoraro, R.E., Reiber, G.E., and Burgess, E.M. (1990). Pathways to diabetic limb amputation. Basis for prevention. *Diabetes Care* 13: 513–521.

Prompers, L., Huijberts, M., Apelqvist, J. et al. (2007). High prevalence of ischaemia, infection and serious comorbidity in patients with diabetic foot disease in Europe. Baseline results from the Eurodiale study. *Diabetologia* 50: 18–25.

Schaper, N.C. (2004). Diabetic foot ulcer classification system for research purposes: a progress report on criteria for including patients in research studies. *Diabetes Metab. Res. Rev.* 20 (Suppl. 1): S90–S95.

Schaper, N.C., Andros, G., Apelqvist, J. et al. (2012). Diagnosis and treatment of peripheral arterial disease in diabetic patients with a foot ulcer. A progress report of the International Working Group on the Diabetic Foot. *Diabetes Metab. Res. Rev.* 28 (Suppl 1): 218–224.

Tentolouris, N., Achtsidis, V., Marinou, K., and Katsilambros, N. (2008). Evaluation of the self-administered indicator plaster neuropad for the diagnosis of neuropathy in diabetes. *Diabetes Care* 31: 236–237.

The International Working Group on the Diabetic Foot (1999). *International Consensus on the Diabetic Foot.* Amsterdam: International Working Group on the Diabetic Foot.

Wagner, F.W. (1981). The dysvascular foot: a system for diagnosis and treatment. *Foot Ankle* 2: 64.

2

Diabetic Neuropathy

K. Makrilakis

First Department of Propaedeutic Medicine, National and Kapodistrian University of Athens Medical School, Laiko General Hospital, Athens, Greece

According to the International Consensus Group on Neuropathy, diabetic neuropathy (DN) is defined as "the presence of symptoms and/or signs of peripheral nerve dysfunction in people with diabetes, after exclusion of other causes." Diabetic neuropathy is a heterogeneous group of conditions that affect different parts of the nervous system and presents with diverse clinical manifestations. Among its various forms, distal symmetric polyneuropathy (DSPN) is the most prevalent one (around 75% of diabetic neuropathies), occurring in at least 20% of people with type 1 diabetes after 20 years of disease duration and at least 10–15% of newly diagnosed persons with type 2 diabetes, with rates increasing to 50% after 10 years of disease duration. It may even be present in up to 10–15% of people with impaired glucose tolerance (pre-diabetes).

Together with peripheral vascular disease, anatomic deformity and trauma, peripheral neuropathy is one of the most important contributing factors to the development of foot ulcerations in people with diabetes. The lifetime risk for a foot ulcer in people with (type 1 or 2) diabetes may be as high as 25%. Neuropathy is present in over 80% of them; it promotes ulcer formation by decreasing pain sensation and perception of pressure and touch, by causing muscle imbalance that can lead to anatomic deformities, and by impairing the microcirculation and integrity of the skin. Once ulcers form, healing may be delayed or difficult to achieve, particularly if any infection penetrates to deep tissues and bone and/or there is diminished local blood flow.

Since more than 50% of affected persons are asymptomatic, if DN is not properly recognized and if preventive foot care is not appropriately implemented, patients are at risk for injuries to their insensate feet and subsequent ulcer formation. Diabetic neuropathy is also a major contributor to falls and fractures through loss of protective sensation (LOPS), proprioception, temperature discrimination, and pain, all ultimately leading to unsteadiness, recurrent minor injuries, and an increased risk of falls.

2.1 Methods of Assessing the Foot at Risk

All people with diabetes should be examined at least annually for the presence of peripheral neuropathy, so that those at risk for ulceration can be identified. An abbreviated history, combined with physical examination, can usually establish the presence and severity of DN and peripheral arterial disease, two of the most important risk factors for developing foot ulcers. In routine clinical practice, however, the clinical exam recommended, is designed to identify LOPS with simple tests, rather than diagnose early neuropathy with sophisticated techniques.

The history should include questions about the usual symptoms of peripheral neuropathy (a burning sensation, pins and needles in the lower extremities, shooting, sharp or stabbing pains, muscle cramps), their distribution in the extremities (the typical picture being a symmetric sensory [or sensorimotor] polyneuropathy in a "stocking-and-glove" distribution), their duration and the time of occurrence (usually neuropathic symptoms are worse during the night, at rest).

The earliest signs of DN probably reflect the gradual loss of integrity of both large myelinated and small myelinated and unmyelinated nerve fibers. Loss of vibratory sensation and altered proprioception (affecting balance and causing numbness and tingling) and light touch reflect large-fiber loss, whereas impairment of pain and temperature sensation occur secondary to the loss of small fibers. Decreased or absent ankle reflexes occur

Atlas of the Diabetic Foot, Third Edition. Ioanna Eleftheriadou, Alexandros Kokkinos, Stavros Liatis, Konstantinos Makrilakis, Nicholas Tentolouris, Anastasios Tentolouris, and Panagiotis Tsapogas.

Companion website: www.wiley.com/go/tentolouris/atlas_diabetic_foot

early in the disease, while a more widespread loss of reflexes and motor weakness are somewhat uncommon late findings.

There are many tests for peripheral neuropathy, some quite sophisticated and performed only in specialized centers. Nevertheless, the tests used to characterize and distinguish patients with a LOPS are simple, fast and easily performed at an outpatient setting – some even at home by the patients themselves, for example the indicator plaster Neuropad® (miro Verbandstoffe, Wiehl-Drabenderhöhe, Germany; see Chapter 12). A routine neurologic examination is the first step. More sophisticated tests include the performance of electromyography and nerve conduction velocity studies, considered only in situations where the clinical features are atypical, the diagnosis is unclear, or a different etiology is suspected. Atypical features that warrant referral include motor more than sensory neuropathy, asymmetry of symptoms and signs, and rapid progression.

2.2 Physical Examination

Five simple clinical tests are considered useful in the diagnosis of LOPS in the diabetic foot (Table 2.1): the 10-g monofilament for evaluation of light touch (pressure sensation) should always be performed, followed by at least one of the other four. Abnormalities in two of these tests render the patient at increased risk for foot ulceration because they signify LOPS in the feet.

First, examine for the presence of light touch and pressure, and then proceed to the examination of pinprick (pain), vibration (using the 128-Hz tuning fork), vibration perception threshold (VPT) (using a biothesiometer, if available) and ankle reflexes.

Although not routinely recommended, the sensation of temperature discrimination is also useful and can be easily performed, as well as examination of proprioception (position sense).

- Examination of light touch (pressure perception) using the 10-g monofilament. This is tested with the Semmes–Weinstein 5.07 monofilament (the filament bending with the application of a 10-g force). The filament should be applied perpendicular to the skin surface of the sole, with sufficient force so that it buckles. The sites of application are not universally agreed, but most propose that the sites of examination should be on the plantar surfaces of the big toe and the first, third and fifth metatarsal heads, bilaterally (Figures 2.1–2.3). Areas of ulceration, calluses, scars and necrotic tissues should always be avoided. The patient is asked to say whether he or she can feel the pressure applied (yes/no) and at which site. The sensation of pressure using the buckling 10-g monofilament should first be demonstrated to the patient on a proximal site (e.g. upper arm). A normal protective sensation of pressure is considered to be present when the test is correct on at least two out of the four sites on each foot, and there should be at least one

Table 2.1 Neurological assessment for identification of loss of protective sensation.

10-g monofilament (plus at least 1 of the following 4):
Pinprick sensation
Vibration using 128-Hz tuning fork
Vibration perception threshold (VPT)
Ankle reflexes

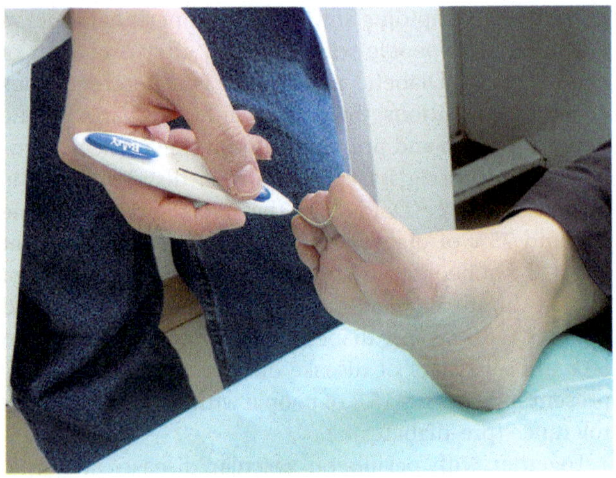

Figure 2.1 Application of the Semmes–Weinstein 5.07 monofilament on the plantar surface of the big toe. When the filament bends, a 10g force has been applied.

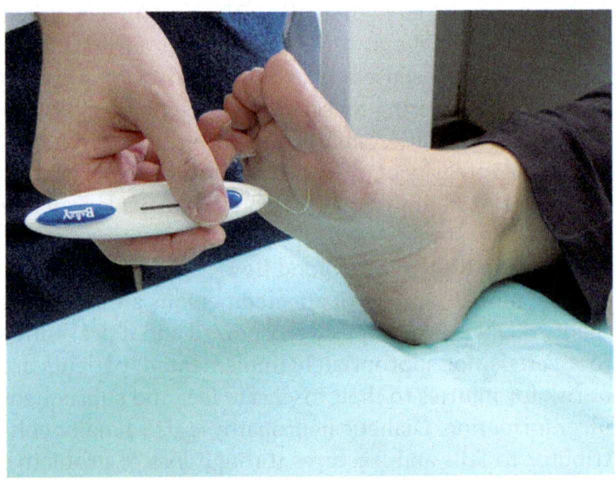

Figure 2.2 Application of the Semmes–Weinstein 5.07 monofilament to the plantar surface of the first metatarsal head.

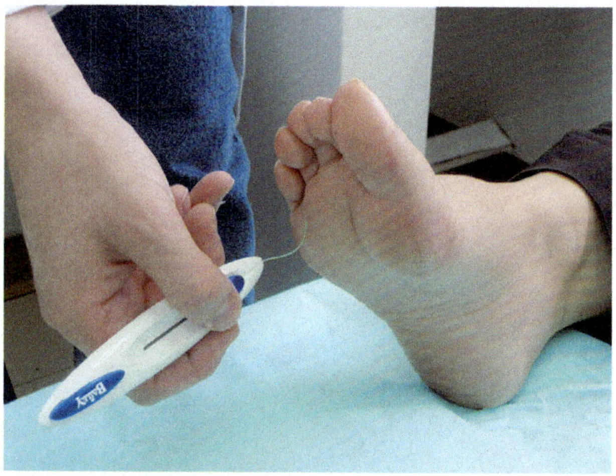

Figure 2.3 Application of the Semmes-Weinstein 5.07 monofilament to the plantar surface of the fifth metatarsal head.

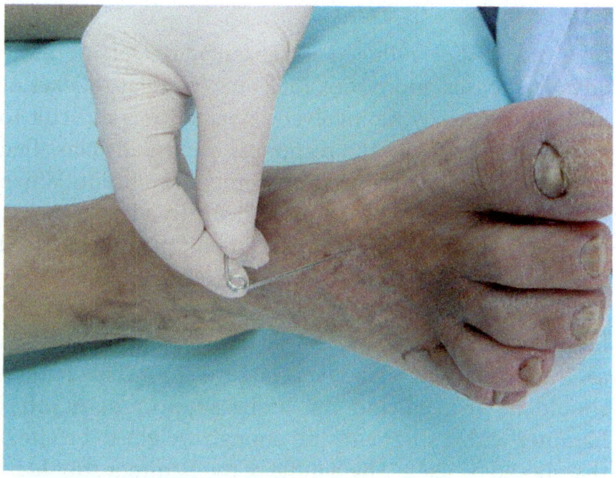

Figure 2.4 The pinprick examination.

"sham" application per site. Many studies have shown that an inability to perceive pressure with the monofilament is associated with a several-fold (around 10-fold) increased risk for foot ulceration.

- <u>Examination of superficial pain (pin-prick sensation)</u>. A disposable pin should be applied just proximal to the toenail on the dorsal surface of the hallux, with just enough pressure to deform the skin. The pin can have a sharp and a dull edge and the patient is asked to recognize if the sharp or the dull edge is touching him and at what site (Figure 2.4). An inability to perceive the pinprick correctly over either hallux is regarded as an abnormal test result. The pinprick should be performed starting from the toe and advancing toward the knee, on the anterior surface of both legs. Patients should not be allowed to watch during the examination. Documentation of the level at which the sensation goes from dull to sharp is made for both sides.

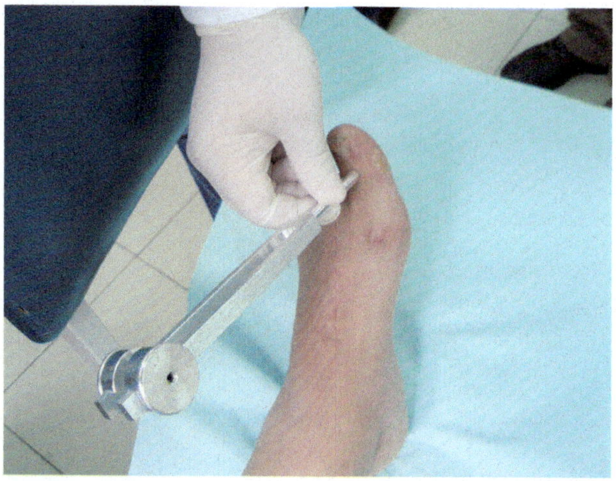

Figure 2.5 Examination of vibration perception using a tuning fork on the dorsal side of the distal phalanx of the great toe, just proximal to the nail bed.

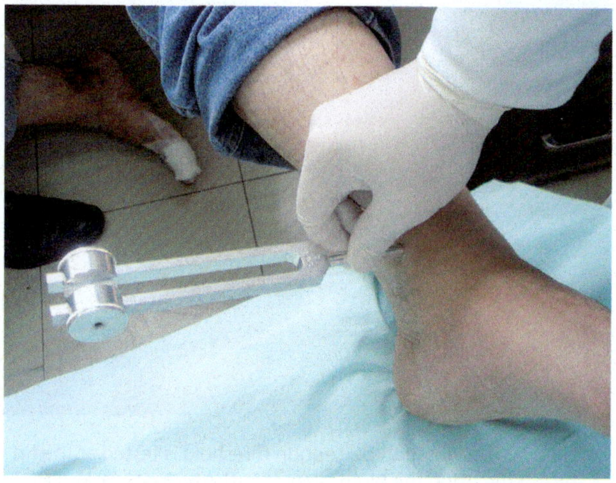

Figure 2.6 Examination of vibration perception using a tuning fork on the medial malleolus.

- <u>Examination of vibration perception (using the 128-Hz tuning fork)</u>. This is tested on the dorsal side of the distal phalanx of the great toes, just proximal to the nail bed (Figure 2.5). It can also be tested at the medial malleolus (Figure 2.6). The tuning fork should be placed perpendicular to the foot at a constant pressure with the patient's eyes closed. The examination is repeated twice, and there should be at least one "sham" application in which the tuning fork is not vibrating. The patient is asked to report his or her perception of both the start and the end of the vibration. An abnormal response is defined when the patient loses the vibratory sensation but the examiner still perceives it while holding the fork on the tip of the toe, or the patient still feels the instrument vibrating while the examiner has stopped it by touching its edge. Normal

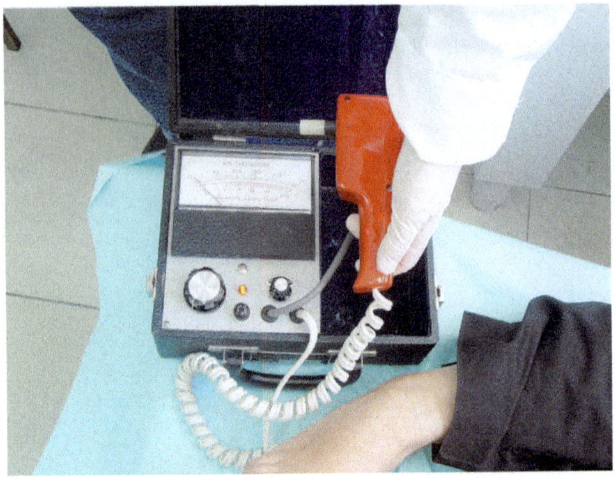

Figure 2.7 The biothesiometer.

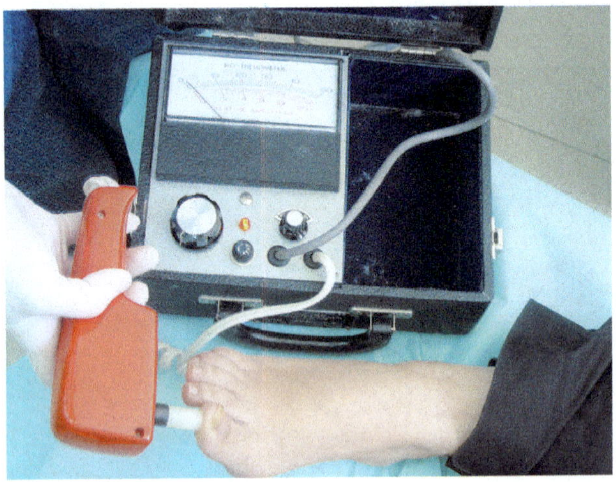

Figure 2.8 The vibration perception threshold is tested at the tip of the big toe using the biothesiometer. The patient is asked to identify when the vibration starts while the voltage of the instrument is gradually increased.

sensation is considered to be present when the patient is correct on two out of three tests.

- Examination of VPT (using the Biothesiometer). The biothesiometer can quantitatively determine the threshold of vibration perception (Figure 2.7). This is measured at the tip of the great toes with the vibrating head of the device balanced under its own weight (Figure 2.8). The vibration stimulus is increased until the patient feels it; the stimulus is then withdrawn and the test repeated. It is usually carried out three times on each side, and the mean value is calculated. A value of over 25 V is usually considered abnormal, since studies have shown that this is associated with a four to sevenfold increased risk for foot ulceration.

Next, the deep tendon reflexes are examined. The ankle (Achilles tendon) reflexes are the first to be

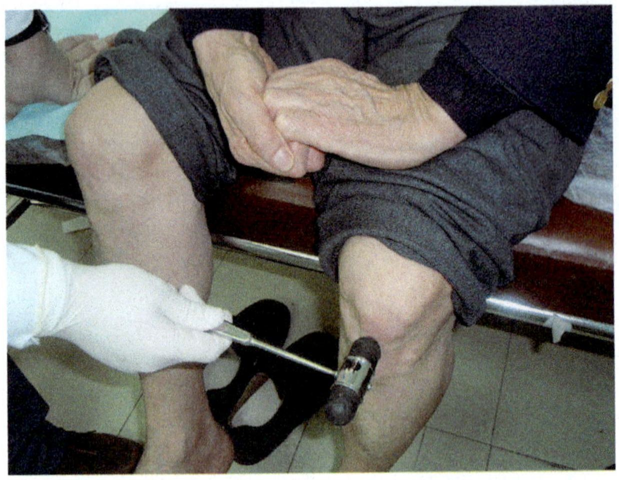

Figure 2.9 The Jendrassik maneuver. While the patellar reflexes are being tested, the patient is asked to hook together the flexed fingers of both hands and pull.

involved (either reduced or absent) in DN. In more advanced cases, more proximal sites (patellar reflexes or arm reflexes) may be involved. Normality is difficult to assess, and therefore the responses are usually classified as present, present with reinforcement or absent. When a patient has reflexes that are difficult to elicit, they can be amplified by using reinforcement procedures: the patient is asked to clench his or her teeth or (when testing the lower extremity reflexes) to hook together the flexed fingers of both hands and pull. This is also known as the Jendrassik maneuver (Figure 2.9). The patient should be relaxed and the limbs supported. A reflex hammer with a soft head and enough weight to be effective should be used. The handle of the hammer should be held between the thumb and index finger and the tendon should be struck firmly, using the wrist (not the arm) to swing the hammer.

- Ankle (Achilles tendon) reflex. Have the patient kneel on the edge of a stable chair, with his or her back toward you. Gently apply pressure to the sole of the foot (causing some dorsiflexion and muscle stretching). Strike the Achilles tendon (Figure 2.10) and observe for plantar flexion of the foot via muscle contraction of the gastrocnemius and soleus muscles. On a lying patient the test is performed by having the knee of the examined leg bent and the leg cross over the other leg, forming the same dorsiflexed position of the sole (Figure 2.11).
- Knee (patellar) reflex. Have the patient sit with the knee flexed at a right angle and hanging freely. Strike the patellar tendon (Figure 2.12). Observe the extension of the lower leg and contraction of the quadriceps muscles. Normal responses may vary from a flicker of the quadriceps muscles to a jump of the lower legs.

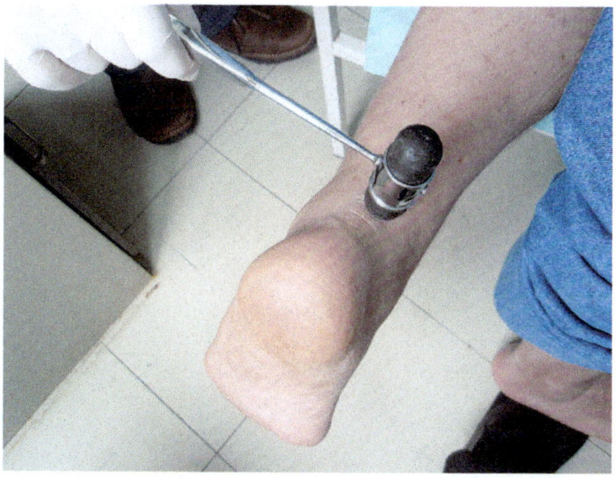

Figure 2.10 The ankle (Achilles tendon) reflex with the patient kneeling on a chair.

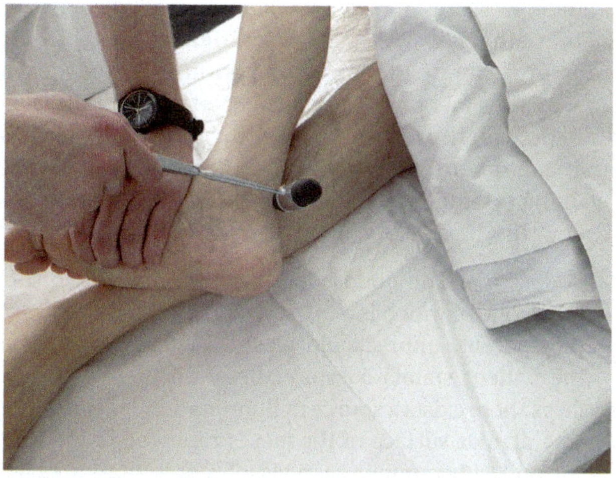

Figure 2.11 The ankle (Achilles tendon) reflex in lying position.

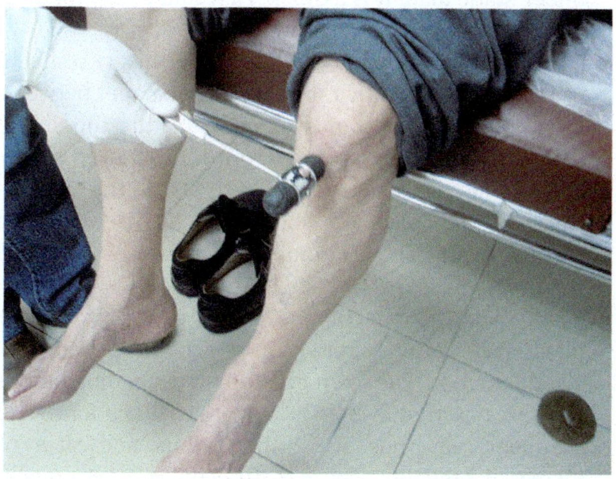

Figure 2.12 The knee (patellar) reflex.

- Examination of temperature sensation. Using two metal rods, one at a temperature of 4° C and the other at 40° C, the dorsum of the feet and legs is touched alternately and the patient (with the eyes closed) is asked to identify whether the rod is cold or hot. A reasonable stimulus is the flat portion of a tuning fork after it has been immersed in cold (or hot) water and dried. Figures 2.13 and 2.14 show the examination of a patient for the perception of temperature differences, using a rod with two different edges, one metal (cool) and the other plastic (warmer). The examination sites are similar to those for pain, as described above.

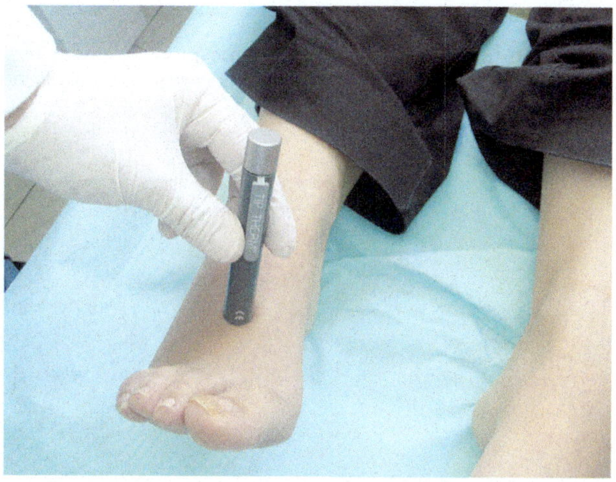

Figure 2.13 Examination of temperature sensation by applying the plastic part of a rod to the dorsal surface of the foot. The patient is expected to feel this side as warmer than the metallic side of the rod.

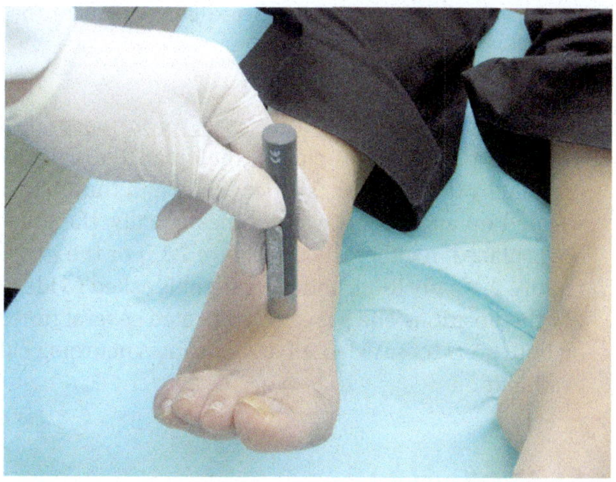

Figure 2.14 Examination of temperature sensation by applying the metal part of a rod on the dorsal surface of the foot. The patient is expected to feel this side as cooler than the plastic side of the rod.

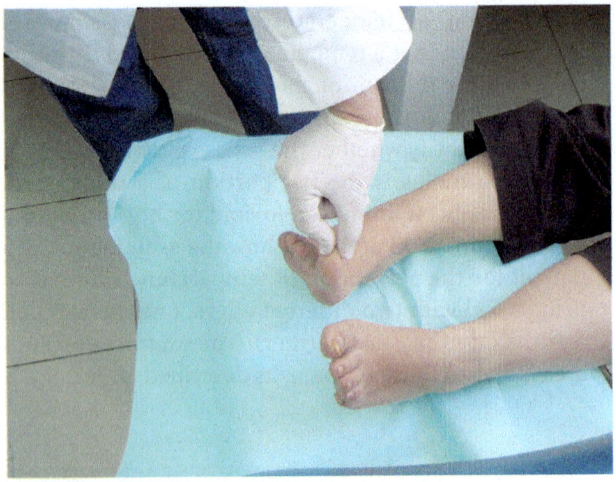

Figure 2.15 Examination for position sense (proprioception). The great toe is placed in the up position, and the patient is asked to identify the direction of movement.

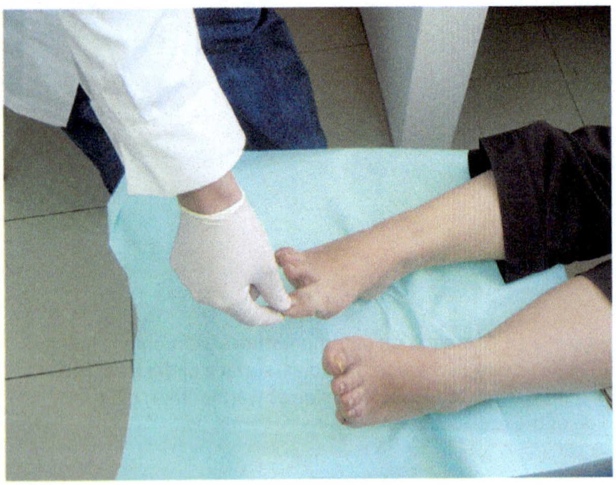

Figure 2.16 Examination for position sense (proprioception). The great toe is placed in the down position.

- Then examine for position sense (proprioception). With the patient's eyes closed, the great toe is firmly grasped by the examiner's index finger and thumb and wiggled up and down several times. Finally, the great toe is placed in either the up (Figure 2.15) or the down (Figure 2.16) position, and the patient is asked to identify the position. The process is repeated several times on both great toes. Video 2.1 demonstrates neurological examination.

2.2.1 Ancillary Tests

Measurement of plantar pressures is usually used to help in manufacturing proper footwear insoles and not to diagnose presence of neuropathy, since abnormal

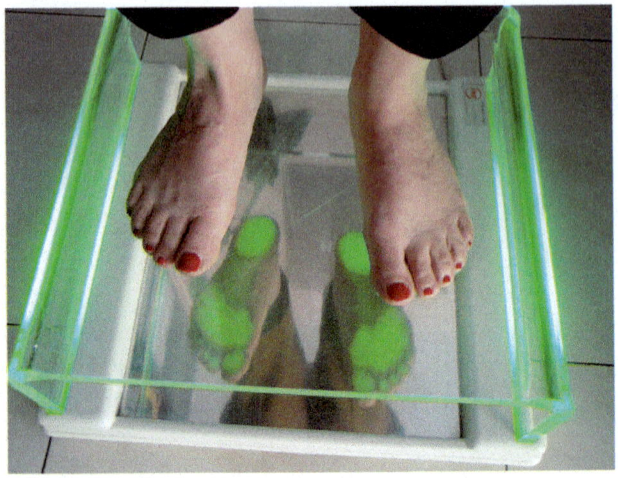

Figure 2.17 The podoscope. The patient stands barefoot on a transparent, unbreakable, plastic surface, and the plantar pressures are visualized in an illuminated mirror underneath.

plantar pressures may be present even in people without neuropathy, but with anatomical deformities. Plantar pressures can be measured by various methods, each of which has its pros and cons. The feet can be evaluated for high-pressure points by means of devices that can quantify the pressures under the foot during walking or standing. There are various techniques for doing this:

- Podoscope. The podoscope is composed of two surfaces, one of which is a mirror and the other is made of transparent, unbreakable plastic material, on which the patient stands barefoot. Between these two surfaces there exists a source of illumination (Figure 2.17). The plantar surface of the feet is reflected in the mirror, and the examiner has a visual representation of the patient's plantar pressures during standing. This method is used for functional examination of the feet under static load. It is a quick, easy and cheap method of foot pressure examination.
- Carbon paper imprint of the foot. For this, two sheets of paper are used with a sheet of carbon paper between them. The patient stands barefoot on the top sheet, and the feet are imprinted onto the lower sheet. Depending on the pressures exercised, the various sites of the soles are shown as intense or faint (Figure 2.18). The examiner can thus see areas of increased pressures or disfiguration.
- Foam mark. This technique uses a box (Figure 2.19) filled with foamy material, on which the patient can stand barefoot. The foam goes down depending on the pressures exerted at the various areas of the foot. The examiner can thus see disfigurations and sites of increased pressure (Figure 2.20). This is a very quick, portable and cheap method of foot pressure examination

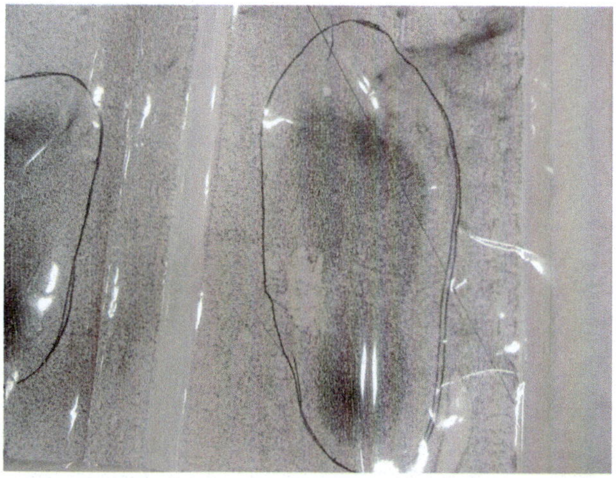

Figure 2.18 A carbon-paper representation of the sole of a diabetic patient, with areas of increased pressure at the heel and the third toe.

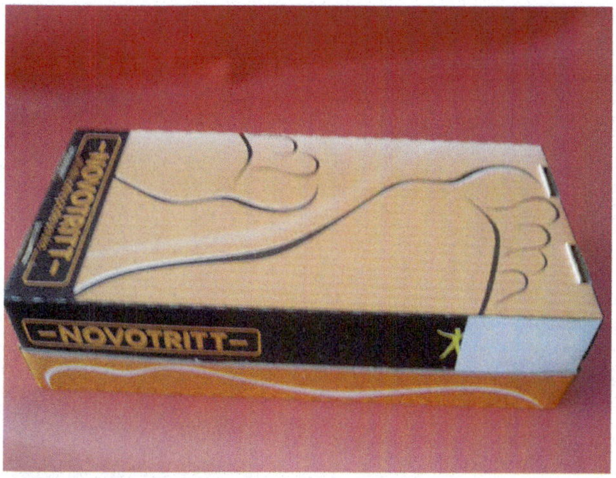

Figure 2.19 The foam-mark box (Novotritt; Acuive, Ruinerwold, The Netherlands), filled with foamy material.

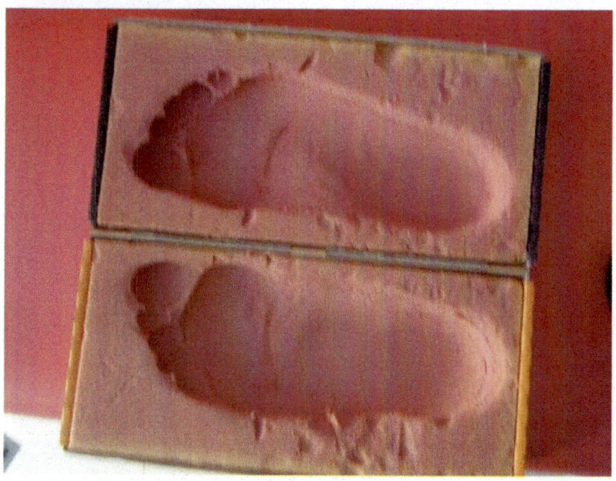

Figure 2.20 The foam-mark made by the soles of a diabetic patient.

that can be used in the doctor's office and can also serve for custom-made insole manufacturing, since by filling the footmark inside the box with plaster, an accurate copy of the footprint is taken.

- Measurement platforms – treadmills. Measurement platforms enable an analysis of the static and dynamic distribution of forces underneath the feet while standing (Figure 2.21) or walking (Figure 2.22). The pressure distribution sensor matrix is integrated underneath the surface of the platform or treadmill (Figure 2.23). During the analyses, the data interpretations occur directly after the measurements, and the results are immediately available in the form of a report. The pressure measurement system enables an analysis of the dynamic force/pressure distribution while standing (Figure 2.24), walking (Figure 2.25) or even running. A

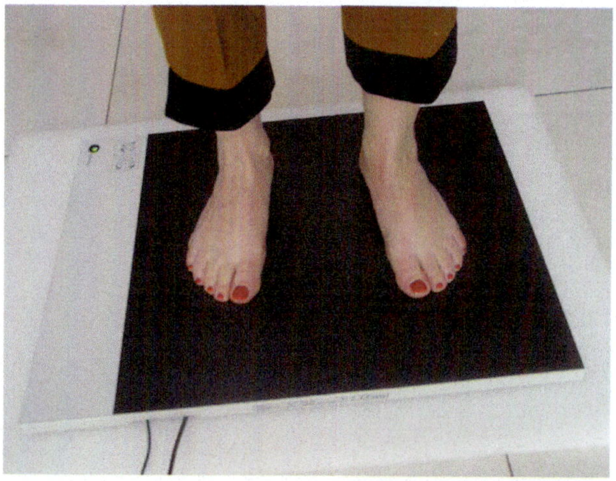

Figure 2.21 A measurement platform while the patient is standing on it.

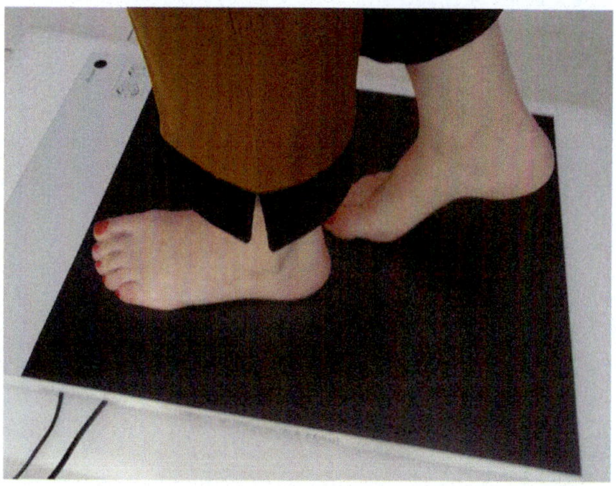

Figure 2.22 A measurement platform while the patient is walking on it.

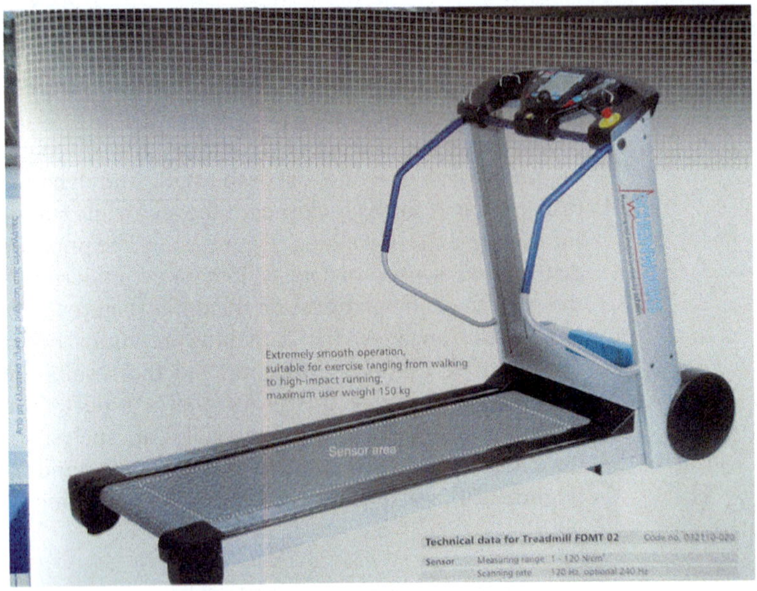

Figure 2.23 A measurement treadmill. The patient can walk or run on it and the plantar pressures are transferred to a computer, where they are analyzed and depicted on a screen.

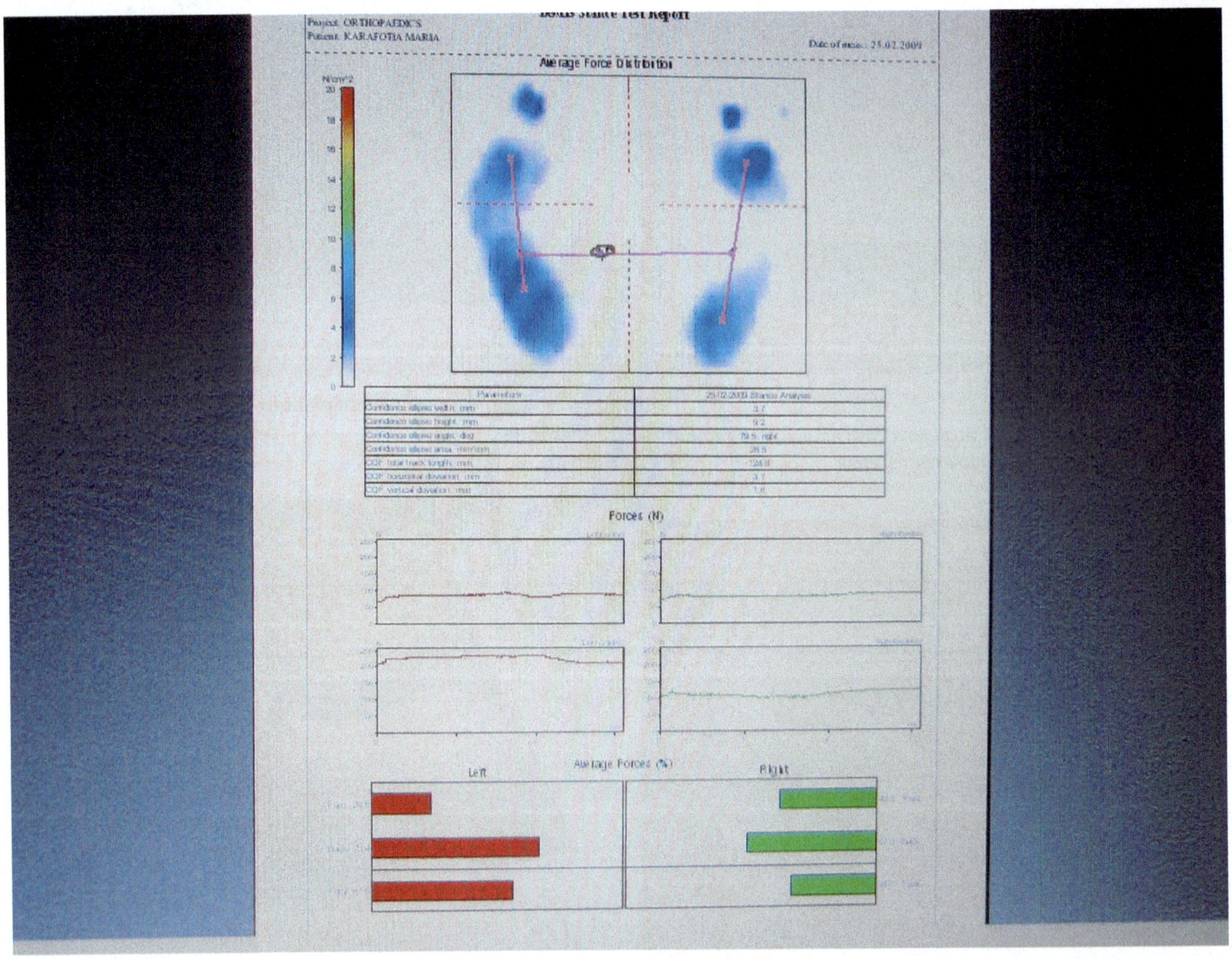

Figure 2.24 Analysis of the dynamic force/pressure distribution from the measurement platform while standing. The forces exerted from the fore-, mid-, and hindfoot are depicted separately for each foot on the lower part of the report.

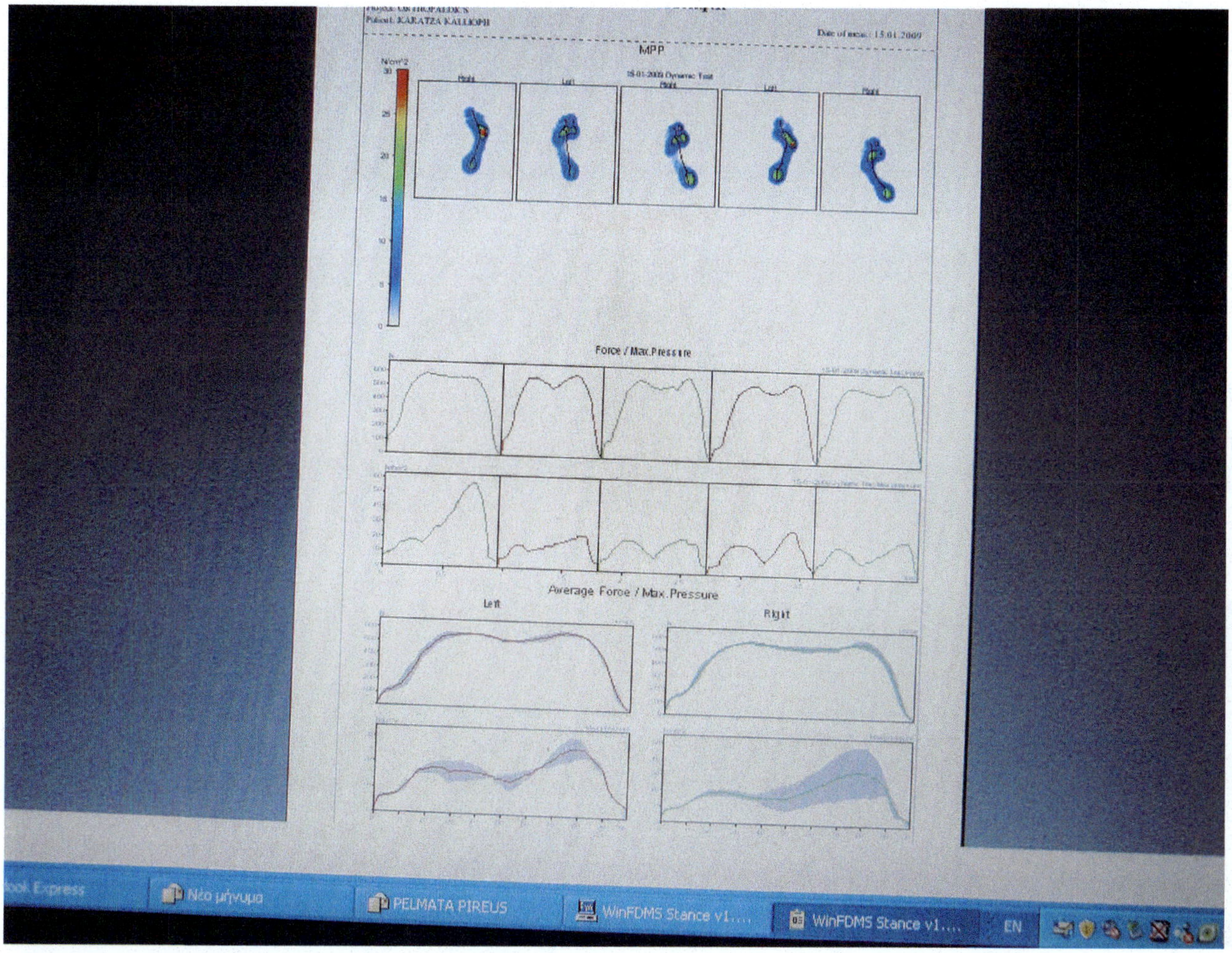

Figure 2.25 Analysis of the dynamic force/pressure distribution from the measurement platform while walking. Notice that three steps have been analyzed on the upper part of the report, while the pressure graphs for each foot are given on the lower part.

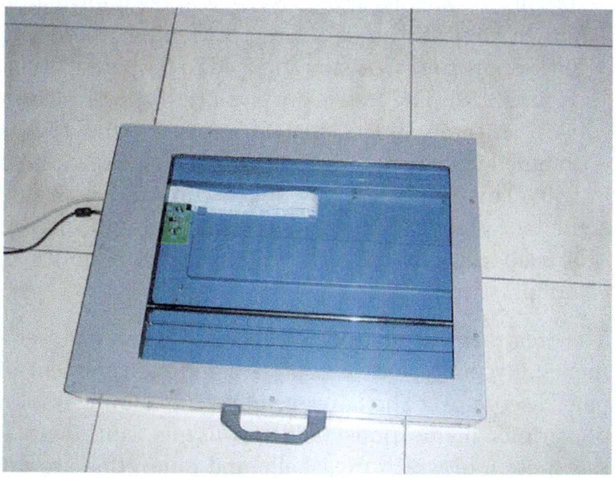

Figure 2.26 A scanner. The patient stands on the scanner surface barefoot, while the instrument scans the plantar surfaces of the feet and gives an analysis on a computer screen.

sensor plate with high-quality calibrated capacitive force sensors supplies the required data to an external computer via a USB interface. This is a more complex, sophisticated and expensive method of foot pressure assessment, suitable for specialized centers.

- Scanners. These scan the feet (Figure 2.26) and provide a view of the exerted forces on a monitor in real time (Figure 2.27). The software included can then process the picture and give information in different colors (depending on pressure sites), dimensions (two- or three-dimensional), visual angle and size. The software also has the capability to guide the automatic manufacturing of custom-made shoe arch supports for a patient's specific foot problem. This is a sophisticated and expensive system of foot pressure measurement.
- In-shoe measurement system. This comprises insoles with attached pressure sensors. The insoles are

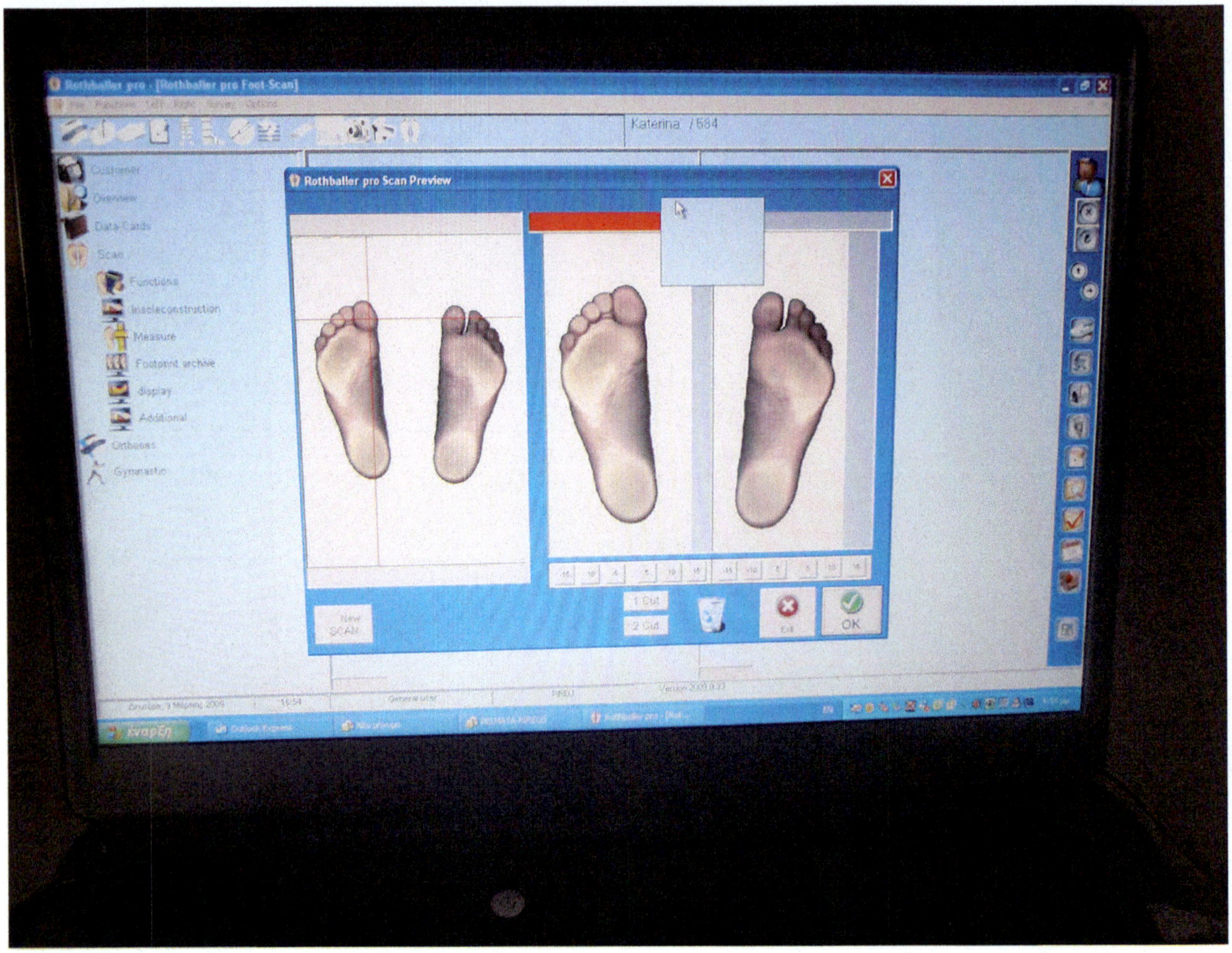

Figure 2.27 The report of the scanned feet of a diabetic patient as seen on the monitor screen. Notice the different shades of gray depending on the pressures exerted by different areas of the soles.

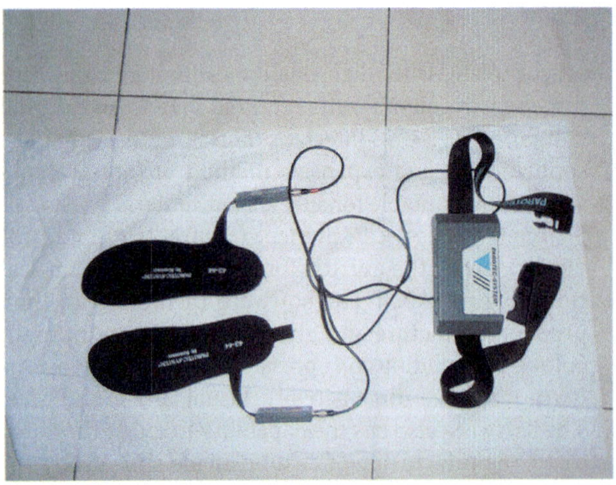

Figure 2.28 The in-shoe measurement system. This comprises insoles with attached pressure sensors that transmit the information (either wirelessly or via a wire, as in this photograph) to a central recorder of the foot pressures, usually attached to the patient's belt.

inserted into the patient's shoes while the patient is standing or walking and then transmit the information (either wirelessly or via a wire) to a central recorder of the foot pressures, usually attached to the patient's belt (Figure 2.28). The results are given retrospectively in a two- or three-dimensional form, as for the results obtained from scanners or platforms (Figures 2.29 and 2.30). This is the best way of detecting and analyzing the foot pressures in everyday circumstances and can be used to see the effect of treatment with orthotics on foot pressures.

The treatment of neuropathy includes three main elements: glycemic control, foot care and management of pain/discomfort. The latter involves the administration of various medications (anticonvulsants, anti-depressants, etc.), of which pregabalin and duloxetine are the only ones formally approved by the European Medicines Agency and the US Food and Drug Administration for the treatment of painful diabetic polyneuropathy.

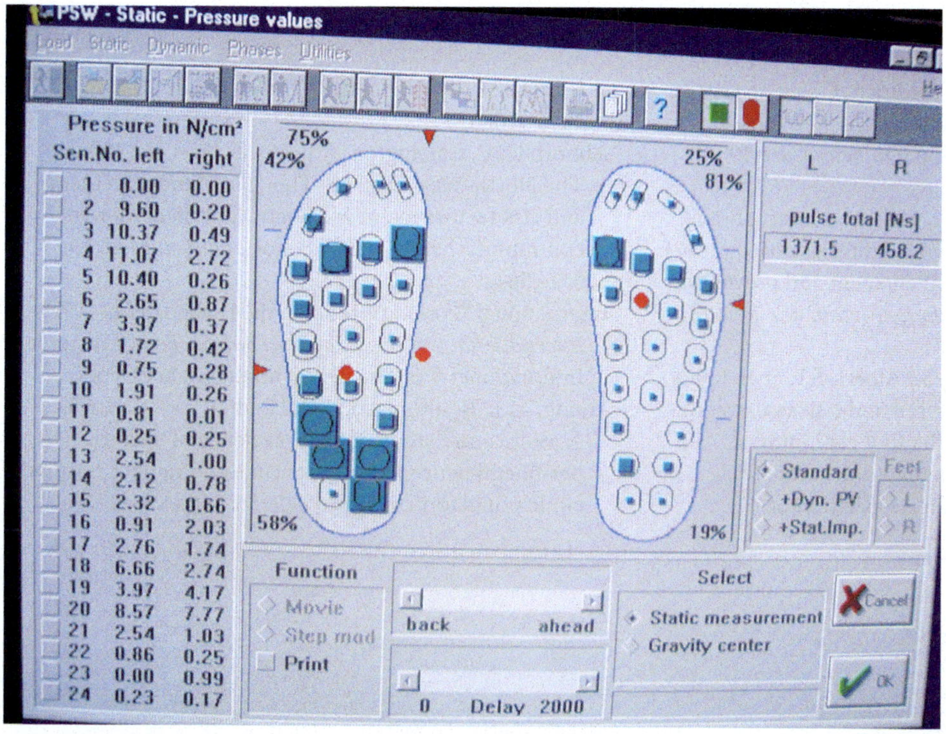

Figure 2.29 Results of an analysis of in-shoe pressure measurement during standing. The pressures at the various sites of the sole are depicted in Ncm^{-2}, separately for the left and right feet.

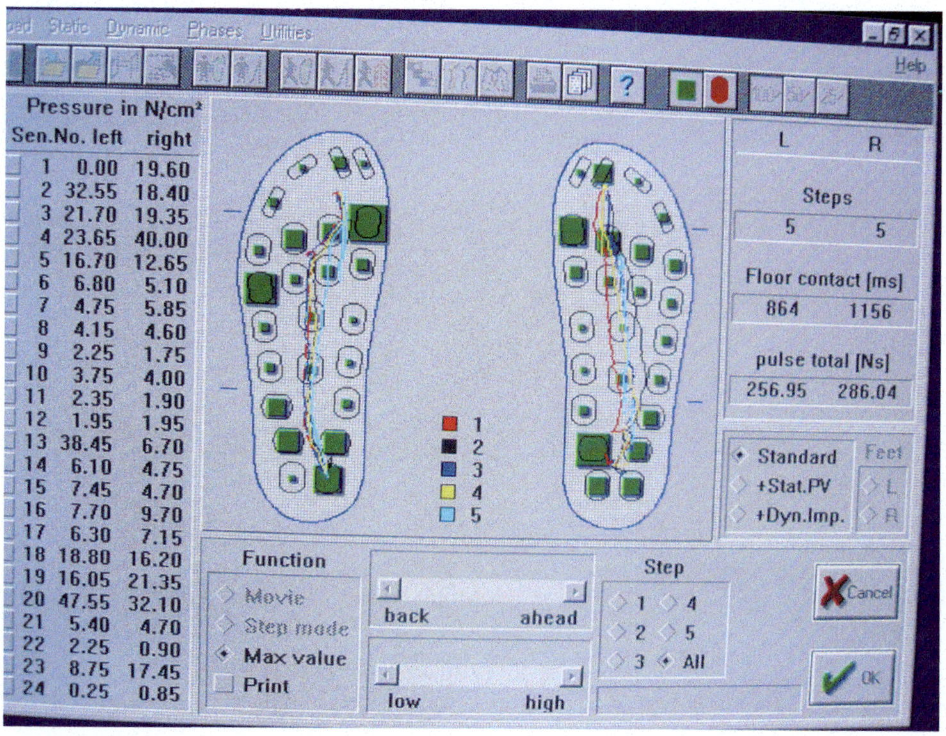

Figure 2.30 Results of an analysis of in-shoe pressure measurement during walking. The patient has taken five steps, and the pressures at the various sites of the sole are depicted in Ncm^{-2}.

Further Reading

Pop-Busui, R., Boulton, A.J.M., Feldman, E.L. et al. (2017). Diabetic neuropathy: a position statement by the American Diabetes Association. *Diabetes Care* 40: 136–154.

Bakker, K., Apelqvist, J., Schaper, N.C., and International Working Group on Diabetic Foot Editorial Board (2012). Practical guidelines on the management and prevention of the diabetic foot 2011. *Diabetes Metab. Res. Rev.* 28: (Suppl 1): 225–231.

Boulton, A.J.M., Armstrong, D.G., Albert, S.F. et al. (2008). Comprehensive foot examination and risk assessment. A report of the task force of the foot care interest Group of the American Diabetes Association, with endorsement by the American Association of Clinical Endocrinologists. *Diabetes Care* 31 (8): 1679–1685.

Abbott, C.A., Carrington, A.L., Ashe, H. et al. (2002). The North-West Diabetes Foot Care Study: incidence of, and risk factors for, new diabetic foot ulceration in a community-based patient cohort. *Diabet. Med.* 19: 377–384.

International Working Group on the Diabetic Foot (1999). *International Consensus on the Diabetic Foot.* Amsterdam: International Working Group on the Diabetic Foot.

Young, M.J., Boulton, A.J., MacLeod, A.F. et al. (1993). A multicentre study of the prevalence of diabetic peripheral neuropathy in the United Kingdom hospital clinic population. *Diabetologia* 36: 150–154.

3

Anatomic Risk Factors for Diabetic Foot Ulceration

P. Tsapogas

Center for Diabetes and Metabolism, Henry Dunant Hospital Center, Athens, Greece

3.1 Pes Planus or Adult-Acquired Flatfoot Deformity (Flatfoot)

Pes planus or flatfoot is the commonest foot deformity, its prevalence being about 20% in the adult population and increasing with age. The majority of flat feet are considered to be variations of normal. The "too many toes" sign refers to a position of the foot that allows the examiner to see all four toes when looking at the foot from behind.

Pes planus is characterized by diminished longitudinal and transverse concavities of the foot (Figures 3.1–3.5). Diminished plantar transverse concavity is associated with an increase in the frontal transverse convexity of the tarsometatarsal joint line (Lisfranc joint line) and a divergence of the five metatarsal bones. The load transfer is displaced to the medial border of the mid-tarsal region. Hindfoot valgus may ensue due to "shortening" of the lateral column, plantar inclination of the talar head and lateral subluxation of the navicular on the talar head (Figure 3.5).

There is evidence that flat feet protect against loading of the metatarsal heads, although they are poor shock absorbers. Pes planus may cause bunionette formation (Figures 3.2 and 3.3) and plantar heel spur pain. Insufficiency or dysfunction of the posterior tibial tendon is thought to be the commonest cause of pes planus.

Midfoot collapse secondary to Charcot neuroarthropathy results in a rocker-bottom foot and will certainly require treatment (Figures 3.4 and 3.5; see also Chapter 10).

A painless deformity that can be accommodated by proper footwear and allows for normal gait does not require surgical treatment. Nevertheless, foot orthotics and arch supports do not alter the osseous relationships and are ineffective in many patients. Indications for the surgical treatment (rarely indicated in diabetic adults) of posterior tibial tendon dysfunction are disabling pain and difficulty with ambulation.

3.2 Bunion

A bunion is an enlargement of bone or tissue around the first metatarsophalangeal joint (Figures 3.6–3.14), or a swollen bursal sac and/or osseous (bony) deformity that has grown on this joint. Hallux valgus is the deformity most commonly associated with a bunion. Bunions are caused by a failure of the tendons and ligaments supporting the first metatarsal. Flatfoot, diabetic neuropathy and/or excessive ligamentous flexibility may produce a bunion. Some of these factors may be genetic. Poorly fitting footwear may exacerbate a bunion; the higher prevalence of bunions in women is probably attributed to this condition.

3.3 Hallux Valgus and Convex Triangular Foot

Hallux valgus is considered to be a medial deviation of the first metatarsal and a lateral deviation and/or rotation of the hallux, with or without medial soft tissue enlargement of the first metatarsal head. Hallux valgus and the associated varus posture of the first metatarsal bone cause various deformities of the other toes, such as varus, clawing and valgus formation (see Figures 3.10–3.13).

The long and short extensor tendons of all the toes shrink like bowstrings, causing subluxation of the phalangeal bases. Contractures of tendons and joint capsules then result in fixation of the deformity. The heads

Atlas of the Diabetic Foot, Third Edition. Ioanna Eleftheriadou, Alexandros Kokkinos, Stavros Liatis, Konstantinos Makrilakis, Nicholas Tentolouris, Anastasios Tentolouris, and Panagiotis Tsapogas.

Companion website: www.wiley.com/go/tentolouris/atlas_diabetic_foot

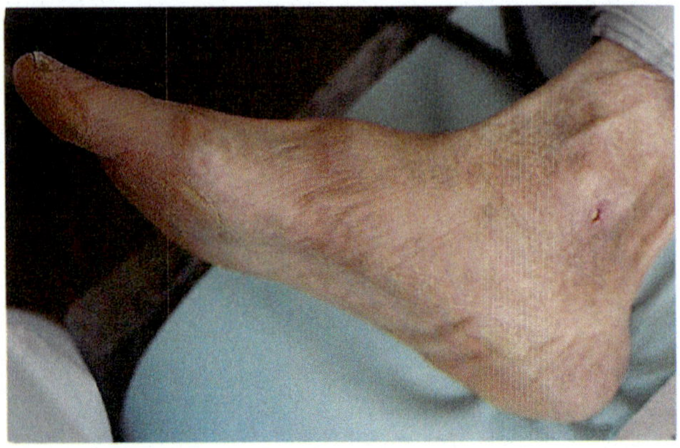

Figure 3.1 Pes planus.

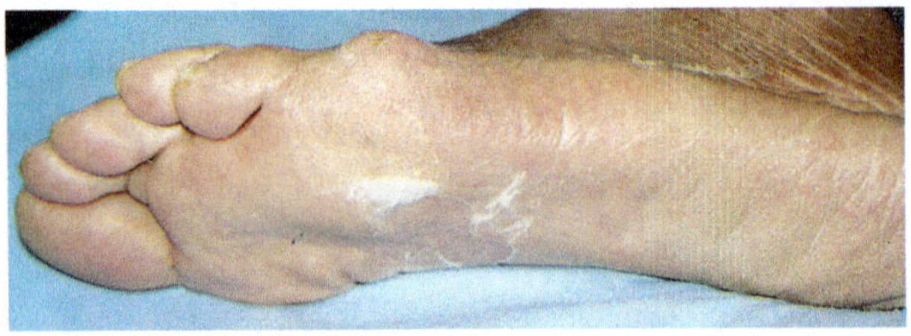

Figure 3.2 Pes planus, with mild callus formation over the plantar and lateral areas of the fifth metatarsal head – a bunionette.

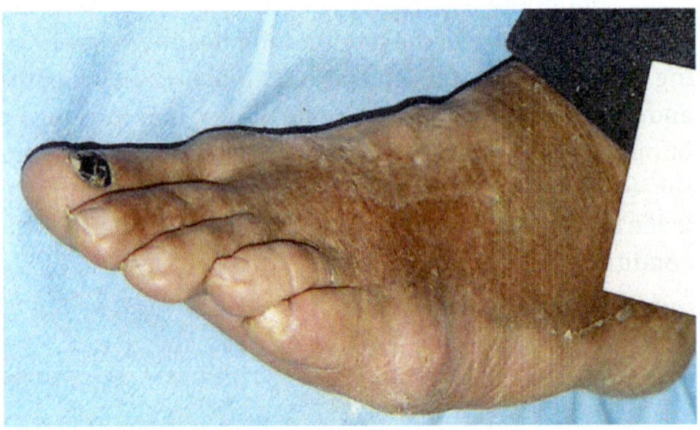

Figure 3.3 Pes planus with bunionette and a subungual hematoma seen at the hallux. This is the dorsal aspect of the foot shown in Figure 3.2.

of the three central metatarsal bones become lowered due to the deformity of the third and fourth toes, resulting in their exposure and callus formation. In more severe involvement, the line of load is displaced progressively toward the medial side of the foot, and the longitudinal arch lowers, leading to pes planovalgus.

According to some experts, hallux valgus is a twofold deformity: valgus of the proximal phalanx of the great toe and varus of the first metatarsal. The forefoot is splayed (Figures 3.15–3.17, and see Figure 3.14), not through stretching of the adductor structures, but

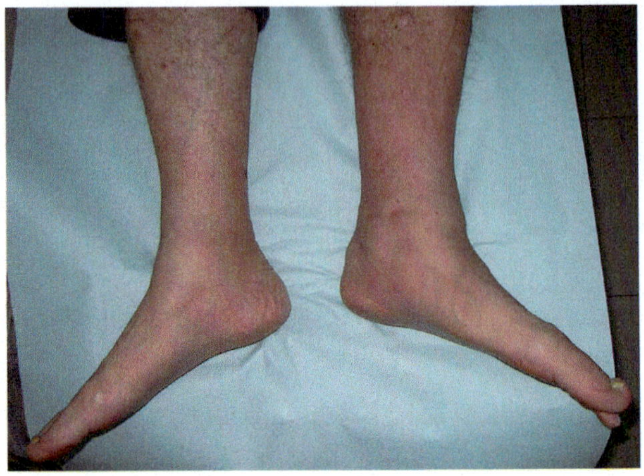

Figure 3.4 Pes planus (acquired left flatfoot) in a 60-year-old gentleman with type 1 diabetes who was on renal dialysis. The acute onset of the condition prompted magnetic resonance imaging investigation for acute Charcot of the midfoot, which was positive.

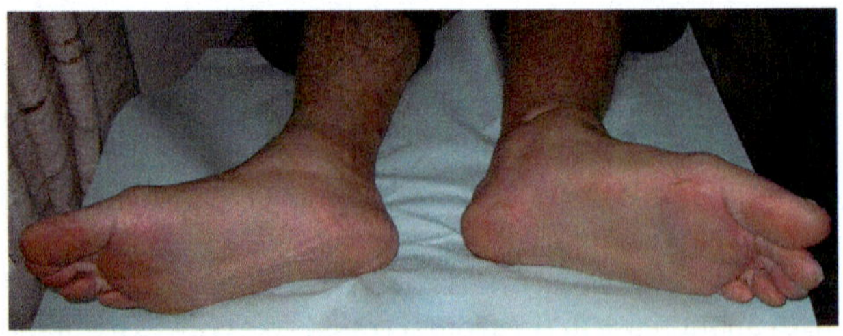

Figure 3.5 Pes planus (plantar aspect) of the left foot of the patient shown in Figure 3.4. Acute neuropathic osteoarthropathy (Charcot foot) is diagnosed with magnetic resonance imaging (see Chapter 10).

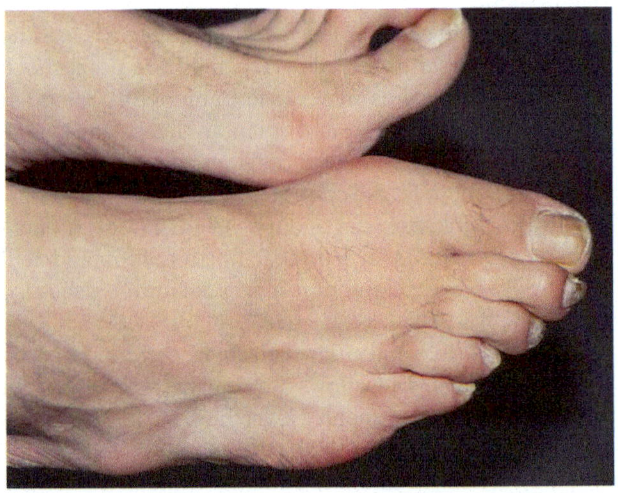

Figure 3.6 A bunion and bunionette with claw toes, muscle atrophy and prominent veins on the dorsum of the foot.

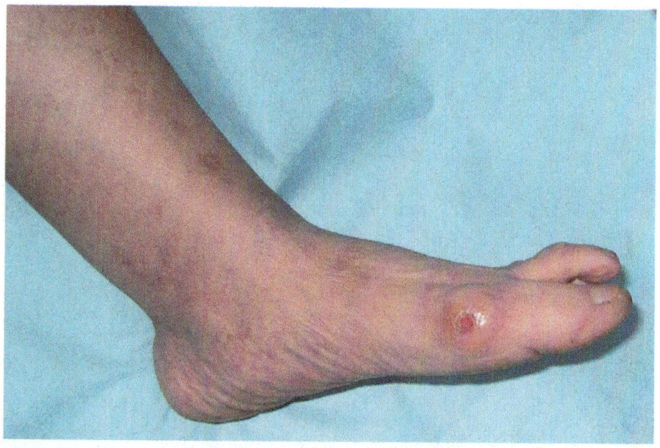

Figure 3.7 An infected neuropathic ulcer and bursitis over a bunion with hallux valgus and claw toes.

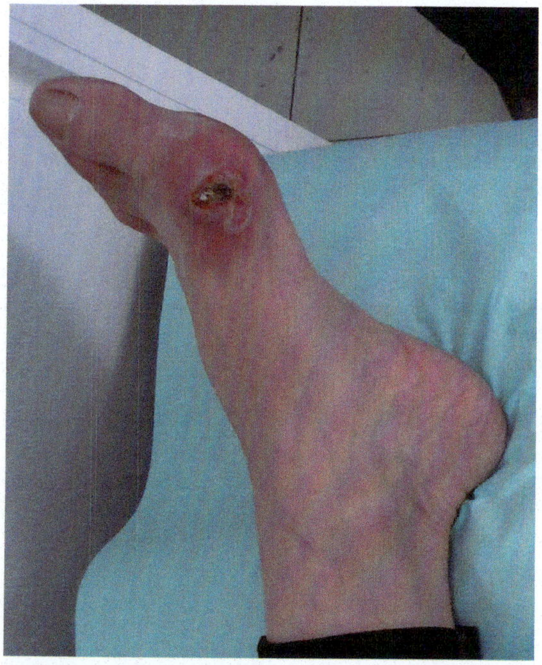

Figure 3.8 An infected neuropathic ulcer and bursitis over a bunion seen on the left foot of a 59-year-old lady with type 2 diabetes and hallux valgus. This lady worked as a tour guide and refused to use proper off-loading shoes or have an operation.

because the first metatarsal head escapes from the control exercised by the base of the proximal phalanx, into which these muscles are inserted. The phalanx and sesamoids remain held by the adductors, while the first metatarsal head drifts away out of control.

A convex triangular foot is characterized by convergence of the first and fifth toes, and claw deformities of the central three toes (see Figures 3.10, 3.11 and 3.13). The first and fifth metatarsals are short and diverge. Both the longitudinal and transverse plantar concavities are accentuated, and the second and third metatarsals

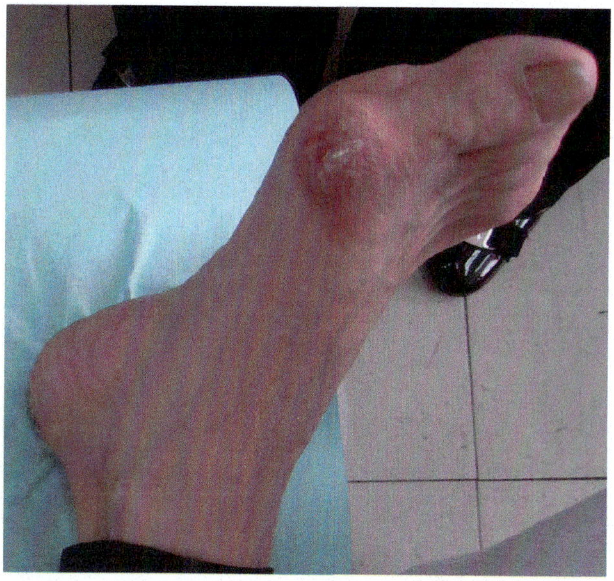

Figure 3.9 A bunion on the right foot of the patient whose left foot is shown in Figure 3.8.

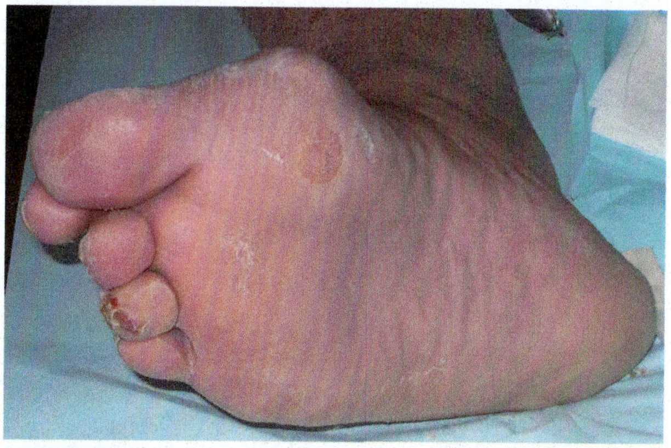

Figure 3.10 Convex triangular foot with hallux valgus, bunion and bunionette. The second toe is overriding the third toe. Painless calluses are seen under the first metatarsal head and on the fourth toe.

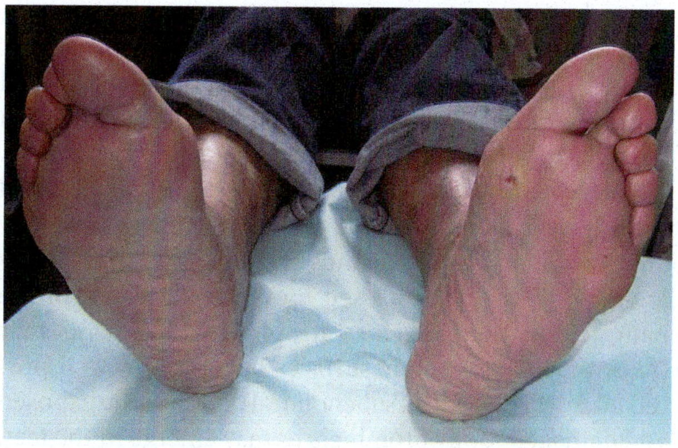

Figure 3.11 Triangular forefeet with bunionette. Callus and a neuropathic ulcer are seen under the first metatarsal head.

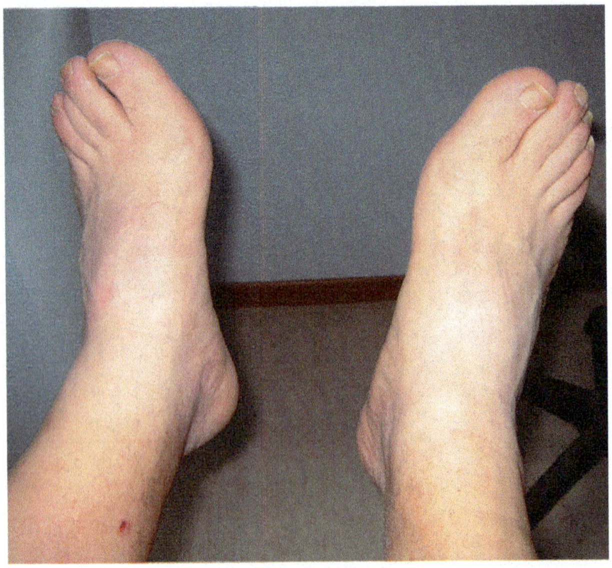

Figure 3.12 Familial convex triangular feet (hallux valgus and quintus varus).

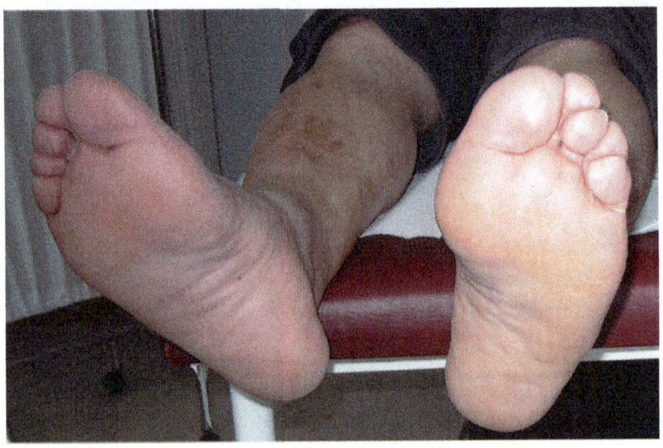

Figure 3.13 Familial convex triangular feet. The second and the fourth left toes override the third and the fifth toes, while the second right toe overrides the third toe. This is the plantar aspect of the feet shown in Figure 3.12.

are fixed in excessive equinus from this level. Cavus feet balance on the heel and the central part of the metatarsal paddle (Figure 3.18). This deformity may cause high pressures over the metatarsal paddle during walking.

Osteoarthritis, the most common form of painful arthritis, can affect any joint, although it most commonly affects the joints of the hands (Figure 3.19), hips, knees and spine. Due to decreased movement because of the pain, regional muscles may atrophy, and ligaments may become more lax, bony surfaces become less well protected by cartilage, and subchondral bone may be exposed and damaged. Bony prominences may emerge in the feet, predisposing to callus and ulceration due to friction and pressure in the shoes (see also Figures 3.14–3.17).

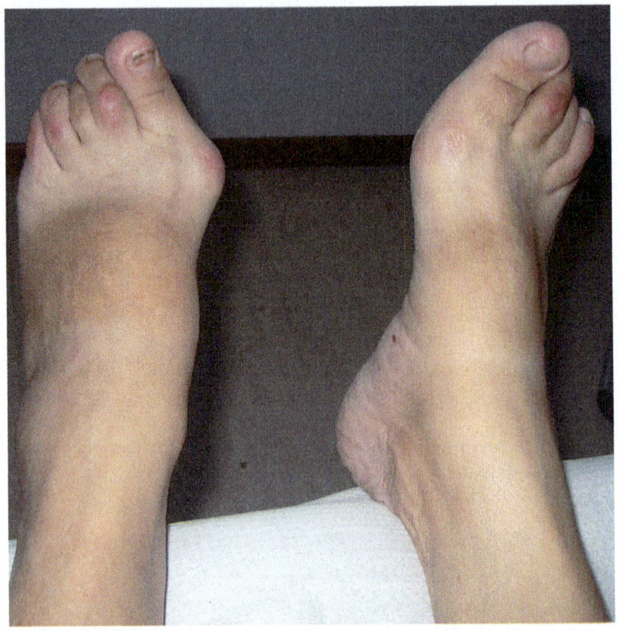

Figure 3.14 Triangular forefeet with overriding toe. Hallux valgus and a bunion of the left foot, as well as claw toes, cab be seen. Corns are present on the phalangophalangeal joints.

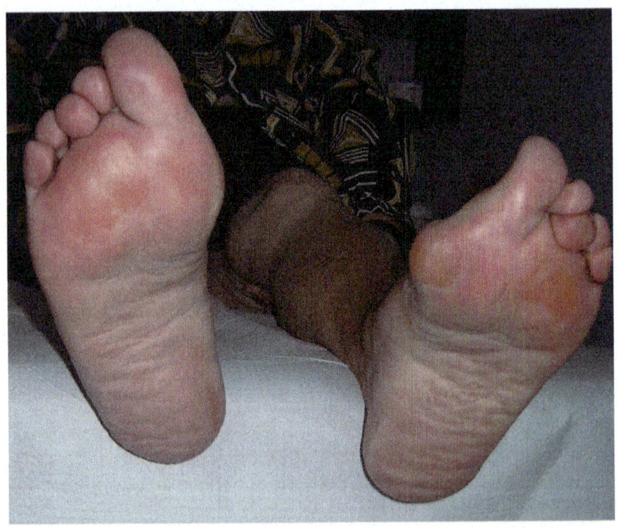

Figure 3.15 Triangular forefeet with the second toe overriding the third toe bilaterally. Callosity has formed under the metatarsal heads of this lady, the dorsal aspect of whose feet is shown in Figure 3.14.

3.4 Bunionette (Tailor's Bunion)

A bunionette is an acquired lesion of the lateral aspect of the fifth metatarsal head. The name "tailor's bunion" originates from the traditional cross-legged sitting posture of

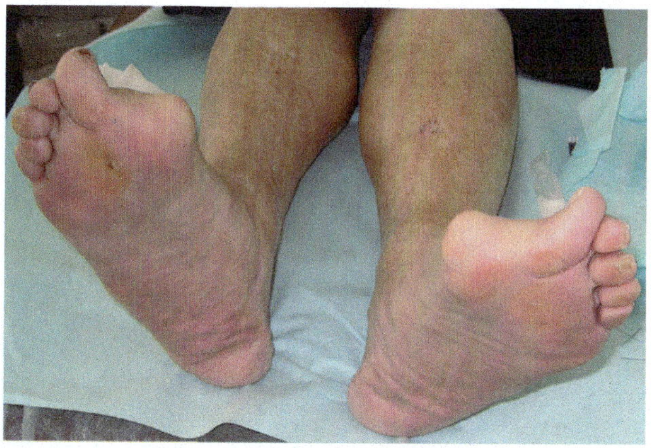

Figure 3.16 Bunions and boutonnière deformity. The proximal interphalangeal joint of the hallux is flexed, and the distal interphalangeal joint is hyperextended. Callus is seen under the metatarsal heads and tips of the toes. A neuropathic ulcer is present under the left second metatarsal head.

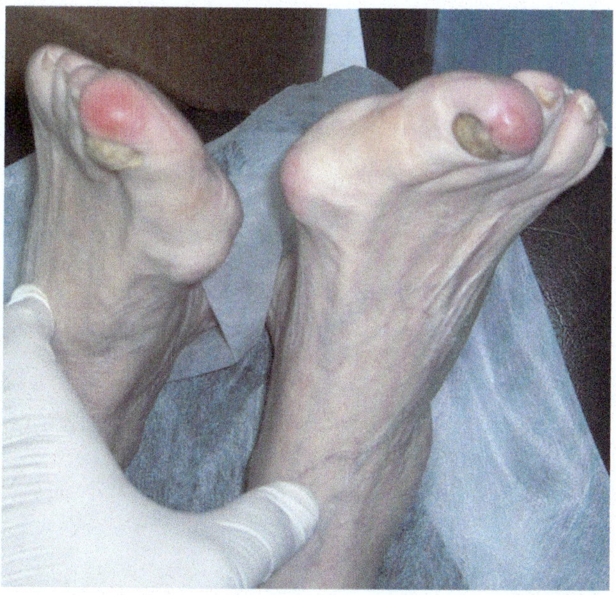

Figure 3.17 Bilateral hallux valgus, bunions and muscle atrophy are seen on both feet of an 80-year-old lady with type 2 diabetes. Claw toes and onychomycosis are also present. Friction within her shoes and rubbing against her bedding caused inflammation of the tip of the great toes bilaterally, which resolved with scaling but no ulceration. This was a stage 1 pressure ulcer.

tailors, pressing the lateral aspects of their fifth metatarsal heads onto sturdy benches.

A bunionette is often associated with a varus deformity of the lesser toe (quintus varus). Ulceration over a bunionette may occur in a patient who has no feeling of pain, and an infection of the ulcer may spread to the bursa and the underlying bone (Figures 3.20 and 3.21).

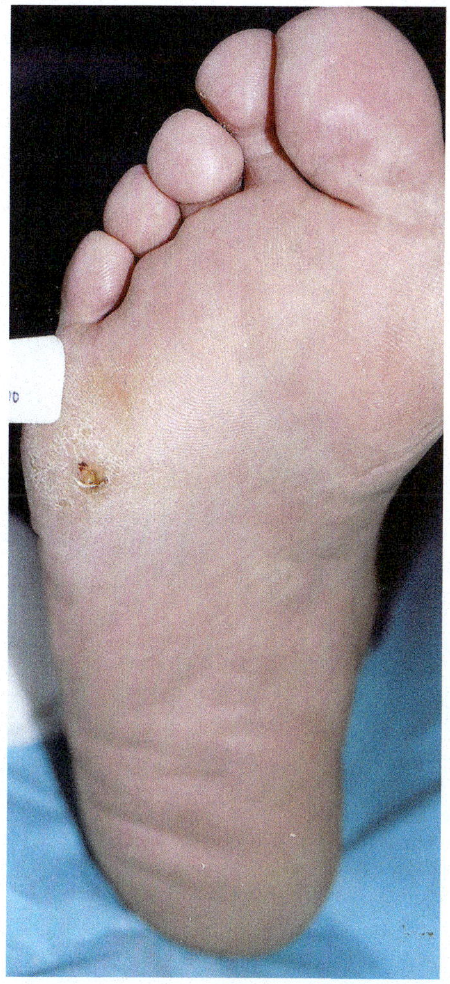

Figure 3.18 Hallux valgus, quintus varus (convex triangular foot), bunionette and claw toes are seen, together with a healing neuropathic ulcer under the fifth metatarsal head.

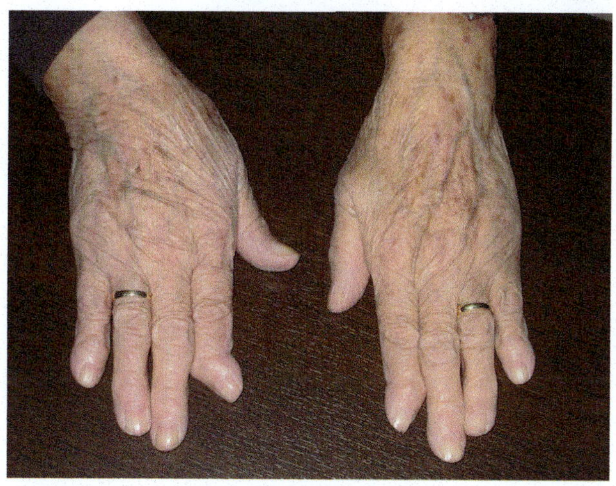

Figure 3.19 Osteoarthritis of the hands of the patient whose feet are shown in Figures 3.14 and 3.15.

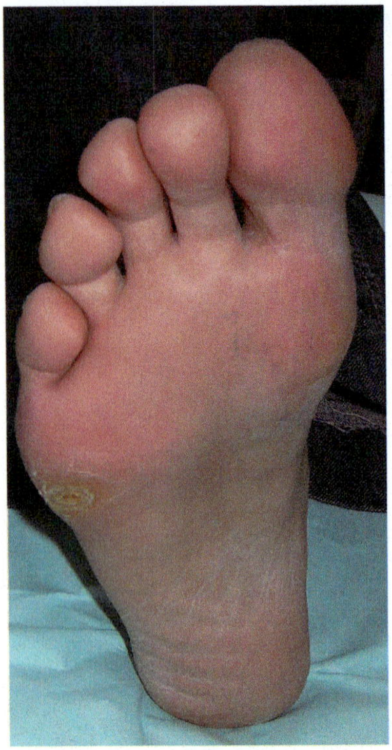

Figure 3.20 An infected neuropathic ulcer over a bunionette is seen on the right foot of a 60-year-old gentleman with type 2 diabetes, with over 2 cm of cellulitis on the dorsal aspect of the forefoot. A hammer deformity of the second toe is present. Osteomyelitis was diagnosed under this bunionette ulcer.

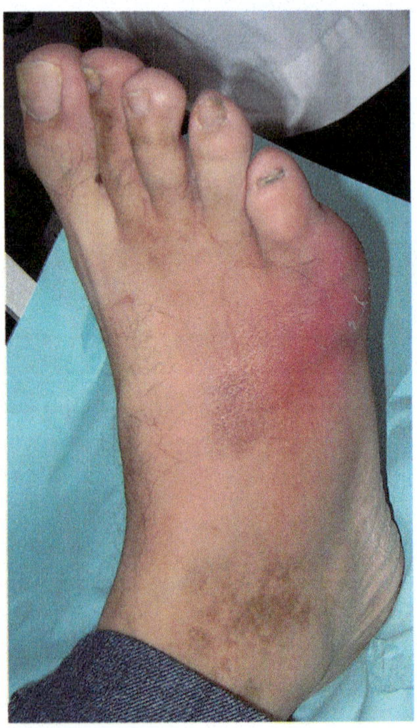

Figure 3.21 Quintus varus and bunionette with an infected neuropathic ulcer and cellulitis.

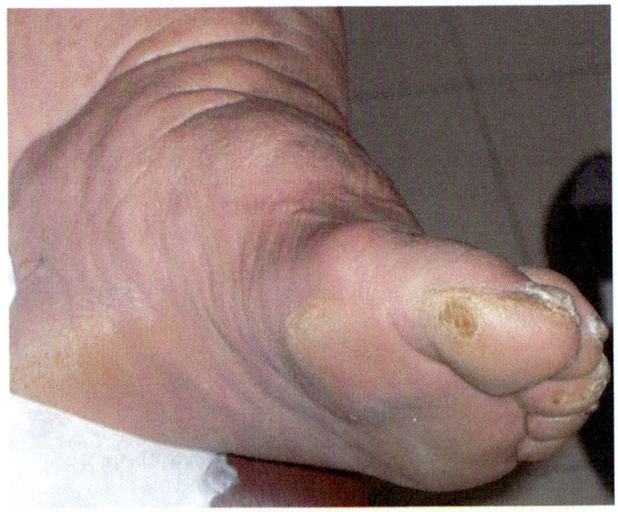

Figure 3.22 A callus over the medial aspect of the second interphalangeal joint of the great toe, caused by friction in the shoe.

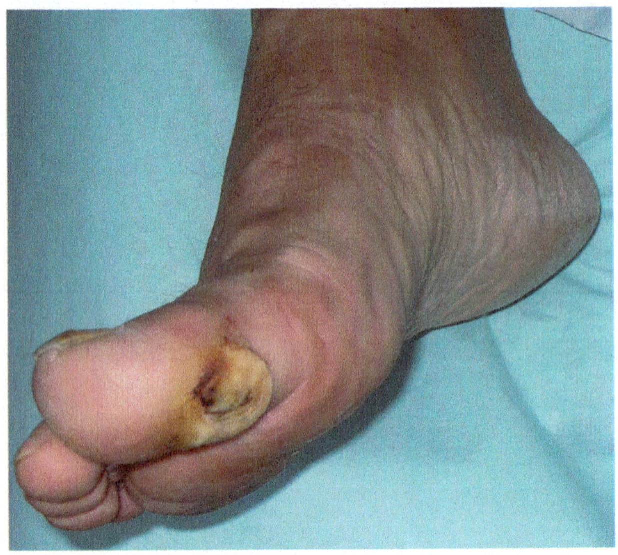

Figure 3.23 A callus over the medial aspect of the second interphalangeal joint of the great toe, caused by friction in the shoe.

3.5 Protruding Interphalangeal Joints

A callus over a tuberosity of a phalanx of the great toe (Figures 3.22–3.27), or a painful end-corn on the crown of a protruding interphalangeal joint of a lesser toe (Figures 3.28–3.34), a consequence of chronic pressure in the shoe, is a frequent complication even in feet with normal sensation. The corn leads to ulceration in neuropathic feet.

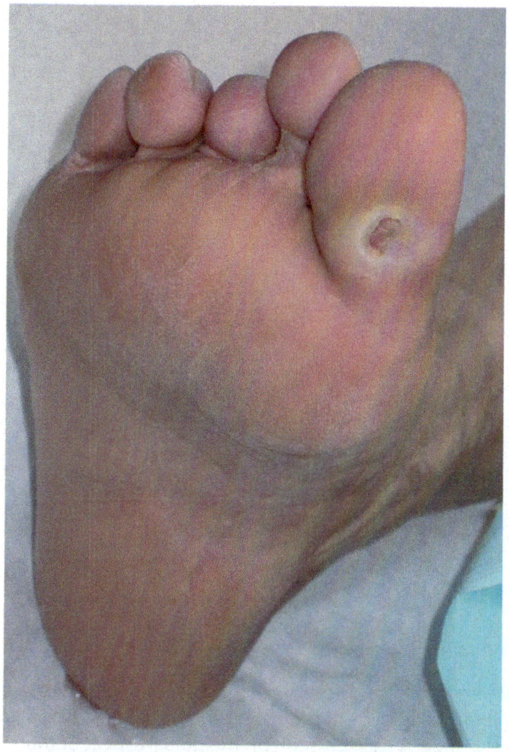

Figure 3.24 A debrided callus over the medial aspect of the second interphalangeal joint of the great toe, caused by friction in the shoe.

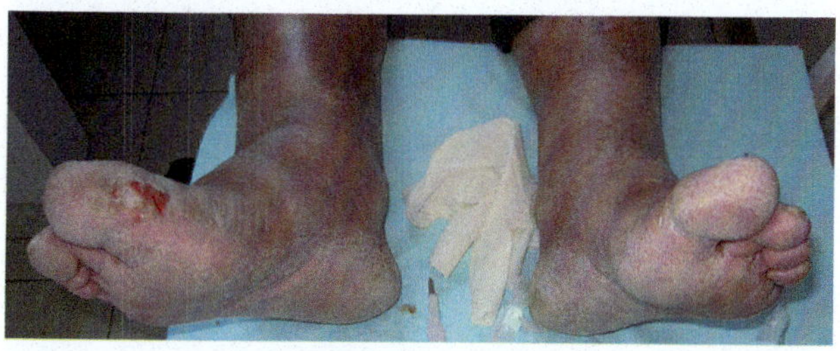

Figure 3.25 A friction ulcer over the medial aspect of the right great toe is seen on the right foot of this 70-year-old gentleman with type 2 diabetes. This ulcer has caused septic arthritis and osteomyelitis of the hallux (see Figures 3.26 and 3.27), which is shortened. Claw toes and dry skin are evident on both feet.

Treatment directed toward the wound alone may be counterproductive, and the ultimate goal must be correction of the underlying etiology caused by the toe deformity. Some orthopedic surgeons suggest flexor tenotomy. The main contraindication to this procedure is small-vessel vascular compromise in the setting of peripheral vascular disease. Neuropathic osteoarthropathy (Charcot foot) as a result of any operation on the foot is also a concern. Callus removal pads or plasters are contraindicated in neuropathic feet because they may erode the skin and create an ulcer (Figure 3.34).

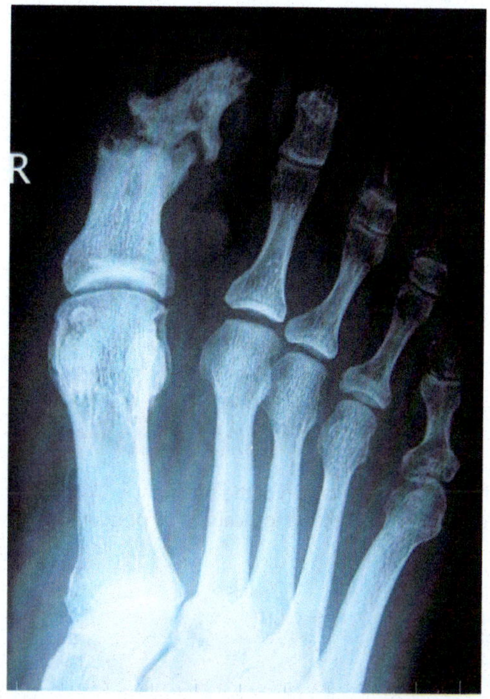

Figure 3.26 Splaying of the forefoot/triangular forefoot and osteomyelitis of the hallux are shown in this plain radiograph of the right foot of the patient shown in Figure 3.25.

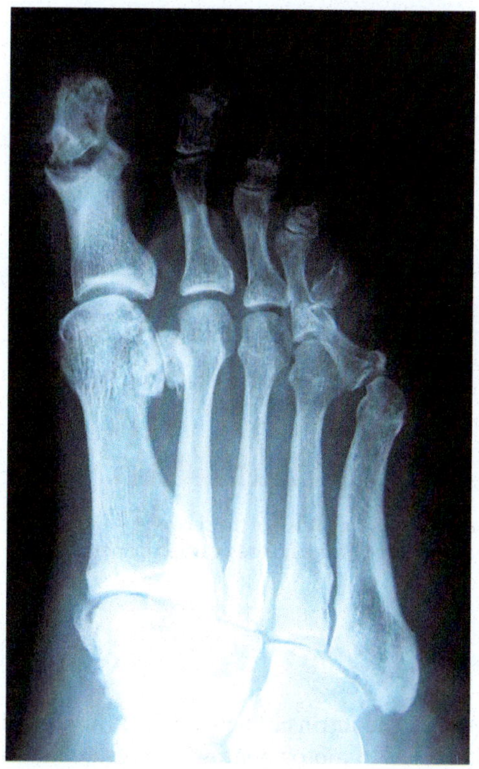

Figure 3.27 Quintus varus, claw toes and osteomyelitis of the hallux are shown on this plain radiograph of the right foot of the patient shown in Figure 3.25.

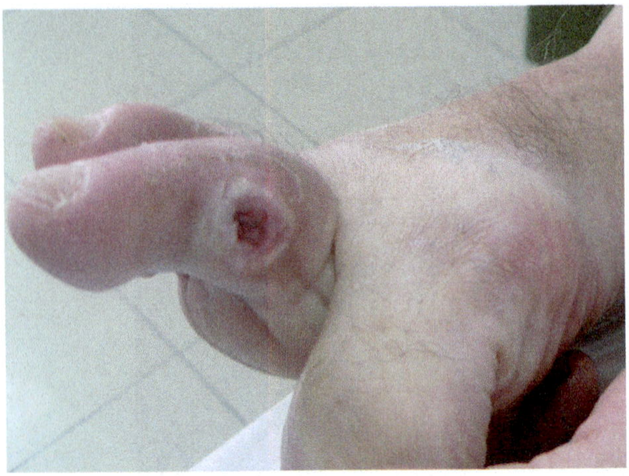

Figure 3.28 A callus over the crown of the second interphalangeal joint of the second toe, caused by pressure in the shoe.

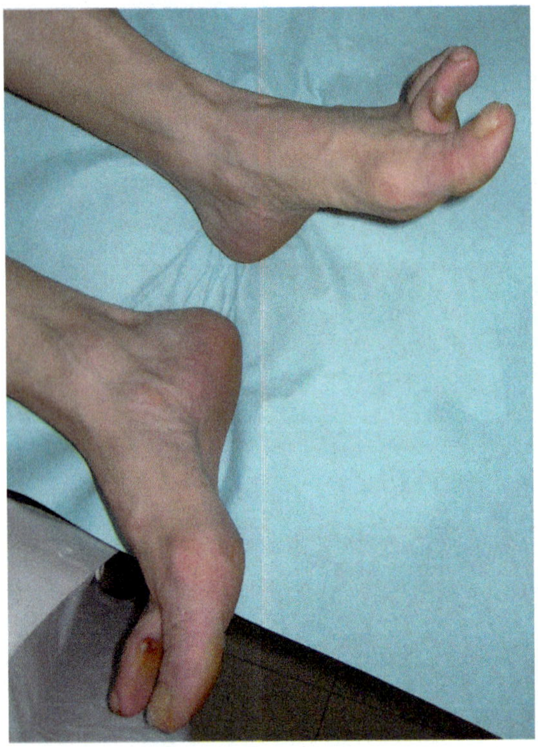

Figure 3.29 Calluses over the crown of the second interphalangeal joint of both second toes, caused by pressure in the shoe.

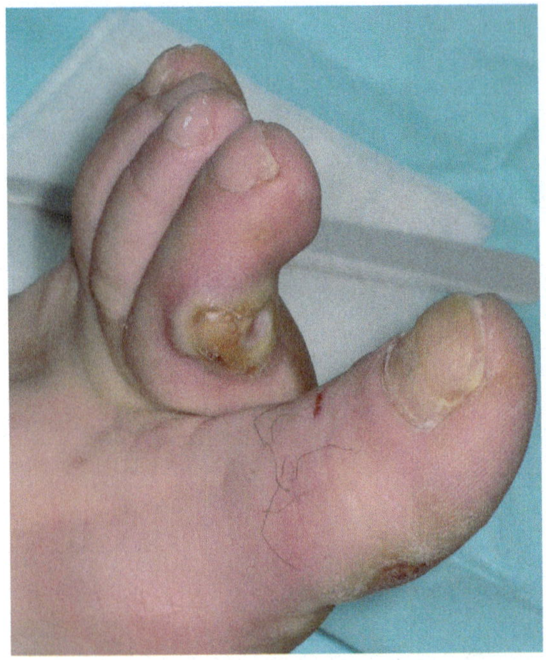

Figure 3.30 A neuropathic ulcer developed over the crown of the second interphalangeal joint of the second toe, caused by pressure in the shoe. A callus is seen on the dorsal aspect of the great toe. The patient's right foot is shown in Figure 3.29.

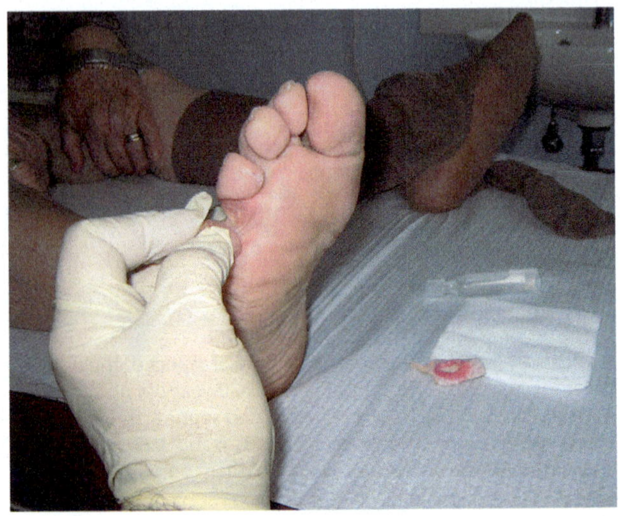

Figure 3.31 An ulcer developed after the application of a callus removal plaster over the fourth metatarsal head. A painful corn was removed before the plaster was applied.

3.6 Claw Toes

Severe atrophy of the intrinsic foot muscles (lumbrical and interossei), due to motor neuropathy, results in an imbalance of the foot muscles and cock-up toes (claw toes; Figures 3.35 and 3.36). This is a typical appearance of a neuropathic foot.

A claw toe, the most common deformity in diabetic patients (Figures 3.37–3.40, and see Figures 3.6, 3.7, 3.10, 3.15, 3.16, 3.24, 3.25, 3.31, 3.50, 3.56 and 3.59), consists of dorsiflexion of the metatarsophalangeal joint, while the proximal interphalangeal and distal interphalangeal joints are in plantar flexion (Figure 3.41). Shifting of the fat pads underneath the metatarsal heads to the front

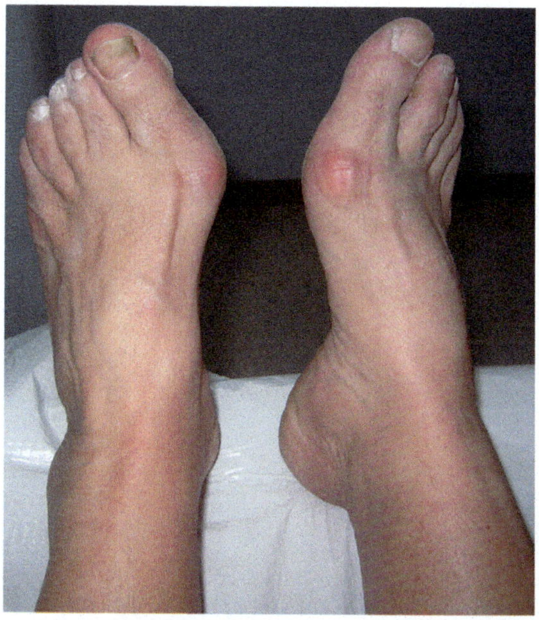

Figure 3.32 Bilateral bunion and convex triangular feet.

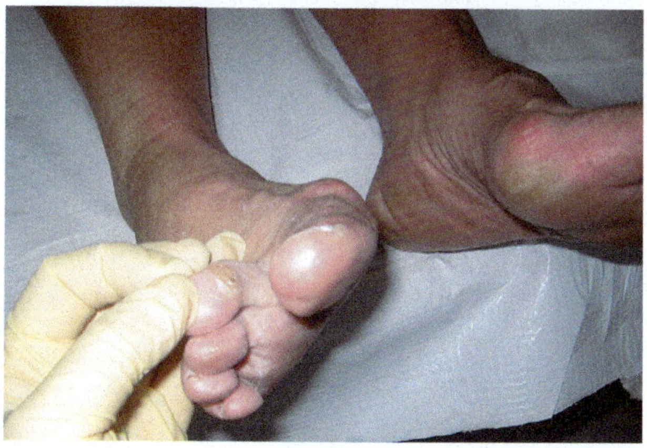

Figure 3.33 A painful corn of the second right toe and callus formation under the first metatarsal head of the patient shown in Figure 3.32.

leaves the metatarsal heads exposed (Figure 3.42 and 3.43), and high plantar pressures develop under the metatarsal heads and no longer along a wide base. The tips of the toes are also at risk for ulceration (see Figure 3.51).

3.7 Prominent Metatarsal Heads

Claw toe deformities may cause prominence of the metatarsal heads (see Figure 3.46) with subsequent callus formation and ulceration. Ulcers and eventual osteomyelitis (Figure 3.44) may develop under the metatarsal heads (Figure 3.45, left foot) or at the tips of the claw

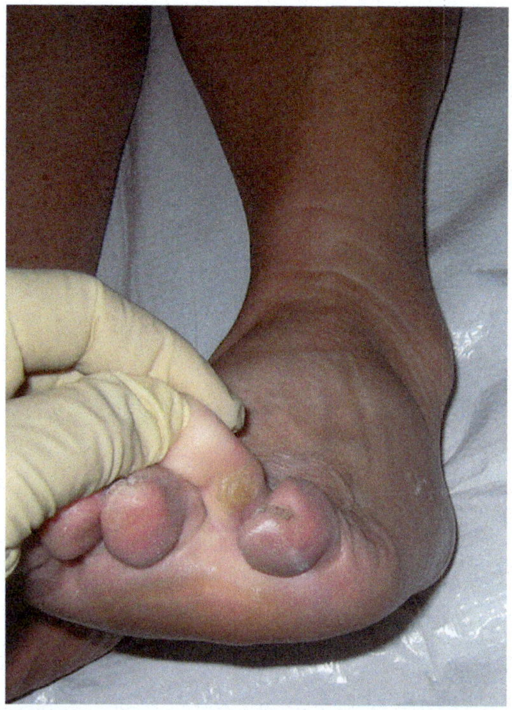

Figure 3.34 A painful corn of the fourth left toe on the left foot of the patient shown in Figure 3.32,

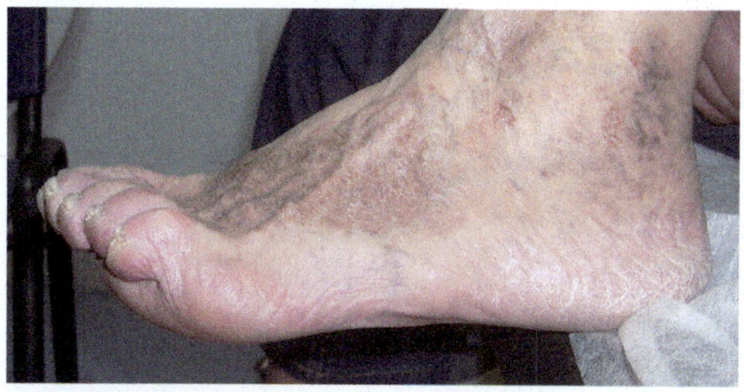

Figure 3.35 Claw toes with overriding second toe and onychogryphosis of the fourth and fifth toenails.

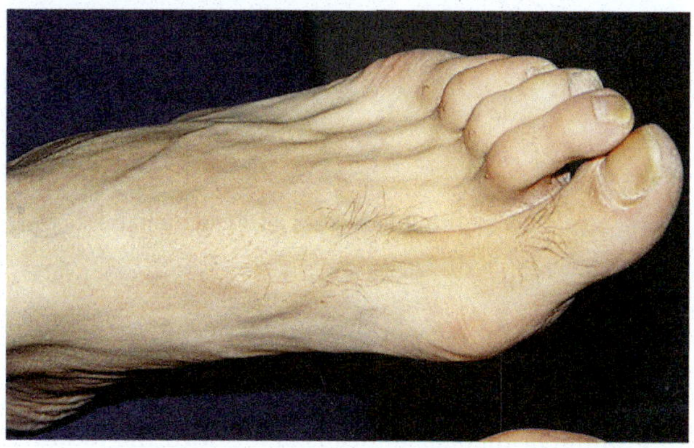

Figure 3.36 Muscle atrophy with claw toes and hallux valgus with quintus varus and bunionette.

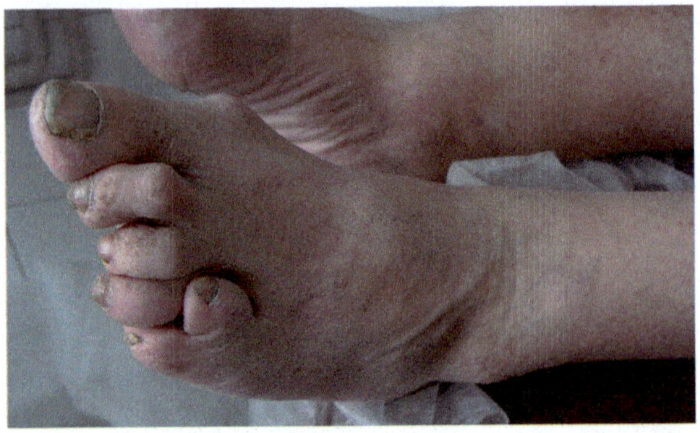

Figure 3.37 Splaying of the right forefoot and bilateral polydactyly.

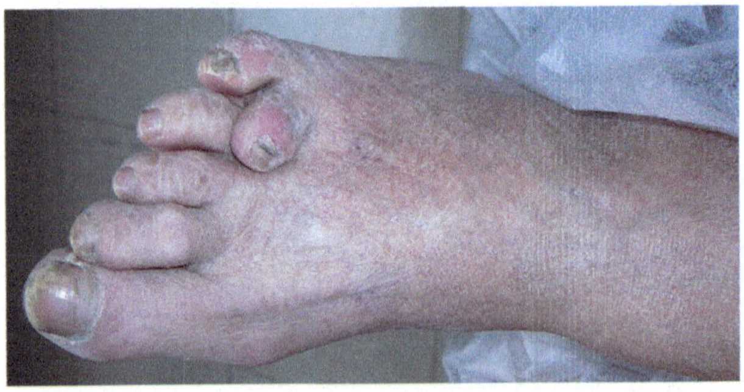

Figure 3.38 Splaying of the forefoot and claw toes of the right foot of the patient whose left foot is shown in Figure 3.37.

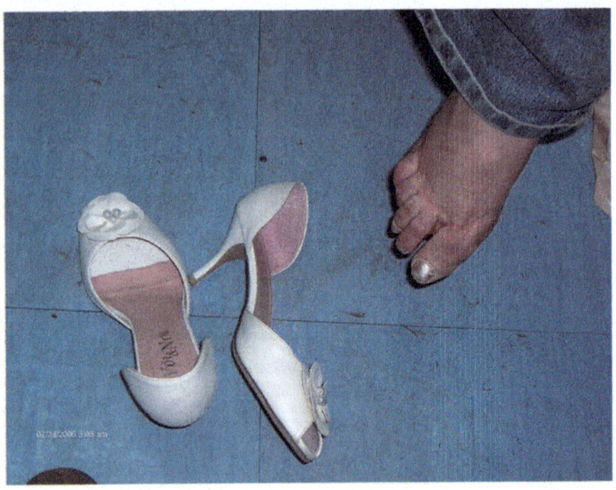

Figure 3.39 Claw fourth and fifth toes resulting from unfitting shoes.

toes, since they are abnormally exposed to pressure during walking.

Even without toe-clawing, hyperextension contributes to prominent metatarsal heads along with migration of the plantar fibrofatty padding distally and dorsally, further exposing the metatarsal heads to increased pressure

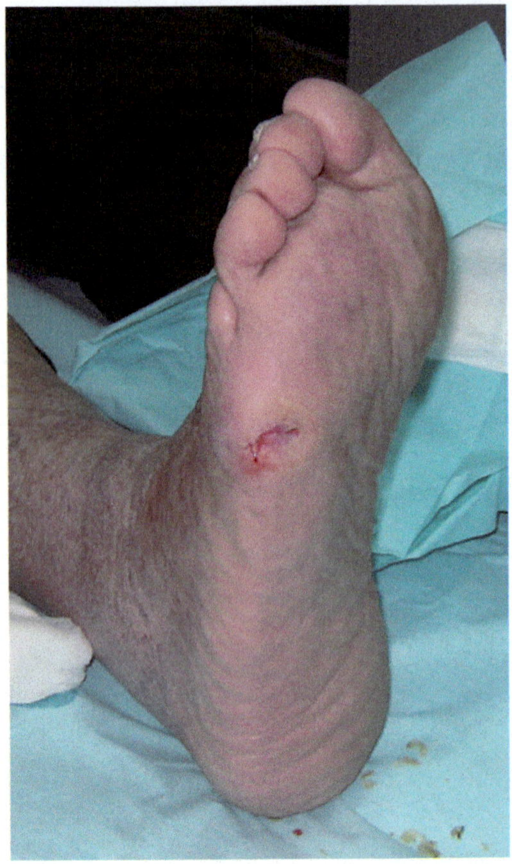

Figure 3.40 Claw toes with overlapping fifth toe and bunionette. There is also a neuropathic ulcer under the fifth metatarsal head.

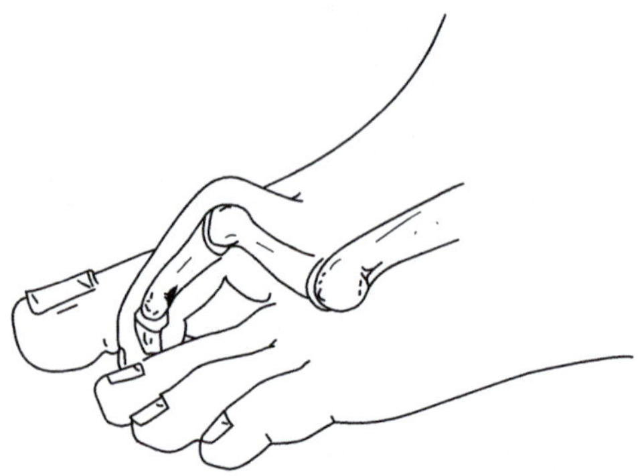

Figure 3.41 Claw toe.

(Figure 3.46, and see Figures 3.18, 3.38, 3.43 and 3.44). Exposed prominent metatarsal heads can be clinically felt by palpation.

3.8 Pes Cavus

Pes cavus is a deformity not necessarily related to diabetes; it may also be a familial trait (Figure 3.47). Normally, the inner edge of the midfoot is raised off the floor, forming an

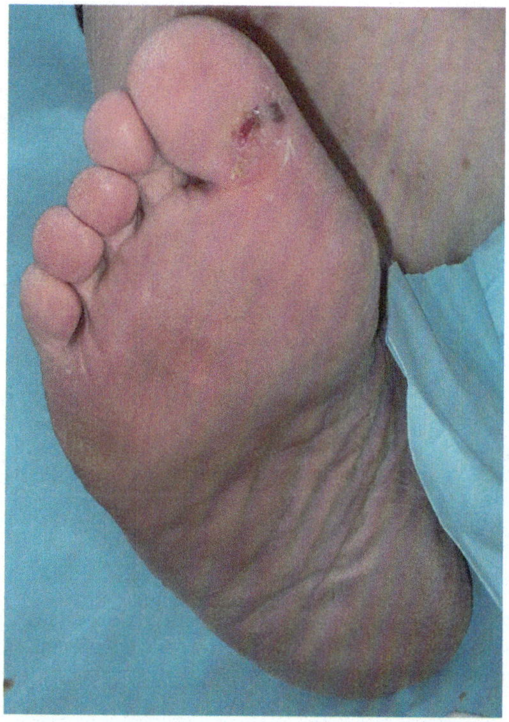

Figure 3.42 Claw toes and pes cavus (a high plantar arch). The metatarsal heads are exposed due to shifting of the fat pads underneath the metatarsal heads. A neuropathic ulcer is healing under the hallux.

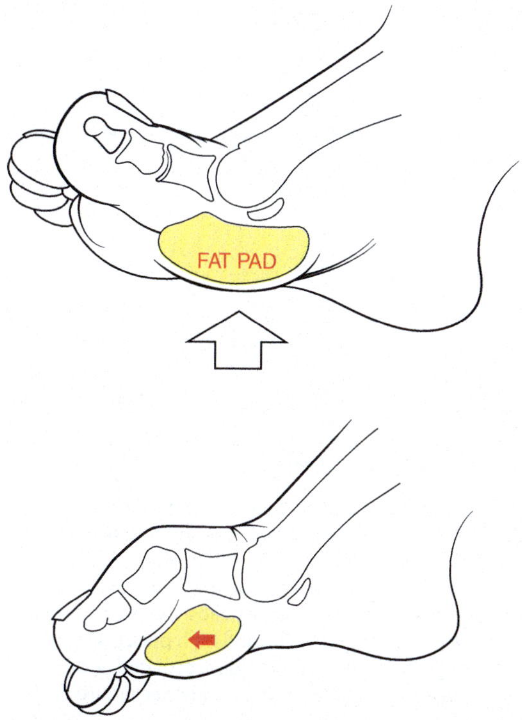

Figure 3.43 The development of claw toes and protruding metatarsal heads. Shifting of the fat pads underneath the metatarsal heads to the front leaves the metatarsal heads exposed to high pressures. *Source:* Adapted from Bowker & Pfeifer (2001).

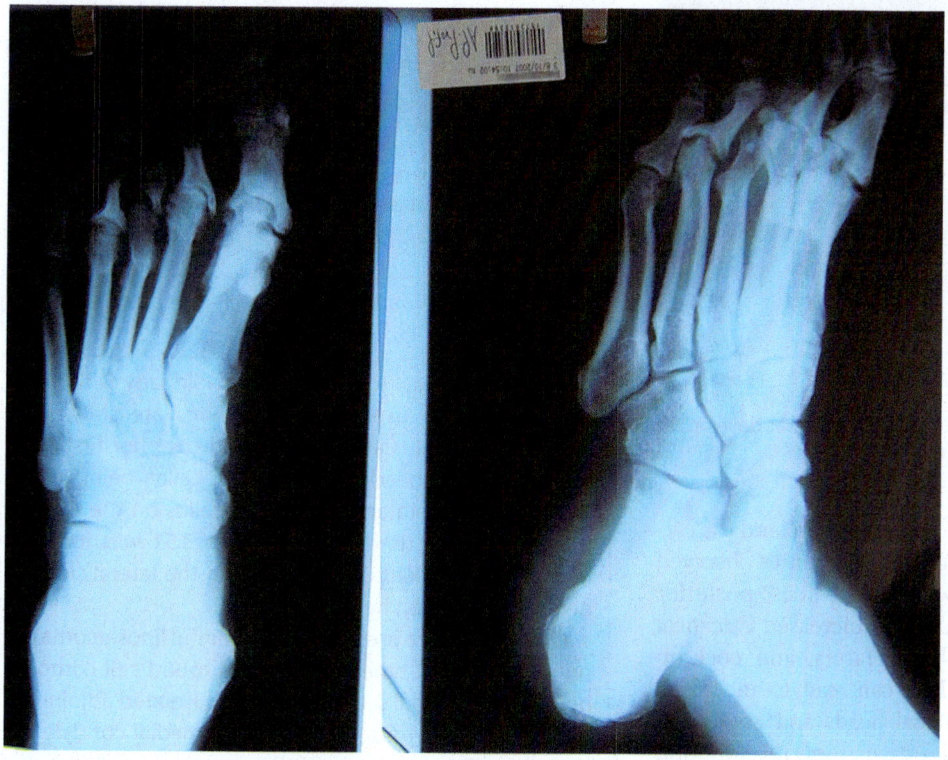

Figure 3.44 A radiograph of the left foot of the patient whose feet are shown in Figure 3.45. Toe-clawing and prominent metatarsal heads are evident, and osteomyelitis of the third toe can be seen.

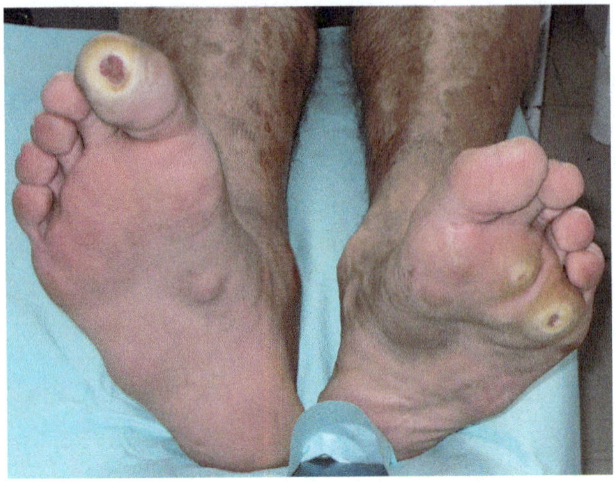

Figure 3.45 Prominent metatarsal heads on the left foot of a 49-year-old gentleman with type 2 diabetes and significant neuropathy. Hallux valgus and bunionettes are present, and typical neuropathic ulcers can be seen on the right hallux and under the left third and fifth metatarsal heads. An ulcer under the hallux is associated with a rigid hallux and high peak pressures on this area. Osteomyelitis of the left third (disarticulated and shortened) toe is present on plain radiography (see Figure 3.44).

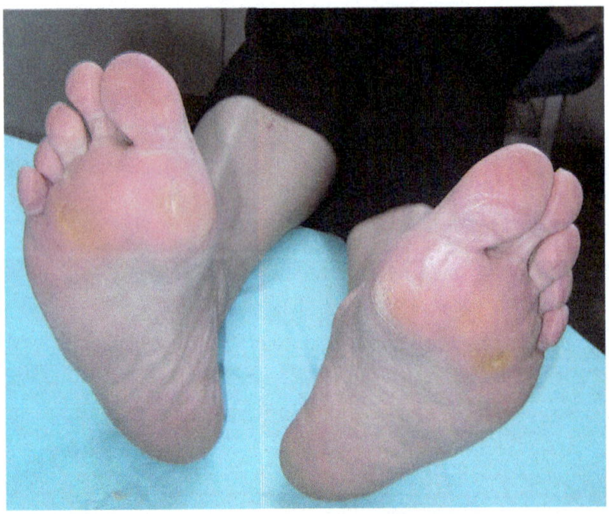

Figure 3.46 Prominent metatarsal heads. Callosity has developed bilaterally under this lady's fourth metatarsal heads.

arch that extends between the first metatarsal and the calcaneus. The spectrum of associated deformities observed with pes cavus includes clawing of the toes, posterior hindfoot deformity (described as an increased calcaneal angle), contracture of the plantar fascia, and cock-up deformity of the great toe. This can lead to increased weight-bearing for the metatarsal heads and associated metatarsalgia and calluses. In a cavus foot, the forefoot, especially the first ray, is drawn downward, and an abnormal distribution of plantar pressure upon standing and

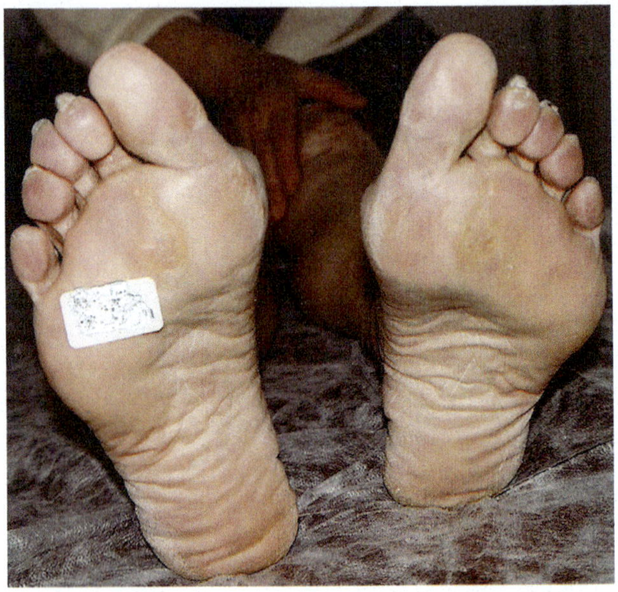

Figure 3.47 Pes cavus, which is probably familial. Hallux valgus, claw toes and callus of the second metatarsal head are present, as are dry skin and onychogryphosis.

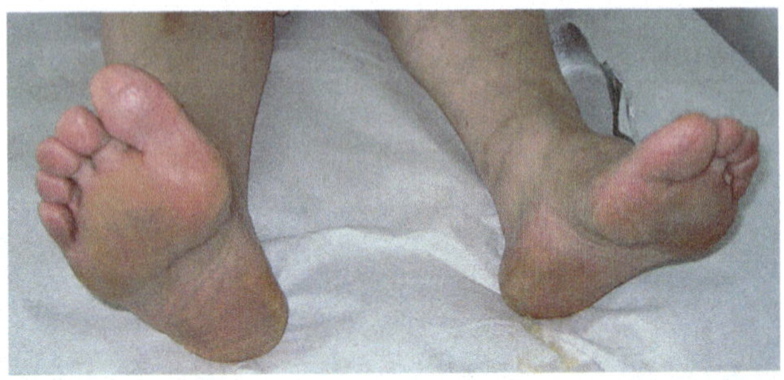

Figure 3.48 Case 3.1: Pes cavus with claw toes. Extensive callosity is seen over the metatarsal heads and heels.

Case 3.1 Pes Cavus and Prominent Metatarsal Heads in a Patient with Liposarcoma

Pes cavus and claw toes in a 50-year-old lady with type 2 diabetes who used improper shoes are shown in Figures 3.48–3.51. Callus has formed over her first and fifth metatarsal heads, hemorrhagic callus being seen over the fifth metatarsal head. The callus on the tips of the second and third toes in Figure 3.51 was formed because this patient used to walk on the lateral side of her left foot and on her right forefoot.

One year before presentation, a painful liposarcoma of primarily myxoid type and a partial round cell component (FNCLCC, total score 3) had been isolated adjoining her right gracilis muscle, next to the medial condyle of her tibia. The histology of liposarcoma is shown in Figures 3.52–3.55.

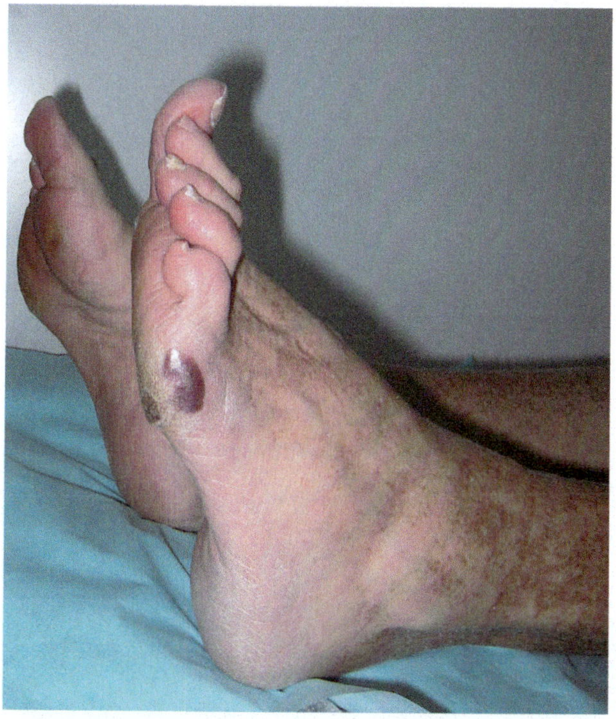

Figure 3.49 Case 3.1: Pes cavus and claw toes. Hemorrhagic callus has formed over a callus on the lateral aspect of the fifth metatarsal head.

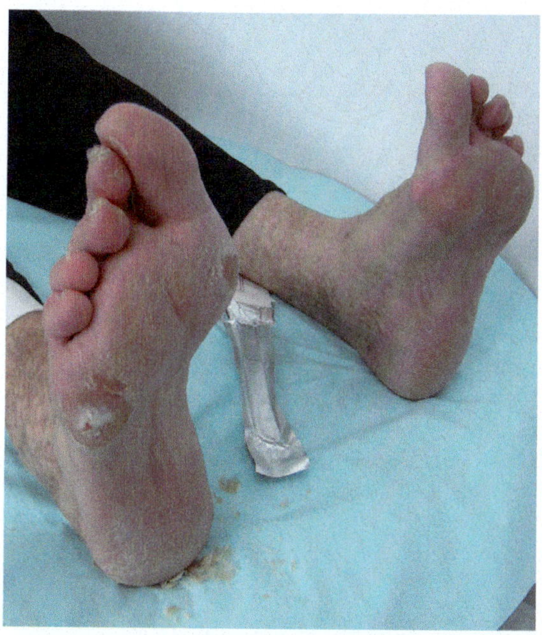

Figure 3.50 Case 3.1: Pes cavus and claw toes. A neuropathic ulcer has formed under the fifth metatarsal head.

walking leads to callus formation under the metatarsal heads (see Figures 3.38, 3.40 and 3.71).

Cavus feet tend to be stiffer than normal; some patients may get ankle strains easily. Patients should be

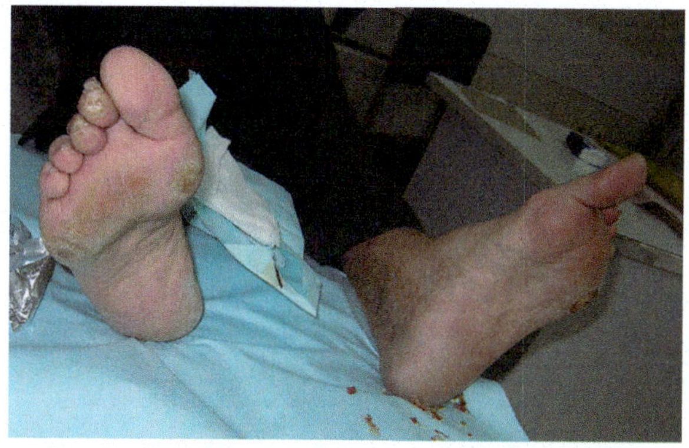

Figure 3.51 Case 3.1: Pes cavus with claw toes. Calluses have formed under the right fourth and fifth metatarsal heads, as well as on the right second and third toe tips.

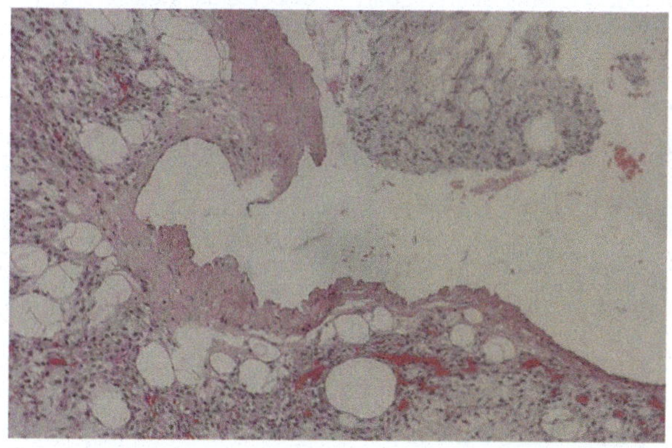

Figure 3.52 Case 3.1: Liposarcoma. A medium-sized vessel has been infiltrated by tumor cells (hematoxylin & eosin ×200). This condition is most frequent in middle-aged and older adults (age 40 and above), liposarcomas being the most common of all soft tissue sarcomas. The reported annual incidence of liposarcoma is in the range of 2.5 per million. *Source:* Courtesy of O. Tzaida, Metaxa Cancer Hospital, Piraeus.

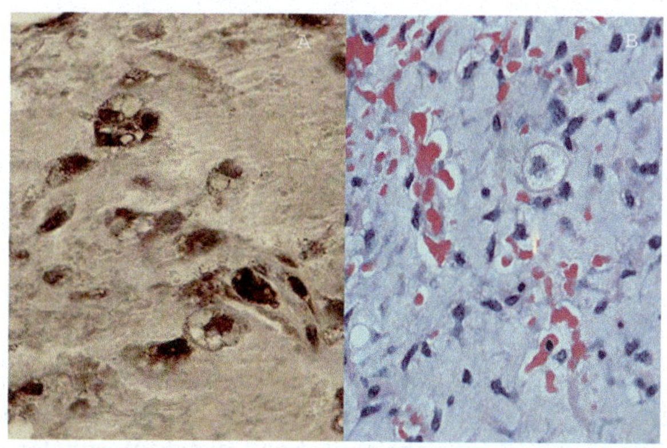

Figure 3.53 Case 3.1: Liposarcoma. Lipoblasts at different stages of maturation (S100 protein ×400) These cells are undifferentiated embryonic precursors of adipocytes. They are round cells that contain one or more large cytoplasmic vacuoles and intracellular glycogen. *Source:* Courtesy of O. Tzaida, Metaxa Cancer Hospital, Piraeus.

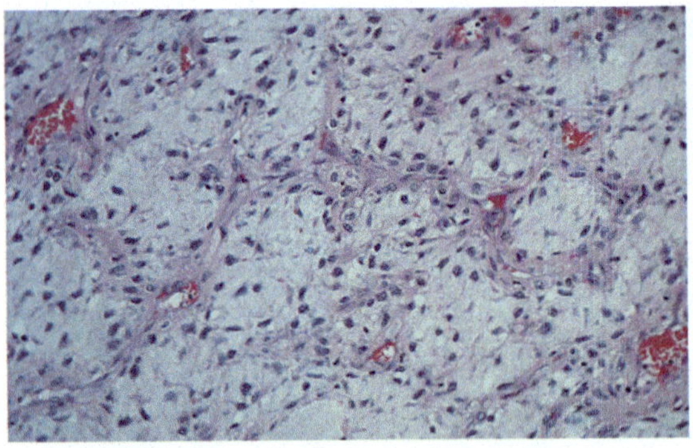

Figure 3.54 Case 3.1: Liposarcoma. The myxoid component with the characteristic arborizing plexiform (chicken-wire) pattern vasculature (hematoxylin & eosin ×200). Pure myxoid tumors have a hypocellular spindle cell proliferation set in a myxoid background with mucin pooling, resembling a pulmonary edema. *Source:* Courtesy of O. Tzaida, Metaxa Cancer Hospital, Piraeus.

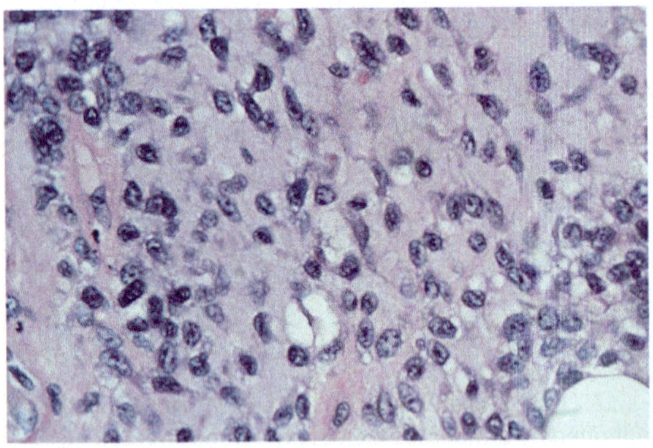

Figure 3.55 Case 3.1: Liposarcoma. The round cell component that constitutes the minority of the illustrated tumor (hematoxylin & eosin ×400). Pure round cell tumors are hypercellular, with over 80% being composed of round cells, with frequent transitions to myxoid areas. *Source:* Courtesy of O. Tzaida, Metaxa Cancer Hospital, Piraeus.

advised to use proper shoes (with extra depth, and broad at the toe box) and orthotic, shock-absorbing insoles. Surgery for the correction of the abnormality is rarely recommended.

3.9 Curly Toe

A curly toe consists of a neutral position or plantar flexion of the metatarsophalangeal joint, and plantar flexion of the proximal interphalangeal and distal interphalangeal joints, of more than 5° each (Figures 3.56 and 3.57). A curly toe is a common congenital malformation (with the third or fourth toe overlapping the adjacent toe; Figure 3.58). Inward or outward rotation may be present. Curly toes may be either fixed or flexible.

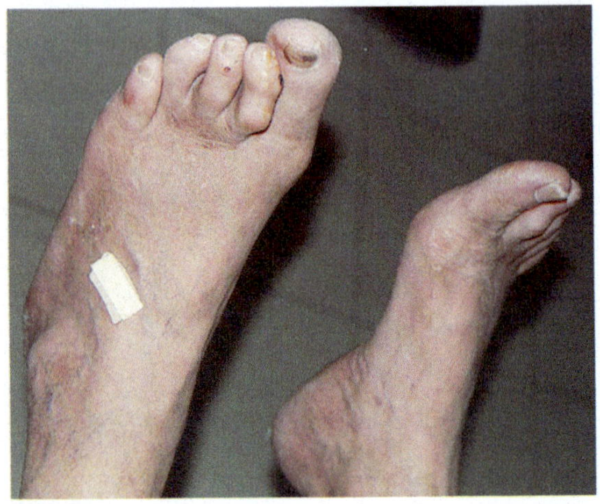

Figure 3.56 Curly fourth left toe, with claw toes and a hammer deformity of the second right toe.

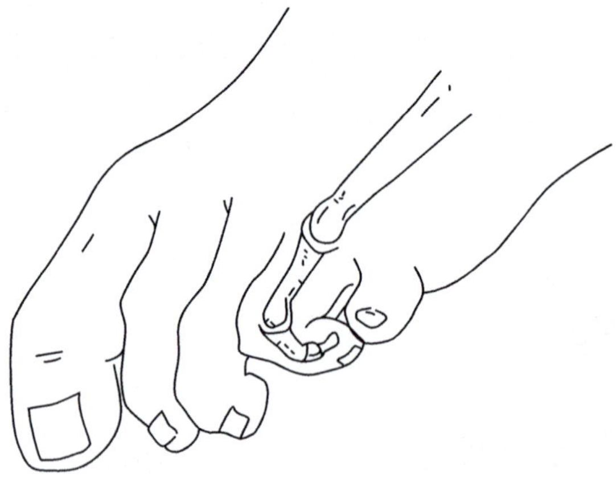

Figure 3.57 Curly fourth toe.

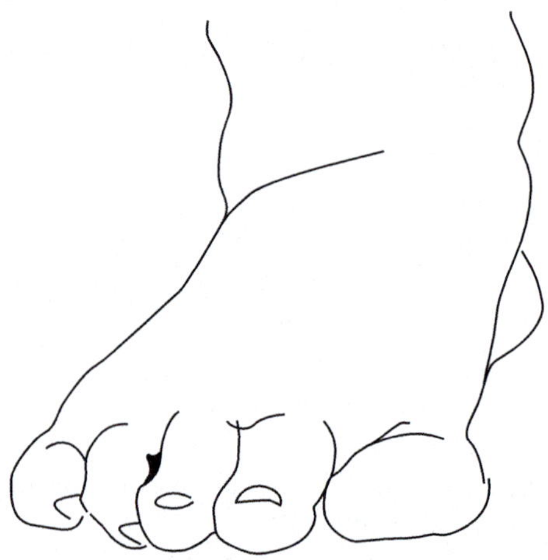

Figure 3.58 Curly fourth toe with medial malrotation.

3.10 Varus Deformity of the Toes

In varus deformity of the toes, the third, fourth and fifth toes drift medially. The toenails of the involved toes may cause superficial ulcers on the adjacent toes (Figure 3.59). Varus deformity often coexists with a bunionette.

3.11 Talipes Equinus (Clubfoot)

Congenital talipes equinus (talipes equinovarus: hindfoot equinus, hindfoot varus and forefoot varus) is a relatively common deformity with an incidence of 1–4 cases per 1000 live births. Its pathology is controversial. It involves many bones, articulations and soft tissue structures. The foot is extremely plantar flexed, with the forefoot swung medially and the sole facing inward (Figure 3.60). Plain radiography is the standard method of evaluation, while ultrasonography, computed tomography and magnetic resonance imaging can also be exploited.

Treatment with orthotics should begin shortly after birth. Surgical treatment is complementary to conservative treatment and is indicated for late presentations (after six months of age),when conservative treatment fails or leaves residual deformities, and in cases of recurrence after conservative treatment.

3.12 Hammer Toe Deformity

Hammer toe is a complex deformity consisting of contraction (hyperflexion) of the proximal interphalangeal joint, while the metatarsophalangeal joint is either

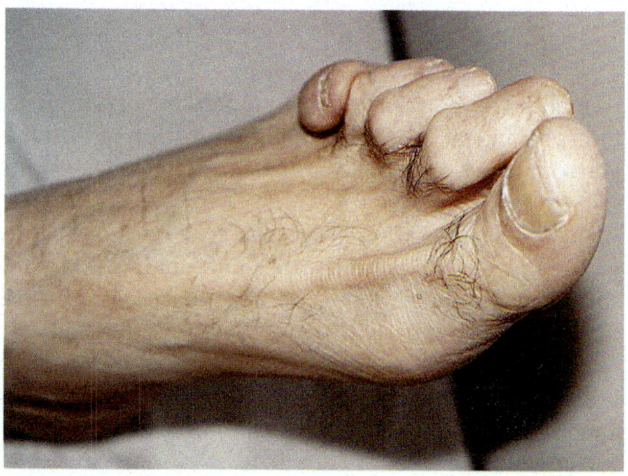

Figure 3.59 Varus deformity of the toes, without ulcerative pathology. Claw toes and an overlapping fifth toe can also be seen.

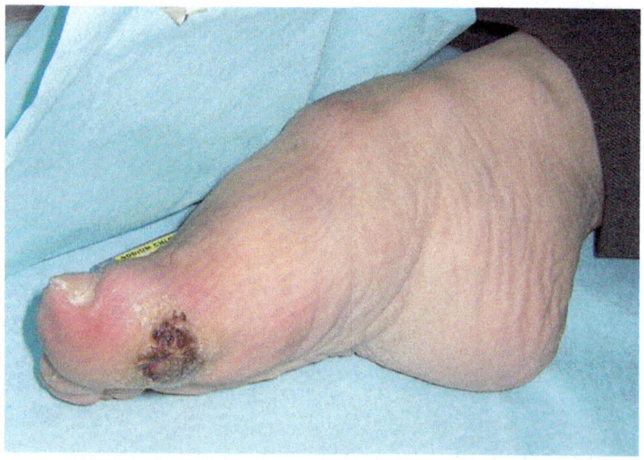

Figure 3.60 Congenital talipes equinus in a 57-year-old gentleman with type 2 diabetes. A neuropathic ulcer can be seen under a hemorrhagic callus over his hallux. No osteomyelitis has been diagnosed. This is the right foot of a non-ambulatory, intellectually disabled patient who is living in an institution. His left foot is equally deformed (a bilateral talipes clubfoot), without any ulcerative pathology.

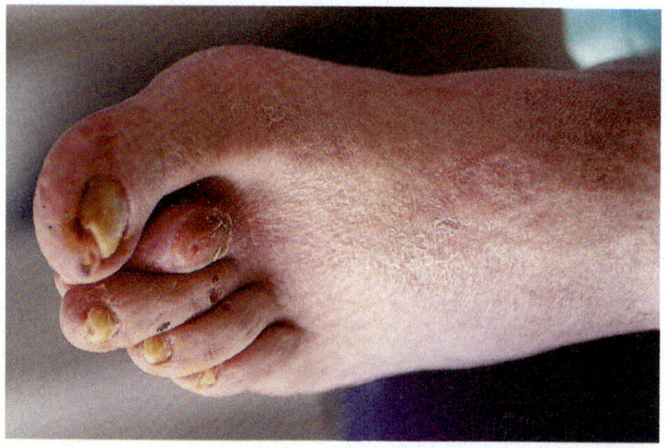

Figure 3.61 An underlapping second hammer toe. Hallux valgus and sheer pressure ulcers are seen on the dorsum of the toes. This is the left foot of the patient whose right foot is shown in Figure 3.64.

dorsiflexed or in a neutral position (Figures 3.61 and 3.62). The distal interphalangeal joint may be in a neutral position, hyperextended or in plantar flexion (Figure 3.63). Hammer toe may be flexible or rigid, and other toe deformities may also be present (Figure 3.64).

3.13 Overriding Toe

The cause of a second overriding toe is acquired and multifactorial. Elongation and laxity of the plantar synovial bursa of the metatarsal joint result in dorsal subluxation of the affected joint. The second toe lacks plantar interossei muscles, and therefore lumbrical muscles predominate,

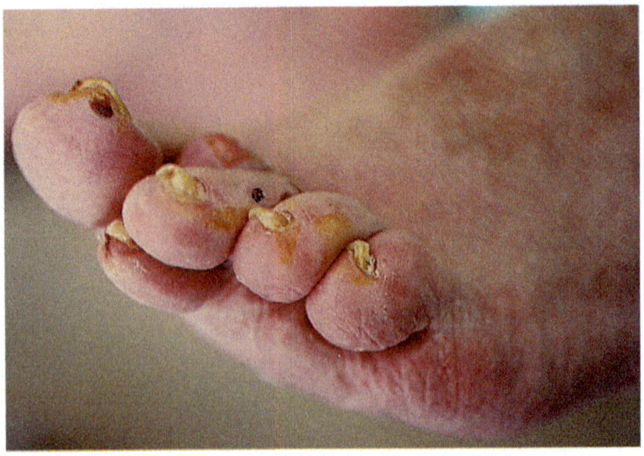

Figure 3.62 An underlapping second hammer toe, with hallux valgus and sheer pressure ulcers on the dorsum of the toes. This is the left foot of the patient whose right foot is shown in Figure 3.64.

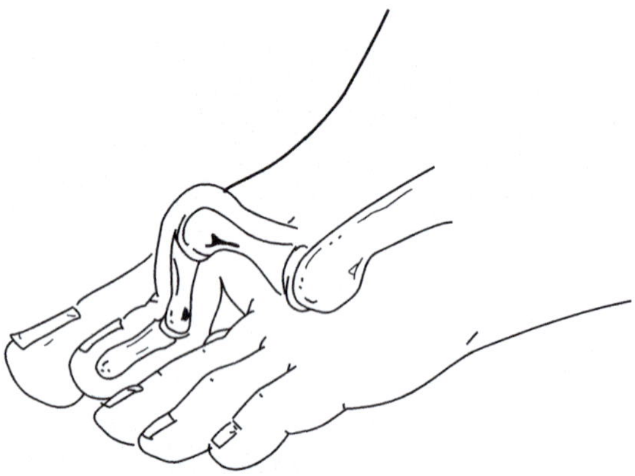

Figure 3.63 Hammer toe.

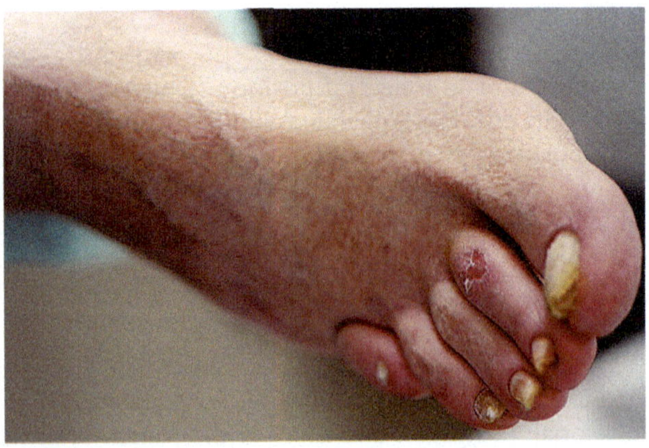

Figure 3.64 Congenital sixth overriding toe. Sheer pressure ulcers are seen on the dorsum of the toes, together with onychomycosis of the toenails.

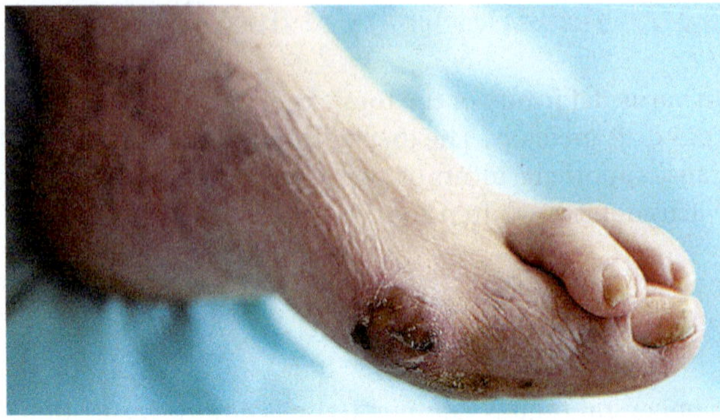

Figure 3.65 An overriding second toe (clawing of the second toe in supraductus). There is a bunion and hallux valgus with fixed varus deformity.

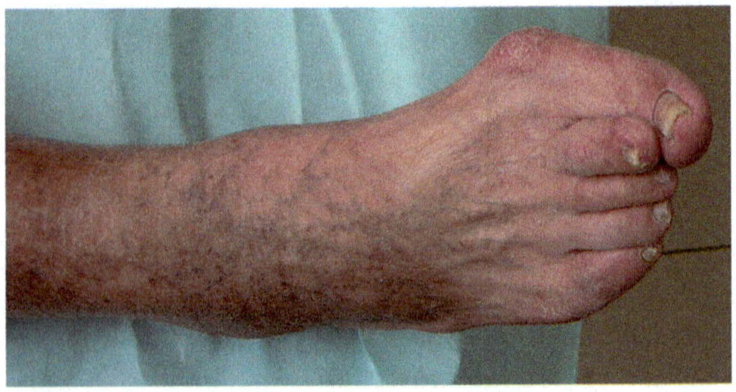

Figure 3.66 An overriding second toe due to hallux valgus.

causing dorsiflexion of the toe. Subluxation of the metatarsophalangeal joint results in shrinkage of the dorsal synovial bursa and the dorsal interosseus muscles. Further atrophy of the intrinsic muscles contributes to the development of the deformity, which may be fixed or flexible (Figures 3.65 and 3.66).

3.14 Mallet Toe

A mallet toe consists of plantar flexion of the distal interphalangeal joint, and a neutral position of the metatarsophalangeal and proximal interphalangeal joints (Figure 3.67).

Toe deformities (hammer toe, claw toe, curly toe, mallet toe, overriding of the toes) are unknown in non-shoe-wearing populations. Their incidence varies from 2 to 20% and increases with age. Women are affected four to five times more often than men. Most people have no underlying disease, although neuromuscular diseases and inflammatory arthropathies may be accompanied by such toe deformities.

Toe deformities are more common in people with diabetes due to muscle atrophy and limited joint mobility. Deformities such as the above, when present in patients

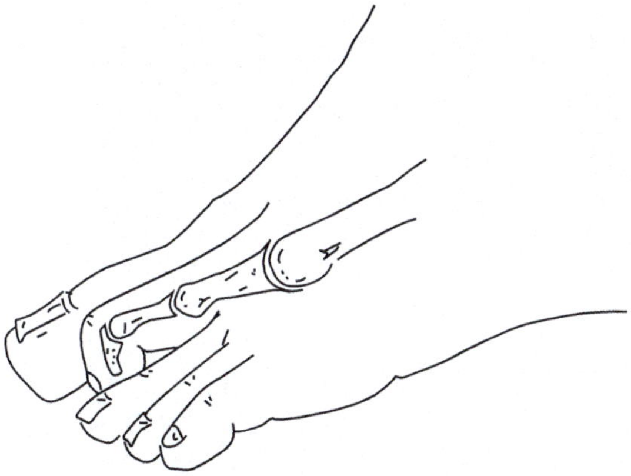

Figure 3.67 Mallet toe.

with a loss of sensation due to diabetic neuropathy, pose a risk for the development of neuropathic ulcers, as prominences are susceptible to skin-on-shoe friction. Patients are instructed to check their feet every day. Shoes with a high toe box protect the deformed toes from ulceration.

3.15 Charcot Foot

The rigid rocker-bottom of chronic Charcot foot predisposes to ulceration (Figure 3.68). Collapse of the midfoot joints results in a rocker-bottom deformity and ulceration at the apex of the collapsed bones (see Chapter 10).

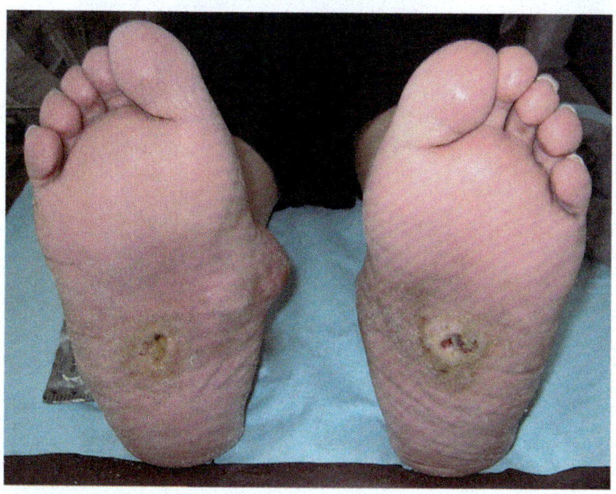

Figure 3.68 Bilateral Charcot foot with neuropathic ulcers at the apex of the collapsed midfoot joints. The bony prominence seen on the medial aspect of the right foot is a frequent finding in Charcot feet, and also predisposes to ulceration.

3.16 The Consequences of Minor Amputation

An amputation or disarticulation due to infection following full-thickness ulceration penetrating into the bones or joints, or wet gangrene, is the first step in restoring the patient's quality of life. Preservation of end-weight-bearing along normal proprioceptive pathways, as well as a limited disruption of body image, is a goal in unavoidable amputations. Nevertheless, any type of amputation alters the biomechanics of the foot, and is considered as a risk factor both for a recurrence of foot ulceration and for a new amputation. Several studies have shown that previous amputations account for 30–50% of new amputations on the same or the contralateral foot within the following five years.

3.17 Postsurgical Consequences of Hallux Surgery

Case 3.2 Correction of Hallux Valgus

The convex triangular feet of a 64-year-old lady with type 2 diabetes are shown in Figures 3.69–3.71. A previous right hallux valgus operation caused shortening of the hallux and exposure of the tip of the second right toe to sheer pressure in her shoe; a painless healing neuropathic ulcer is seen medially to the nail. Modest edema is present, probably due to the use of the antihypertensive amlodipine.

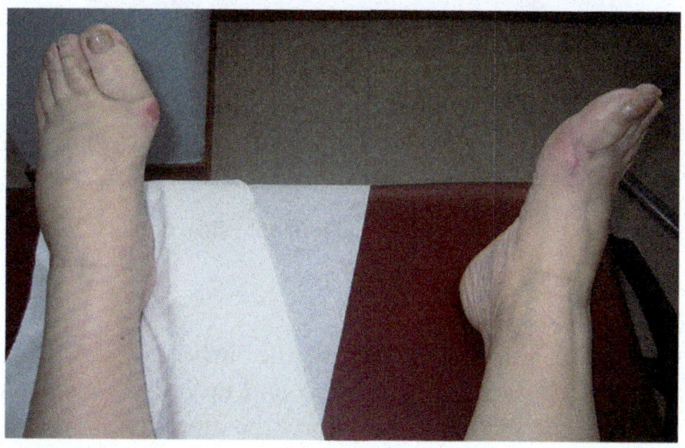

Figure 3.69 Case 3.2: Left hallux valgus and bunion. The right foot has a surgically corrected hallux valgus.

3.18 Toe Disarticulations

Hallux disarticulation (Figure 3.72) may lead to a bony prominence proximal to the metatarsal head due to the presence of the medial sesamoid bone; therefore, the sesamoids should be removed, together with their

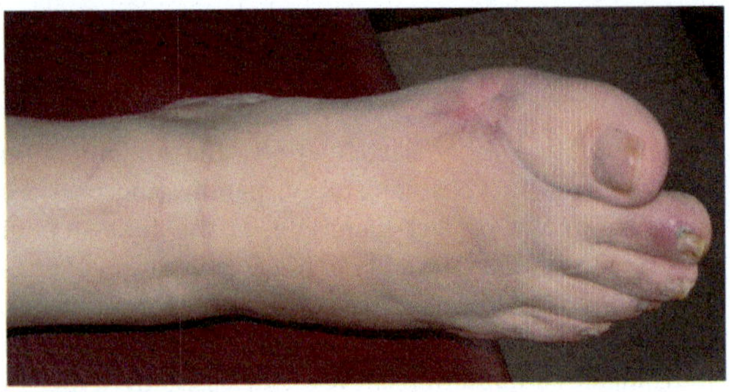

Figure 3.70 Case 3.2: A postsurgical short hallux valgus.

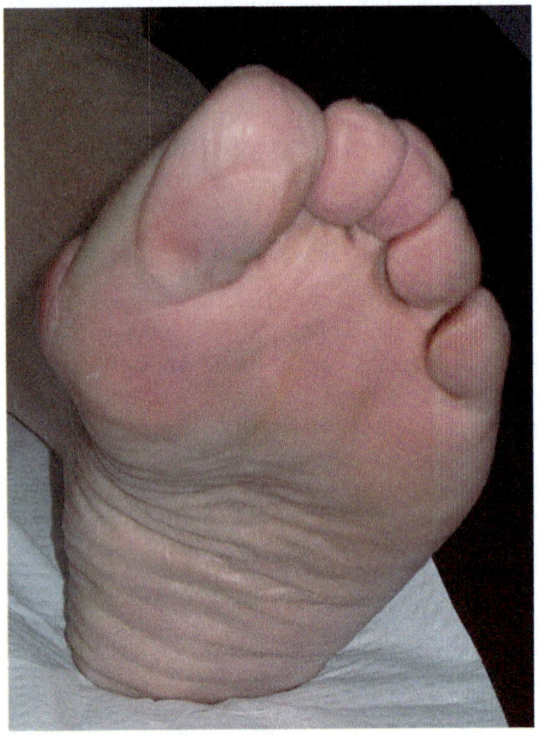

Figure 3.71 Case 3.2: A triangular forefoot with a bunion.

fibrocartilaginous plate and the articular cartilage. Second toe disarticulation may end up in hallux valgus because the second toe supports the great toe, or disarticulation may lead to an ulcer under the second metatarsal head (Figures 3.73 and 3.74).

Third or fourth toe disarticulations are better tolerated since the remaining adjacent toes close the space, with good results. Fifth toe disarticulation may expose the skin under the fifth metatarsal head to high pressures and ulceration. One should avoid leaving a lesser toe isolated by removing the toes on either side, since it has no function and is exposed to high pressures and injury (Figure 3.75, and see Figure 3.78).

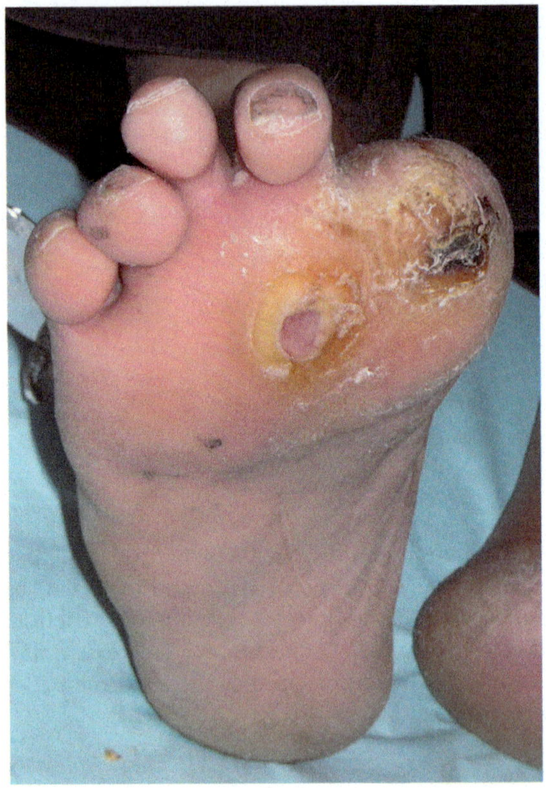

Figure 3.72 Disarticulation of the first toe. Neuropathic ulcers can be seen under the first and second metatarsal heads, and hemorrhagic callus and claw toes are also apparent.

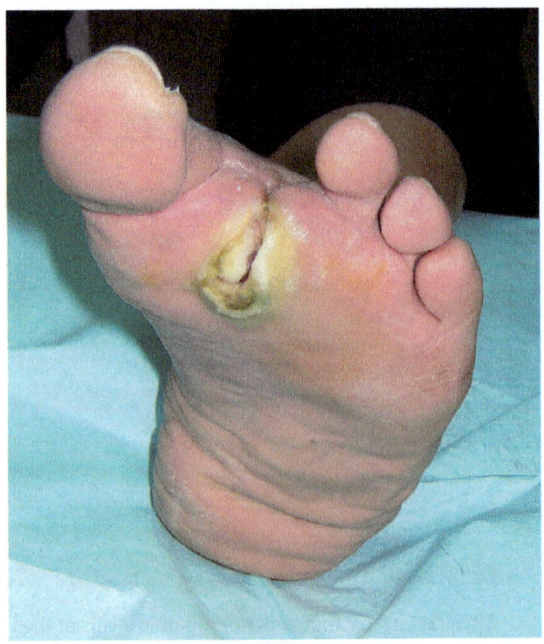

Figure 3.73 A neuropathic ulcer three months after second toe disarticulation.

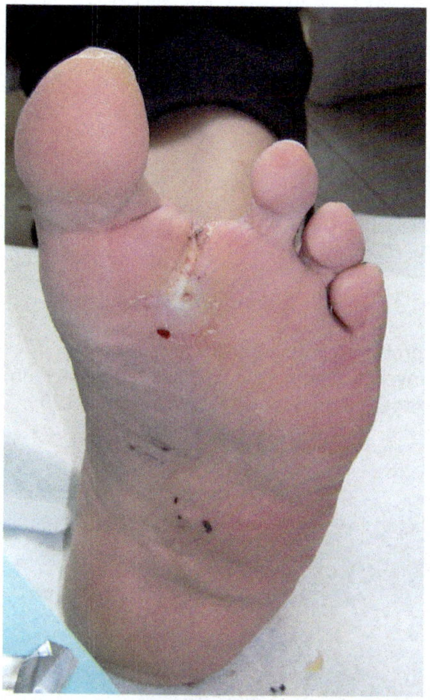

Figure 3.74 Disarticulation of the second toe. A neuropathic ulcer after six months of proper shoe use.

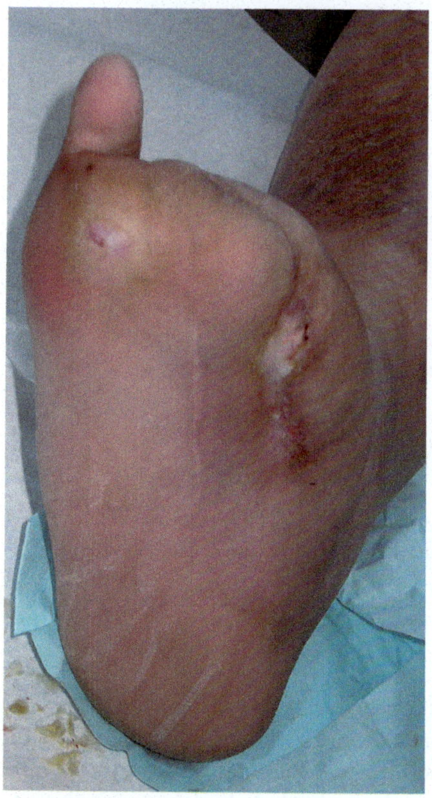

Figure 3.75 A neuropathic ulcer after amputation of the first four toes with first ray amputation. Leaving a single toe in place is not recommended since this toe is highly vulnerable to pressure ulcers and is liable to subsequent amputation (see also Figure 3.78).

3.19 Ray Amputations

Ray amputation is the removal of a toe together with its metatarsal bone. First ray amputation (Figures 3.76–3.78) results in dysfunction of the foot during both stance and propulsion. This disability is related to the length of the removed metatarsal shaft. Most surgeons preserve the longest metatarsal shaft possible.

The base of the proximal phalanx has to be preserved in order to keep the attachment of the short flexor of the hallux intact, thus keeping the sesamoids in place and maintaining the windlass mechanism. This mechanism protects the first metatarsal head from overloading during the propulsion phase of gait. In the case of an obligatory removal of the hallux due to osteomyelitis of the proximal phalanx, the surgeon should preserve all uninvolved portions of the metatarsal bone except the avascular sesamoids and their fibrocartilaginous plate.

A hallux disarticulation at the metatarsophalangeal joint exposes the head of the third metatarsal to abnormally high pressure during stance, and may displace the second toe medially. The loss of support of the hallux for the adjacent toes may cause deformities, fractures or neuropathic osteoarthropathy and eventual ulceration on the latter (Figures 3.79 and 3.80, and see Figure 3.77).

Single lesser ray amputations are better tolerated (Figures 3.81–3.84, and see Figures 3.87–3.91). Multiple lateral ray amputations are sometimes required in cases of extended infection (Figures 3.85 and 3.86).

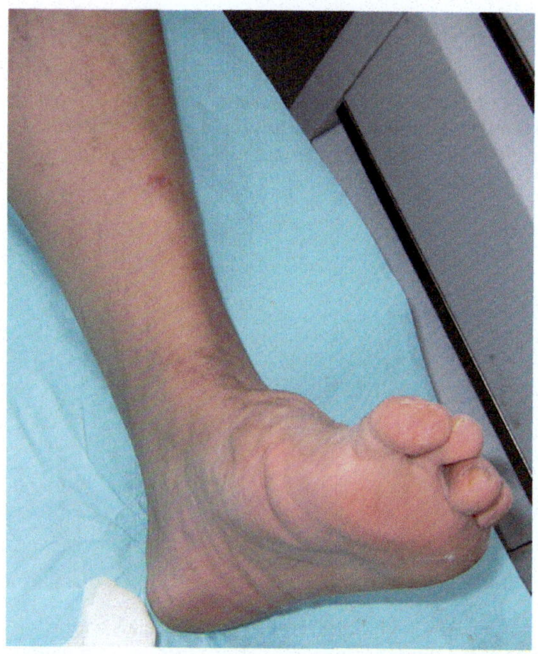

Figure 3.76 First ray amputation of the foot shown in Figures 3.79 and 3.80.

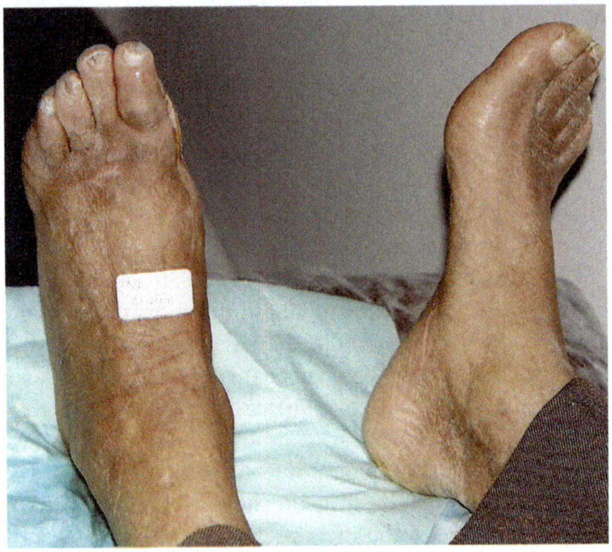

Figure 3.77 First ray amputation.

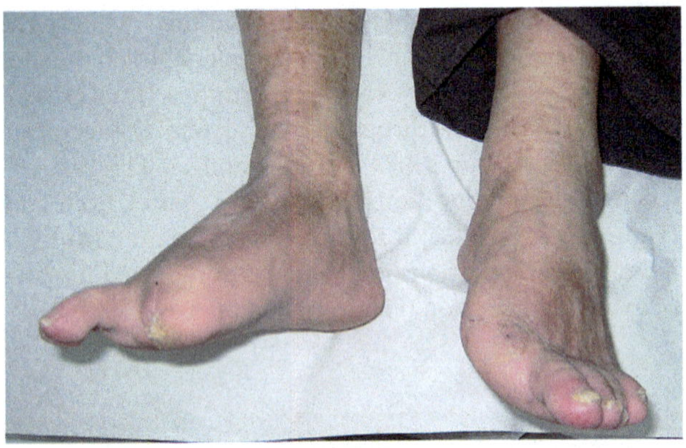

Figure 3.78 The left foot shows first ray amputation, and the right foot first, second and fifth toe disarticulations. Leaving a single toe in place is not recommended since this toe is highly vulnerable to pressure ulcers and subsequent amputation (see also Figure 3.75).

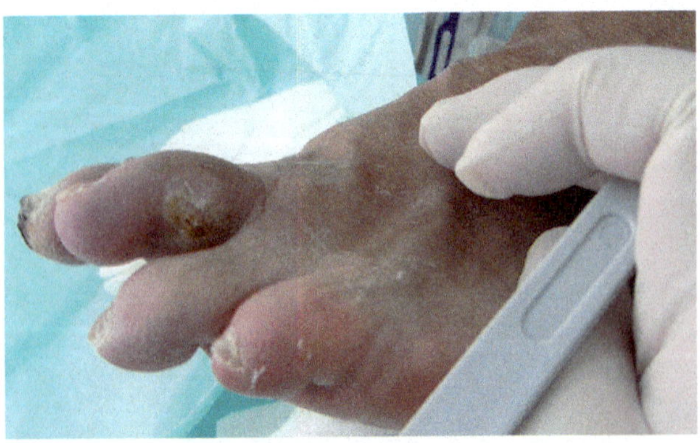

Figure 3.79 A neuropathic ulcer is seen under a callus on the lateral side of the third toe six months after a first ray amputation. The absence of the great toe resulted in displacement of the last phalanx of the second and the third toes, and a corn over the interphalangeal joint of the third (now second) toe.

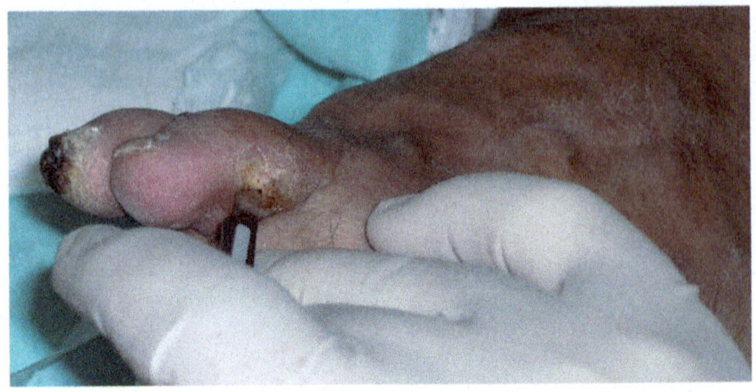

Figure 3.80 Gentle probing through a callus reveals bony exposure and osteomyelitis. A hemorrhagic callus can be seen on the tip of the second toe. This foot is also shown in Figure 3.79.

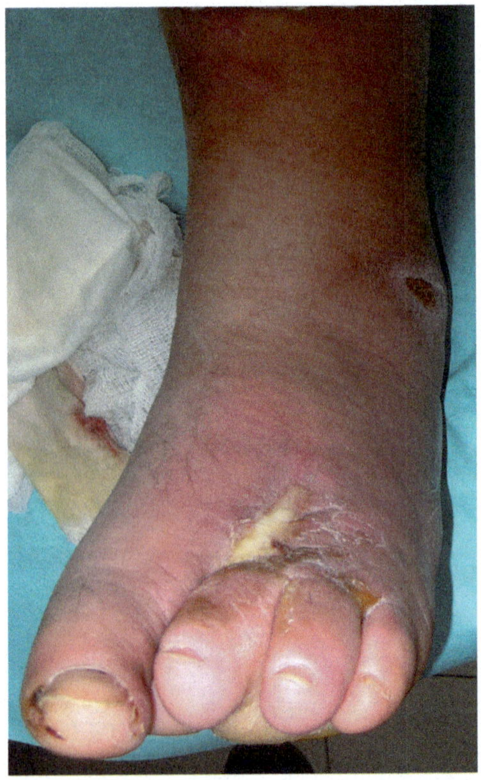

Figure 3.81 Second ray amputation. Claw toes are evident, together with a neuro-ischemic ulcer over the lateral side of the heel.

Sole incisions pose a risk for ulceration. Incisions should be performed on the dorsum or the side of the foot (see Figures 3.81 and 3.83) and not on the plantar surface. Scar tissue over a healed ulcer may contribute to a new ulceration in a similar way as callus does. Improper footwear may expose the base of the amputated metatarsal or adjacent metatarsals to increased forces and lead to a new ulcer (see Figures 3.81–3.84).

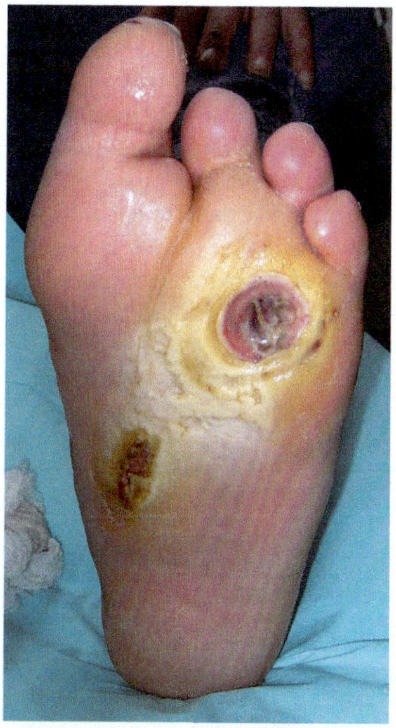

Figure 3.82 Second ray amputation. A full thickness neuro-ischemic ulcer with osteomyelitis is present under the fourth metatarsal base of this foot, also shown in Figure 3.81.

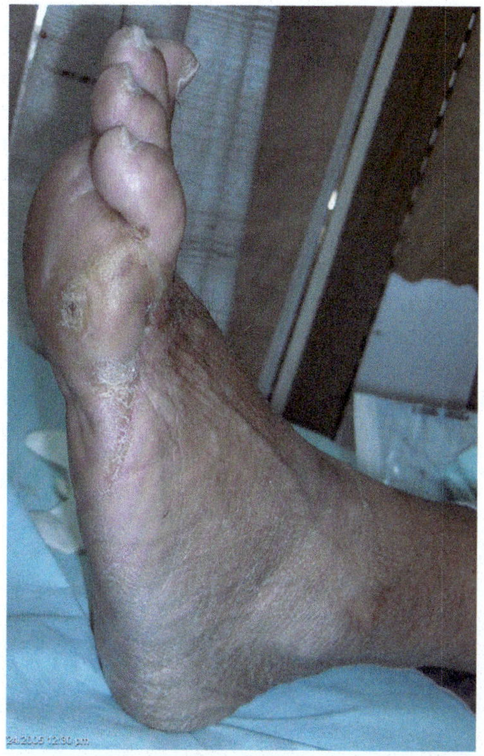

Figure 3.84 Fifth ray amputation. Claw toes and prominent veins are evident. Debridement of a callus under the fourth metatarsal head revealed a full-thickness ulcer.

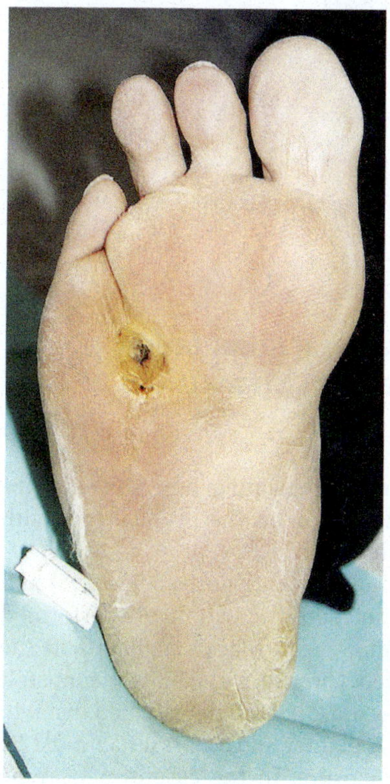

Figure 3.83 Fourth ray amputation with a neuropathic ulcer under the base of the fourth transmetatarsal residuum. A fourth ray amputation may have an adequate functional and cosmetic result as long as proper footwear is used.

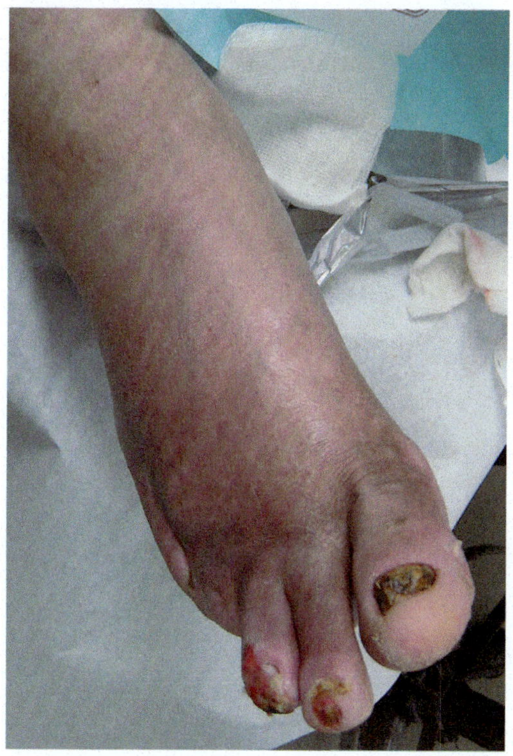

Figure 3.85 Fourth toe disarticulation and fifth ray amputation.

Case 3.3 Alignment of a Postsurgical Hallux Valgus, Due to a Second Toe Disarticulation

After removal after of her second toe, postoperative hallux valgus developed in a 55-year-old lady with type 1 diabetes who had been a professional dancer. After removal of the toe, her left great toe gradually dislocated to a valgus posture, under riding the adjacent (third) toe (Figure 3.87). Gross callus formation developed on the medioplantar aspect of the first metatarsal head (Figure 3.88), which caused constant discomfort on walking and dancing. Callus was also noticed over the third metatarsal head.

A plain X-ray film showed disarticulation of the left second toe, dislocation of the metatarsophalangeal joint of the great toe, medial pronation of the first metatarsal head, and hallux valgus deformity with rotation, together with dislocation of the sesamoids, and arthritis; necrosis of the head of the third metatarsal bone was also seen (Figure 3.89).

She was referred to the orthopedic department and had her second metatarsal removed. Hallux valgus deformity was corrected by arthrodesis of the metatarsophalangeal joint. After the operation, no significant callus developed within the next three months (Figure 3.90). Six years after the arthrodesis, the postsurgical hallux valgus was present again, still with minor callosity and no ulcer (Figure 3.91). The third toe was again overlapping.

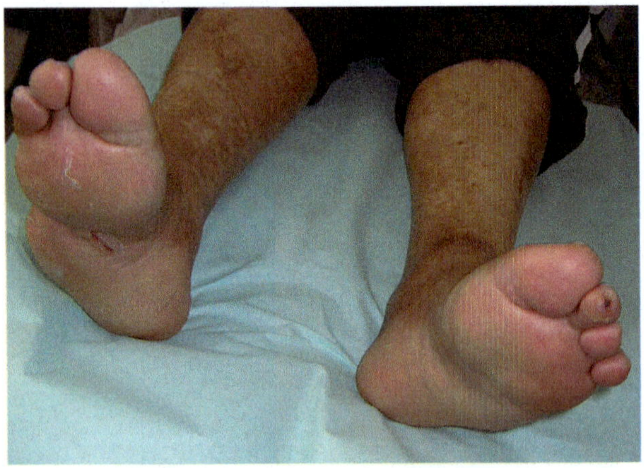

Figure 3.86 Right fourth and fifth ray amputation, with claw toes.

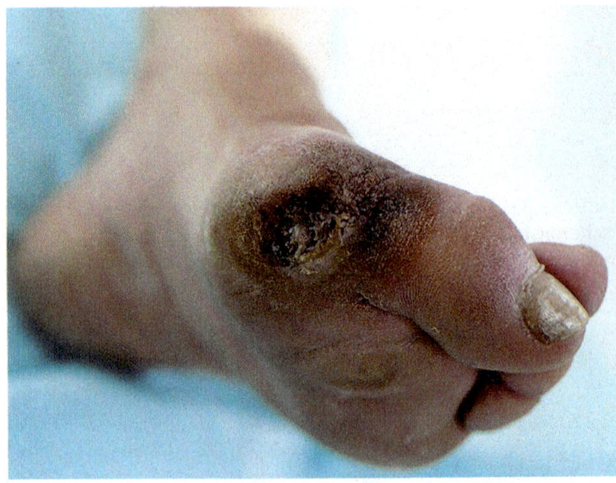

Figure 3.88 Case 3.3: Postsurgical hallux valgus after second toe amputation – 2.

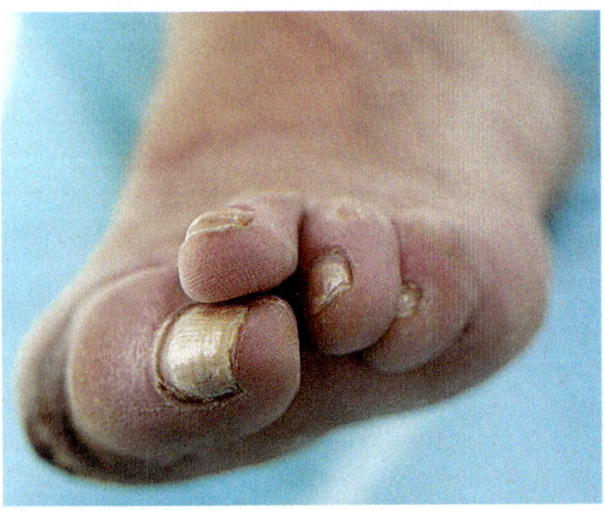

Figure 3.87 Case 3.3: Postsurgical hallux valgus after second toe amputation – 1.

3.20 Transmetatarsal Amputation and Tarsometatarsal (Lisfranc) Disarticulation

With at least the hindfoot remaining, a person can continue to bear weight directly on the residual foot with adequate proprioceptive feedback.

Transmetatarsal amputations (Figures 3.92–3.94) and tarsometatarsal (Lisfranc) disarticulations are performed when infection or gangrene is more extended and the toes cannot be salvaged. Circulatory viability is a must. If gangrene is present, it must be well demarcated distal to the amputation site. A plantar and a dorsal flap must be viable for successful closure. In the case of a Lisfranc amputation, usually the first, third and fourth metatarsals are disarticulated, whereas the base of the second metatarsal should be left in place to help preserve the

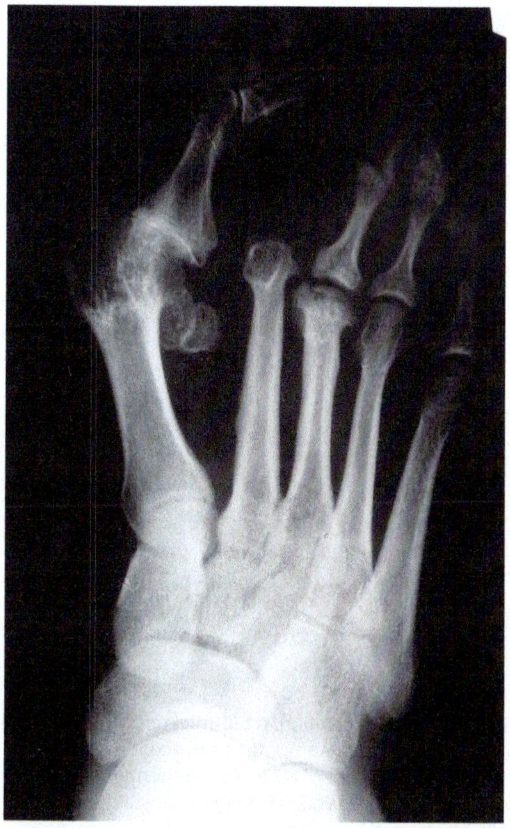

Figure 3.89 Case 3.3: Postsurgical hallux valgus after second toe amputation – 3.

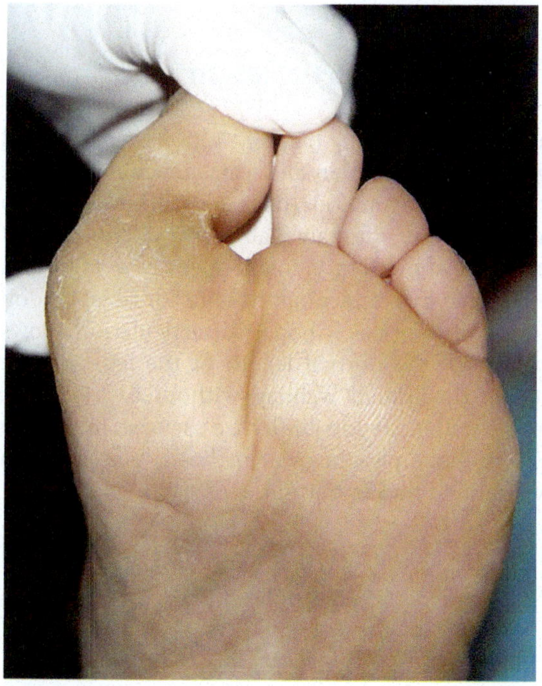

Figure 3.90 Case 3.3: Corrected postsurgical hallux valgus (after second toe amputation) – 1.

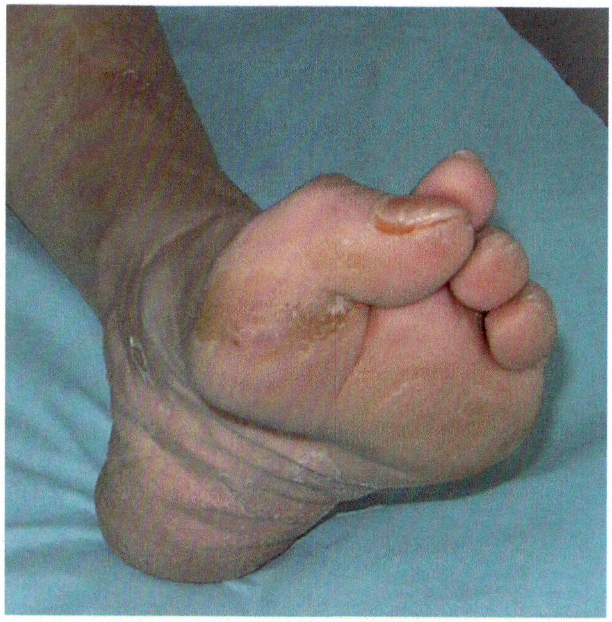

Figure 3.91 Case 3.3: Corrected postsurgical hallux valgus (after second toe amputation) – 2.

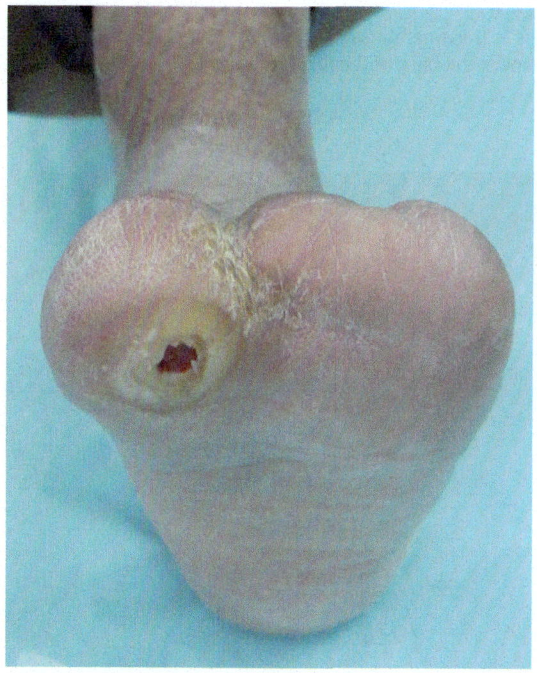

Figure 3.92 Transmetatarsal amputation. A neuropathic ulcer has formed under the first metatarsal base.

proximal transverse arch. A portion of the fifth metatarsal base is also retained to preserve the insertion of the peroneus brevis tendon.

Distal pressure and shear from improper footwear may cause ulceration on an insensate or dysvascular residuum, resulting in reamputation to a more proximal level.

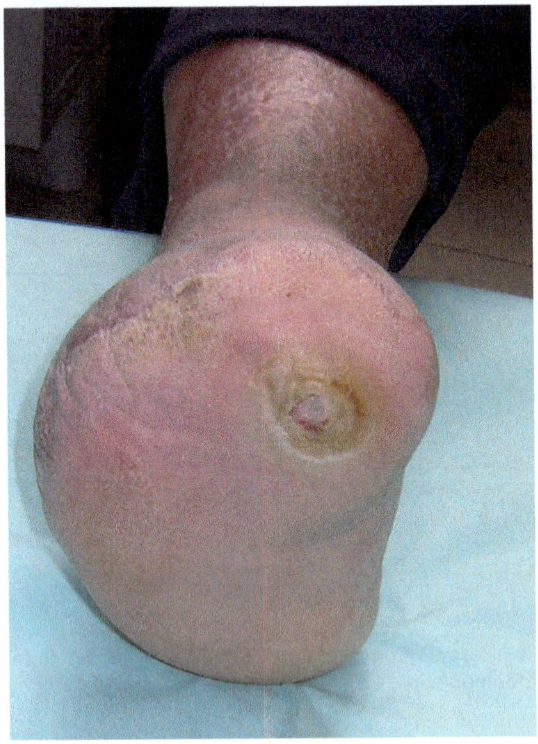

Figure 3.93 Transmetatarsal amputation. A neuropathic ulcer has formed under the base of the first metatarsal.

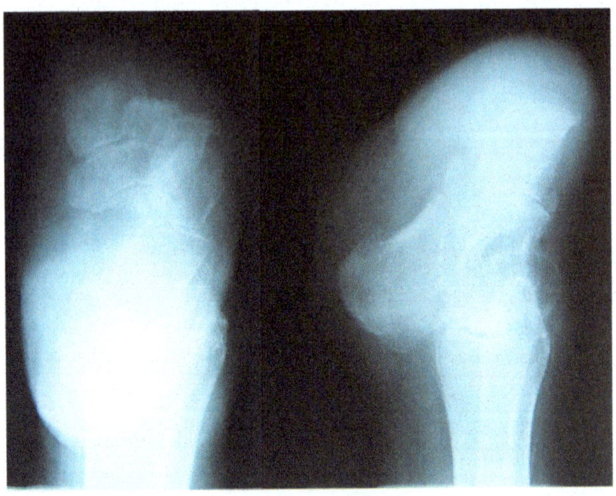

Figure 3.94 Transmetatarsal amputation seen on a radiograph of the foot shown in Figure 3.93.

Reference

Bowker, J.H. and Pfeifer, M.A. (2001). *Levin and O'Neal's The Diabetic Foot*, 6e. Mosby.

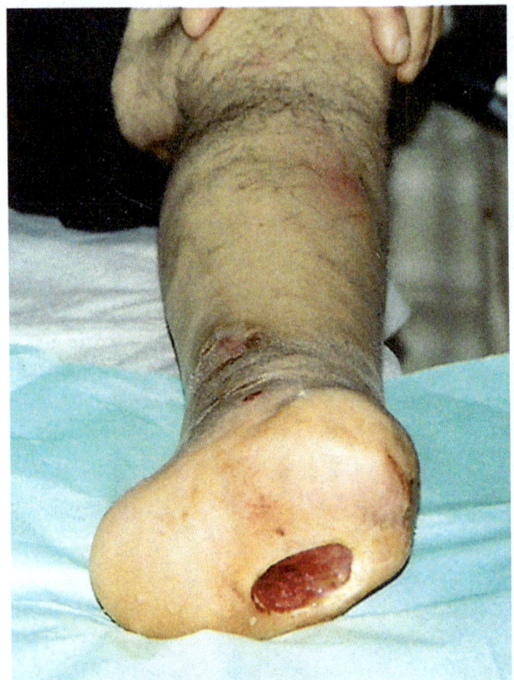

Figure 3.95 Chopart disarticulation. A full-thickness neuropathic ulcer, which remained after the amputation procedure, is seen on the plantar area of the left foot of a 73-year-old gentleman with type 2 diabetes. This patient, who was severely unstable when trying to walk, never used any ankle prosthesis or orthosis, as indicated. The ulcer healed for a period of two months when the patient was hospitalized because of a hip fracture, but reappeared afterwards.

3.21 Chopart Disarticulation

Chopart disarticulation (Figure 3.95) is performed through the talonavicular and calcaneocuboid joints, preserving only the hindfoot (talus and calcaneus). As no muscles insert onto the talus, all active dorsiflexion of the remaining short foot is lost. However, dorsiflexion can be restored by reattaching the anterior tibial tendon to the neck of the talus. Chopart disarticulation allows preservation of the normal length of the leg, and the patient can do limited walking without a prosthesis. Reasonable walking is possible by the use of an intimately fitting fixed-ankle prosthesis or orthosis, placed into a shoe with a rigid rocker-bottom.

Further Reading

Bowker, J.H. (2007). Partial foot amputations and disarticulations: surgical aspects. *J. Prosthet. Orthot.* 19 (3S): 62–76.

Bowker, J.H. and San Giovanni, T.P. (2001). Minor and major lower limb amputation in persons with diabetes mellitus. In: *Levin and O'Neal's the Diabetic Foot*, 6e (ed. J.H. Bowker and M.A. Pfeifer), 607–635. St Louis: Mosby.

Brodsky, J.W., Kourosh, S., Stills, M., and Mooney, V. (1988). Objective evaluation of insert material for diabetic and athletic footwear. *Foot Ankle* 9: 111–116.

Burns, J., Crosbie, J., Hunt, A., and Ouvrier, R. (2005). The effect of pes cavus on foot pain and plantar pressure. *Clin. Biomech. (Bristol, Avon)* 20: 877–882.

Chairman, E.L. (2000). Amputation of the foot. In: *Textbook of Hallux Valgus and Forefoot Surgery* (ed. V.J. Hetherington), 471–480. Cleveland, OH: VJ Hetherington Available at: http://www.ocpm.edu/hallux/index.asp (accessed September 2009).

Deland, J.T., de Asla, R.J., Sung, I.H. et al. (2005). Posterior tibial tendon insufficiency: which ligaments are involved? *Foot Ankle Int.* 26: 427–435.

Frey, C., Thompson, F., Smith, J. et al. (1993). American orthopedic foot and ankle society women's shoe survey. *Foot Ankle* 14: 78–81.

Girdlestone, G.R. and Spooner, H.J. (1937). A new operation for hallux valgus and hallux rigidus. *J. Bone Joint Surg. Am.* 19: 30–37.

Ikeda, K. (1992). Conservative treatment of idiopathic clubfoot. *J. Pediatr. Orthop.* 12: 217–223.

Klaue, K., Hansen, S.T., and Masquelet, A.C. (1992). Clinical, quantitative assessment of first tarsometatarsal mobility in the sagittal plane and its relation to hallux valgus deformity. *Foot Ankle Int.* 15: 9–13.

Lountzis, N., John Parenti, J., Cush, G. et al. (2007). Percutaneous flexor tenotomy – office procedure for diabetic toe ulcerations. *Wounds* 19: 64–68.

Mayfield, J.A., Reiber, G.E., Sanders, L.J. et al. (1998). Preventive foot care in people with diabetes. *Diabetes Care* 21: 2161–2177.

Mueller, M.J. (1997). Therapeutic footwear helps protect the diabetic foot. *J. Am. Podiatr. Med. Assoc.* 87: 360–364.

Pomeroy, G.C., Pike, R.H., Beals, T.C., and Manoli, A. (1999). Acquired flatfoot in adults due to dysfunction of the posterior tibial tendon. *J. Bone Joint Surg. Am.* 81: 1173–1182.

Tanenberg, R.J., Schumer, M.P., Greene, D.A., and Pfeifer, D.A. (2001). Neuropathic problems of the lower extremities in diabetic patients. In: *Levin and O'Neal's the Diabetic Foot*, 6e (ed. J.H. Bowker and M.A. Pfeifer), 33–64. St Louis: Mosby.

4

Other Foot-Related Risk Factors

N. Tentolouris

First Department of Propaedeutic Internal Medicine, National and Kapodistrian University of Athens, Medical School, Laiko General Hospital, Athens, Greece

In this chapter, we describe the contribution of foot-related risk factors to the development of diabetic foot problems. Topics such as callus formation over various sites, dry skin, corns, nail deformities, edema, diabetic bullae and diabetic thick skin are included. The cause of these problems, their diagnosis and management are also discussed.

4.1 Callus

4.1.1 Callus Under Bone Prominence and Dry Skin

A 72-year-old male patient with type 2 diabetes and severe neuropathy attended the outpatient diabetes clinic for his regular follow-up. Callus under the head of his right third metatarsal and a bony prominence were seen at the outer aspect of his fifth metatarsal head (Figure 4.1). Claw toes, onychomycosis and dry skin were also present. The cause of the callus in this patient was high plantar pressure under the areas of callosities together with dryness of the skin. The patient was prescribed extra-depth shoes with orthotic insoles. A lubricating cream was also prescribed to prevent the skin cracking.

Dry skin of the feet is a consequence of diabetic peripheral autonomic neuropathy. The sweat glands are innervated by the thin, unmyelinated, postganglionic, sudomotor, cholinergic sympathetic C-fibers. Sudomotor dysfunction has a high sensitivity for the detection of distal small-fiber neuropathy and can be detected early in diabetes, even in subjects with normal nerve conduction. Recent cross-sectional data suggest that dry skin is associated with an increased risk for foot ulceration.

4.1.2 Callus over Prominent Metatarsal Heads

A 70-year-old female patient who had had type 2 diabetes since the age of 50 attended the foot clinic for regular podiatry treatment. She complained of numbness in both feet, deep aching pain of her calves and painful heel cracks.

On examination, her peripheral pulses were palpable but weak, and her ankle–brachial pressure index was 0.8 on the left and 0.7 on the right. The vibration perception threshold was 30 V in both feet. Achilles tendon reflexes were absent, and pain, temperature, light touch and vibration sensation were severely diminished.

Pes cavus and hallux valgus were present on both feet (most prominent on the left), together with obvious prominence of her metatarsal heads and callus formation. The fat pads of her metatarsal heads were translocated toward the toes. The skin of her feet was dry (Figure 4.2). The calluses were debrided on a regular basis, but her heel cracks (Figure 4.3) resisted recovery despite debridement. In Figure 4.4, the heel cracks of another neuropathic patient are shown.

Callus develops in areas of high pressure on the feet, as a physiologic reaction of the skin against loading. Dry skin due to anhidrosis is another contributing factor. The callus then adds further pressure to the underlying tissues by functioning as a foreign body under the foot.

Prospective studies have shown that the regular removal of calluses reduces the risk for foot ulceration. Preventive footwear and custom-made insoles can drastically reduce callus formation. Although there are no data in the literature on the effect of lubricating creams to prevent callus formation, clinical experience is that these works if used once or twice daily, preferably after bathing. However, patients tend to show low adherence to this recommendation.

Atlas of the Diabetic Foot, Third Edition. Ioanna Eleftheriadou, Alexandros Kokkinos, Stavros Liatis, Konstantinos Makrilakis, Nicholas Tentolouris, Anastasios Tentolouris, and Panagiotis Tsapogas.

Companion website: www.wiley.com/go/tentolouris/atlas_diabetic_foot

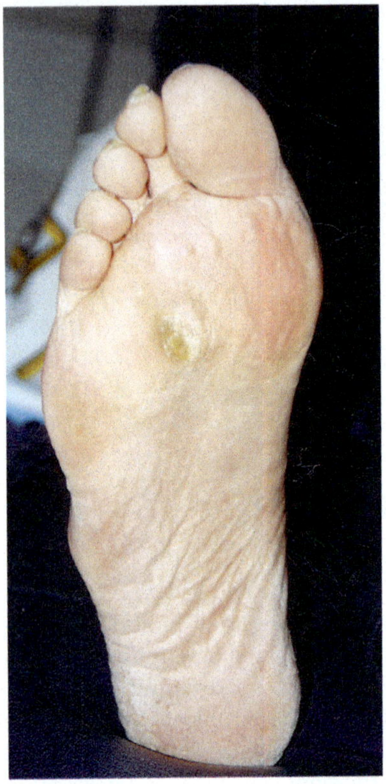

Figure 4.1 Callus over prominent metatarsal heads.

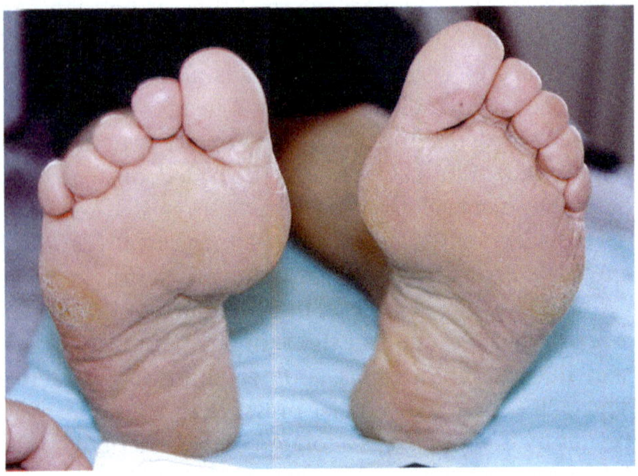

Figure 4.2 Callus over a prominence of the metatarsal heads. Pes cavus and hallux valgus can also be seen.

4.1.3 Hemorrhagic Callus

A 64-year-old male patient with type 2 diabetes diagnosed at the age of 47 attended the outpatient diabetic foot clinic because of an ulcer under his right foot.

On examination, a painless ulcer surrounded by hemorrhagic callus was seen under his third metatarsal head (Figure 4.5). Claw toe deformity, a curly fourth toe and a heloma molle in his fourth interdigital space were also

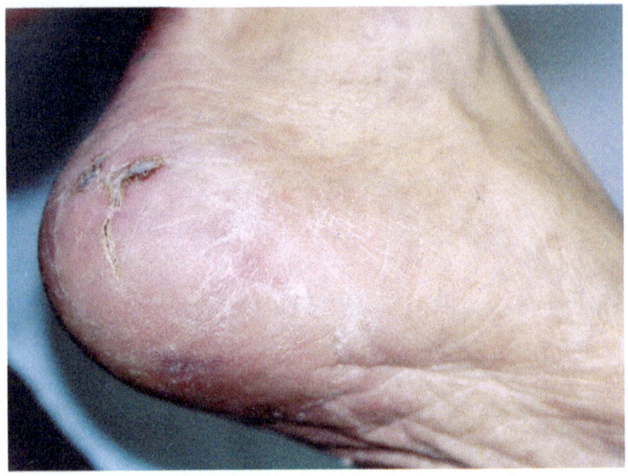

Figure 4.3 Heel cracks due to a combination of dry skin and ischemia in the patient shown in Figure 4.2.

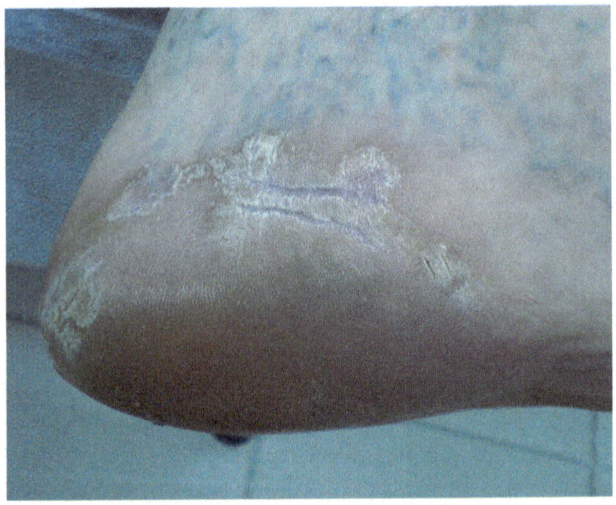

Figure 4.4 Heel cracks due to dry skin.

noticed. The patient had bounding peripheral pulses and severe peripheral neuropathy.

The ulcer was debrided, and the patient was educated about foot care. Off-loading of the ulcer area was achieved using an "almost-half" shoe (see Chapter 13) and a total-contact orthotic insole, with a window under the ulcer area. Such temporary "shoes" cause instability, so the patient was instructed to use a crutch. The ulcer healed completely in eight weeks.

The cause of the ulcer in this patient was high plantar pressure under his prominent metatarsal heads (Figure 4.6). After the ulcer had healed, protective footwear (extra-depth shoes, custom-made insoles) was prescribed to reduce the peak pressure on the third metatarsal head. No relapse of the ulcer occurred in the subsequent months.

In another case, a 65-year-old obese male patient with type 2 diabetes of 12 years' duration was referred to the

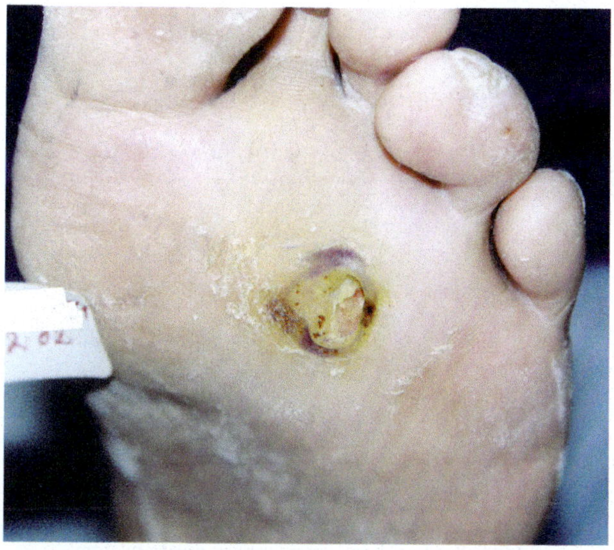

Figure 4.5 A neuropathic ulcer under a hemorrhagic callus.

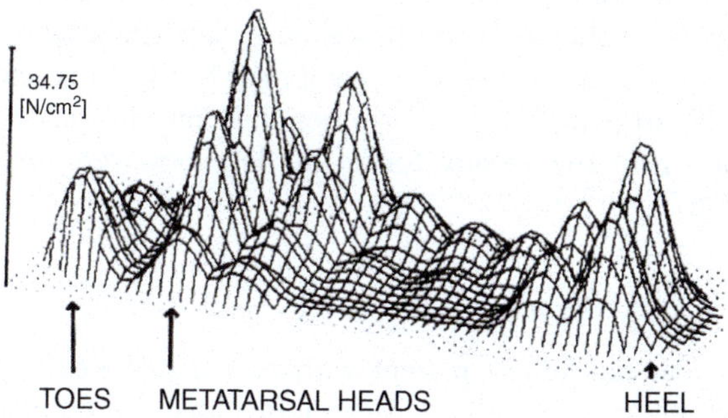

Figure 4.6 Plantar pressures recorded by a pedobarograph for the patient shown in Figure 4.5.

foot clinic by his family physician. The patient had noticed a painless black area on his left great toe and was afraid that it was gangrene, but he was unaware of the injury and ulcer on his right foot.

On examination, he had severe peripheral neuropathy and palpable pedal pulses. A large, hard hemorrhagic callus was noticed at the inner, lower aspect of the left great toe, and a large hyperkeratotic hemorrhagic area with a small ulcer under the fourth metatarsal head of the right foot (Figure 4.7). Hallux valgus and a claw toe deformity were present. Hyperpigmentation of the skin of the left calf due to venous insufficiency can be seen in the figure. The callus was removed, and proper footwear was prescribed.

4.1.4 Ulcer Under a Callus Area

A 70-year-old male patient with long-standing type 2 diabetes attended the outpatient diabetic foot clinic for the removal of a callus from his right foot. On examination, a

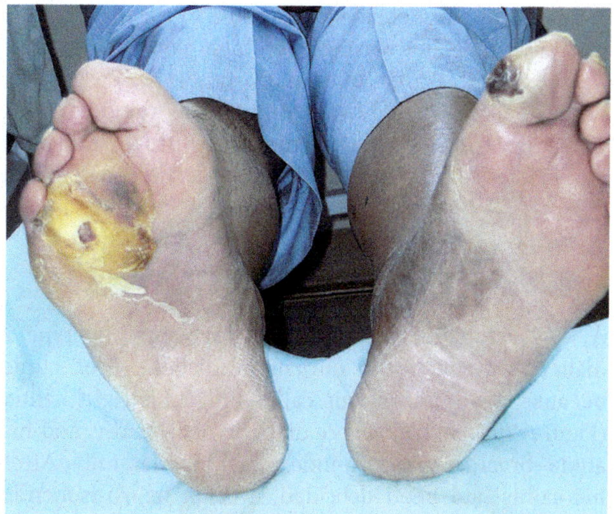

Figure 4.7 Gross callus formation on the right forefoot, and hemorrhagic callus on the left great toe.

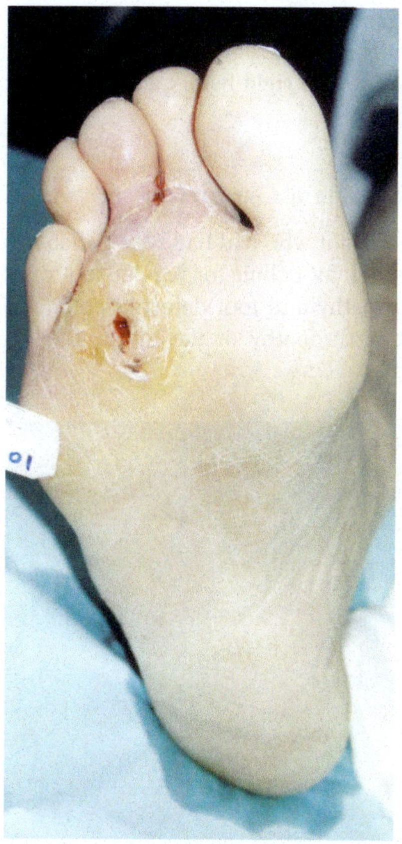

Figure 4.8 A neuropathic ulcer under a callus.

neuropathic ulcer surrounded by callus was noticed under his fourth metatarsal head (Figure 4.8). Claw toes, varus deformity of the foot and prominent metatarsal heads on his right foot were noticed. Discoloration of the skin of his lower tibia due to venous insufficiency was also seen.

The callus was debrided. The cause of the ulcer in this man was the callus arising from high plantar pressures. High peak pressures accompany almost all cases with prominent metatarsal heads due to claw toe deformity. The prevention of callus formation by proper footwear and insoles is necessary to avoid the recurrence of such ulcers.

4.1.5 Callus Under a Hallux

A 70-year-old male patient with long-standing type 2 diabetes attended the outpatient diabetic foot clinic because of a hemorrhagic callus under his right hallux (Figure 4.9). He had severe diabetic neuropathy, and his ankle–brachial pressure index was 0.7 bilaterally. After his callus had been debrided, a clean neuro-ischemic ulcer was revealed.

The forefoot is a common site for ulceration. In one series, ulcers of the forefoot accounted for 93% of all foot ulcers. Almost 20% of the ulcers developed under the hallux, 22% over the metatarsal heads, 26% at the tips of the toes and 16% on the dorsum of the toes. Ulcer under a hallux is associated with a rigid hallux and high peak pressures on this area.

4.1.6 Callus Due to Bilateral Charcot Foot

A 52-year-old male patient who had had type 1 diabetes for 34 years attended the foot clinic for regular foot care. He had severe neuropathy and foot deformities due to bilateral neuro-osteoarthropathy of the midfoot. Even though he always wore custom-made shoes and insoles, he needed callus removal monthly. A superficial ulcer was noticed under the fifth metatarsal head of his left foot (Figure 4.10). Claw deformities and callus formation at the tip of the second toe of his left foot were also present.

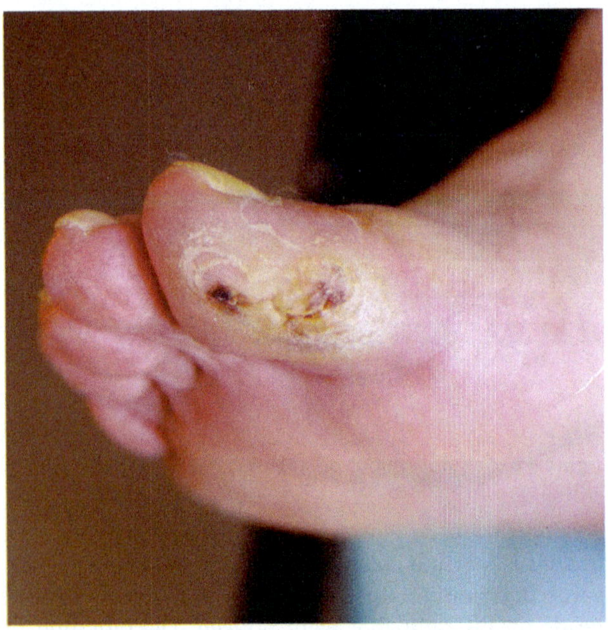

Figure 4.9 Hemorrhagic callus under a hallux.

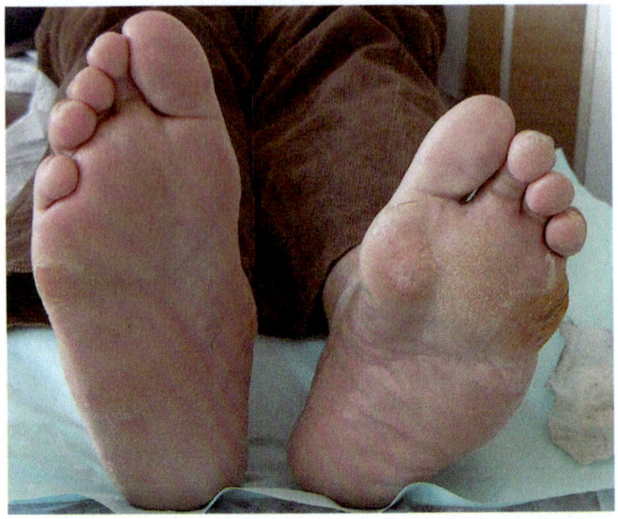

Figure 4.10 Callus over bony prominences due to bilateral Charcot neuro-osteoarthropathy.

4.1.7 Callus over the Heel

A 58-year-old female patient with type 2 diabetes and severe neuropathy attended the foot clinic for regular foot care. She had suffered trauma from a nail in her left heel two years previously, which had been complicated by an infection that had completely healed. Although she wore proper shoes and insoles, she still needed regular removal of callus from her left heel (Figure 4.11). Hallux valgus, claw toes and an overriding second toe deformity were also present.

The heel is an uncommon site of callus development. The cause of callus in this case was scar formation from the healed ulcer. Hard tissue may develop over healed ulcers or surgical scars, and ulcers may recur in such areas.

Another case of gross callus formation together with cracking of the skin of the left heel is shown in Figure 4.12. In this case, the callus was caused by high plantar pressures together with improper footwear.

4.1.8 Bilateral Callus Formation

A 48-year-old male patient with long-standing type 1 diabetes was referred to the foot clinic. The patient had gross callus formation on the inner aspect of his great toes and under his fifth metatarsal heads (Figure 4.13).

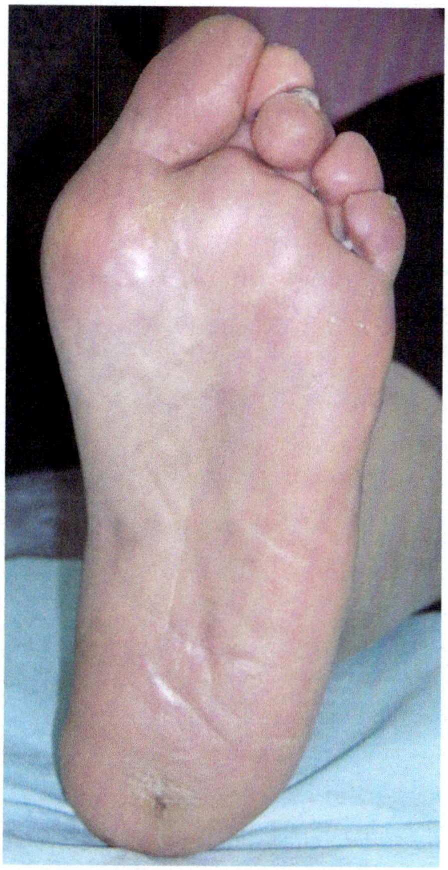

Figure 4.11 Callus over the heel.

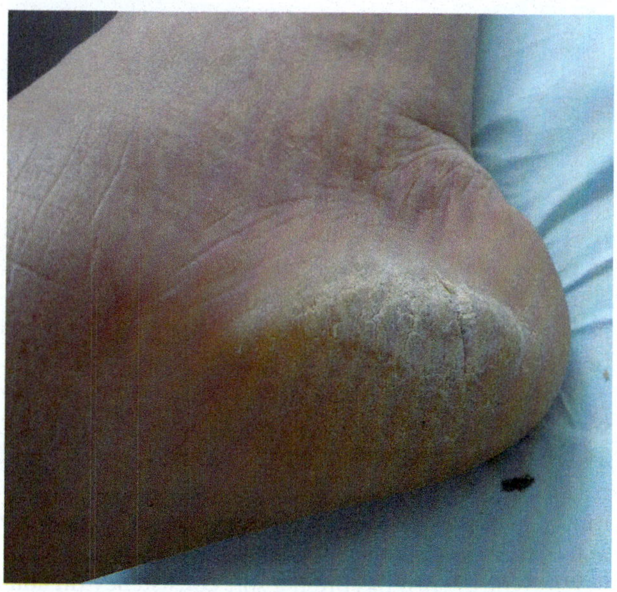

Figure 4.12 Gross callus formation with cracking of the skin of the left heel.

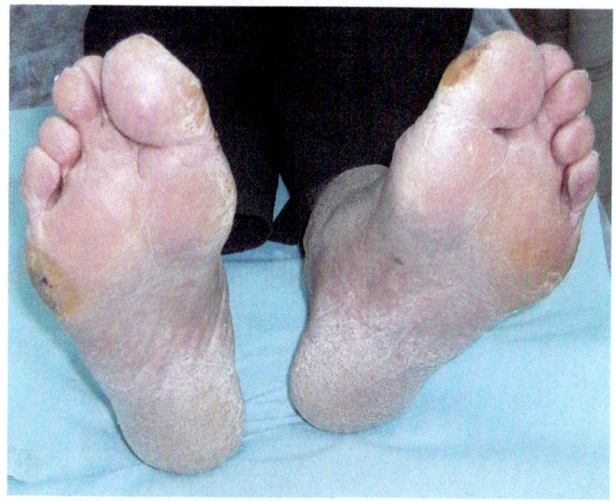

Figure 4.13 Bilateral callus formation.

An overriding second toe, bilateral claw toe deformities and dry skin were present. On examination, the patient demonstrated severe neuropathy. The calluses in this patient were caused by inappropriate footwear and prominent fifth metatarsal heads. The calluses were removed, and proper footwear and a lubricating cream were prescribed.

4.1.9 Callus Under the Great Toe

A 54-year-old male patient with type 2 diabetes of 14 years' duration was referred to the foot clinic. On examination, he had severe neuropathy. Gross callus formation with a painless ulcer at its center was noticed. Smaller amounts of callus were seen under his first, third and fourth metatarsal heads (Figure 4.14). Hyperpigmentation of the skin due to venous insufficiency and a scar from saphenectomy for coronary artery bypass grafting to treat coronary artery disease were seen. The cause of the callosities was inappropriate footwear and prominent metatarsal heads. The ulcer was debrided and dressed.

4.2 Corns

4.2.1 Heloma Durum (Hard Corn)

A 67-year-old male patient with type 2 diabetes attended the outpatient diabetic foot clinic because of painless hyperkeratosis on the dorsum of his toes.

On examination, he had severe neuropathy and normal peripheral pulses. Significant muscle atrophy was seen on the dorsum of his feet. Mild hallux valgus and a claw toe deformity were also present. Because of bunions, due to hallux valgus deformity, a red and swollen

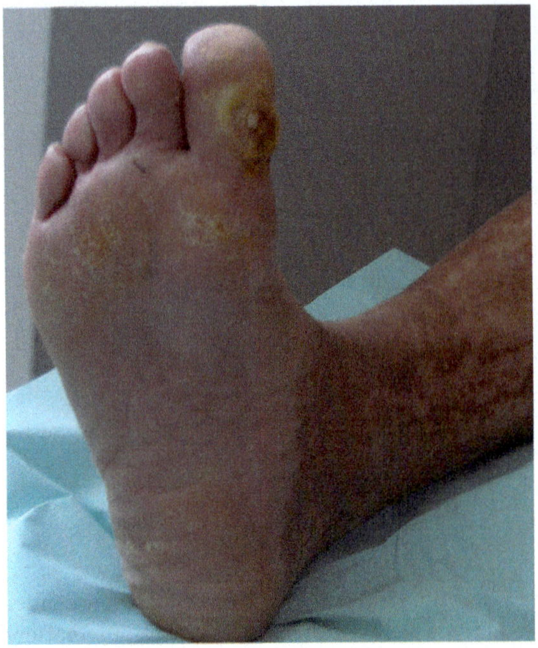

Figure 4.14 Gross callus on the great toe.

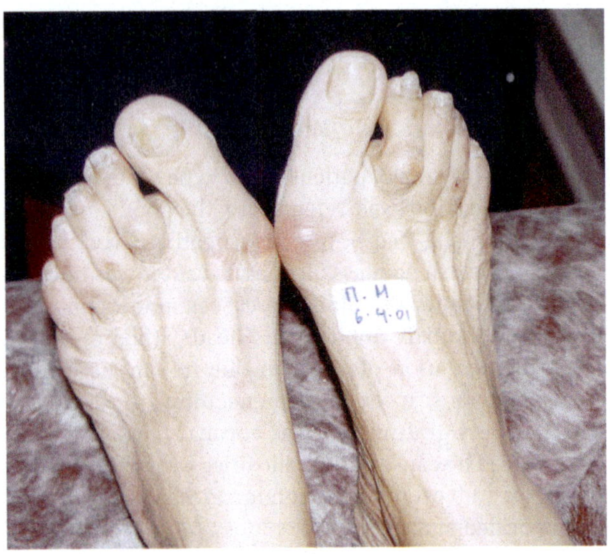

Figure 4.15 Heloma durum (hard corn), bunion, bursitis and claw toes.

bursa had developed on the medial aspect of both first metatarsal heads, caused by pressure and friction on these areas from his shoes. Painless corns were also present on the dorsum of the toes (Figure 4.15).

Such corns – called heloma durum or hard corns (Figure 4.16) – are caused by pressure and friction on the deformed toes from low toe box shoes. Proper shoes (shoes with a broad and high toe box) were prescribed to this patient to accommodate the deformity. The heloma durum and bursitis did not relapse.

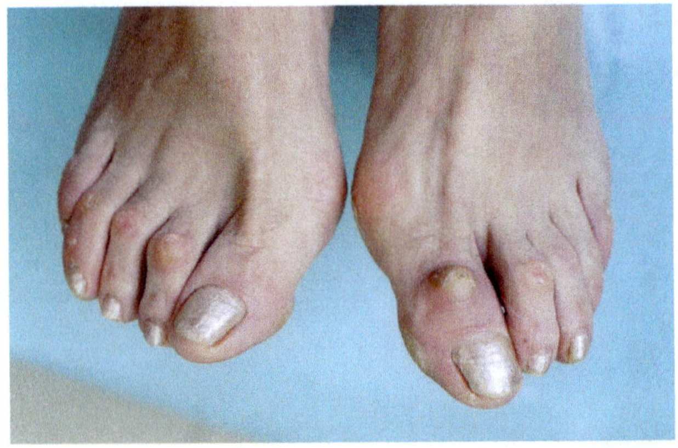

Figure 4.16 Multiple heloma durum (hard corns).

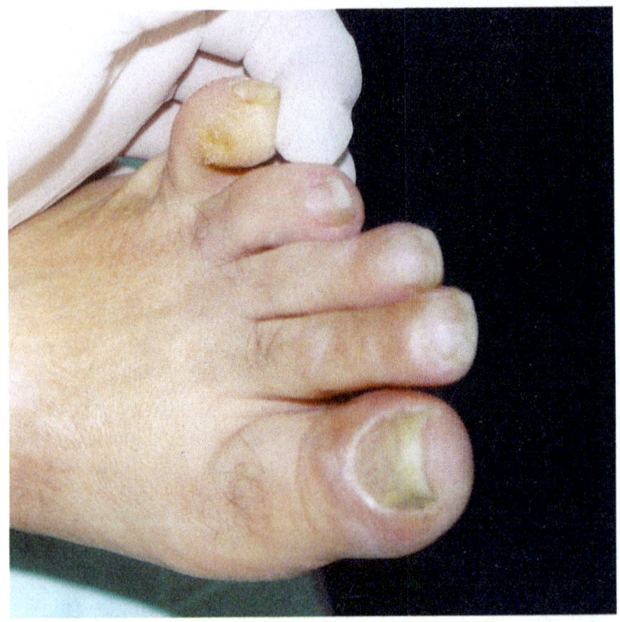

Figure 4.17 Heloma molle (soft corn).

4.2.2 Heloma Molle (Soft Corn)

A 54-year-old male patient with type 2 diabetes diagnosed at the age of 48 attended the outpatient diabetic foot clinic. He had severe diabetic neuropathy and was complaining of a mild pain in his left little toe. On examination, a painful corn was seen at this location (Figure 4.17).

Corns are circular hyperkeratotic areas that may be soft or hard. They have a polished or translucent center and may become painful due to persistent pressure and friction. Soft corns develop in the interdigital spaces; they are called heloma molle and are caused by pressure and friction from the bones of the adjacent toe.

This type of corn has often a soft consistency (in contrast to a heloma durum) owing to moisture retention in the interdigital space. The most common location of

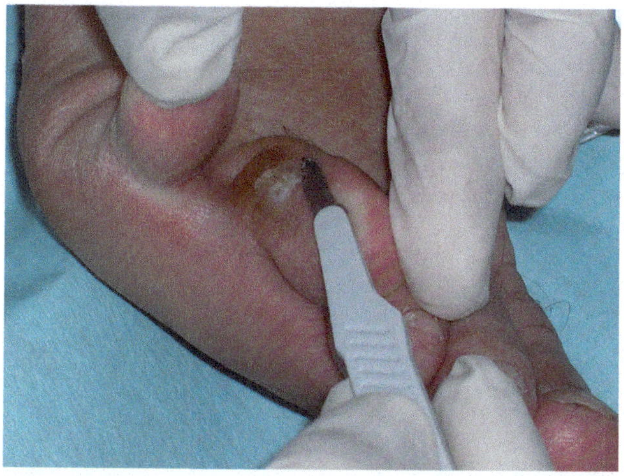

Figure 4.18 Typical site of a heloma molle.

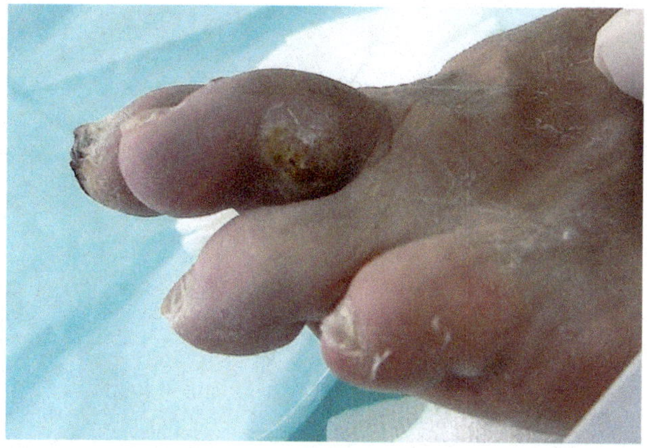

Figure 4.19 An infected heloma molle.

a heloma molle is the lateral side of the fourth toe (Figure 4.18), being caused by pressure and friction from the adjacent head of the proximal phalanx of the fifth toe; it may, however, occur in the other interdigital spaces as well. Osteoarthritic changes in the distal interphalangeal joints often cause heloma molle. Kissing heloma molle results when the ends of the phalanges are too wide.

Tight shoes aggravate the problem. This condition is especially common in women who wear high-heel shoes, which shift the body's weight to the front of the foot, squeezing the toes into a narrow, tapering toe box.

Heloma molle, like heloma durum, may cause discomfort, and this may be complicated by infection. Wide shoes or shoes with a high toe box prevent recurrence. Permanent treatment involves the surgical removal of a small part of the bones or exostoses that are involved in the pathogenesis of the heloma molle.

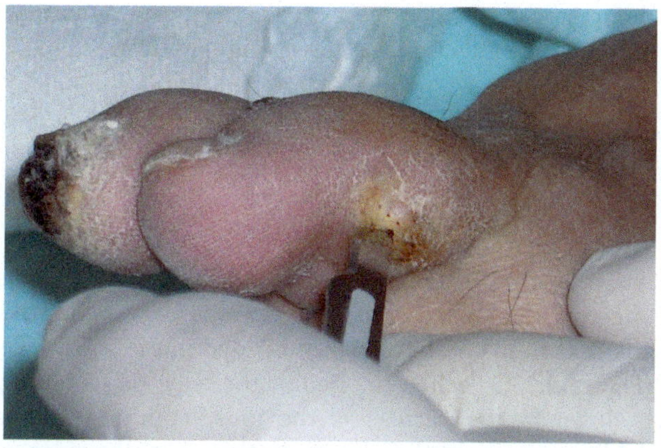

Figure 4.20 An ulcer under a heloma molle in the patient shown in Figure 4.19.

4.2.3 Heloma Molle Complicated by Infection

This 62-year-old female with long-standing type 2 diabetes was referred to the foot clinic. She had dense peripheral neuropathy. She was complaining of moderate discomfort of the third toe of her left foot, which was swollen and warm with a "sausage-like" appearance, a finding typical in osteomyelitis. Heloma molle (Figure 4.19) and an ulcer (Figure 4.20) under the hyperkeratotic area were present at the outer aspect of her third toe. A hemorrhagic callus was also present at the tip of her second toe.

The hyperkeratotic tissue was removed, and the ulcer was dressed (Figure 4.21). Swabs taken from the base of the ulcer after debridement revealed *Staphylococcus aureus*. A plain X-ray at that time was normal, but as she had osteomyelitis, the patient was managed based on

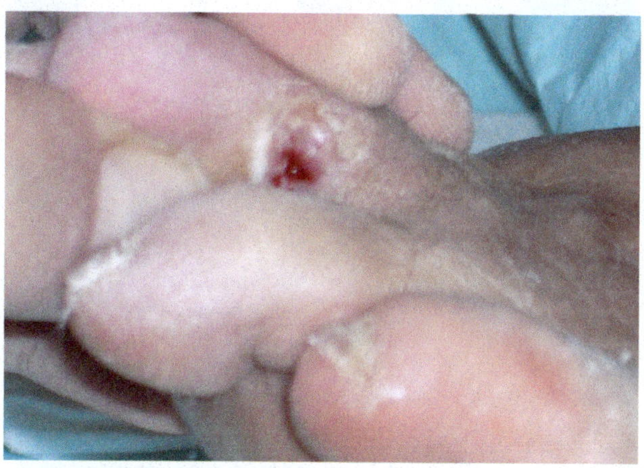

Figure 4.21 An infected heloma molle after debridement, in the same patient as shown in Figure 4.19.

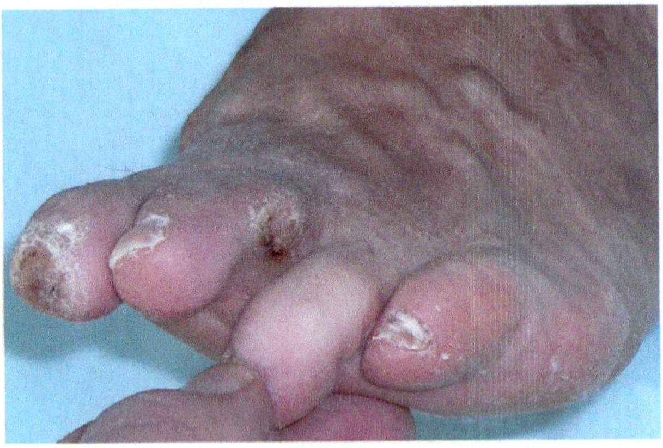

Figure 4.22 An infected heloma molle three weeks after debridement and treatment with antibiotics, in the same patient as shown in Figure 4.19.

the results of the swab culture with trimethoprim–sulfamethoxazole. Three weeks later, the ulcer was smaller, although the infection was persisting (Figure 4.22).

4.3 Nail Deformities

4.3.1 Ingrown Nails (Onychocryptosis)

An ingrown toenail is a common condition usually affecting the hallux. A section of a nail curves into the adjacent flesh and becomes embedded in the soft tissue (Figure 4.23). Peeling the nail at the edge or trimming it down at the corners is the most common cause. Additionally, tight shoes or socks that press the sides of the nail and make it curve into the skin, as well as congenital or traumatic reasons, may cause an ingrown nail.

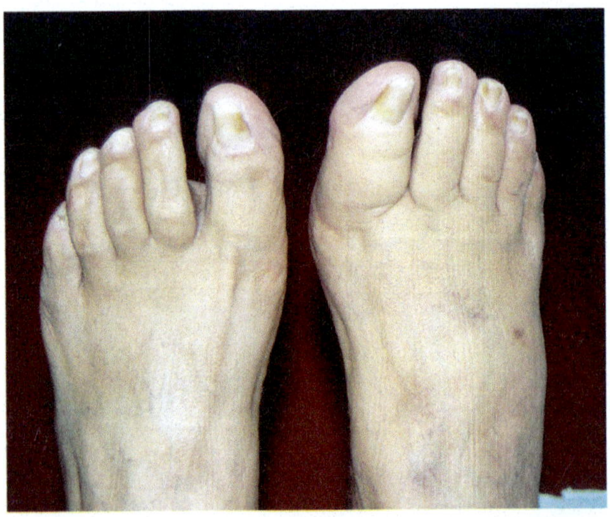

Figure 4.23 Onychocryptosis (ingrowing toenail) of both halluxes. Note the brown discoloration caused by chronic infection with *Candida albicans*. Claw toe deformity of the second, third and fourth toes can also be seen.

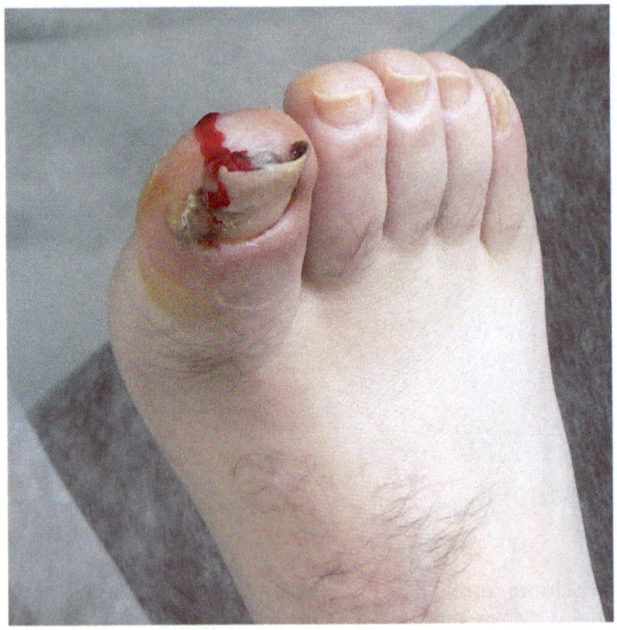

Figure 4.24 Paronychia caused by onychocryptosis.

An ingrown nail predisposes to local infection (paronychia) as it provides an entry point for pathogens (Figures 4.24 and 4.25); therefore, it should be treated as soon as it is recognized. Nails should be trimmed in a straight line.

Infection with *Candida albicans* is another cause of chronic paronychia, especially when patients' feet are exposed to moisture for long periods. The nail is usually affected, and it becomes ridged, deformed and brown.

4.3.2 Onychodystrophy

Onychodystrophy is a widely used term. It refers to nail changes apart from changes involving the color seen in nail dyschromia. Toenails undergo changes much more than do fingernails, as a consequence of trauma, the environment of the shoe or sock, and the forces associated with ambulation. The toenails may undergo degeneration and become thickened in response to repeated microtrauma. Partial or complete disruption of the various keratinous layers of the nail plate is most relevant.

Onychodystrophy represents various pathologic processes of the nails such as infections, mainly onychomycosis, and non-infectious disorders including psoriasis, allergic and irritant dermatitis, and severe peripheral arterial disease. Nail changes may also be a clue to other dermatologic or systemic diseases, and the use of antimicrobial and antineoplastic chemotherapeutic agents (docetaxel), antimalarials, penicillamine and the human immunodeficiency virus protease inhibitor indinavir.

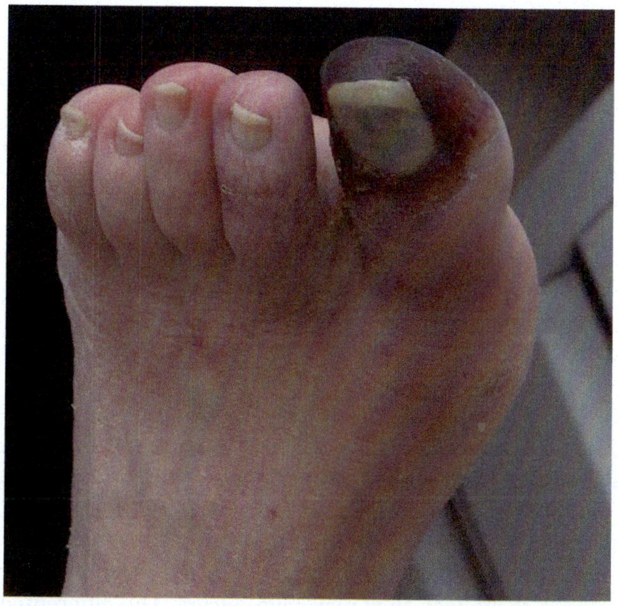

Figure 4.25 Paronychia caused by onychocryptosis in a patient with peripheral arterial disease. In addition to infection affecting the great and second toes, hematoma due to unnoticed trauma can be seen.

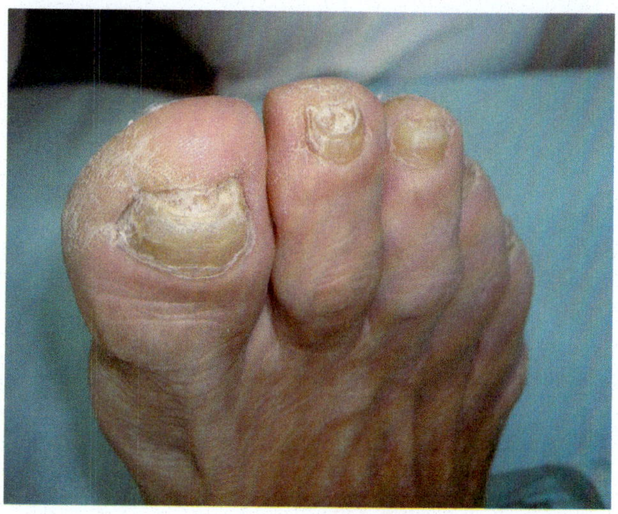

Figure 4.26 Onychodystrophy in a patient with peripheral neuropathy.

Whether onychodystrophy is more common among patients with diabetes is not known. The foot of a diabetic patient with onychodystrophy as a result of repetitive trauma caused by peripheral neuropathy and improper footwear is shown in Figure 4.26.

4.3.3 Onychogryphosis

A 75-year-old male patient with type 2 diabetes was referred to the foot clinic for foot care. He was a psychiatric patient treated on an outpatient basis. The patient had findings of peripheral neuropathy. Claw toes and extreme onychogryphosis were noticed (Figure 4.27). His nails were cut using a special nail trimmer. Education on foot care was given, and extra-depth shoes were provided to accommodate the deformity. The man visited the clinic monthly and had his nails cut without any other foot problems developing.

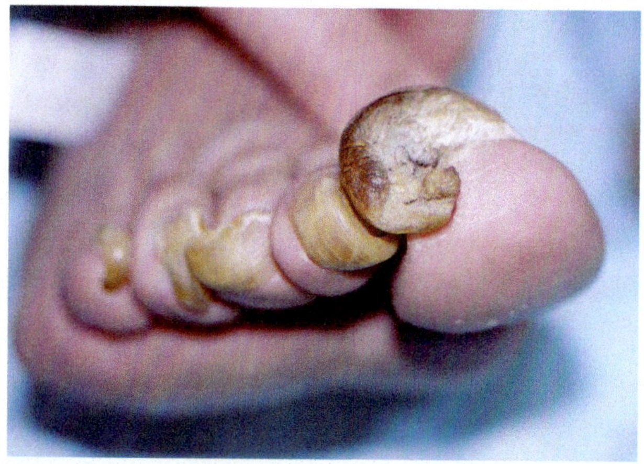

Figure 4.27 Onychogryphosis.

Onychogryphosis, an extreme form of onychodystrophy, is a severe deformation of the nail, most often affecting the great toes. The nail becomes very thick, discolored, hard and elongated, resembling a ram's horn. The nail bed can become hypertrophied. Onychogryphosis is most commonly caused by infrequent nail-cutting and impaired peripheral circulation, but it may also be caused by repetitive trauma. The deformed nail can press against another toe, causing ulcerations. When the patient does not wear shoes, the deformed toenail often grows vertically. When socks or shoes are being worn, the deformed toe nails tend to develop in such a way as to accommodate this activity.

4.4 Edema

4.4.1 Edema in a Patient with a Foot Ulcer

A 72-year-old female patient attended the outpatient foot clinic for a painless, clean neuropathic ulcer under the head of her third metatarsal. Gross edema was seen at the left ankle due to treatment with amlodipine for hypertension. The ulcer was debrided and dressed (Figure 4.28).

Edema of the lower legs may accompany systemic disorders such congestive heart failure, liver insufficiency or nephrotic syndrome (Figure 4.29) or may be related to use of calcium channel blockers. In such cases, the edema is bilateral. Localized edema is related to

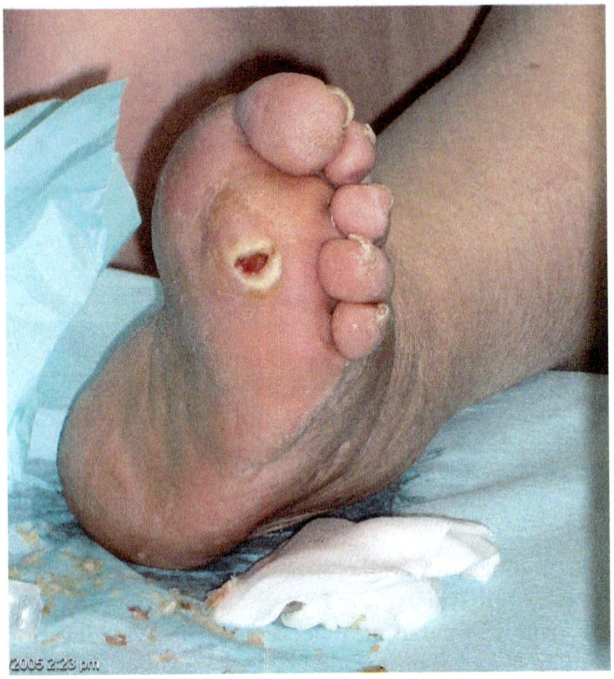

Figure 4.28 Ankle edema in a patient with a foot ulcer.

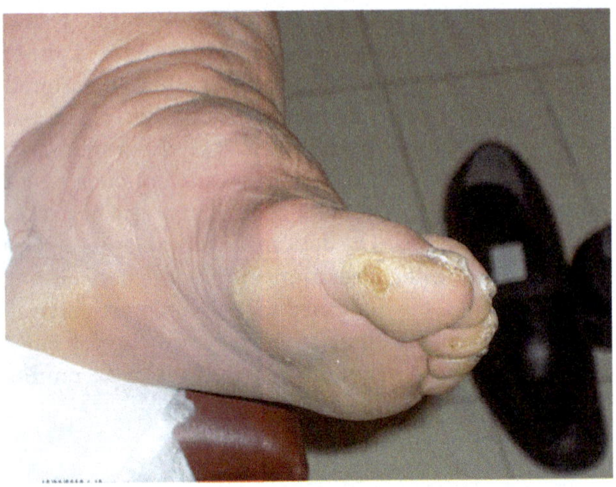

Figure 4.29 Gross ankle edema in a patient with advanced diabetic nephropathy. Callus formation is seen on the great toe, over the first metatarsal head and at the tip of the third toe due to inappropriate footwear. A claw toe deformity is also present.

infections, venous insufficiency, joint subluxation, arthritis, fractures or crystal deposit disorders. Mild foot edema may also accompany active ulcers, even in the absence of infection. Gross edema in patients with a foot ulcer may aggravate the blood supply and retard healing, particularly in patients with peripheral arterial disease. Additionally, edema may fluctuate during the day and may expose skin to friction and breakdown if shoes with inadequate room are used. Patients with edema should buy new footwear at the end of the day, when their edema is usually more severe. Edema has been associated with an increased risk for foot ulceration.

4.5 Diabetic Bullae (Bullosis Diabeticorum)

A 64-year-old man attended the foot clinic because of a ruptured bulla over his tibia (Figure 4.30). The bulla evolved acutely without any predisposing factor and ruptured in a few days. The patient did not complain of pain or discomfort.

Diabetic bullae present as tense blisters on a non-inflammatory base, appearing rapidly and healing in a few weeks. They affect men more commonly than women. The most common locations are the feet and lower legs, followed by the hands. They may go unnoticed by patients with neuropathy, and if they are located on the toes or the plantar aspect of the feet, they may cause ulcers. The differential diagnosis includes the autoimmune blistering diseases porphyria cutanea tarda, pseudoporphyria and bullous impetigo. Acutely developed diabetic bullae in another diabetic patient are shown in Figure 4.31.

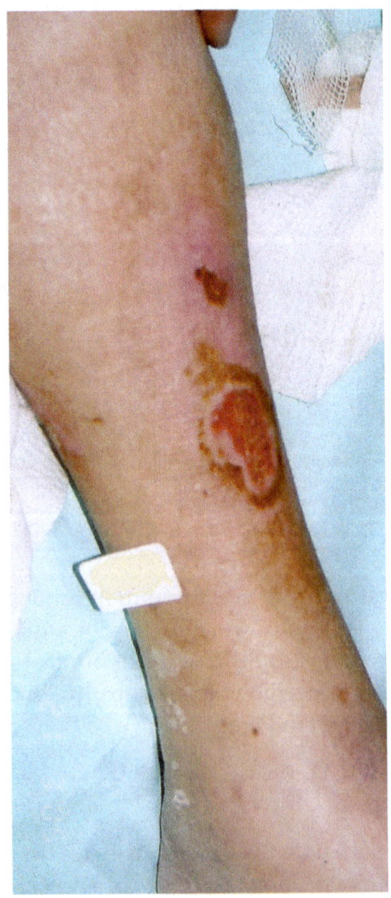

Figure 4.30 A ruptured diabetic bulla.

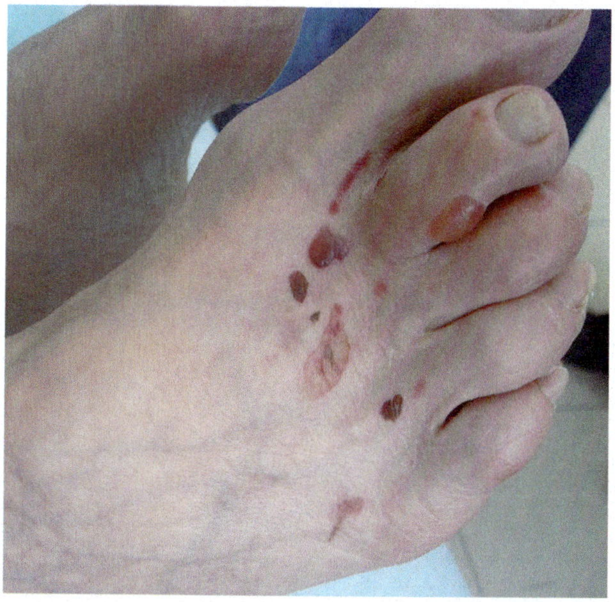

Figure 4.31 Diabetic bullae.

4.6 Diabetic Thick Skin

The skin of diabetic patients is thicker and less elastic in comparison with that of healthy subjects: Figure 4.32 shows a patient with long-standing type 2 diabetes, and Figure 4.33 a non-diabetic subject of a similar age and gender. Collagen bundles in the dermis of patients with diabetes are thickened and disorganized as a result of irreversible glycation of the collagen. Collagen has a low turn-over rate, and the formation of advanced glycation end-products damages the protein itself and reduces the ability of collagenase to remodel the collagen fibers. The combination of thickened skin and limited joint mobility due to the glycation of periarticular tissues – so-called cheiroarthropathy (Figure 4.34) – is seen in 30% of patients with long-standing type 1 diabetes.

Limited joint mobility of the hand can be demonstrated by the inability to flatten the affected hand on a table top and by a failure to approximate the palms with the fingers fanned and the wrist maximally flexed (the prayer sign). The most accurate sign is a limitation of extension when the examiner passively tests the interphalangeal and metacarpophalangeal joints.

Limited joint mobility of the hallux (hallux limitus) of the same patient is shown in Figure 4.35. When joint mobility is severely limited or the hallux is rigid, the term

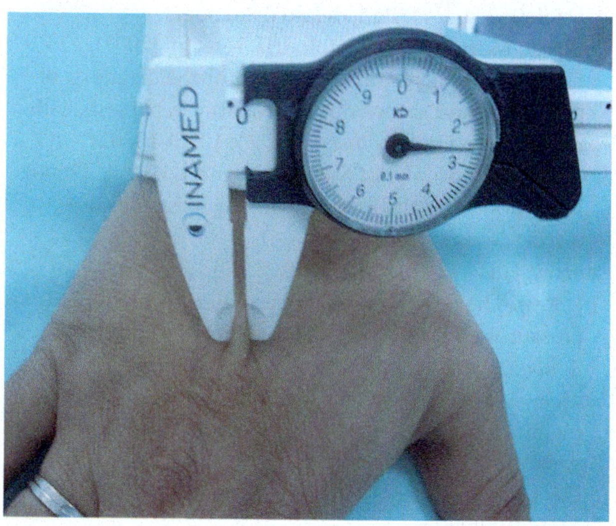

Figure 4.33 Normal skin thickness of the hand of a non-diabetic subject of similar gender and age to the patient shown in Figure 4.32.

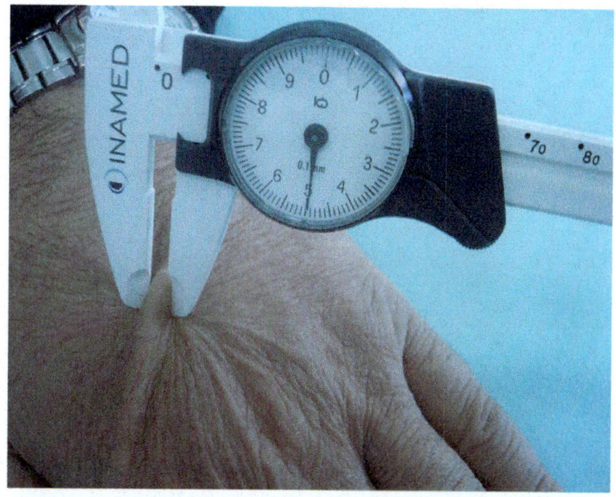

Figure 4.32 Increased skin thickness of the hand in a patient with long-standing type 2 diabetes.

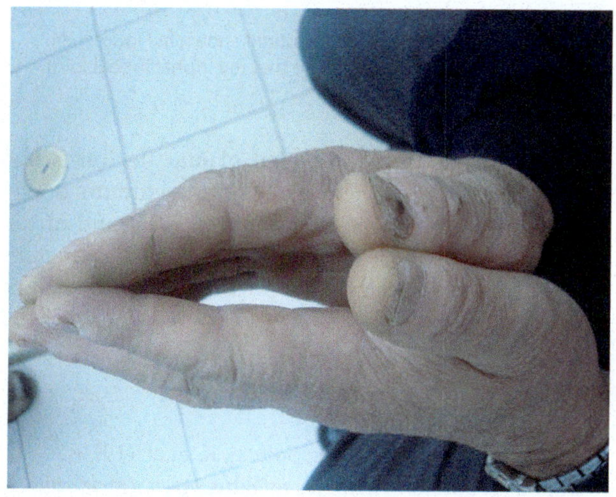

Figure 4.34 Cheiroarthropathy. Failure to approximate the palms with the fingers fanned and the wrist maximally flexed (the prayer sign) is typical.

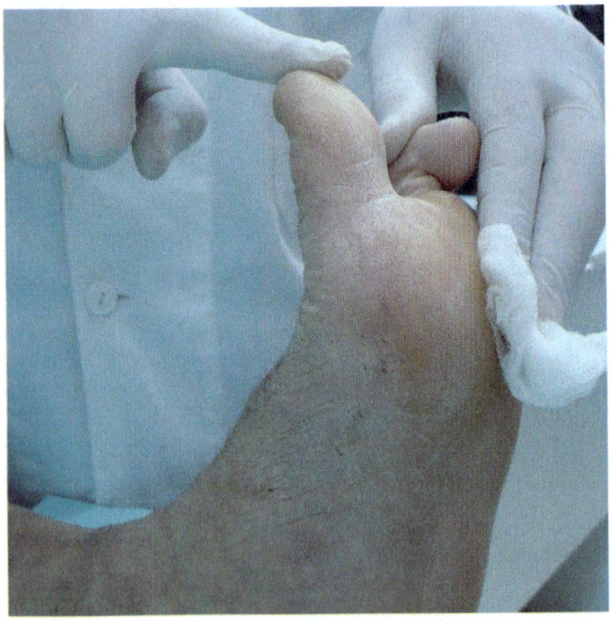

Figure 4.35 Hallux limitus in the patient shown in Figure 4.34. Note the limited dorsiflexion of the metatarsophalangeal joint.

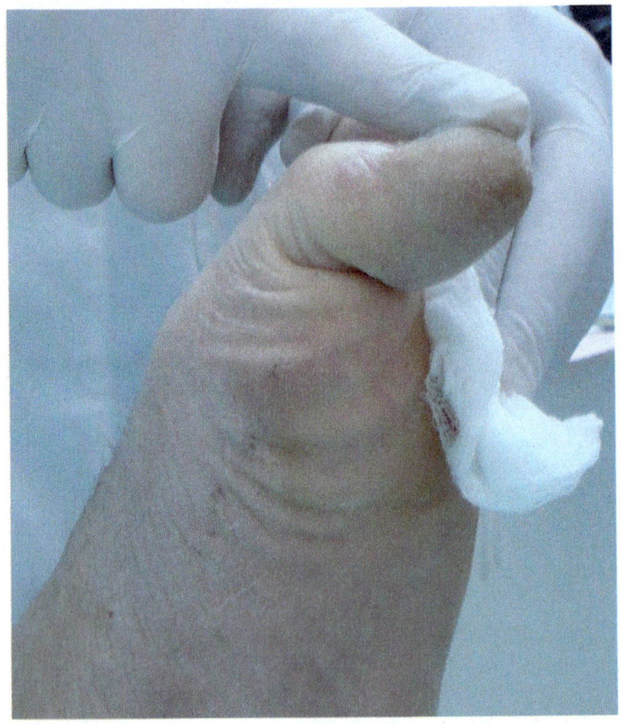

Figure 4.36 Preservation of plantar flexion in patients with hallux limitus.

hallux rigidus is used. Note that plantar flexion is not affected (Figure 4.36). Normally, the maximum dorsiflexion of the first metatarsal joint is 65–75° and maximum plantar flexion less than 15°. The presence of hallux limitus causes the peak plantar pressure under the hallux to build up significantly more quickly and to a greater degree than that under the first metatarsal head.

Further Reading

Bernstein, J.E., Medenica, M., Soltani, K. et al. (1979). Bullous eruption of diabetes mellitus. *Arch. Dermatol.* 115: 324–325.

Daniel, C.R. and Scher, R.K. (1984). Nail changes secondary to systemic drugs or ingestants. *J. Am. Acad. Dermatol.* 10: 250–258.

Dawber, R.P.R., de Berker, D.A.R., and Baran, R. (2001). Science of the nail apparatus. In: *Baran and Dawber's Diseases of the Nails and their Management*, 3e (ed. R. Baran, R.P.R. Dawber, D.A.R. de Berker, et al.), 1–47. Oxford: Blackwell Science.

Hoeldtke, R.D., Bryner, K.D., Horvath, G.G. et al. (2001). Redistribution of sudomotor responses is an early sign of sympathetic dysfunction in type 1 diabetes. *Diabetes* 50: 436–443.

Huntley, A.C. and Walter, R.M. (1990). Quantitative evaluation of skin thickness in diabetes mellitus: relationship to disease parameters. *J. Med.* 21: 257–264.

Jelinek, J.E. (1994). Cutaneous manifestations of diabetes mellitus. *Int. J. Dermatol.* 33: 605–617.

Kern, D.G. (1990). Occupational disease. In: *Nails: Therapy, Diagnosis, Surgery* (ed. R.K. Scher and C.R. Daniel), 224–243. Philadelphia: Saunders.

Liatis, S., Marinou, K., Tentolouris, N. et al. (2007). Usefulness of a new indicator test for the diagnosis of peripheral and autonomic neuropathy in patients with diabetes mellitus. *Diabet. Med.* 24: 1375–1380.

Low, V.A., Sandroni, P., Fealey, R.D., and Low, P.A. (2006). Detection of small-fiber neuropathy by sudomotor testing. *Muscle Nerve* 34: 57–61.

Murray, H.J., Young, M.J., Hollis, S., and Boulton, A.J. (1996). The association between callus formation, high pressures and neuropathy in diabetic foot ulceration. *Diabet. Med.* 13: 979–982.

Nathan, M. (1993). Long-term complications of diabetes mellitus. *N. Engl. J. Med.* 305: 1676–1685.

Norman, A. (2001). Dermal manifestations of diabetes. In: *Geriatric Dermatology* (ed. R. Norman), 143–154. New York: Parthenon.

Perez, I. and Kohn, R. (1994). Cutaneous manifestations of diabetes. *J. Am. Acad. Dermatol.* 30: 519–531.

Sibbald, G.R., Landolt, S.J., and Toth, D. (1996). Skin and diabetes. *Endocrinol. Metab. Clin. N. Am.* 25: 463–472.

Singer, W., Spies, J.M., McArthur, J. et al. (2004). Prospective evaluation of somatic and autonomic small fibers in selected autonomic neuropathies. *Neurology* 62: 612–618.

Tentolouris, N., Marinou, K., Kokotis, P. et al. (2009). Sudomotor dysfunction is associated with foot ulceration in diabetes. *Diabet. Med.* 26: 302–305.

Toonstra, J. (1985). Bullous diabeticorum. *J. Am. Acad. Dermatol.* 13: 799–805.

Tosti, A. and Piraccini, B.M. (2000). Treatment of common nail disorders. *Dermatol. Clin.* 18: 339–348.

Young, M.J., Cavanagh, P.R., Thomas, G. et al. (1992). The effect of callus removal on dynamic plantar foot pressures in diabetic patients. *Diabet. Med.* 9: 55–57.

5

Skin and Systemic Diseases with Manifestations in the Feet

S. Liatis and N. Tentolouris

First Department of Propaedeutic Internal Medicine, National and Kapodistrian University of Athens, Medical School, Laiko General Hospital, Athens, Greece

5.1 Necrobiosis Lipoidica (Necrobiosis Lipoidica Diabeticorum)

A 50-year-old lady with well-controlled type 1 diabetes who was diagnosed at the age of 38 has been visiting the outpatient clinic for her diabetes control on a regular basis. She has been free of micro- or macroangiopathy. Two years after her diabetes was diagnosed, the patient noticed a few small, red, irregular, violaceous papules on the dorsum of her feet. These papules slowly enlarged, coalesced and became scaly, irregular plaques, with minimal central atrophy and a red advancing border (Figure 5.1). New lesions appeared on her left ankle and her right leg. Apart from cosmetic problems, the plaques were asymptomatic.

A biopsy of these lesions showed necrobiosis lipoidica (NL, formerly known as necrobiosis lipoidica diabeticorum), a rare disease (a prevalence of 0.3% in diabetic populations) of unknown mechanism, strongly associated with diabetes mellitus but also found in subjects with normal or abnormal glucose tolerance.

Typically, such lesions occur on the anterior shins of both lower legs, but they may be also located on the arms, hands, or head. Affected areas may be partially or completely anesthetic. They may precede the diagnosis of diabetes, and are sometimes pruritic, dysesthetic or painful. They ulcerate – usually after trauma (Figure 5.2, another patient) – in approximately 25–35% of cases and may heal with scarring. Occasionally, the ulcerated lesions may be infected as shown in Figure 5.3. That was the case in a 17-year old woman with type 1 diabetes since the age of 8, who presented with a long-standing and extensively ulcerated and infected NL lesion on her left shin. The lesion had been present for almost two years and had deteriorated over the past three months, while the patient's diabetes was very poorly controlled (HbA1c: 13.5%). Pseudomonas aeruginosa was isolated from the exudate and treated accordingly (Figure 5.4, after a 15-day course with antibiotics).

Another case of necrobiosis lipoidica is shown in Figure 5.5, where extensive atrophy of the affected area can be noted. Histology of the lesions consists of collagen degeneration (necrobiosis; Figure 5.6) and fibrosis, histiocyte infiltration (Figure 5.7) and granuloma formation (Figure 5.8). Capillary walls appear thickened (Figure 5.7).

The treatment of this condition is unsatisfactory, and tight control of the diabetes does not cause regression of the lesions. The topical application of corticosteroids may improve early lesions but should not be used for chronic lesions as it may worsen skin atrophy. Various other agents have been tried, such as aspirin or pentoxifylline, with mixed results; cyclosporine and mycophenolate mofetil have been reported to be beneficial in some cases. A small study has shown that approximately 50% of patients responded to the topical application of 8-methoxypsoralen (methoxsalen) to the skin prior to treatment with ultraviolet A light. There are also some case reports in the literature in which NL patients have been successfully treated with infliximab and other anti-TNF-α (tumor necrosis factor-alpha) agents, as in the case of Figures 5.3–5.4, where, after antibiotic treatment, and since the patient had been treated unsuccessfully with several agents during the previous years, treatment with the anti-TNF-α monoclonal antibody infliximab was offered with significant improvement (Figure 5.9).

Atlas of the Diabetic Foot, Third Edition. Ioanna Eleftheriadou, Alexandros Kokkinos, Stavros Liatis, Konstantinos Makrilakis, Nicholas Tentolouris, Anastasios Tentolouris, and Panagiotis Tsapogas.

Companion website: www.wiley.com/go/tentolouris/atlas_diabetic_foot

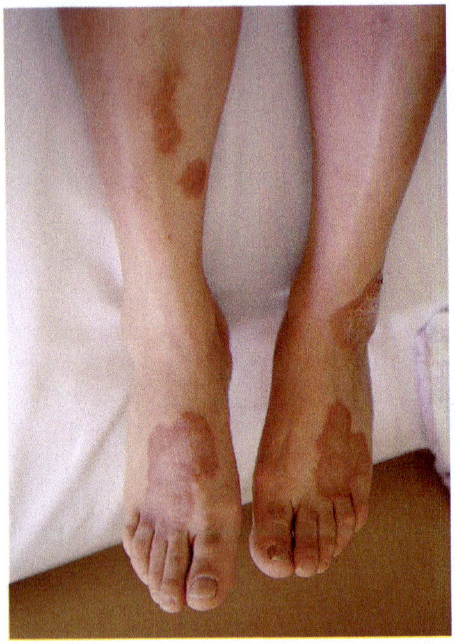

Figure 5.1 Necrobiosis lipoidica. Scaly, irregular plaques with minimal central atrophy and an advancing red border can be seen.

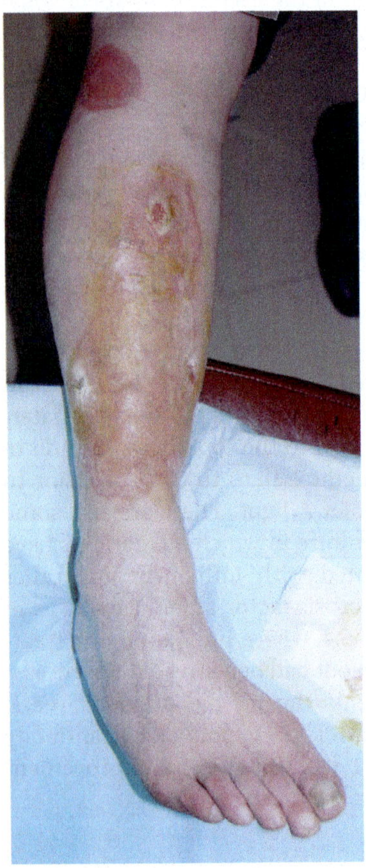

Figure 5.2 Ulcerated lesions of necrobiosis lipoidica. Note a lesion that is not ulcerated over the epiphysis of the fibula.

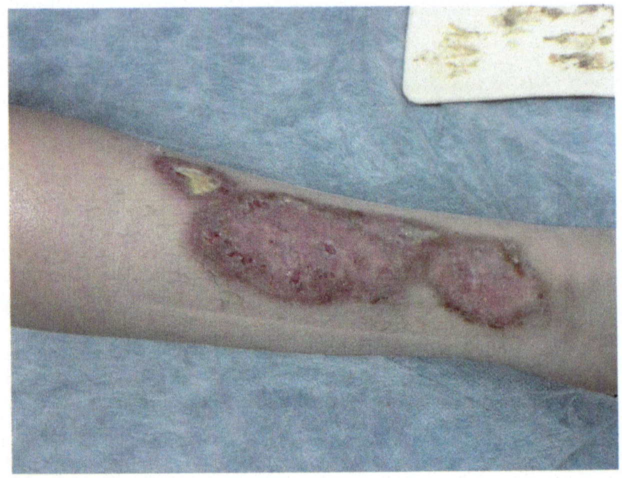

Figure 5.3 Lesions of ulcerated necrobiosis lipoidica, infected with pseudomonas aeruginosa.

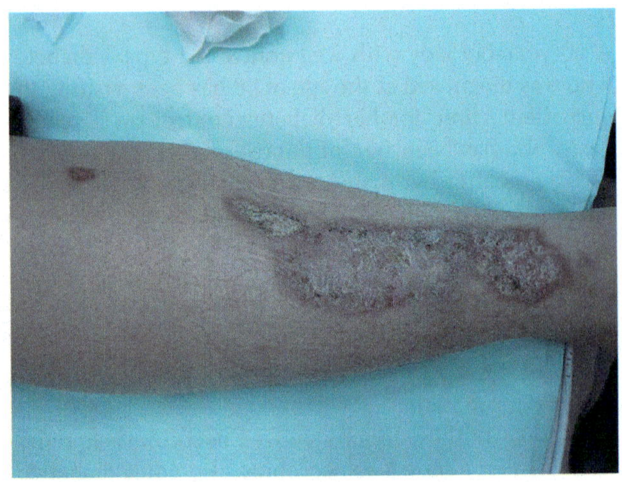

Figure 5.4 The lesion of Figure 5.3 after a 15-day course of antibiotic therapy.

5.2 Diabetic Dermopathy

A 58-year-old patient who had had type 2 diabetes for 18 years attended the outpatient diabetes clinic. He had background retinopathy and microalbuminuria. On examination, he had brown, scar-like atrophic lesions on his legs (Figure 5.10), consistent with diabetic dermopathy.

Diabetic dermopathy (Figure 5.11 – another patient) is the most common (approximate prevalence 50%) dermatologic condition associated with diabetes, but it is not specific to diabetes. It affects patients older than 50 years with a long duration of diabetes and is associated with microvascular complications of the disease.

Diabetic dermopathy is an inflammatory condition that begins as a cluster of erythematous papules that coalesce. Histologic examination of the early lesions

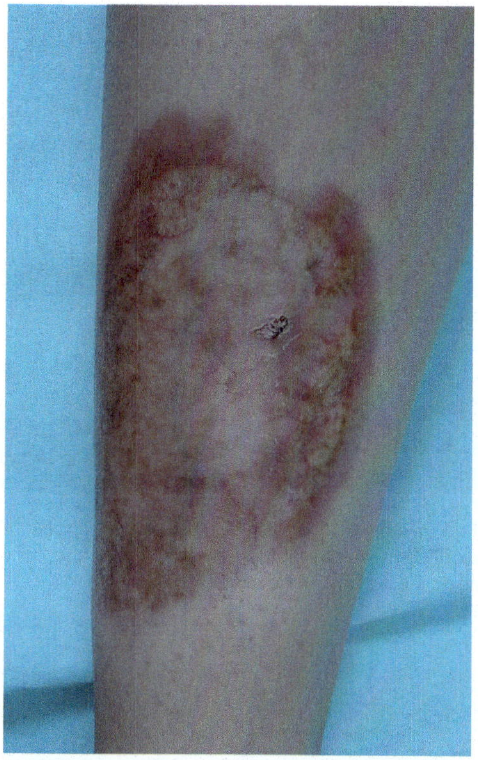

Figure 5.5 Necrobiosis lipoidica. There are irregular plaques with severe atrophy, yellow areas, and an advancing red border.

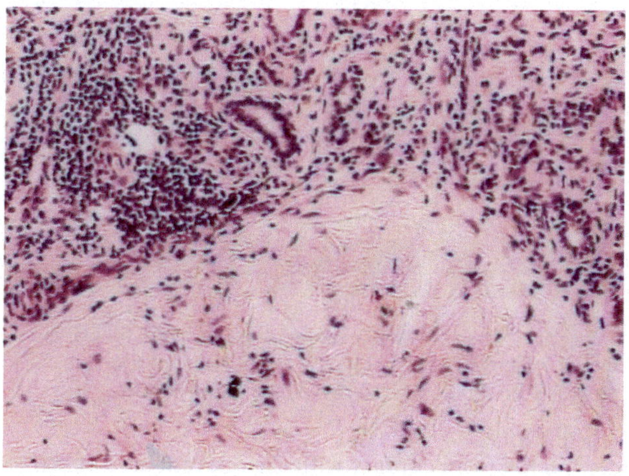

Figure 5.6 Histology of the patient shown in Figure 5.1, with necrobiosis lipoidica. There are foci of "hyalinized" collagen bundles (necrobiosis), fibrosis and histiocyte infiltration. The walls of the capillaries appear thickened (arrow) (hematoxylin and eosin ×00).

shows thickening of the blood vessels with perivascular lymphocyte infiltrates. The lesions appear as brown, scar-like and slightly elevated early in the disease, with atrophic later lesions. They are usually bilateral, and many appear in crops. Common sites are the shins, forearms and legs. The brown appearance is due to

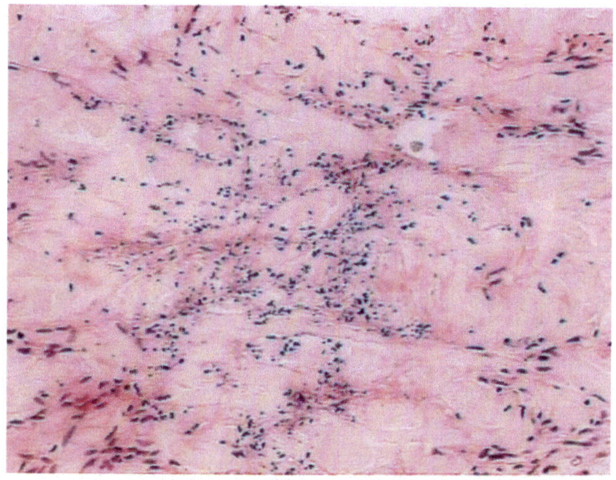

Figure 5.7 Histology of the patient from Figure 5.1, with necrobiosis lipoidica, also showing foci of "hyalinized" collagen bundles (necrobiosis), fibrosis, and histiocyte infiltration (hematoxylin and eosin ×100).

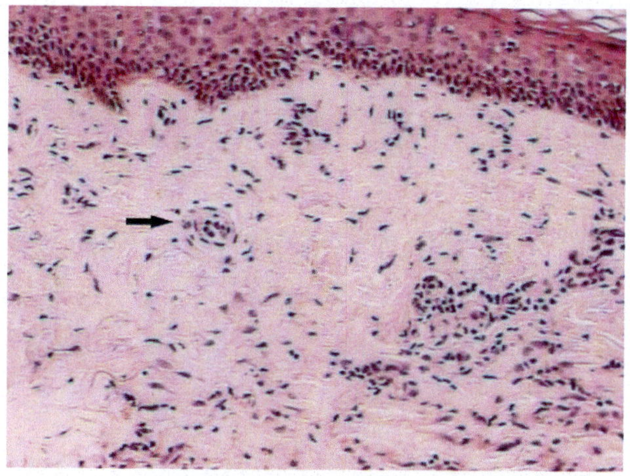

Figure 5.8 Histology of the patient shown in Figure 5.1, with necrobiosis lipoidica. Note the presence of a granuloma (arrow) (hematoxylin and eosin ×100).

hemosiderin-laden histiocytes and extravasated erythrocytes in the superficial dermis. No treatment is required, and the problem is cosmetic only.

5.2.1 Warts

This diabetic patient attended the outpatient diabetic foot clinic because of a painful callus (Figure 5.12) over the outer aspect of her heel of about six months' duration. After removal of the callus, multiple black specks in the center of the callus were apparent (Figure 5.13), an appearance typical of warts.

Warts are common, and are caused by a viral infection, specifically by the human papillomavirus. They can be

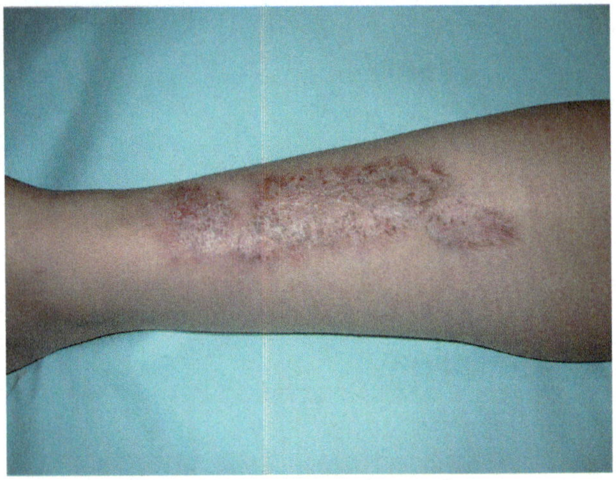

Figure 5.9 Necrobiosis lipolytica (patient shown in Figures 5.3 and 5.4) after treatment with infliximab.

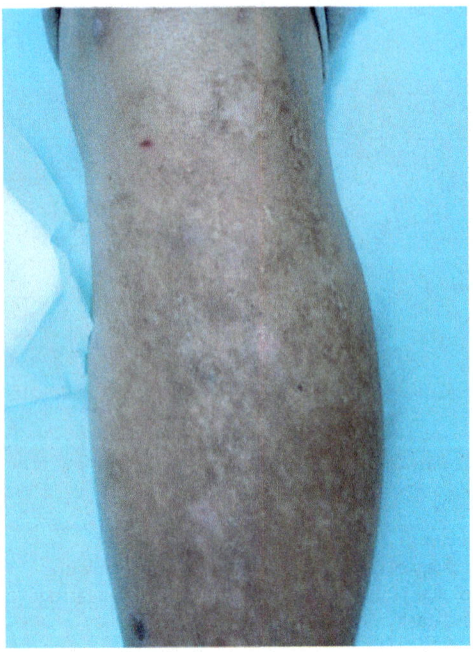

Figure 5.10 Diabetic dermopathy.

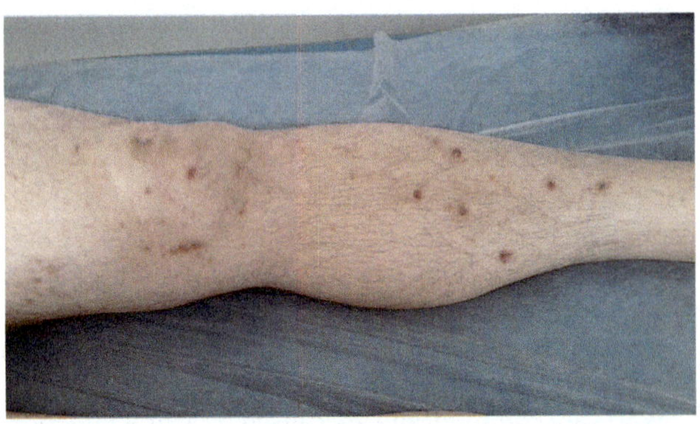

Figure 5.11 Diabetic dermopathy in another patient.

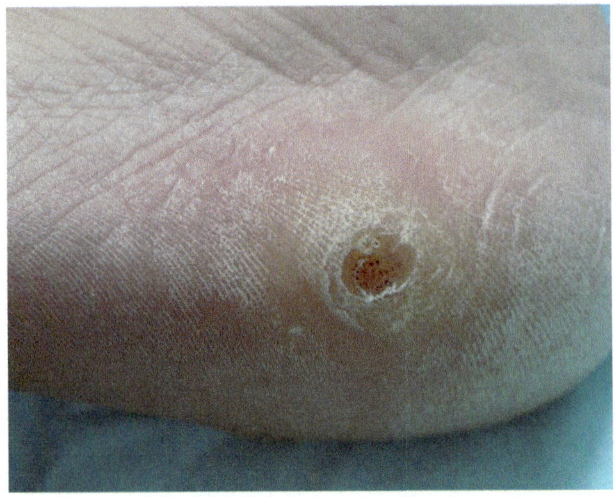

Figure 5.12 Plantar wart (verruca, verruca pedis), which appears as a hard and painful lump, with multiple black specks in the center. These warts are usually found on pressure points on the soles of the feet.

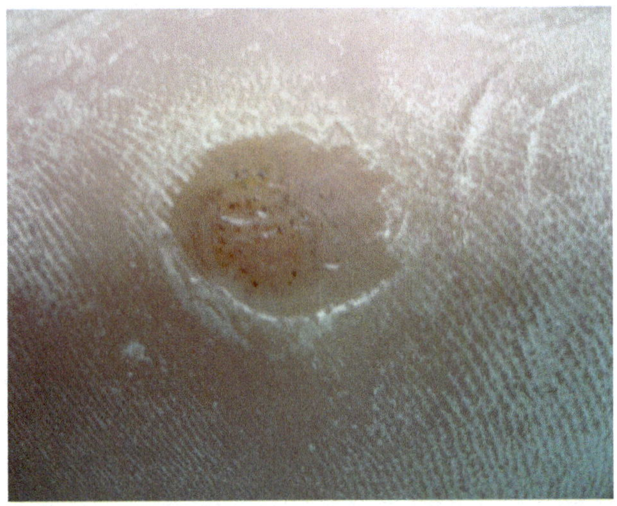

Figure 5.13 The appearance of the plantar warts of the patient shown in Figure 5.10 after callus removal. Note the multiple black specks in the center, which are typically found in warts.

contracted from contact with the relevant area of skin of an infected person. It is also possible to get warts from using towels or other objects used by an infected person. They typically disappear after a few months but can last for years and can recur.

There are approximately 100 strains of human papillomavirus. Types 1, 2 and 3 causes most common warts. Type 1 is associated with deep plantar (sole of the foot) and palmar (palm of the hand) warts (Figure 5.14). Type 2 causes common warts, plantar warts and mosaic plantar warts. Type 3 causes flat warts. A plantar wart (also known as a verruca or verruca pedis) manifests as a hard, sometimes painful lump with multiple black specks in

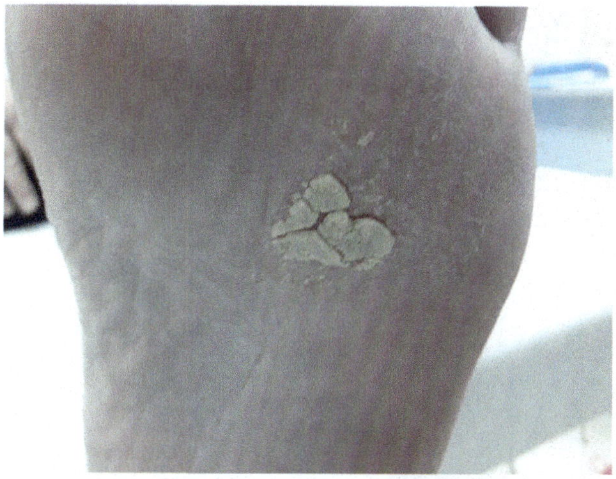

Figure 5.14 Plantar warts.

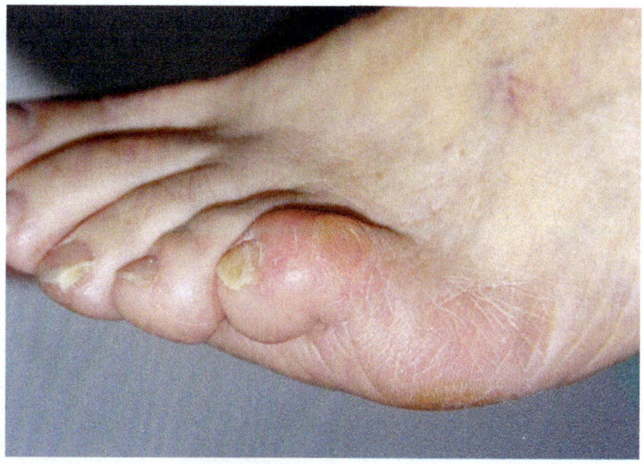

Figure 5.15 A painful inflammatory lesion of the fifth toe, due to calcium pyrophosphate dihydrate deposition disease.

the center, and is usually found on pressure points on the soles of the feet.

One systematic review of 52 clinical trials of various cutaneous wart treatments concluded that topical treatments containing salicylic acid were the best supported, with an average cure rate of 75%, compared with 48% for the placebo. Various other treatment modalities exist with potential benefit, such as the topical application of fluorouracil, bleomycin, cryotherapy and laser therapy.

5.3 Calcium Pyrophosphate Dihydrate Deposition Disease

A 74-year-old woman with type 2 diabetes was referred to the outpatient diabetic foot clinic for possible osteomyelitis of her fifth left toe. She had intense pain at this site both at rest and on walking. The pain started after the patient had used a tight pair of shoes for a few hours. On examination, redness, edema and callus formation were noticed on the outer aspect of the left fifth toe (Figure 5.15). She had findings of diabetic neuropathy, and her peripheral pulses were palpable.

Debridement of the callus revealed a cheesy material exuding from the base of a superficial ulcer. A culture of this material did not reveal microorganisms. A plain radiograph showed radio dense deposits in the articular bursae of the distal interphalangeal joint, but no osteomyelitis was apparent (Figure 5.16). Examination of this material by compensated polarized light microscopy showed rhomboid-shaped and weakly positive birefringent crystals, which is typical of calcium pyrophosphate dihydrate (CPPD) deposition disease.

The patient was advised to rest, and she had to visit the foot clinic on a weekly basis for callus debridement. The ulcer had completely healed after three weeks.

CPPD deposition disease (or pseudogout) of the foot joints is common in patients with diabetes and may pose a differential diagnosis problem when the location is atypical. The knee is the joint most frequently affected by pseudogout, followed by the wrist, shoulder, ankle, elbow and hands, although every joint can be affected. Treatment includes rest, aspiration of the joint fluids and the systemic use of non-steroidal anti-inflammatory medication.

5.4 Psoriasis

A 65-year-old patient with type 2 diabetes was referred to the foot clinic because of painless, non-itching skin lesions on both feet (Figure 5.17 and 5.18) and palms (Figure 5.19).

Psoriasis is a common dermatologic disease affecting 1–2% of the population. It is a chronic inflammatory skin disorder characterized by erythematous, sharply demarcated papules and rounded plaques, covered by silvery micaceous scale (Figures 5.17–5.19). Other patterns of psoriasis appear as shiny, red patches in areas of friction, such as in the folds of skin in the groin, the armpits or under the breasts, or as pustular (blisters of noninfectious pus on red skin) or "erythrodermic" (reddening and scaling of most of the skin). Pustular psoriasis is a rare form characterized by small pustules (whitehead-like lesions) found all over the body or confined to the palms, soles and other isolated areas of the body (Figure 5.20, showing a different patient). Lesions tend to be symmetric.

About 50% of patients have fingernail involvement, appearing as a punctuate pitting, longitudinal striations, brownish discoloration, nail thickening or subungual hyperkeratosis (Figures 5.21, 5.22 and 5.24). In such cases,

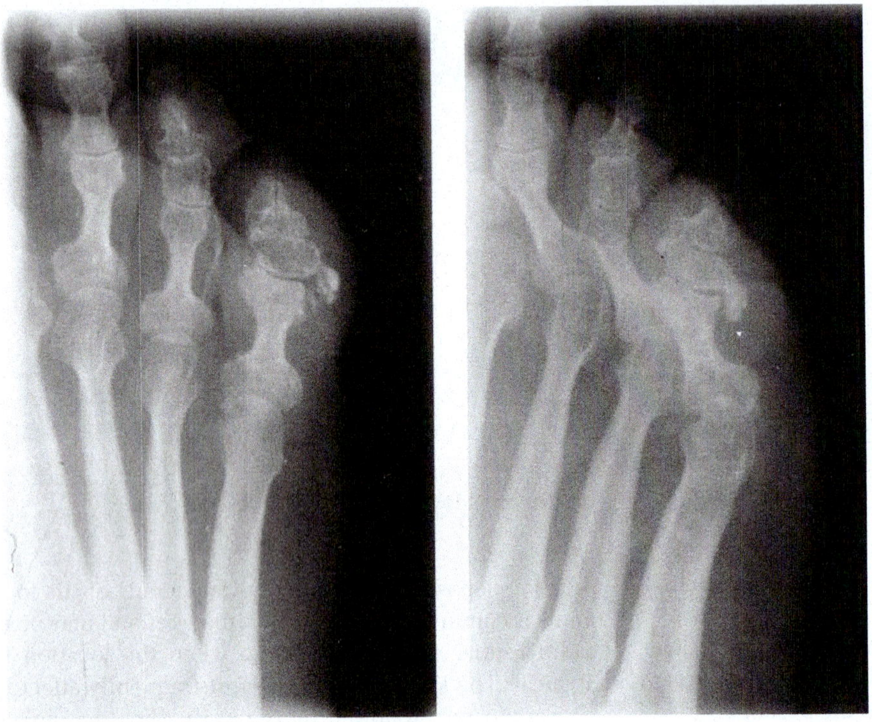

Figure 5.16 Radiodense deposits in the articular bursae of the distal interphalangeal joint of the fifth toe, due to calcium pyrophosphate dihydrate deposition disease.

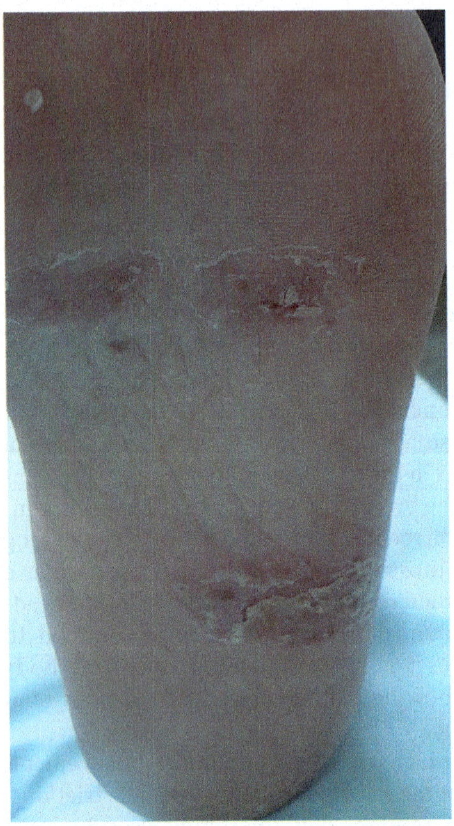

Figure 5.17 Plaque psoriasis (or psoriasis vulgaris) on the sole.

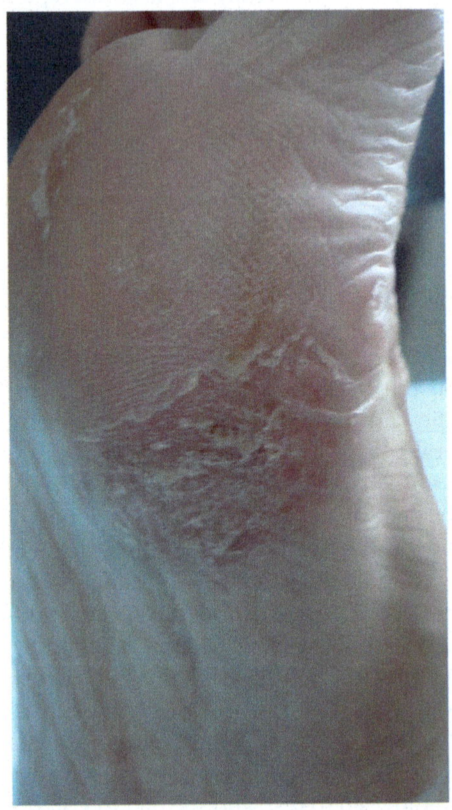

Figure 5.18 Plaque psoriasis (or psoriasis vulgaris) on the sole of the patient shown in Figure 5.14.

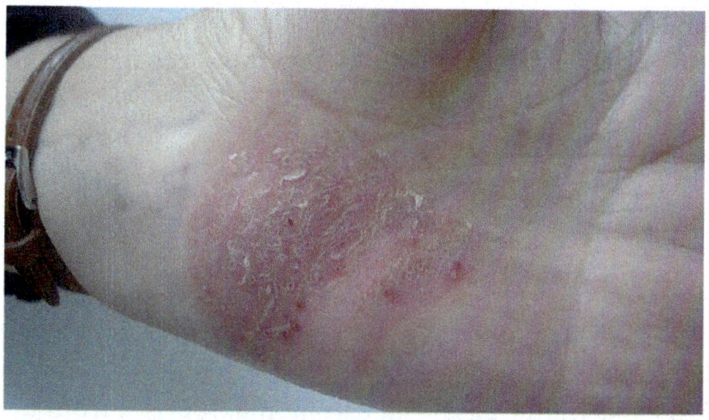

Figure 5.19 Plaque psoriasis (or psoriasis vulgaris) on the palm of the patient from Figure 5.14.

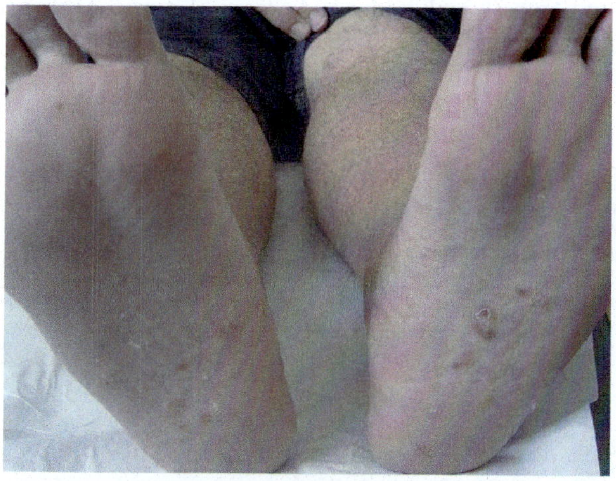

Figure 5.20 Pustular psoriasis of the sole.

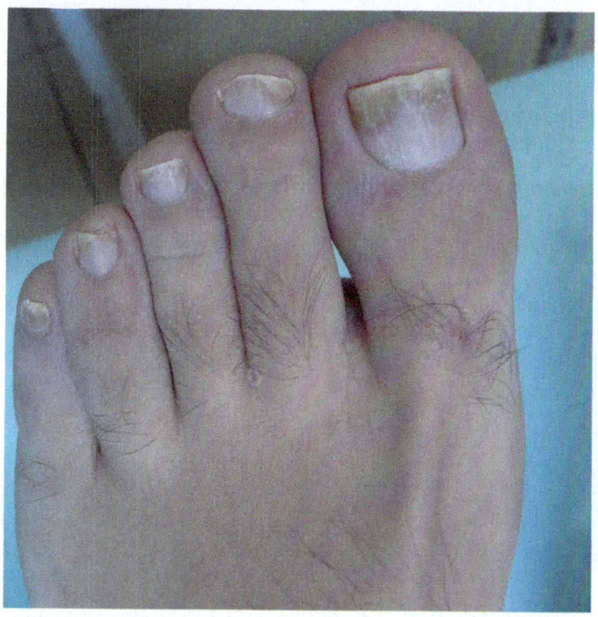

Figure 5.21 Nail involvement in psoriasis. Note the longitudinal striations, the brownish discoloration at the distal edge and the nail thickening.

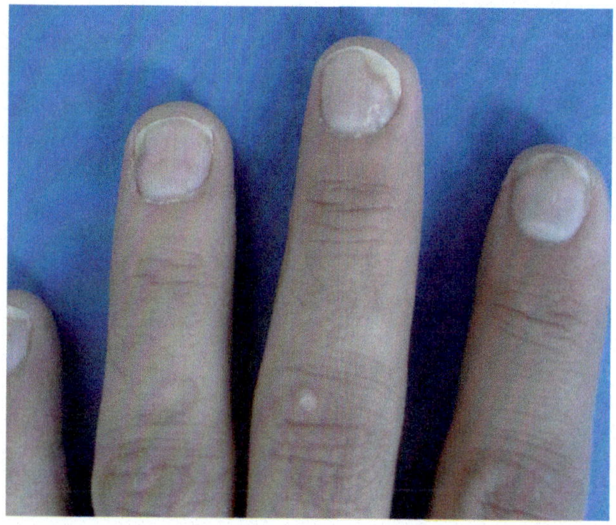

Figure 5.22 Fingernail involvement in psoriasis in the patient shown in Figure 5.17. Notice the longitudinal striations and the brownish discoloration at the distal edge and lateral nailfold. Punctuate pitting is also present.

onychomycosis, lichen planus, alopecia areata and pityriasis rubra pilaris should be included in the differential diagnosis. Approximately 5–10% of patients have joint involvement.

Treatment depends on the type, location, and extent of the disease. Topical lesions are managed with topical glucocorticoids, coal tar, calcipotriene (a synthetic, activated form of vitamin D_3) and/or ultraviolet light. For widespread disease, methotrexate, and antitumor necrosis factors can be used.

5.5 Palmoplantar Keratoderma

A 64-year-old male patient with type 2 diabetes diagnosed at the age of 55 attended the foot clinic for foot care and education because of palmoplantar keratoderma. On examination, diffuse thickening of the palmar and plantar skin, together with hyperkeratosis, was noticed (Figure 5.23). Nail deformities were also seen. He had findings of peripheral neuropathy, while his peripheral arteries were palpable.

The patient was instructed on foot care. Local debridement with keratolytics was prescribed. Protection from friction with soft insoles may also be helpful in this condition.

Palmoplantar keratoderma is an autosomal dominant trait characterized by diffuse, thickened hyperkeratosis of the palms and soles. Hyperkeratosis may become so thickened that the skin may crack, especially in dry, cold weather. Tinea pedis frequently develops as fissures allow a portal of entry for the fungus. The nails of

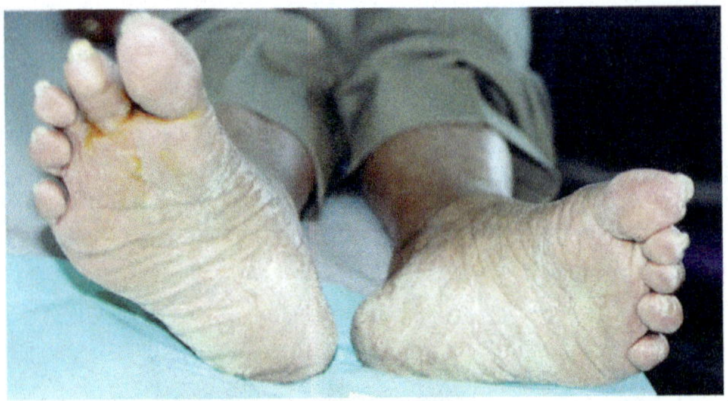

Figure 5.23 Palmoplantar keratoderma.

the hands and toes may be dystrophic and become fungally infected.

5.6 Hyperkeratotic Eczema

A 65-year-old male patient with long-standing diabetes visited the outpatient diabetic foot clinic for a chronic pruritic lesion of his left foot.

On examination, he had severe diabetic neuropathy, and his peripheral pulses were palpable. A hyperkeratotic lesion with dense yellowish scales over a red skin patch was seen at the plantaro-lateral aspect of his left foot (Figure 5.25). The scales were firmly adherent to the epidermis and not easily debrided. In addition, dry skin was present at the heel. The patient was referred to the dermatology department for treatment.

This situation occurs on the palms and soles, almost exclusively in men. It may result from irritation or allergy, although the cause is usually unknown. Topical moisturizers with lactic acid or urea are applied after 20 minutes' soaking in water. Topical coal tar preparations may be applied daily under occlusion if severe lichenification is present. Oral antihistamines low-dose corticosteroids may be of some help for short periods.

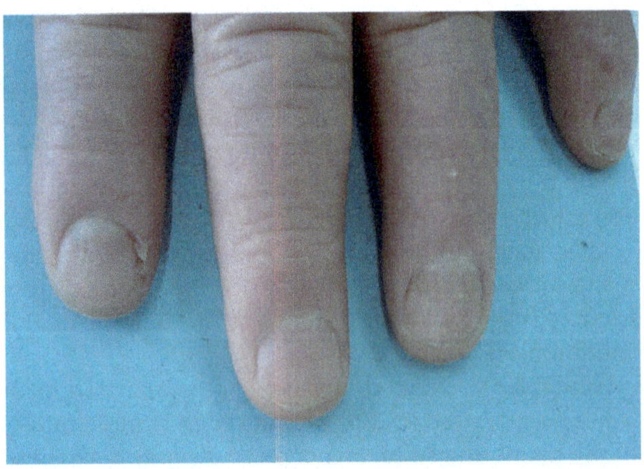

Figure 5.24 Fingernail involvement in psoriasis in a patient with both type 2 diabetes mellitus and psoriasis. On the fourth finger, punctuate pitting and brownish discoloration predominate.

5.7 Squamous Cell Carcinoma

A squamous cell carcinoma (SCC) developed on the neglected burn scar of a 48-year-old male patient with diabetes (Figure 5.26). SCC is the second most common skin cancer after basal cell carcinoma. It arises from the dermis and is most common in areas exposed to the sun. It is an aggressive and invasive cancer; it may penetrate underlying tissues, and it gives rise to metastases in distant tissues, lymph nodes and organs. (Figure 5.27 shows another patient before surgery and Figure 5.28 a further patient after fifth ray amputation.)

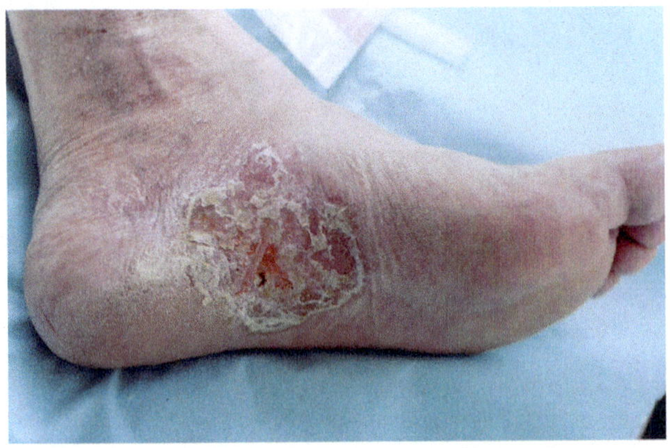

Figure 5.25 Hyperkeratotic eczema: a hyperkeratotic lesion with dense yellowish scales over a red skin patch. The scales are firmly adherent to the epidermis and cannot easily be debrided with a blade. There is dry skin on the heel.

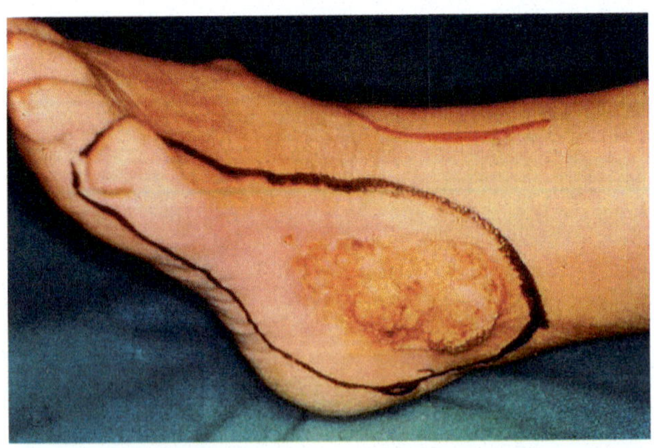

Figure 5.26 Squamous cell carcinoma presented as an ulcer on the lateral aspect of the foot of a diabetic patient. The design of the excision and the recipient vessels are depicted. *Source:* Courtesy of O. Papadopoulos.

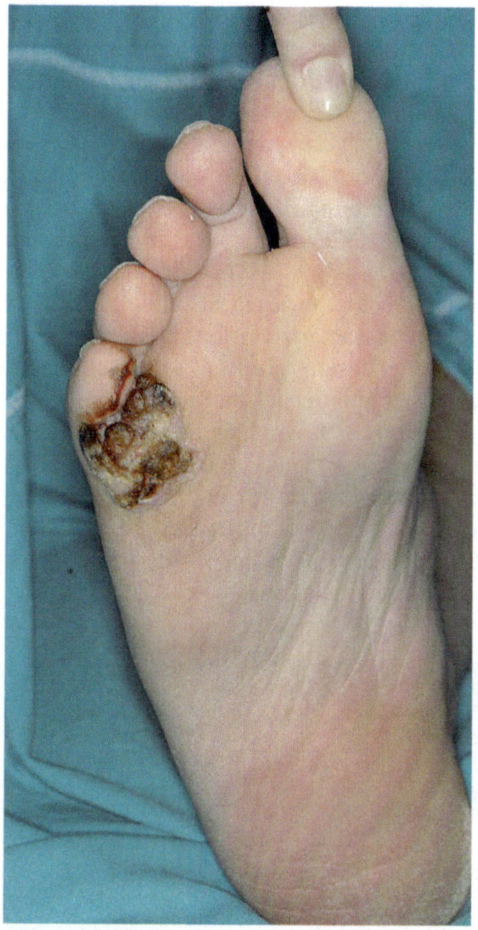

Figure 5.27 Squamous cell carcinoma presenting as an ulcer over the fifth metatarsal head. Notice the irregular borders and the absence of callus. *Source:* Courtesy of O. Papadopoulos.

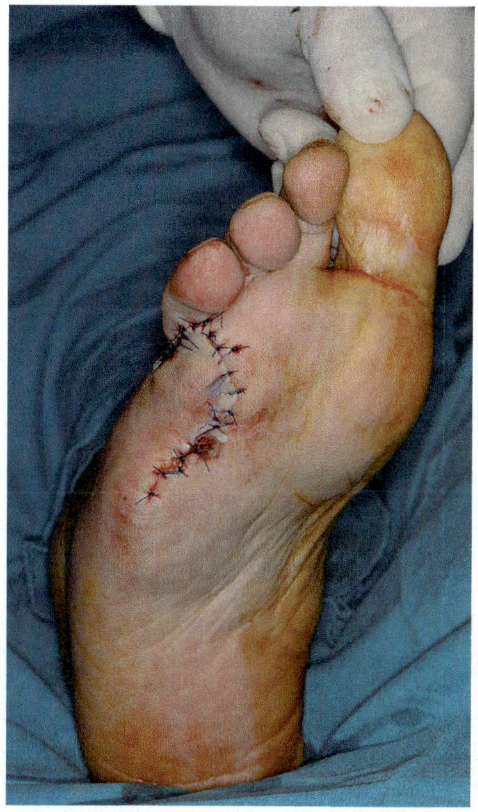

Figure 5.28 The result after a fifth ray amputation in the patient shown in Figure 5.24. *Source:* Courtesy of O. Papadopoulos.

Presentations vary, so the neoplasm is difficult to diagnose. Pink, red or tan plaques, ulcers or erosions and scaling can be seen. Secondary SCC arises in areas of old scars, especially burn scars, chronic non-healing wounds and radiation lesions (Marjolin's ulcers). SCC should be included in the differential diagnosis when lesions with atypical characteristics are seen on the feet.

5.8 Dermatofibrosarcoma Protuberans

Recurrent dermatofibrosarcoma protuberans (DFSP) occurred in a 71-year-old male diabetic patient. DFSP is an uncommon aggressive soft tissue sarcoma of low malignant potential, arising in the dermis of young to middle-aged adults, and it is slightly more frequent in men than women (57% versus 43%). It is most commonly located on the trunk and proximal extremities. Initially, it presents as asymptomatic bluish, red or flesh-colored nodules on top of plaque-like lesions, of a few millimeters to more than 20cm in size, or as a superficial ulceration of some of these nodules. It infiltrates the surrounding tissues and, if untreated, may ulcerate (Figure 5.29). It may recur after surgical excision and give rise to metastases.

5.9 Malignant Fibrous Histiocytoma

A 54-year-old diabetic patient presented with a large, rapidly increasing painless tumor with superficial ulceration and redness at the ankle (Figure 5.30). He complained of fever and malaise. A malignant fibrous histiocytoma (MFH) was diagnosed by histologic examination of the tumor.

MFH (fibrous histiocytoma, multinucleate cell angiohistocytoma) is the most common soft tissue sarcoma of late adult life, accounting for 20–24% of soft tissue sarcomas. The tumor occurs with a peak incidence in the fifth and sixth decades, but an age range of 10–90 years has been reported. MFH most commonly occurs in the extremities (70–75%, with the lower extremities accounting for 59%

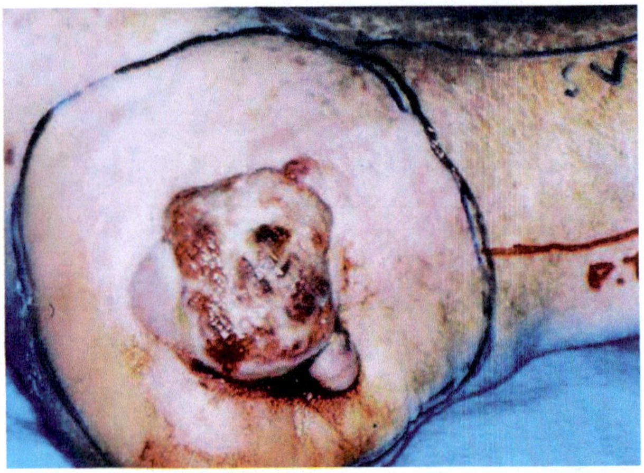

Figure 5.29 Ulceration in recurrent dermatofibrosarcoma protuberans of the heel of a diabetic patient. The design of the excision and the recipient vessels are depicted. *Source:* Courtesy of O. Papadopoulos.

of cases), followed by the retroperitoneum. Tumors typically arise in deep fascia or skeletal muscle. The tumor presents as enlarging painless soft tissue mass with ulceration, typically 5–10cm in diameter; fever, malaise and weight loss are common. The differential diagnosis includes other soft tissue sarcomas, such as liposarcoma and synovial sarcoma.

5.10 Malignant Melanoma

A 75-year-old patient with type 2 diabetes attended the clinic because of a chronic non-healing ulcer on his left midfoot. On examination, a superficial ulcer with irregular borders, pigmented lesions with hues of a tan to brown appearance and satellite pigmented lesions on the left midfoot were seen (Figure 5.31). Callus formation, hallux valgus and a claw toe deformity were also present.

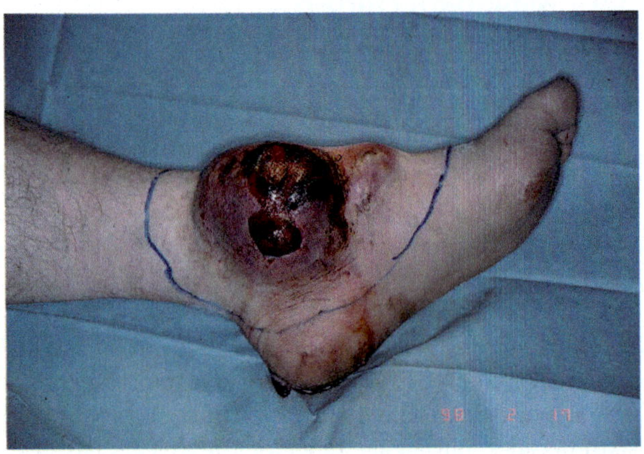

Figure 5.30 Malignant fibrous histiocytoma at the ankle. *Source:* Courtesy of O. Papadopoulos.

The patient underwent surgical removal of the lesion followed by plastic surgical reconstruction (Figure 5.32). The histology was diagnostic of malignant melanoma.

Malignant melanoma is common, with an increasing incidence worldwide. It is commonly noted in sun-exposed areas, but can be found in non-exposed areas such as the soles. A subungual location for a melanoma is not rare (Figure 5.33, showing another patient with Hutchinson's sign – see below). Asymmetry of the lesions, irregular borders, color variegation, and a diameter greater than 6 mm characterize melanomas. In the early stages, flat pigmented lesions are seen in the skin. As the melanoma infiltrates the deeper dermis, the previously flat melanoma becomes elevated, and a papule, nodule, or plaque may arise. Later clinical manifestations include ulceration, epidermal breakdown and/or the development of large fungating cutaneous masses.

The periungual extension of brown-black pigmentation from longitudinal melanonychia onto the proximal

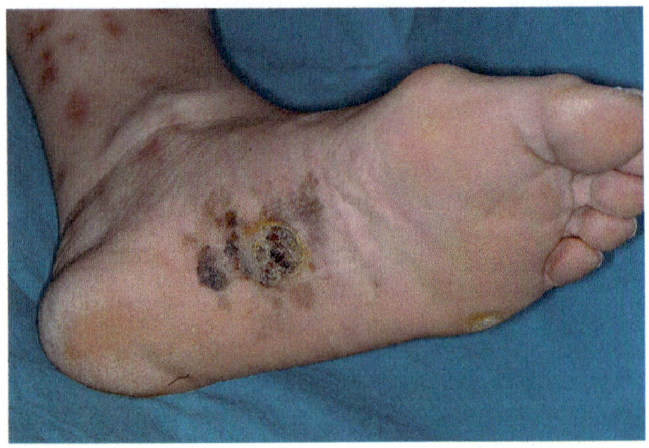

Figure 5.31 Malignant melanoma. *Source:* Courtesy of O. Papadopoulos.

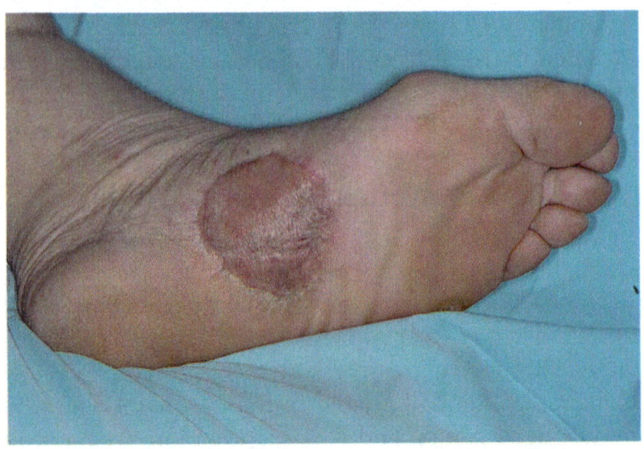

Figure 5.32 The result after removal of the melanoma and reconstructive surgery in the patient shown in Figure 5.28. *Source:* Courtesy of O. Papadopoulos.

and lateral nail folds is called Hutchinson's sign. It is an important indicator but not a diagnostic sign of subungual melanoma, and the ultimate diagnosis must be histologic.

5.11 Necrotizing Vasculitis

Systemic vasculitis may manifest with scattered, discrete, purpuric eruptions on the extremities. A 67-year-old diabetic woman was admitted to the internal medicine ward because of a relapse of polyarteritis nodosa with black necrotic lesions on her lower legs, feet and hands, with kidney and gastrointestinal tract involvement. She had a history two years previously of amputation of four toes (great, third, fourth, and fifth toes) from her left foot due to necrotizing lesions from vasculitis. On examination, large necrotic painless lesions were seen on her feet (Figure 5.34), lower legs (Figures 5.35) and hands (Figure 5.36). Bilateral edema and redness up to the knee joint was also noted. A biopsy from her hand revealed large- and small-vessel cutaneous vasculitis.

Large-vessel vasculitis involves the arterioles and arteries, whereas small-vessel vasculitis involves the postcapillary venules. Cutaneous small-vessel vasculitis often manifests with urticaria-like lesions or palpable purpura on the legs or over dependent areas. Large-vessel vasculitis manifests as ulceration and necrosis of the skin, livedo reticularis, purpura, Raynaud's phenomenon and small nail fold infarcts. The types of large-vessel vasculitis include classic polyarteritis nodosa, Wegener granulomatosis, allergic granulomatous angiitis (Churg–Strauss disease) and giant cell arteritis; with the exception of the last, all have similar cutaneous manifestations Figures 5.35 and 5.36.

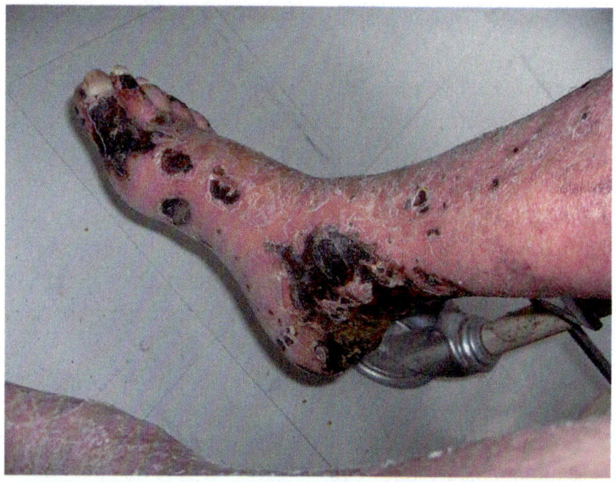

Figure 5.34 Necrotizing vasculitis affecting the feet of a diabetic patient with polyarteritis nodosa.

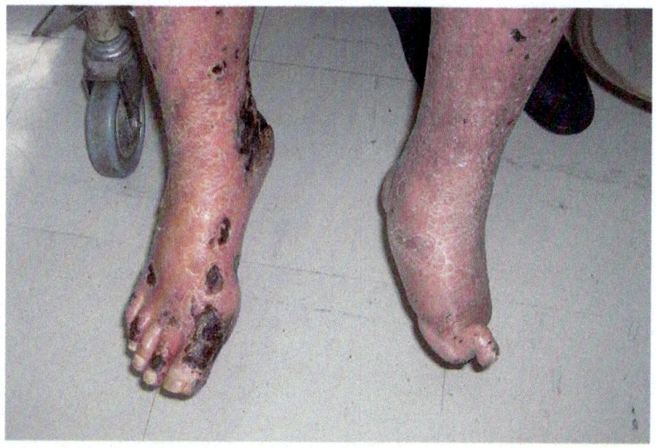

Figure 5.35 Necrotizing vasculitis affecting the lower legs and feet of the patient from Figure 5.31.

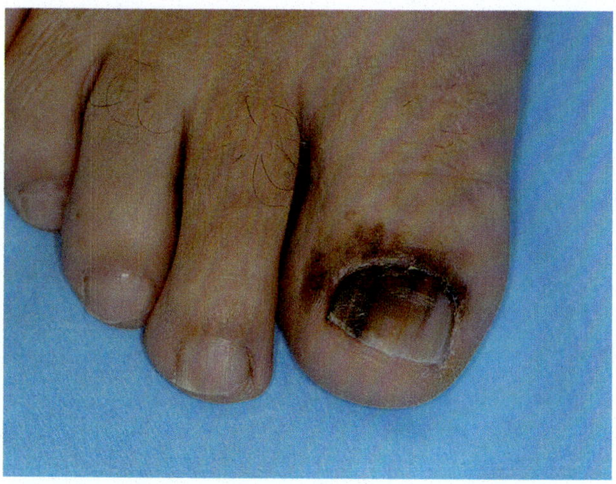

Figure 5.33 Subungual malignant melanoma with Hutchinson's sign. *Source:* Courtesy of O. Papadopoulos.

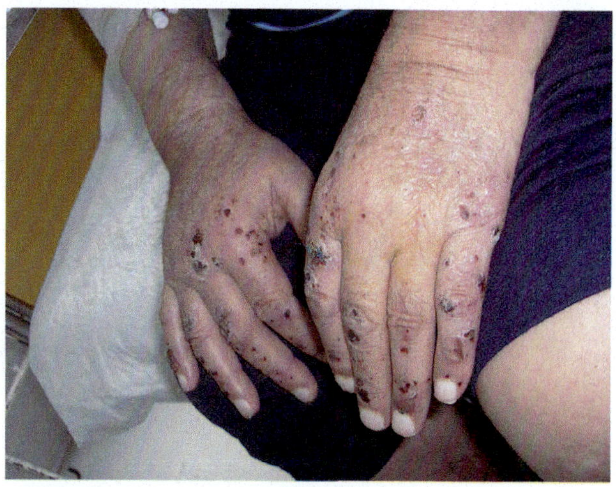

Figure 5.36 Necrotizing vasculitis on the hands of the patient from Figure 5.31.

Further Reading

Basoulis, D., Fragiadaki, K., Tentolouris, N. et al. Anti-TNF-α treatment for recalcitrant ulcerative necrobiosis lipoidica diabeticorum: a case report and review of the literature. *Metabolism* 65: 569–573.

Bikowski, J.B. (1999). Psoriatic nail disease: diagnosis and treatment options. *Cutis* 64: 1–9.

Boulton, A.J.M., Cutfield, R.G., Abouganem, D. et al. (1988). Necrobiosis lipoidica diabeticorum: a clinicopathologic study. *J. Am. Acad. Dermatol.* 18: 530–537.

Frediani, B., Filippou, G., Falsetti, P. et al. (2005). Diagnosis of calcium pyrophosphate dihydrate crystal deposition disease: ultrasonographic criteria proposed. *Ann. Rheum. Dis.* 64: 638–640.

Friedman, R., Rigel, D., and Kopf, A. (1985). Early detection of malignant melanoma: the role of physician examination and self-examination of the skin. *CA Cancer J. Clin.* 35: 130–151.

Gibbs, S., Harvey, I., Sterling, J.C., and Stark, R. (2003). Local treatments for cutaneous warts. *Cochrane Database Syst. Rev.* 3: CD001781.

Kouskoukis, C.E., Scher, R.K., and Ackerman, A.B. (1983). The "oil drop" sign of psoriatic nails. A clinical finding specific for psoriasis. *Am. J. Dermatopathol.* 5: 259–262.

Meurer, M. and Szeimies, R.M. (1991). Diabetes mellitus and skin diseases. *Curr. Probl. Dermatol.* 20: 11–23.

Miller, A. and Mihm, M. (2006). Melanoma. *N. Engl. J. Med.* 355: 51–65.

Norman, A. (2001). Dermal manifestations of diabetes. In: *Geriatric Dermatology* (ed. R. Norman), 143–154. New York: Parthenon.

Rose, J.H. and Belsky, M.R. (1989). Psoriatic arthritis in the hand. *Hand Clin.* 5: 137–144.

Shemer, A., Bergman, R., Linn, S. et al. (1998). Diabetic dermopathy and internal complications in diabetes mellitus. *Int. J. Dermatol.* 37: 113–115.

Sibbald, G.R., Landolt, S.J., and Toth, D. (1996). Skin and diabetes. *Endocrinol. Metab. Clin. N. Am.* 25: 463–472.

Towheed, T.E. and Hochberg, M.C. (1996). Acute monoarthritis: a practical approach to assessment and treatment. *Am. Fam. Physician* 54: 2239–2243.

Weyand, C.M. and Goronzy, J.J. (2003). Medium- and large-vessel vasculitis. *N. Engl. J. Med.* 349: 160–169.

6

Neuropathic Ulcers

A. Kokkinos and K. Makrilakis

First Department of Propaedeutic Internal Medicine, National and Kapodistrian University of Athens, Medical School, Laiko General Hospital, Athens, Greece

Impaired pain sensation, propensity toward hyperkeratosis and callus formation due to sudomotor dysfunction, and the occurrence of areas of increased plantar pressure due to motor neuropathy, as in the case of claw toes, all serve to increase the risk for neuropathic ulcer formation. The most common sites of foot ulcerations due to neuropathy are areas of increased pressure, such as over prominent metatarsal heads or on the toes, interdigital surfaces, heels or bony prominences over various foot deformities. Proper debridement, offloading, and treatment of infection are of paramount importance in the treatment of neuropathic ulcers.

6.1 Over a Callus in Various Sites of the Foot

Case 6.1

A 43-year-old woman with type 1 diabetes presented with a callus under the head of the right first metatarsal, together with prominent metatarsal heads (Figure 6.1). She complained of numbness of the lower extremities, and on physical examination had decreased pinprick, temperature and monofilament sensation. Debridement of the hyperkeratosis was performed on a bi-weekly to monthly basis, and appropriate footwear was advised. Three months later, a small ulcer developed at the site of the callus (Figure 6.2), which greatly improved over the following seven months (Figure 6.3).

Case 6.2

A 48-year-old man with history of type 2 diabetes and severe peripheral neuropathy presented with a large hemorrhagic callus over the head of his first metatarsal (Figure 6.4). Debridement was performed (Figure 6.5), and the patient was advised about appropriate off-loading of the foot by a change in his shoes. Ten weeks later, he returned with continued thick hyperkeratosis (Figure 6.6), debridement of which now revealed an ulcer (Figure 6.7).

Case 6.3

A 74-year-old female with type 2 diabetes was referred to the outpatient diabetic foot clinic because of callus formation on her sole. She was under treatment with insulin and had a history of hypertension and ischemic heart disease.

On examination she was found to have severe peripheral neuropathy and normal peripheral pulses. In addition, significant muscle atrophy of her feet, claw toes and a hemorrhagic callus on the fourth metatarsal head of her right foot were found (Figure 6.8). An impressive finding was the palpation of her metatarsal heads just below the skin, as the fat pads had been displaced anteriorly. After callus removal a superficial ulcer was revealed (Figure 6.9). The patient was advised to rest. Extra depth shoes and orthotic insoles were prescribed in order to accommodate her deformed toes and relieve the load under the

Atlas of the Diabetic Foot, Third Edition. Ioanna Eleftheriadou, Alexandros Kokkinos, Stavros Liatis, Konstantinos Makrilakis, Nicholas Tentolouris, Anastasios Tentolouris, and Panagiotis Tsapogas.

Companion website: www.wiley.com/go/tentolouris/atlas_diabetic_foot

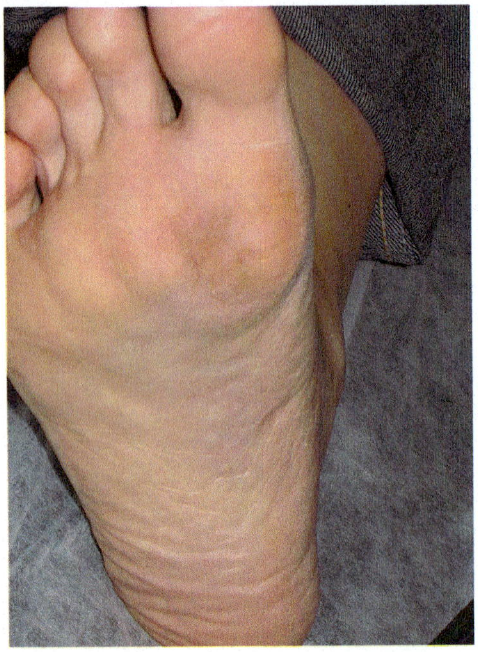

Figure 6.1 A callus over the head of the right first metatarsal, together with prominent metatarsal heads.

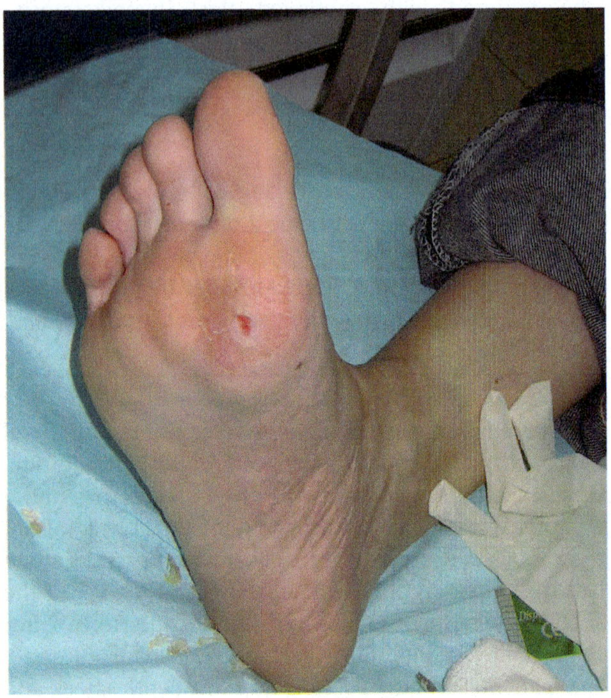

Figure 6.2 A small ulcer developed at the site of the callus, three months after picture in Figure 6.1 was taken.

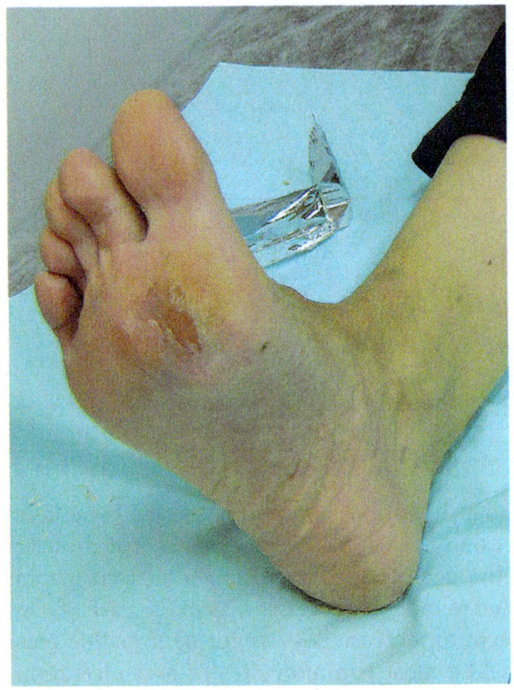

Figure 6.3 Healing of the ulcer shown in Figure 6.2 over the next seven months. Note some remaining hyperkeratosis around the area of the healed ulcer.

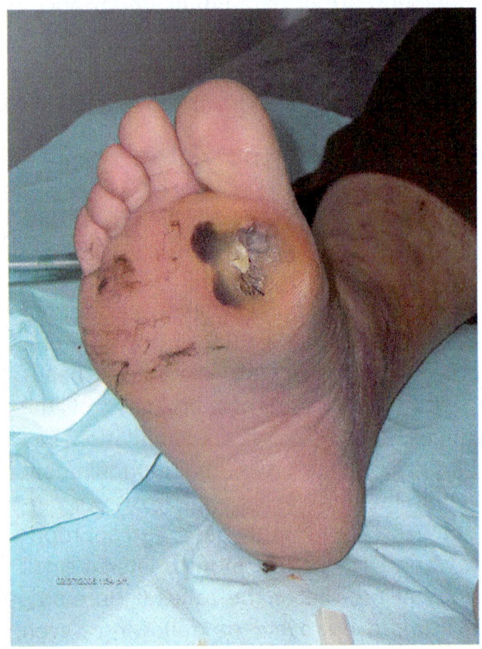

Figure 6.4 A large hemorrhagic callus over the head of the first metatarsal on a patient with prominent metatarsal heads.

metatarsal heads. Post-debridement in-shoe pressures when she used her own shoes showed a significant load under her metatarsal heads (Figure 6.10 Panel A). The maximum pressure in this area was 282 kPa; however, after insertion of an orthotic insole the maximum in-shoe pressure was reduced to 155 kPa (Figure 6.10 Panel B). The ulcer healed in eight weeks.

Reduced thickness of the fat pad is associated with high plantar pressures. Although some authors have

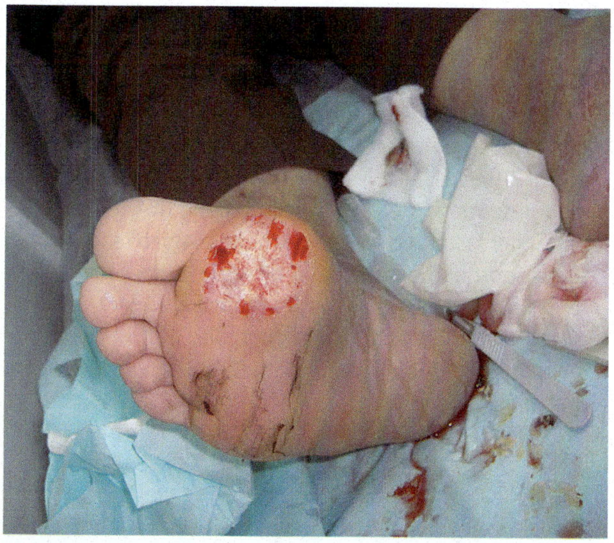

Figure 6.5 Debridement of the callus shown in Figure 6.4.

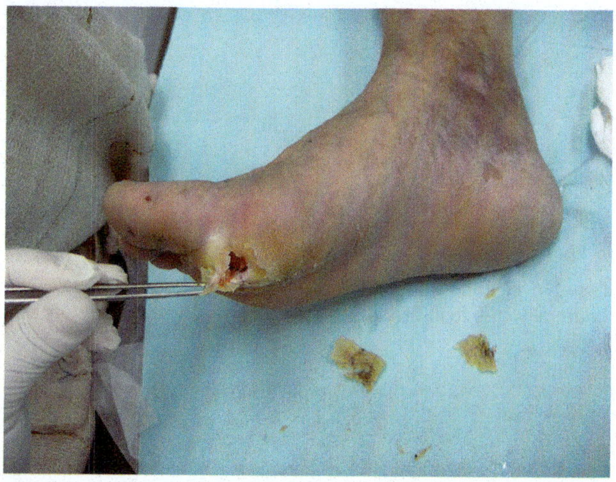

Figure 6.6 Debridement of the thick hyperkeratosis in Figure 6.5 revealed an ulcer underneath.

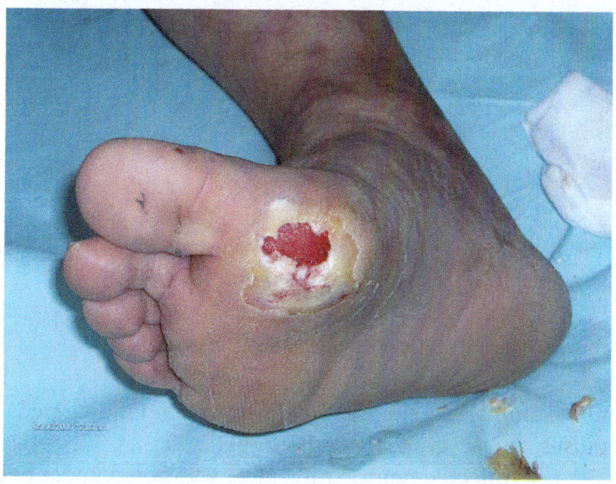

Figure 6.7 The ulcer over the head of the first metatarsal shown in Figure 6.6 after final debridement of the thick hyperkeratosis.

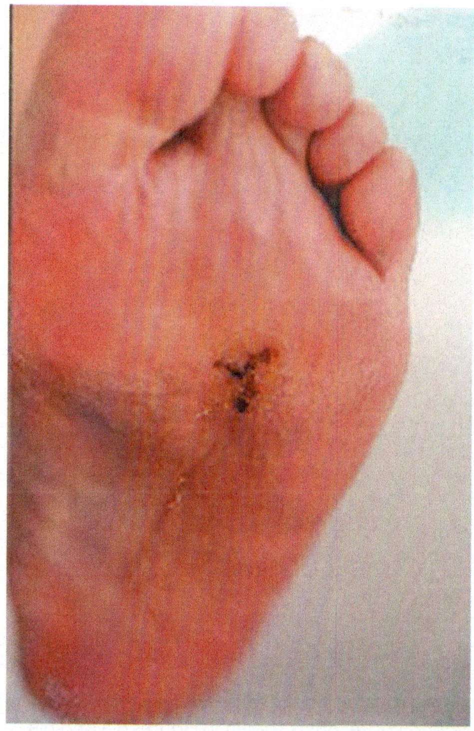

Figure 6.8 Hemorrhagic callus under the fourth metatarsal head. Claw toes and prominent metatarsal heads are also present.

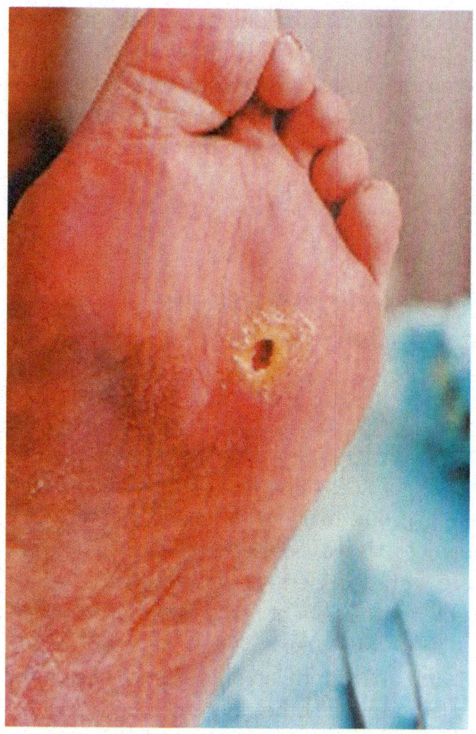

Figure 6.9 A neuropathic ulcer in the same patient whose foot is shown in Figure 6.8.

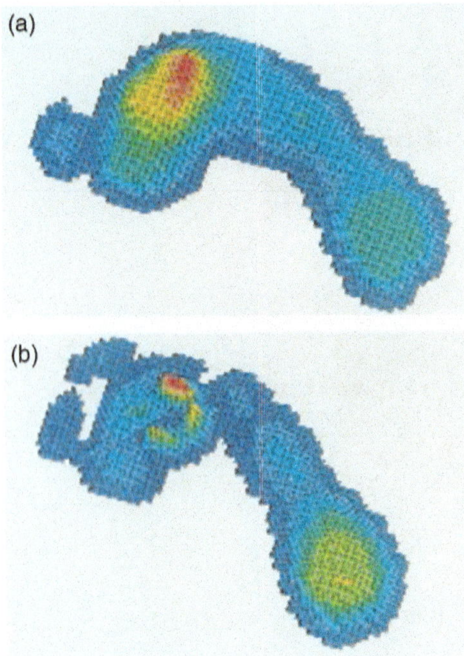

Figure 6.10 Plantar pressures before (a) and after (b) orthotic insoles in the patient whose foot is shown in Figures 6.8 and 6.9.

suggested that threshold pressures of 500–1000 kPa may lead to the development of foot ulceration when walking barefoot, it seems that each patient has an individual threshold. In the present case the maximum pressure was obviously below this threshold. However, high plantar pressures alone do not cause foot ulceration; it is the combination of different risk factors (mentioned in Chapter 1) that is necessary for the development of ulceration.

6.2 Over a Bony Prominence or in Various Foot Deformities

Case 6.4

A 53-year-old man with type 2 diabetes presented with ulcers on the lateral sides of his first metatarsals bilaterally (Figure 6.11), due to ill-fitting shoes pressing on bony prominences. He was advised to change his shoes, and local care with debridement was initiated. Due to financial problems, the patient could not afford special shoes, but he cut the inner sides of his own shoes (Figure 6.12), and one month later his ulcers had significantly improved, especially the right one (Figure 6.13). The left ulcer needed another six months of continued care in order to improve (Figure 6.14).

Case 6.5

This 32-year-old type 1 female diabetic patient, attended the outpatient diabetic foot clinic for chronic neuropathic ulcers of her feet. She had a renal transplant at the age of 30 years, because of end-stage renal failure due to diabetes. Soon after her transplant she noticed a bulla under her last three metatarsal heads, which readily ruptured soon and a superficial ulcer developed. She also reported an ulcer of two years' duration under the third metatarsal head of her right foot. She had never been instructed in foot care and had never worn proper footwear.

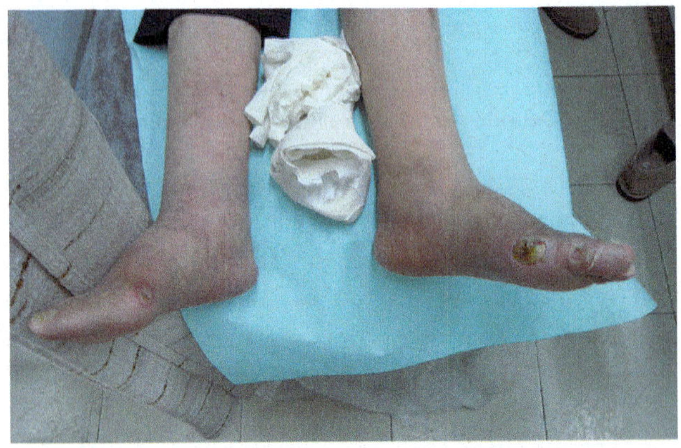

Figure 6.11 Ulcers on the lateral sides of the first metatarsals, bilaterally, due to ill-fitting shoes pressing on bony prominences.

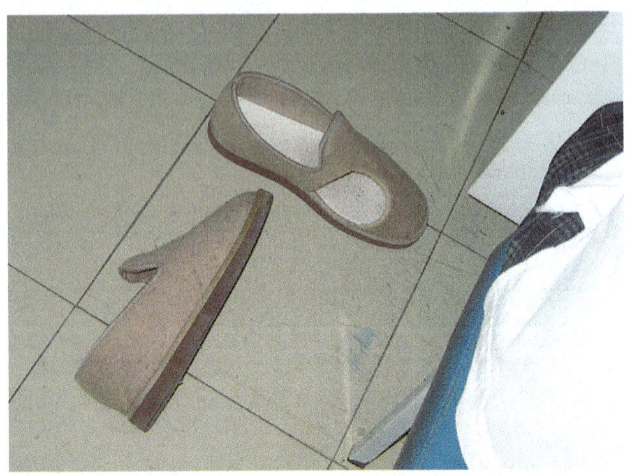

Figure 6.12 The shoes of the patient referred to in Figure 6.11, showing the inner side cut at the site of the ulcer.

On examination, she was found to have bounding pedal pulses, and severe diabetic neuropathy.

A non-infected neuropathic ulcer was noted under her left third, fourth and fifth metatarsal heads. Its dimensions were 3.5 × 4 × 0.4 cm, surrounded by callus. A

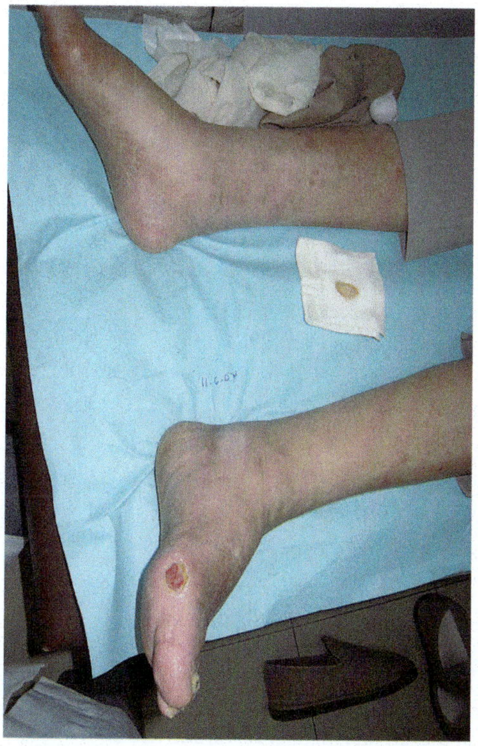

Figure 6.13 Improvement of the ulcers on the lateral sides of the first metatarsals, especially the right one, one month after Figure 6.11 was taken.

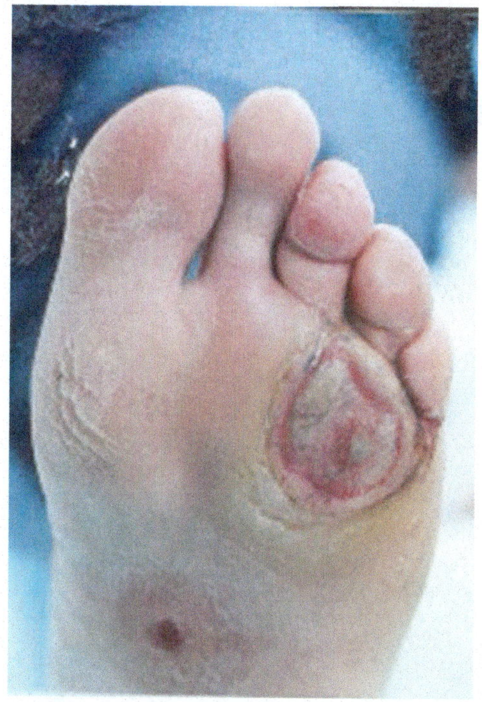

Figure 6.15 Neuropathic ulcers under prominent metatarsal heads, and on the midsole. Claw toes and dry skin are also apparent.

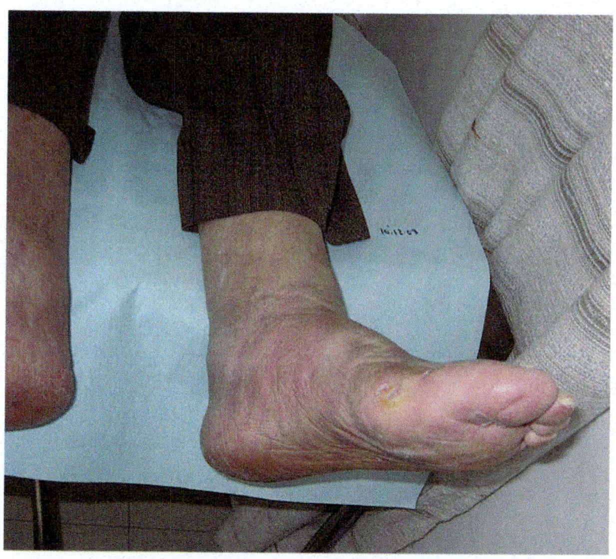

Figure 6.14 Improvement of the ulcer on the lateral side of the left first metatarsal, six months after Figure 6.13 was taken.

smaller neuropathic ulcer was also noticed at the midsole (Figure 6.15). Claw toe deformity of her lesser toes, dry skin and desquamation of the tip of her third toe were also present. Under her right third metatarsal head a neuropathic ulcer was noted in an area of gross callus formation, in addition to claw toe deformity (Figure 6.16).

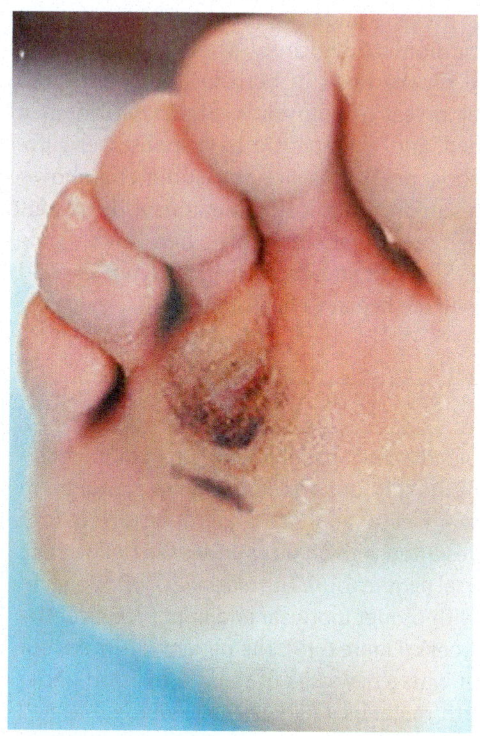

Figure 6.16 Neuropathic ulcer surrounded by callus. Claw toe. Right foot of patient whose left foot is shown in Figure 6.15.

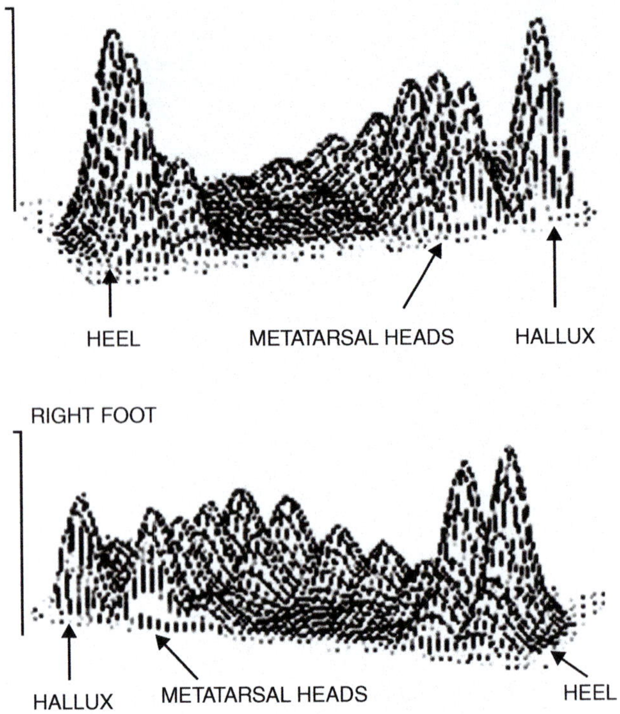

Figure 6.17 Original in-shoe peak plantar pressures at the left (upper panel) and right foot (lower panel) of the patient whose feet are illustrated in Figures 6.15 and 6.16.

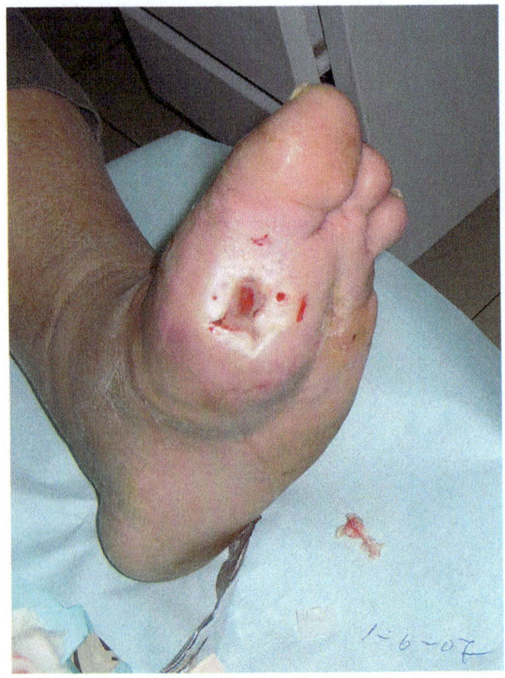

Figure 6.18 A patient with Charcot osteoarthropathy and an ulcer over the head of the left first metatarsal. He also had an amputation of his fifth toe.

A callus was present under her right fifth metatarsal head, over a bunionette deformity. Mild callus formation was observed on the heels of both feet. A plain radiograph did not reveal osteomyelitis. Sharp debridement was performed and therapeutic half shoes were prescribed. In-shoe peak pressure measurement showed high pressures under both heels, metatarsal heads, and halluxes when the patient wore her own shoes (Figure 6.17). She had standard treatment on a weekly basis and the ulcers began to heal slowly.

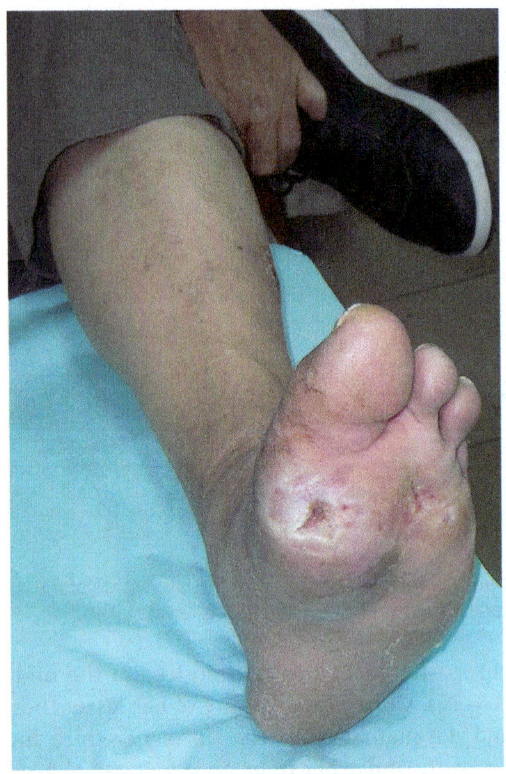

Figure 6.19 The patient in Figure 6.18, three weeks later. Note the improved ulcer over the head of the first metatarsal.

Case 6.6

A 52-year-old diabetic patient with Charcot osteoarthropathy of the left foot and left fifth toe amputation due to osteomyelitis and subsequent distorted foot anatomy, presented with an ulcer under the head of the first metatarsal (Figure 6.18). The ulcer was debrided and off-loaded with proper footwear and improved over the next three weeks (Figure 6.19). The patient returned four months later with a new area of callus formation under the left fourth metatarsal (Figure 6.20), which revealed an ulcer after debridement of the hyperkeratosis (Figure 6.21).

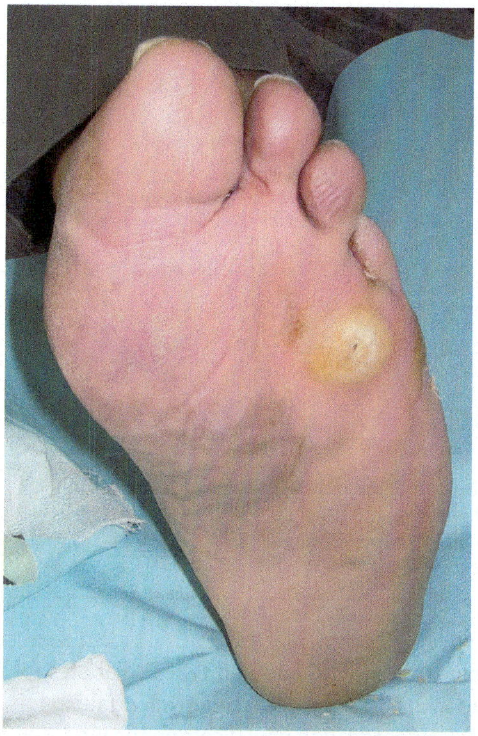

Figure 6.20 The patient from Figure 6.18, four months later. Notice that the ulcer over the left first metatarsal has completely healed, but the patient now has a new area of hyperkeratosis over the head of the fourth metatarsal.

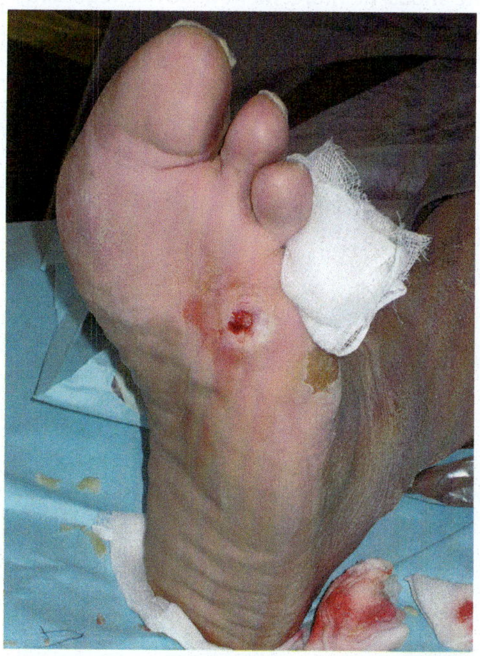

Figure 6.21 The patient from Figure 6.20, revealing an ulcer under the callus of the fourth metatarsal head after debridement.

6.3 On a Toe (Tips, or Dorsum of Phalanges)

Case 6.7

A 40-year-old woman who had had a history of type 1 diabetes since the age of 13 and a history of osteomyelitis of the first phalanx of the right big toe four years previously (Figure 6.22) presented to the diabetic foot clinic with a complaint of glycemic deterioration over the previous few days. She had a chronic callus over the head of her left fifth metatarsal (Figure 6.23), which was being treated with weekly debridement.

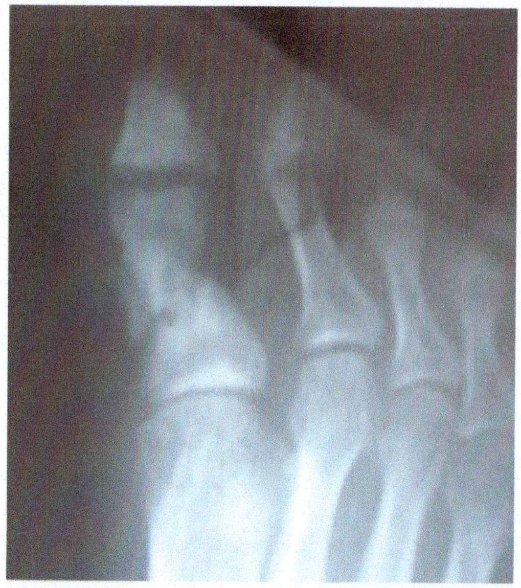

Figure 6.22 An X-ray of the right big toe showing excessive destruction of the first phalanx of the big toe, consistent with osteomyelitis.

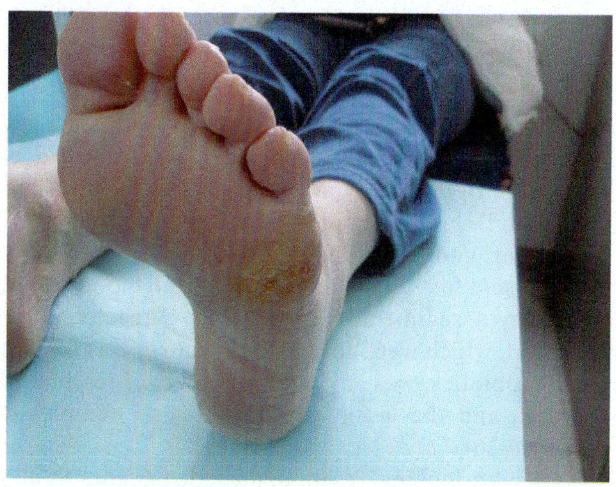

Figure 6.23 Hyperkeratotic callus over the left fifth metatarsal head of the patient shown in Figure 6.22.

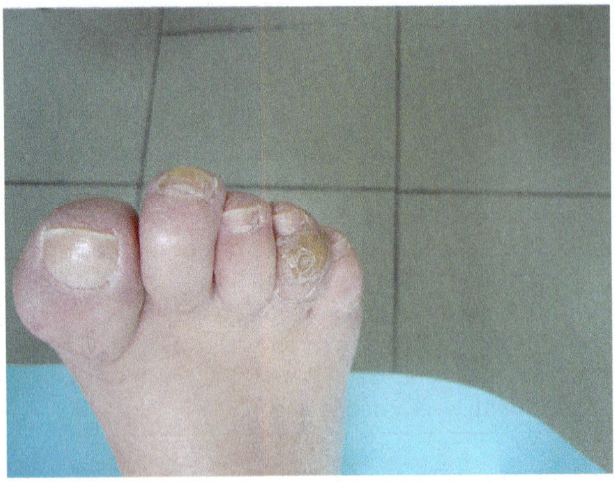

Figure 6.24 A non-inflamed callus on the dorsum of the right fourth toe in the patient from Figure 6.22. Note the claw toe deformity of the toes, especially the second toe.

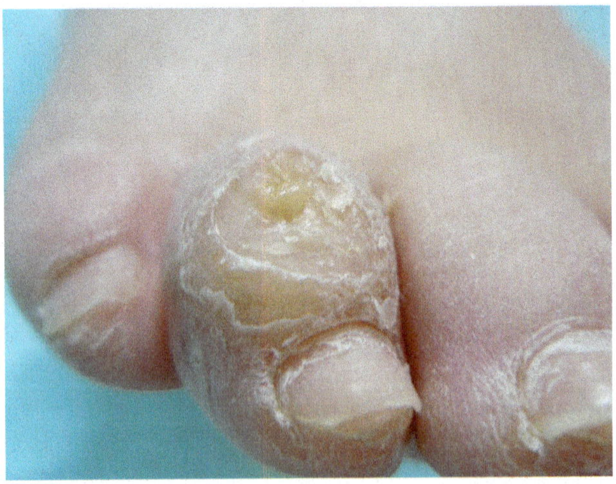

Figure 6.25 Debridement of the hyperkeratotic callus shown in Figure 6.24 revealed the presence of pus on the dorsum of the right fourth toe.

She reported that she had injured her right leg a few days previously and had developed a callus on the dorsum of her right fourth toe (Figure 6.24), which was not inflamed. Debridement of the callus revealed the presence of pus under the skin hyperkeratosis (Figure 6.25). Pus was sent for culture, and blood for full blood count, erythrocyte sedimentation rate and C-reactive protein level, which were normal. The woman was treated with antibiotics, was advised on proper off-loading of the area and the lesion gradually healed completely (Figure 6.26).

A "benign-looking" lesion in diabetic patients should always raise suspicion of an underlying infection, especially in the presence of glycemic deterioration, as in this case.

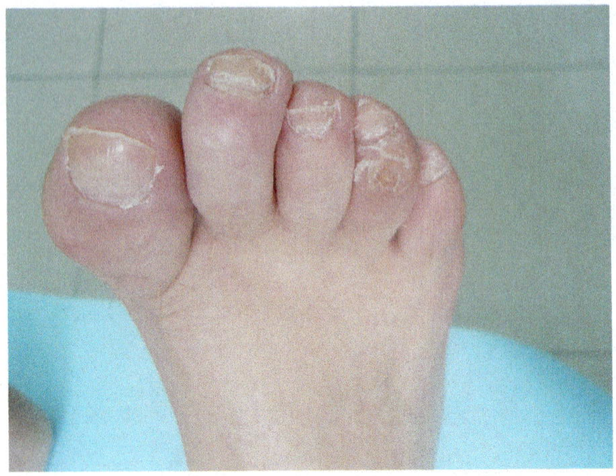

Figure 6.26 The foot of the patient shown in Figure 6.25, one month later. The abscess on the fourth toe has completely healed, with some remaining hyperkeratosis.

Case 6.8

A 62-year-old woman who had had type 2 diabetes for 22 years, and who had a chronic ulcer on her right big toe (Figure 6.27), presented with new ulcers on the inner surfaces of her second toes (between the first and second toes) bilaterally (Figure 6.28) due to ill-fitting shoes. The ulcers showed no signs of inflammation and were debrided (Figure 6.29); in addition, the patient was advised to change her shoes. On follow-up five weeks later, the ulcers had nearly healed (Figure 6.30), but they recurred four months later (Figure 6.31), again due to inappropriate shoes. Reinforcement of advice regarding proper shoes and continued local care led to a marked improvement four months later (Figure 6.32).

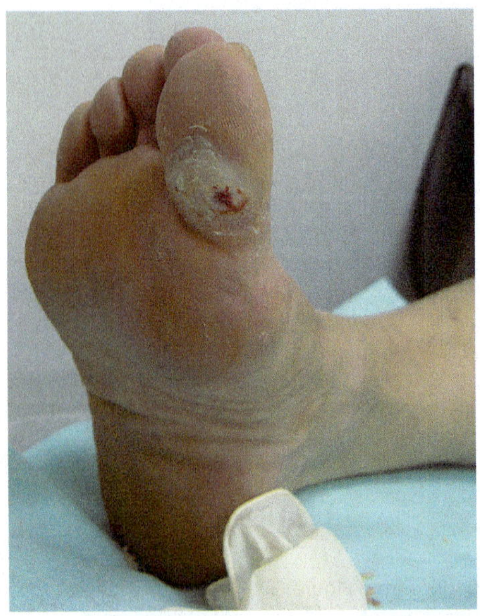

Figure 6.27 Hyperkeratosis at the base of the right big toe.

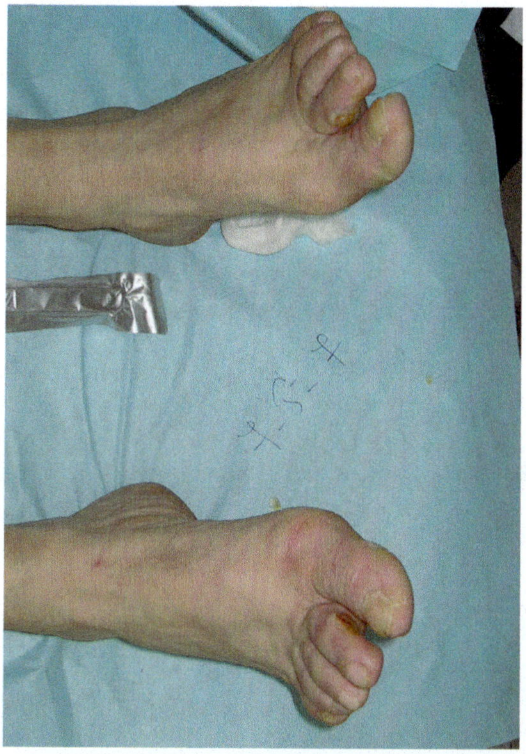

Figure 6.28 Ulcers on the inner surfaces of the second toes bilaterally (between the first and second toes) in the patient shown in Figure 6.27.

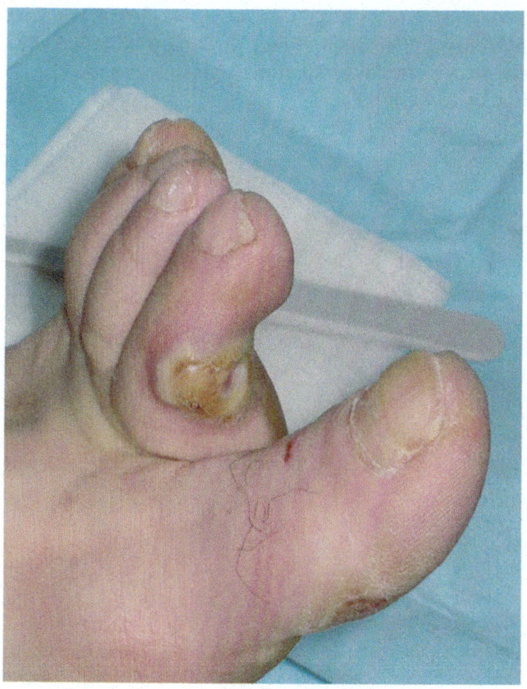

Figure 6.29 An ulcer on the inner surface of the left second toe, without signs of inflammation (the same patient as in Figure 6.27).

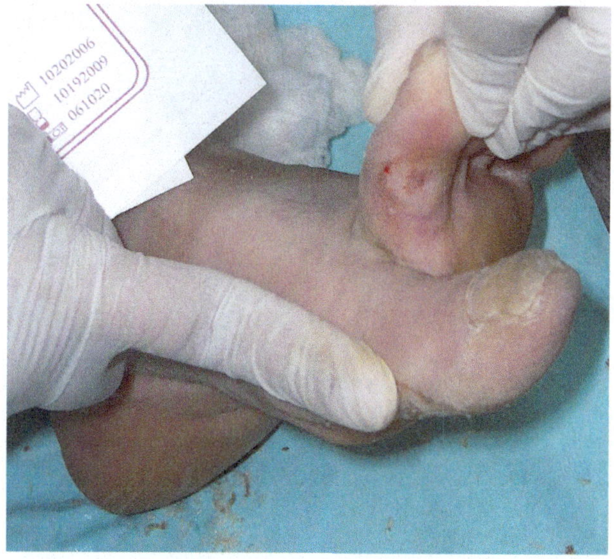

Figure 6.30 A nearly healed ulcer on the inner surface of the left second toe shown in Figure 6.29, five weeks later.

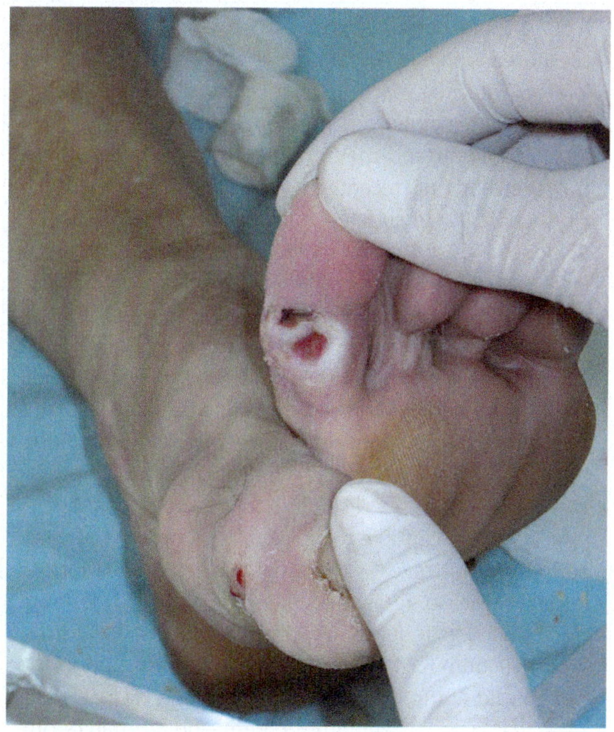

Figure 6.31 Recurrence of the ulcer on the inner surface of the left second toe, four months after the picture in Figure 6.30. Note also a small new ulcer on the outer surface of the first toe, caused by inappropriate shoes.

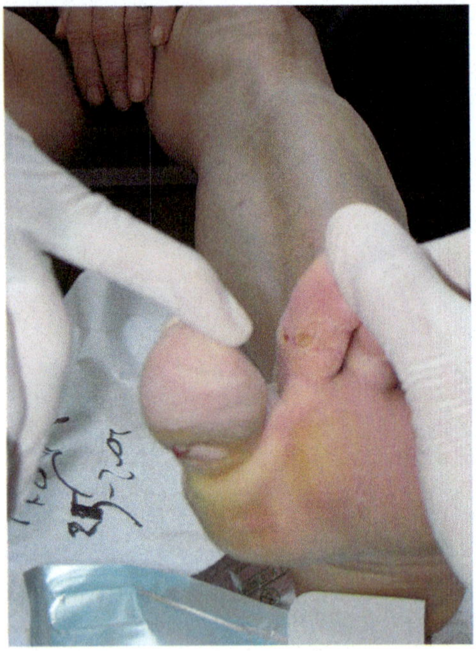

Figure 6.32 A marked improvement of the ulcer shown in Figure 6.31, four months later.

6.4 Over a Metatarsal Head

Case 6.9

A 60-year-old man with type 2 diabetes for the last 16 years presented with a hyperkeratotic lesion he had had on his left foot for three years, which recently had developed an intermittent, malodorous, purulent discharge. He was taking vildagliptin and metformin for his diabetes, which, however, had only recently been properly controlled (last HbA1c: 6.2%). He suffered from diabetic neuropathy, as evidenced by impaired monofilament perception and increased vibration perception threshold bilaterally. He also had bilateral proliferative diabetic retinopathy. After hyperkeratosis removal, a large (1.8cm × 2.2cm), deep (1.4cm) ulcer with a greenish hue on its edges was revealed above the head of the third metatarsal (Figure 6.33). He was given empiric antimicrobial treatment with oral ciprofloxacin and instructions on offloading. Cultures from its discharge yielded a Pseudomonas aeruginosa strain, which was susceptible to ciprofloxacin. An arterial ultrasound did not reveal substantial evidence of peripheral vascular disease. Two weeks later, the area and depth of the lesion were reduced very much, and there was no discharge (Figure 6.34). Twenty days later, even though the patient did not follow offloading instructions closely, the ulcer was even smaller (4mm × 6mm, and 4mm in depth, Figure 6.35), and 40 days after initial presentation it had almost completely healed (Figure 6.36).

Case 6.10

A 43-year-old woman with an 11-year history of type 2 diabetes, severe peripheral neuropathy and a history of osteomyelitis of the left foot presented with an ulcer over the head of her right third metatarsal (Figure 6.37). The ulcer was debrided, and antibiotics were started.

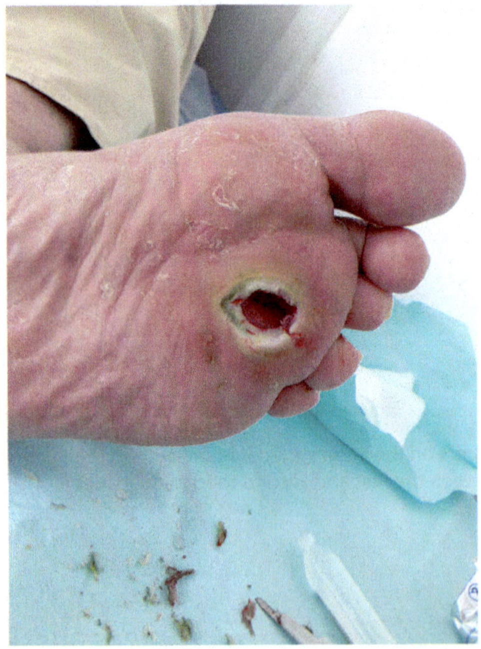

Figure 6.33 A deep, infected ulcer over the head of the third left metatarsal revealed after hyperkeratosis removal. Note the greenish hue on its periphery.

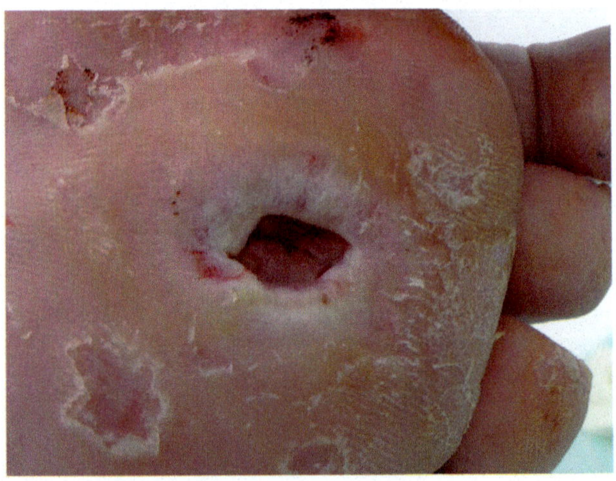

Figure 6.34 Remarkable reduction in the area and depth of the ulcer, with no discharge or further signs of infection.

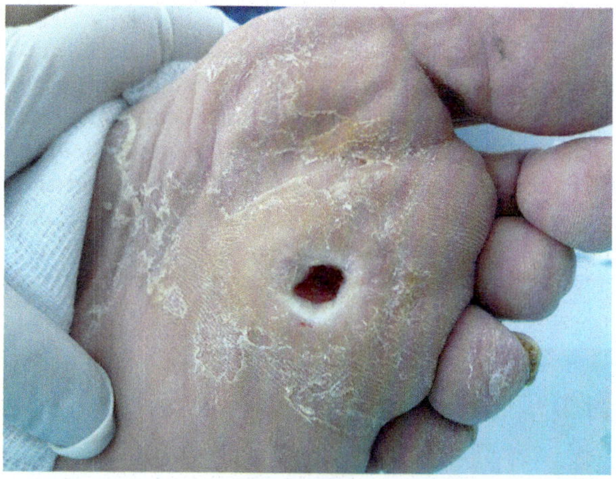

Figure 6.35 Ulcer area even smaller, with a depth of 4 mm.

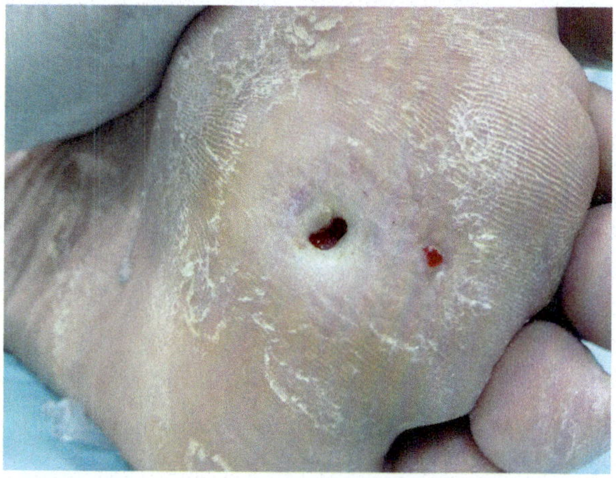

Figure 6.36 Forty days after initial presentation, the ulcer first shown in Figure 6.33 is almost fully healed.

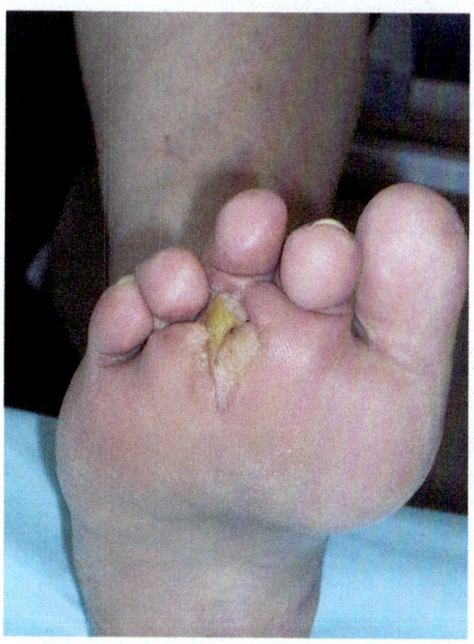

Figure 6.37 An ulcer covered with hyperkeratosis is present over the head of the right third metatarsal. Note the deformity of the third toe.

Two weeks later, she returned with a new lesion on the dorsal aspect of her right second metatarsal head (Figure 6.38), which proved to be a fistula communicating with the previous ulcer on the plantar aspect of the foot (Figure 6.39). She was treated with debridement and antibiotics again, in addition to off-loading, and one month later showed a significant improvement in both lesions (Figures 6.40 and 6.41). She missed her follow-up appointments to the clinic and two years later again presented with a large ulcer under the head of her second metatarsal (Figure 6.42).

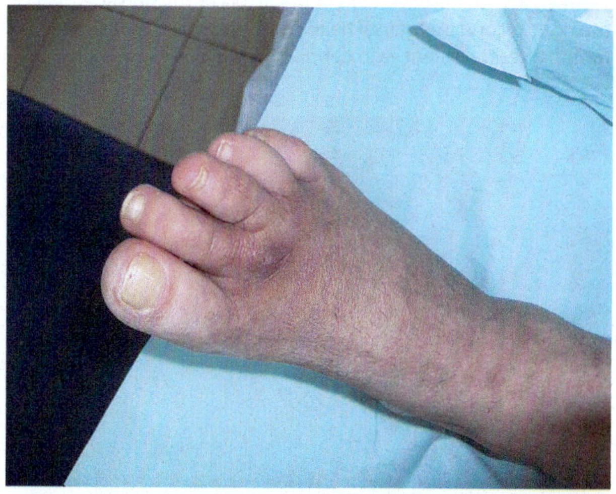

Figure 6.38 A new lesion is present on the dorsal aspect of the right second metatarsal head (the same patient as in Figure 6.37).

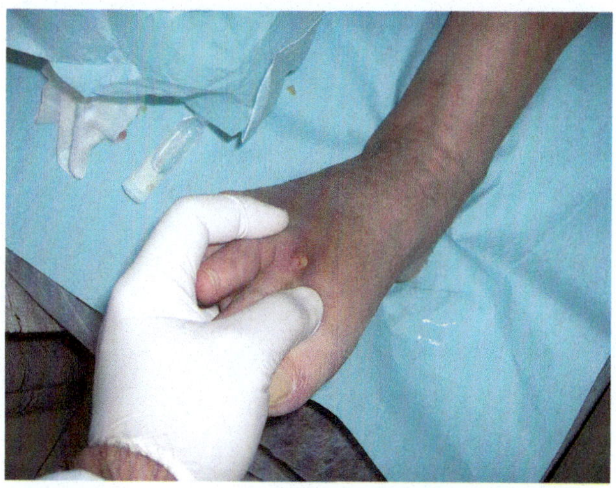

Figure 6.39 Pus is coming out of the lesion over the right second metatarsal head shown in Figure 6.38. This proved to be a fistula communicating with the ulcer on the plantar aspect of the right third metatarsal of the foot (shown in Figure 6.37).

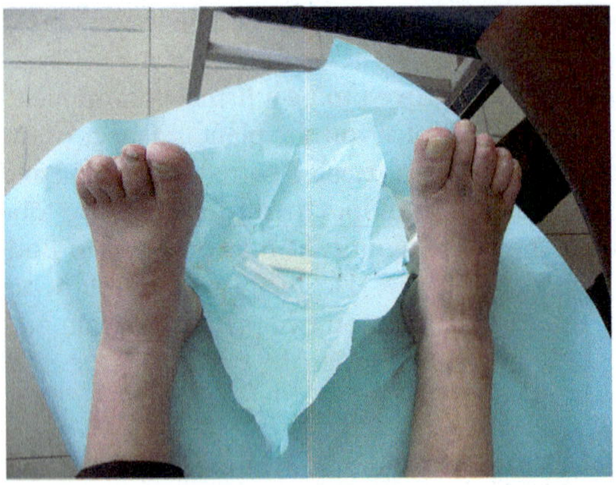

Figure 6.40 An improvement in the fistula of the dorsal aspect of the right second metatarsal head shown in Figure 6.39, one month after treatment with debridement and antibiotics.

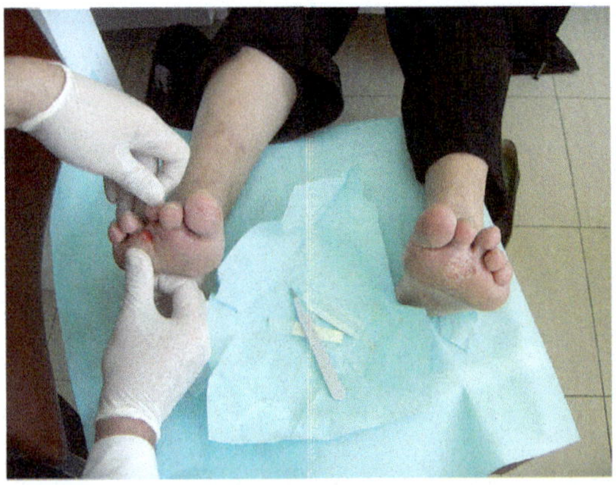

Figure 6.41 An improvement in the ulcer on the plantar aspect of the right third metatarsal shown in Figure 6.37. Note that the hyperkeratoses of the right big toe and the left second metatarsal head have been debrided.

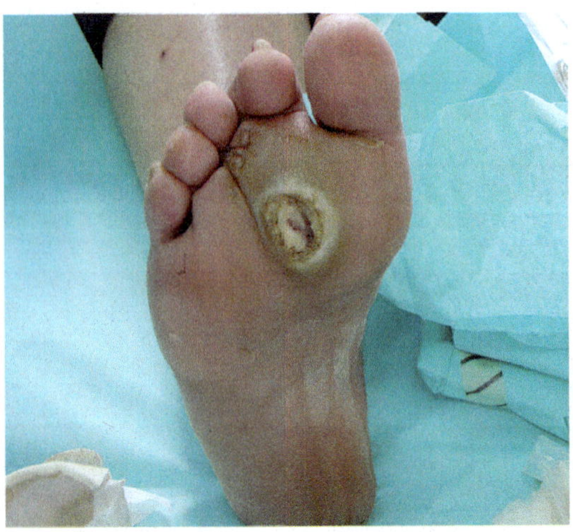

Figure 6.42 A large ulcer has developed over the head of the second metatarsal of the patient shown in the preceding figures, with a thick hyperkeratotic rim, indicating very poor off-loading of the foot. Note the healed old ulcer under the third toe.

Case 6.11

Another patient is shown here with a neuropathic ulcer over the head of his third metatarsal (Figure 6.43), with significant hyperkeratosis around it (Figure 6.44). After three months of repeated sessions of debridement and proper off-loading, the ulcer had undergone significant improvement (Figure 6.45).

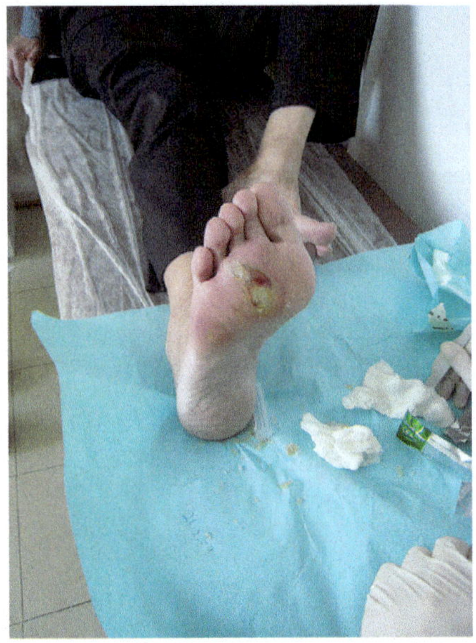

Figure 6.43 A neuropathic ulcer over the head of the third metatarsal. Note the prominent metatarsal heads.

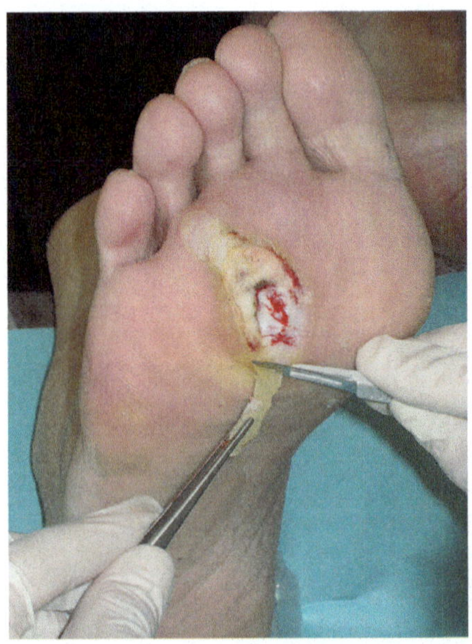

Figure 6.44 Significant hyperkeratosis around the ulcer of the patient in Figure 6.43, which underwent extensive debridement on a weekly basis.

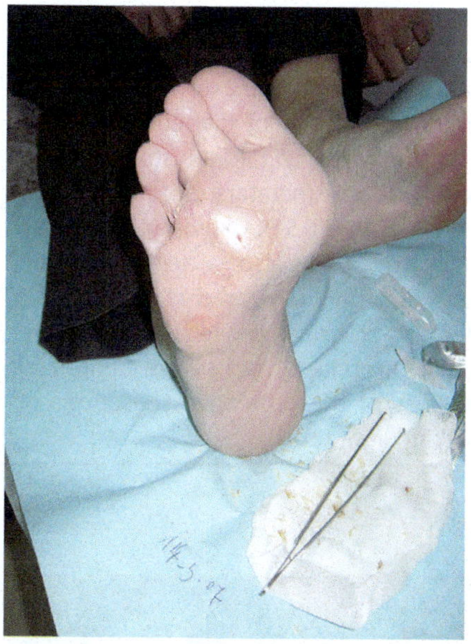

Figure 6.45 The ulcer of the patient in Figure 6.43 had nearly healed three months later.

6.5 Heat Injuries

Case 6.12
A 40-year-old man with type 1 diabetes and severe peripheral neuropathy was being treated at the diabetic foot clinic for a chronic neuropathic ulcer over the head of his right first metatarsal (Figure 6.46). He had also tried a therapeutic ambulatory cast for forefoot off-loading (Figure 6.47), and the ulcer had improved fairly well (Figure 6.48).

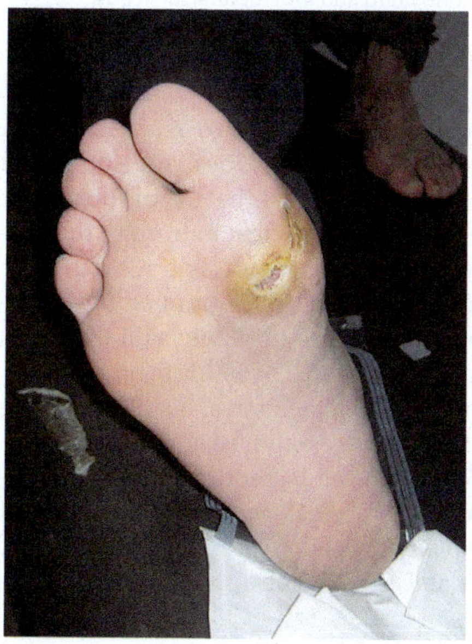

Figure 6.46 A chronic neuropathic ulcer at the head of the right first metatarsal.

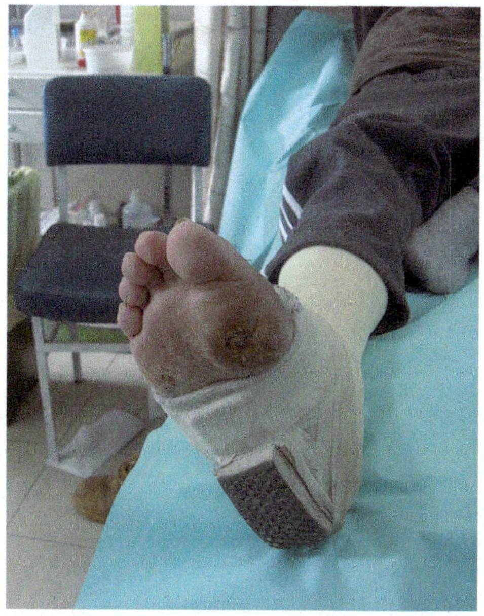

Figure 6.47 A therapeutic ambulatory cast for forefoot off-loading on the patient seen in Figure 6.46, with an ulcer at the head of the right first metatarsal.

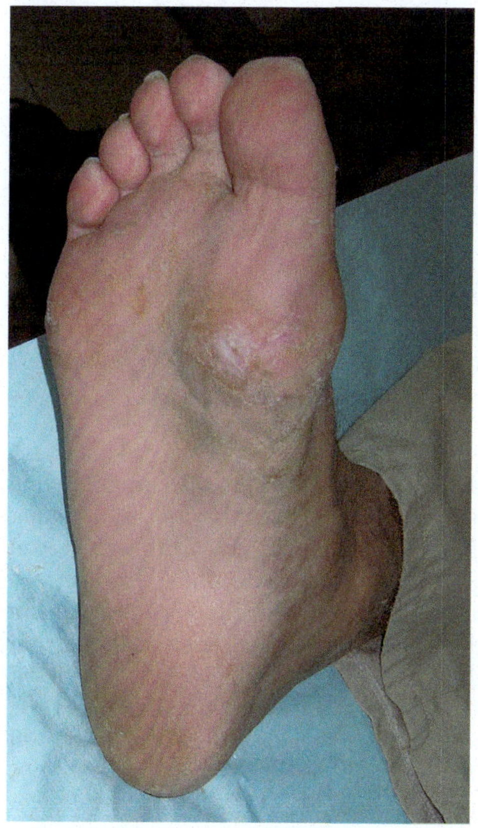

Figure 6.48 The ulcer at the head of the right first metatarsal, shown in Figure 6.47, has nearly healed.

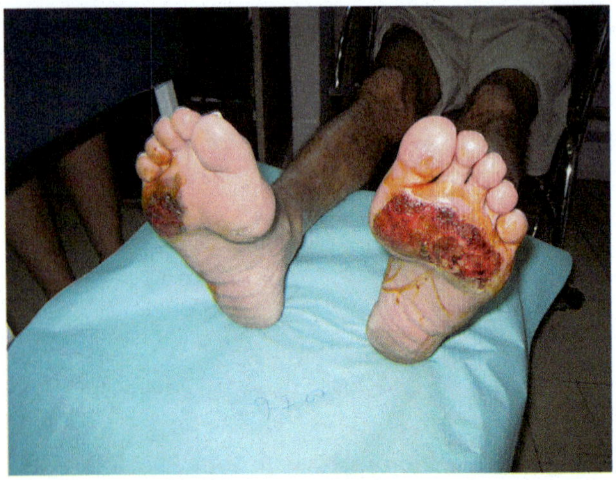

Figure 6.49 The patient from Figure 6.46 with burst blisters on both soles after having walked barefoot on an asphalt road.

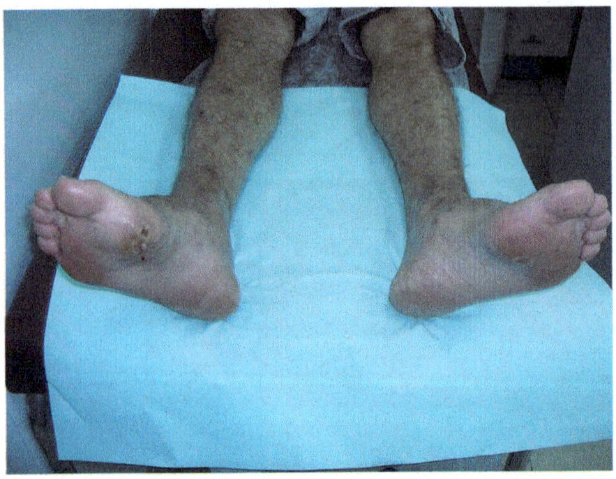

Figure 6.50 Three weeks after local and systemic treatment of the blisters shown in Figure 6.49.

He then suddenly presented to the diabetic foot clinic with huge blisters on both soles (Figure 6.49). He had walked barefoot on a hot summer day on an asphalt road, without realizing that he was burning his feet. He reported that blisters had developed immediately and he had burst them. Local care (antiseptic ointment and cleaning of the blisters) was instituted, together with systemic antibiotics, and bedrest (see Chapter 13). Three weeks later the blisters had healed relatively well (Figure 6.50).

Case 6.13

A 55-year-old male patient with type 2 diabetes since the age of 43 attended the outpatient diabetic foot clinic because of ulcers on his feet. He had a history of a left great toe disarticulated at the metatarsophalangeal joint due to osteomyelitis (Figure 6.51). Osteomyelitis of the fifth right metatarsal head was also evident on a plain radiograph (Figure 6.52). He was treated with antibiotics and local debridement, with an improvement of his condition (Figure 6.53). The patient had severe peripheral neuropathy, with loss of the protective sensations of pain, temperature and light touch.

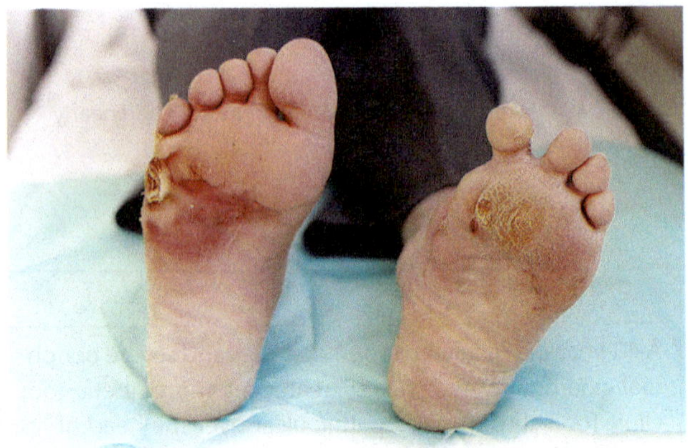

Figure 6.51 Right foot: a neuropathic ulcer over the fifth metatarsal head. Left foot: hallux disarticulation, medial displacement of the second toe with a claw deformity, and callus formation under second, third and fifth metatarsal heads.

The man presented to the clinic two years later with multiple burns over the tips of his toes, and superficial ulcers over the fifth metatarsal heads of both feet (Figure 6.54). He had exposed his feet in front of the fireplace to dry his wet socks. No pain was felt. Although the patient was aware of the burns, he continued his activities for a week before he visited the clinic. Full-thickness burns were present over the tips of all his toes.

Blisters over the right fifth metatarsal head, and on the left fourth and fifth toes were removed, and ulcers developed (Figure 6.55), since the patient still worked regularly despite opposite medical advice. Callus formed around the new plantar ulcers. Amoxycillin–clavulanic acid was started, and the patient attended the diabetic

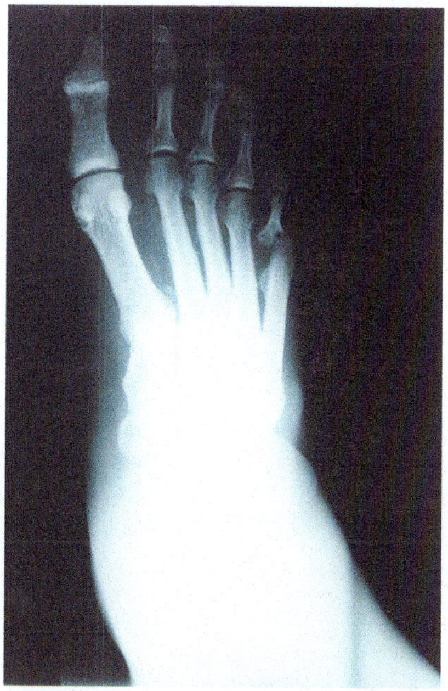

Figure 6.52 A plain radiograph of the right foot of the patient shown in Figure 6.51, showing osteomyelitis of the fifth metatarsal head and the proximal phalanx of the fifth toe. There is also subluxation of the metatarsophalangeal joint. Calcification of the digital artery between the first two metatarsal bones and osteoarthritis of the first distal phalangophalangeal joint can be seen.

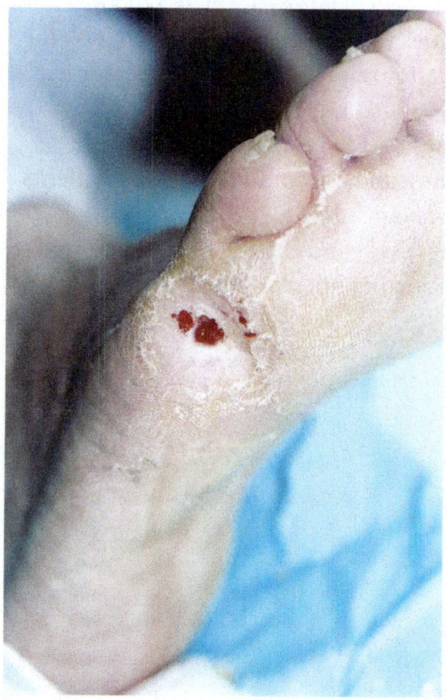

Figure 6.53 Nearly complete healing of the ulcer shown in Figure 6.51.

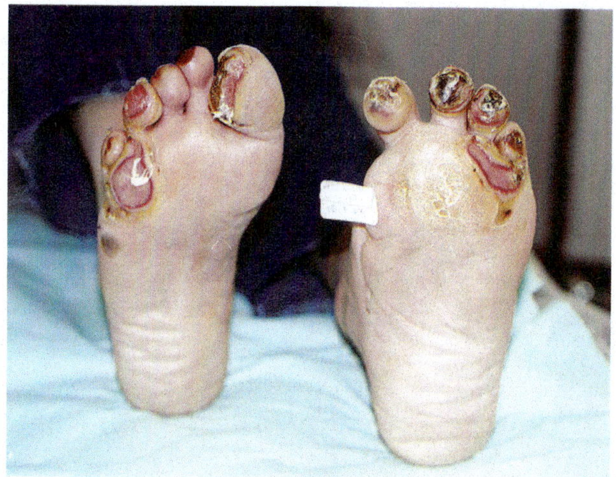

Figure 6.54 Thermal injury of the feet of the patient from Figure 6.51.

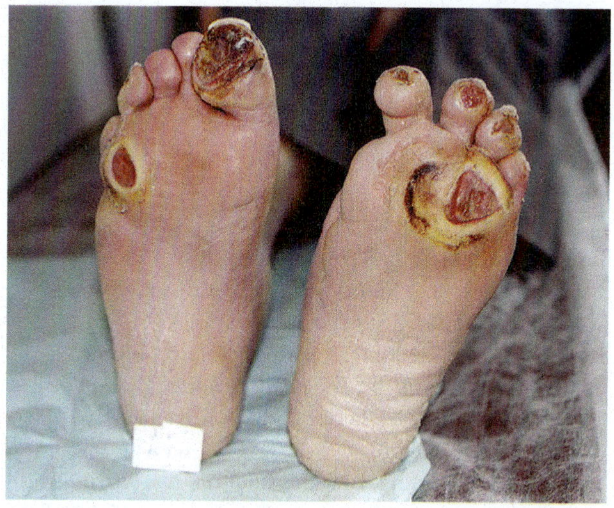

Figure 6.55 Neuropathic ulcers over the fifth metatarsal heads and progression of thermal injury in the patient shown in Figure 6.51. The patient did not comply with the doctors' advice.

foot clinic on a weekly basis. All the ulcers had healed within two months except the one on his right great toe, which was complicated by osteomyelitis and soft tissue infection.

Five months after the burn, his right hallux had to be disarticulated. The patient refused preventive shoes, and four months after this second amputation, new ulcers developed under the fifth metatarsal heads bilaterally (Figure 6.56).

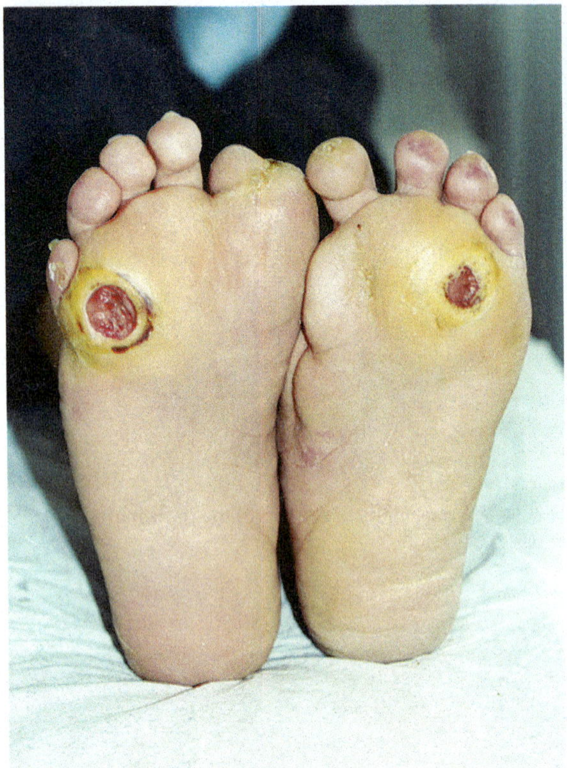

Figure 6.56 Disarticulation of the right hallux at the metatarsophalangeal joint and recurrence of ulcers over the fifth metatarsal heads of the patient shown in Figure 6.51.

Further Reading

Boulton, A.J., Kirsner, R.S., and Vileikyte, L. (2004). Clinical practice. Neuropathic diabetic foot ulcers. *N. Engl. J. Med.* 351: 48–55.

Boulton, A.J.M. (2000). The pathway to ulceration: aetiopathogenesis. In: *The Foot in Diabetes*, 3e (ed. A.J.M. Boulton, H. Connor and P.R. Cavanagh), 61–72. Chichester: Wiley.

Markakis, K., Bowling, F.L., and Boulton, A.J. (2016). The diabetic foot in 2015: an overview. *Diabetes Metab. Res. Rev.* 32 (Suppl 1): 169–178.

Pham, H., Armstrong, D.G., Harvey, C. et al. (2000). Screening techniques to identify people at high risk for diabetic foot ulceration: a prospective multicenter trial. *Diabetes Care* 23: 606–611.

Ramsey, S.D., Newton, K., Blough, D. et al. (1999). Incidence, outcomes, and cost of foot ulcers in patients with diabetes. *Diabetes Care* 22: 382–387.

Singh, N., Armstrong, D.G., and Lipsky, B.A. (2005). Preventing foot ulcers in patients with diabetes. *JAMA* 293: 217–228.

7

Peripheral Vascular Disease

K. Makrilakis

First Department of Propaedeutic Internal Medicine, National and Kapodistrian University of Athens, Medical School, Laiko General Hospital, Athens, Greece

Peripheral vascular disease (PVD) implies the atherosclerotic narrowing of blood vessels in the lower extremities with compromise of blood flow to the extremities. It is pathologically similar in diabetic and non-diabetic patients, although usually more diffuse and multifocal in the latter.

PVD is clinically identified by intermittent claudication and/or the absence of peripheral pulses in the lower legs and feet. Signs of decreased perfusion of the extremities include the absence of foot pulses, a decrease in skin temperature, thin skin, a lack of skin hair and a bluish skin color. The disease may present with typical ischemic pain in one or more muscle groups, atypical pain or no symptoms. Intermittent claudication is defined as a reproducible discomfort of a defined group of muscles that is induced by exercise and relieved by rest (usually within 10 minutes).

This disorder results from an imbalance between the supply and demand of blood flow that fails to satisfy ongoing metabolic requirements. Atherosclerotic lesions responsible for these symptoms are usually found in the arterial segment one level above the affected muscle group. Accordingly, the cramping pain of calf claudication is most frequently due to femoral disease, and less likely due to popliteal and proximal tibioperoneal disease, whereas the aching discomfort and weakness of hip, thigh and buttock claudication is due to aortoiliac disease.

The prevalence of PVD in diabetic patients is 15–30%. The disease progresses with both duration of diabetes and age. The cornerstone of patient evaluation is history and physical examination. A diagnostic work-up is based on a history of intermittent claudication, rest pain, walking distance, palpation of the leg pulses and measurement of the ankle–brachial pressure index (ABI) (See Video 7.1). Palpation of the foot pulses remains the cornerstone of screening for PVD. The absence of two or more pulses on either foot is diagnostic of the disease.

Based on the results of the clinical examination, a decision has to be made on whether the doctor proceeds with more sophisticated methods of examination in order to determine the exact level and degree of the arterial obstruction. A detailed atherosclerotic risk factor assessment should also be performed.

In the differential diagnosis of intermittent claudication, clinicians should consider etiologies such as arthritis, spinal stenosis, radiculopathy, venous claudication, and inflammatory processes.

Two classification systems have been used for lower extremity PVD: the Fontaine system and the Rutherford system. Both are based upon the severity of symptoms and markers of severe disease such as ulceration and gangrene (Table 7.1).

The **Fontaine clinical staging** of peripheral arterial disease includes four stages:

- *Stage I* is asymptomatic. Patients, however, may complain of numbness or that their legs get tired easily, but they do not seek medical help. Usually, the superficial femoral artery is stenosed at the level of the hunterian duct, but the lateral circulation via the deep femoral artery is adequate for the limb's needs.
- *Stage II* patients suffer from intermittent claudication. They are subclassified as *Stage IIa* if they can walk without symptoms for more than 250m, and as *stage IIb* if they have to stop earlier than this.
- *Stage III* patients suffer from rest pain in the limb, which may become constant and very intense, usually during the night; the pain is often resistant to analgesics. The prognosis at this stage is not good: half of these patients will have an amputation within the next five years.

Atlas of the Diabetic Foot, Third Edition. Ioanna Eleftheriadou, Alexandros Kokkinos, Stavros Liatis, Konstantinos Makrilakis, Nicholas Tentolouris, Anastasios Tentolouris, and Panagiotis Tsapogas.

Companion website: www.wiley.com/go/tentolouris/atlas_diabetic_foot

Table 7.1 Classification of peripheral arterial disease: Fontaine's stages and Rutherford's categories.

Fontaine		Rutherford		
Stage	**Clinical description**	**Grade**	**Category**	**Clinical description**
I	Asymptomatic	0	0	Asymptomatic
IIa	Mild claudication	I	1	Mild claudication
IIb	Moderate to severe claudication	I	2	Moderate claudication
		I	3	Severe claudication
III	Ischemic rest pain	II	4	Ischemic rest pain
IV	Ulceration or gangrene	III	5	Minor tissue loss
		III	6	Major tissue loss

Source: Reprinted from Dormandy and Rutherford (2000), with permission.

- *Stage IV* patients have gangrene. Minor trauma, ulcers or paronychias may evolve to gangrene when stage III peripheral artery disease is present. The patient feels pain at rest unless diabetic neuropathy is also present.

The **Rutherford classification** defines claudication categories 0–3 as asymptomatic, mild, moderate and severe, respectively. Categories 4–6 encompass ischemic rest pain and minor and major tissue loss in patients with critical limb ischemia.

In patients with suspected lower extremity PVD based upon the history and physical examination, non-invasive tests are performed first to confirm the clinical diagnosis and to further define the level and extent of obstruction. These include an ABI, exercise treadmill test, segmental limb pressures, segmental volume plethysmography, and ultrasonography. Data suggest that computed tomography angiography (CTA) and magnetic resonance angiography (MRA) may become important non-invasive methods for assessment as well.

It is suggested that all diabetic patients aged over 50 years and those over 40 years old and one more atherosclerotic risk factor are screened for PVD, even if they are asymptomatic. The main value of identifying patients with asymptomatic lower extremity PVD is related to the association of these lesions with an increased risk for myocardial infarction, stroke and cardiovascular mortality. PVD is considered to be a coronary equivalent, and such patients should be treated with risk factor reduction.

7.1 Non-Invasive Vascular Tests

7.1.1 Calculation of the ABI

A relatively simple and inexpensive method to confirm the clinical suspicion of arterial occlusive disease is to measure the resting (and if needed post-exercise) systolic blood pressures in the ankles and arms. This is performed by measuring the systolic blood pressure (by Doppler probe) in the brachial, posterior tibial and dorsalis pedis arteries (Figures 7.1–7.3). The highest of the four measurements in the ankles and feet is divided by the higher of the two brachial measurements. This ratio is referred to as the ankle–brachial (or ankle–arm) index, or ABI (Figure 7.4).

The normal ABI ranges from 0.9 to as high as 1.4, since the pressure is higher in the ankle than in the arm. Values of over 1.3 suggest a non-compressible calcified vessel. An ABI of less than 0.9 is indicative of PVD and is associated with 50% or more stenosis in one or more major vessels. An ABI of 0.40–0.90 suggests a degree of arterial obstruction often associated with claudication. An ABI value below 0.4 or an ankle systolic pressure of less than 50mmHg represents advanced ischemia. A

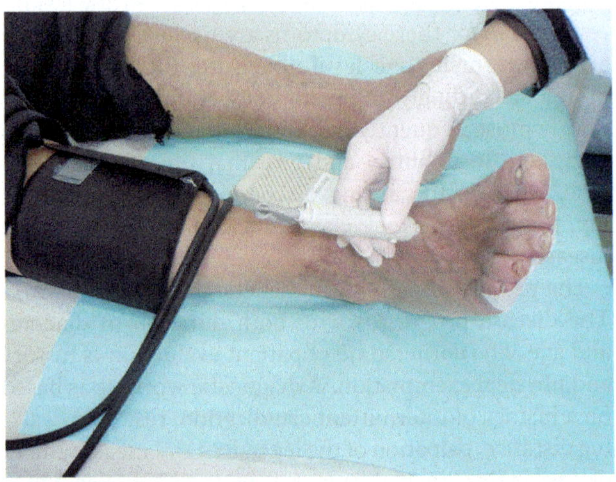

Figure 7.1 Measurement of the dorsalis pedis systolic blood pressure. A blood pressure cuff is placed around the calf, and the blood pressure is measured with a Doppler probe over the dorsalis pedis artery.

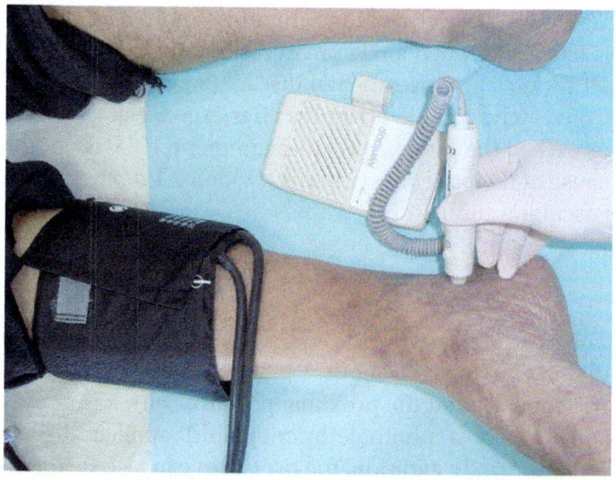
Figure 7.2 Measurement of the posterior tibialis systolic blood pressure. A blood pressure cuff is placed around the calf and the blood pressure is measured with a Doppler probe over the posterior tibialis artery.

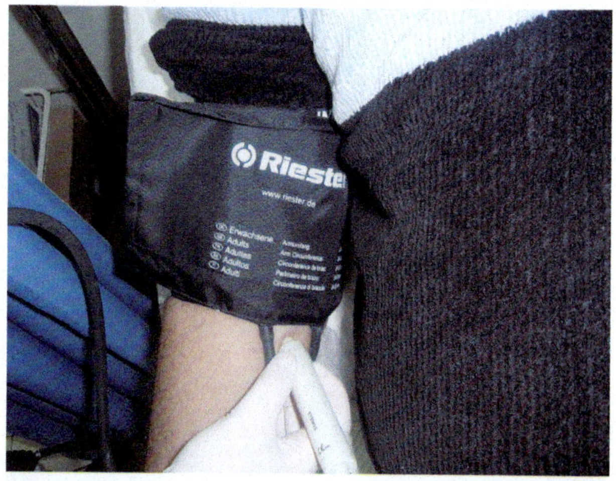
Figure 7.3 Measurement of the brachial systolic blood pressure using a Doppler probe.

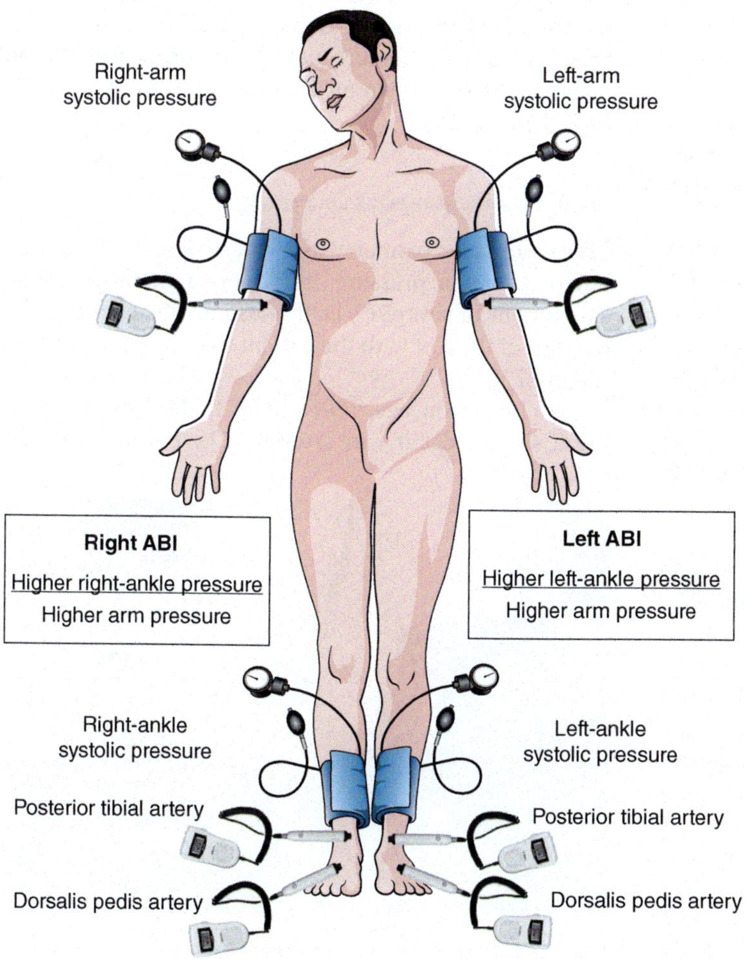

Figure 7.4 The technique of ankle–brachial pressure index measurement.

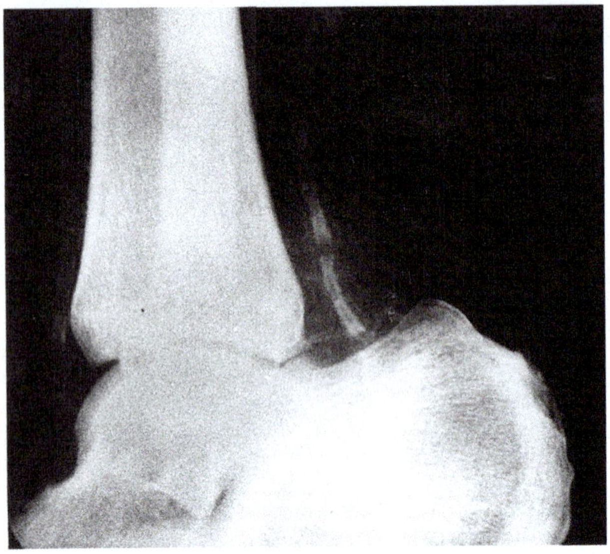

Figure 7.5 Extensive calcification of the posterior tibial artery.

decrease of more than 0.15 in the ABI during follow-up suggests significant narrowing and is an indication for further study with angiography. A spontaneous rise in the ABI is usually attributable to the development of a collateral circulation.

The ABI correlates with clinical measures of lower extremity function such as walking distance, velocity, balance and overall physical activity. In addition, a low ABI has been associated with a higher risk for coronary heart disease, stroke, transient ischemic attack, progressive renal insufficiency, and all-cause mortality.

A potential source of error with the ABI is that calcified vessels may not compress normally, possibly resulting in falsely elevated Doppler signals. Thus, an ABI of over 1.4 is suspicious for calcified vessels (Figure 7.5). In such patients with arterial calcification, an accurate pressure may be obtained by measuring the toe pressure and calculating the toe–brachial index (see below). An abnormally high ABI (over 1.4) is also associated with higher rates of leg pain and cardiovascular risk.

If ABIs are normal at rest but symptoms strongly suggest claudication, ABIs and segmental pressures should be obtained before and after exercise on a treadmill or using active pedal plantar flexion, which involves repeatedly rising up on the toes. This may unmask a hemodynamically significant stenosis that is subclinical at rest but significant on exertion.

In the standard fixed treadmill exercise test, the patient walks at 2 miles per hour on a 12% gradient for five minutes or until symptoms of claudication prohibit continuous exercise. Ankle pressures and/or pulse volume recordings are monitored with the patient in the supine position immediately after exercise and then every minute until the pressures return to pre-exercise levels. When this happens within 5 minutes, single-level disease is likely, but when ankle pressures remain decreased for 10 minutes, multisegmental disease is probably present. Conversely, if ankle pressures after exercise are equal to or exceed the pre-exercise measurement, PVD is not the cause of the patient's symptoms. Video 7.1 demonstrates vascular examination.

7.1.2 Toe Pressures

Toe pressures are measured by a pneumatic cuff with a diameter which is about 1.2 times that of the digit, wrapped around the proximal phalanx, with a flow sensor (usually a photoplethysmograph) applied distally (Figure 7.6). In addition, toe pressures can also be measured using a digital strain gauge.

Normal toe pressures average 90–100mmHg (the lower limit of normal being 50 mmHg) and are usually 20–30 mmHg less than ankle pressures. Rest pain, skin lesions or both are present in approximately 50% of limbs with toe pressures of 30mmHg or less, and in a much lower proportion of patients with toe pressures above this level. Toe pressures are no different between patients with and without diabetes. Falsely high toe pressures due to arterial calcification seldom occur at the toe level. For this reason, toe pressure determination is valuable in diabetic patients when an ankle pressure is abnormally high (Video 7.1).

7.1.3 Transcutaneous Oximetry

Transcutaneous oximetry (the measurement of transcutaneous oxygen pressure, $TcPO_2$) is a method for the assessment of severe PVD. It is usually measured at the dorsum of the feet with the patient in the supine position (Figure 7.7).

With increasing age, $TcPO_2$ tends to decrease, paralleling a similar decline in arterial PO_2. Normal subjects

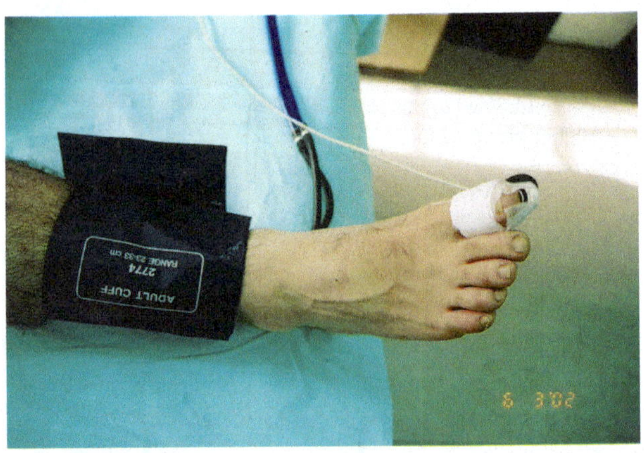

Figure 7.6 Toe pressure measurement.

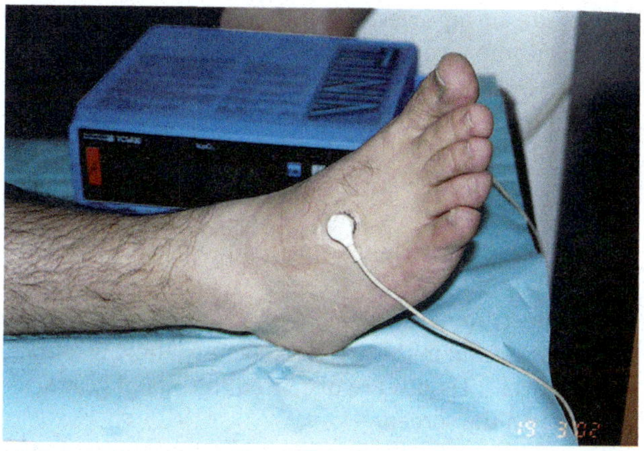

Figure 7.7 Transcutaneous oximetry.

have values of 40–70 mmHg. In general, a resting TcPO_2 over 55 mmHg may be considered normal, regardless of age. Patients with anemia may also have lower values. Patients with rest pain or gangrene have values between 0 and 30 mmHg. In diabetes, TcPO_2 is lower than in age-matched arteriopathic patients. A TcPO_2 below 40 mmHg is associated with a failure of wound healing, whereas an increase after angioplasty or bypass surgery predicts the success of the intervention. Because the results are not affected by arterial calcification, this method is particularly valuable for evaluating diabetic vascular disease (Video 7.1).

7.1.4 Segmental Pressure Measurement

Once the presence of arterial occlusive disease has been verified using ABI measurements at rest or during exercise, the level and extent of PVD can be assessed with segmental limb pressures. To determine segmental pressure in the legs, pressure cuffs 10–12cm wide are applied around the thigh at the groin level, above the knee, below the knee and at ankle level (Figure 7.8). By listening with a Doppler probe over the pedal arteries (posterior tibial or dorsalis pedis), one can measure the pressure at the level of the inflated cuff.

A pressure index can be obtained by dividing the segmental systolic pressure by the brachial pressure. The pressure index should be 1.0 or slightly higher; a normal pressure index at the high thigh level is 1.3. The pressure gradient between any two adjacent levels in the normal leg is normally less than 20mmHg. Gradients above 20mmHg suggest that a significant stenosis is present in the intervening arterial segment. When the gradient exceeds 40 mmHg, the artery is occluded. A 20mmHg or greater reduction in pressure is considered significant if such a gradient is present either between segments along the same leg or when compared with the same level in the opposite leg.

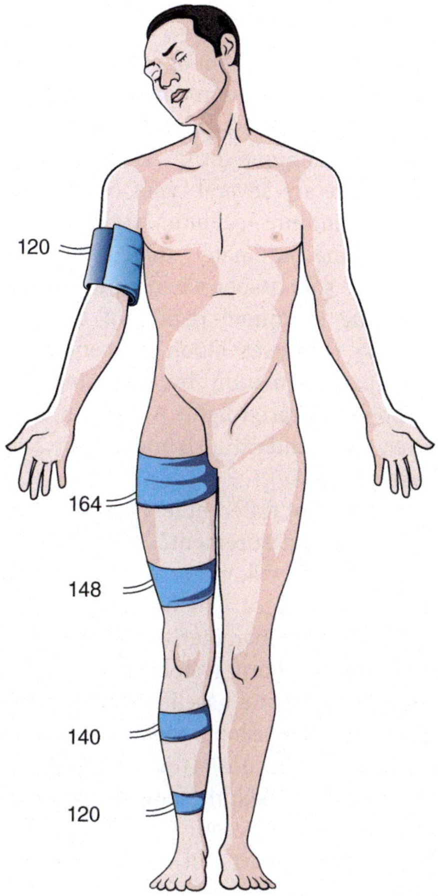

Figure 7.8 Normal segmental pressures (the numbers representing mmHg). The pressure gradient between any two adjacent levels in the normal leg is less than 20–30mmHg. Gradients greater than 30mmHg suggest that a significant stenosis is present at the intervening arterial segment. When the gradient exceeds 40mmHg, the artery is occluded.

The level of peripheral occlusive disease can be detected by such measurements. For example, a significant reduction in pressure between the brachial artery and the upper thigh reflects aortoiliac disease, between the upper and lower thigh reflects superficial femoral artery disease, between the lower thigh and upper calf reflects distal superficial femoral artery or popliteal disease, and between the upper and lower calf reflects infrapopliteal disease. In addition, a toe pressure less than 60% of the ankle pressure indicates digital artery occlusive disease.

It should be taken into account that patients with severe stenosis at a proximal level (e.g. aortoiliac disease) may have falsely normal pressure gradients between the upper and lower thigh in the presence of severe superficial femoral artery stenosis. In addition, obstructions below the knee may not be diagnosed unless the stenosis is severe enough, involving all three tibial arteries.

7.1.5 Segmental Plethysmography

Plethysmography, or the measurement of volume change in an organ or limb, is usually used in conjunction with segmental limb pressures to assess the level of arterial disease. This is a useful technique for the assessment of peripheral arteries. There are several types of plethysmograph (air, mercury, indium–gallium, strain gauge), and all measure the same parameter: the momentary change in volume of the soft tissues when a pulse wave fills the arteries of the examined region of the leg. Photoplythesmography measures blood concentration in the cutaneous microcirculation by detecting the reflection of the applied infrared light. Air plethysmographs are, however, the standard instruments for segmental plethysmography.

Pressure cuffs are applied at different levels of the legs, as in segmental pressure measurement. A plethysmograph records the change in volume as a wave, which reflects the intra-arterial changes. The normal segmental volume pulse contour is characterized by a steep, almost vertical upstroke, a sharp systolic peak, and a downslope that bows toward the baseline during diastole. In the middle of the downslope, there is a prominent dicrotic wave. Distal to a stenosis, the upslope is less steep, the peak becomes rounded, the downslope bows away from the baseline, and the dicrotic wave disappears. Examples of various degrees of arterial stenosis are presented in Figure 7.9.

A plethysmography record is not affected by the presence of arterial calcification; for this reason, it is a valuable method for the assessment of PVD in diabetes.

7.1.6 Ultrasonography

Arterial ultrasound examination has become very popular in recent years. It is a simple and valid method of low cost to determine the site and degree of obstructive lesions, and the patency of a vessel after revascularization. Ultrasonographic equipment used for these tasks include B-mode imaging, pulse-wave Doppler, continuous wave Doppler and color Doppler display.

The site of an arterial stenosis can be identified by serial placements of the Doppler probe along the extremities, the exact site of arterial disease being located by the use of duplex scanning. Duplex scanners use the combination of real-time B-mode ultrasound imaging of the arterial wall together with the pulsed Doppler, and examine flow patterns in a defined area within the artery lumen. The pulsed Doppler technique performs a spectral analysis of the pulse wave, which delineates the complete spectrum of frequencies (that is, blood flow velocities) found in the arterial waveform during a single cardiac cycle. Tissues are displayed in tints of gray scale (duplex) on the screen.

The addition of color frequency mapping (color duplex or triplex) makes the identification of arterial stenosis easier and allows a better description of the atheromatous plaques on the arterial wall. The normal spectrum shows a typical triphasic flow pattern, consisting of a steep systolic upstroke, a systolic peak, a reverse flow component in early diastole and a presystolic zero flow (Figure 7.10). A clear spectral window under the systolic peak is a normal finding, signaling the absence of slow turbulent flow components. If a stenosis is present, this window fills in.

The degree of stenosis can be quantified by analyzing the spectral waveform, and by determining the peak systolic velocity ratio. In general, a cross-sectional reduction of at least 30% must be present to produce a detectable spectral change. The flow velocities may vary, but peak systolic velocities in the arteries above the knee are about 50–100cm second^{-1}, while those below the knee are approximately 50cm second^{-1}.

7.1.6.1 Qualitative Analysis of the Waveform

Inspecting the contour of the spectral waveform is of considerable diagnostic value. Atherosclerotic disease proximal to the site of the probe produces a subtle change in the contour of the systolic peak or in the early deceleration phase (Figure 7.10). With increasing proximal stenosis, the reverse flow component is damped and then disappears entirely.

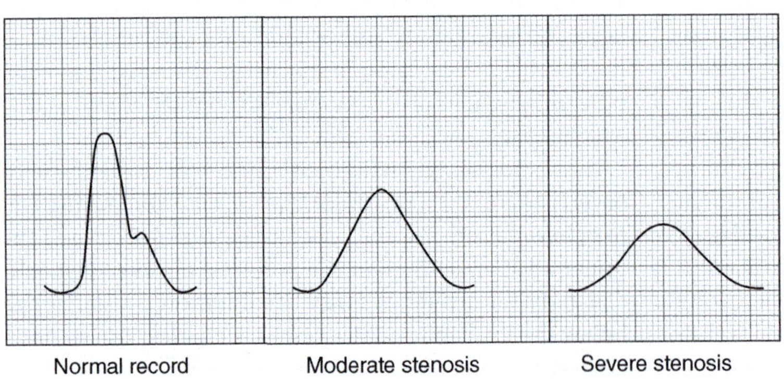

Figure 7.9 Plethysmography pulse volume waveforms associated with different degrees of peripheral vascular disease.

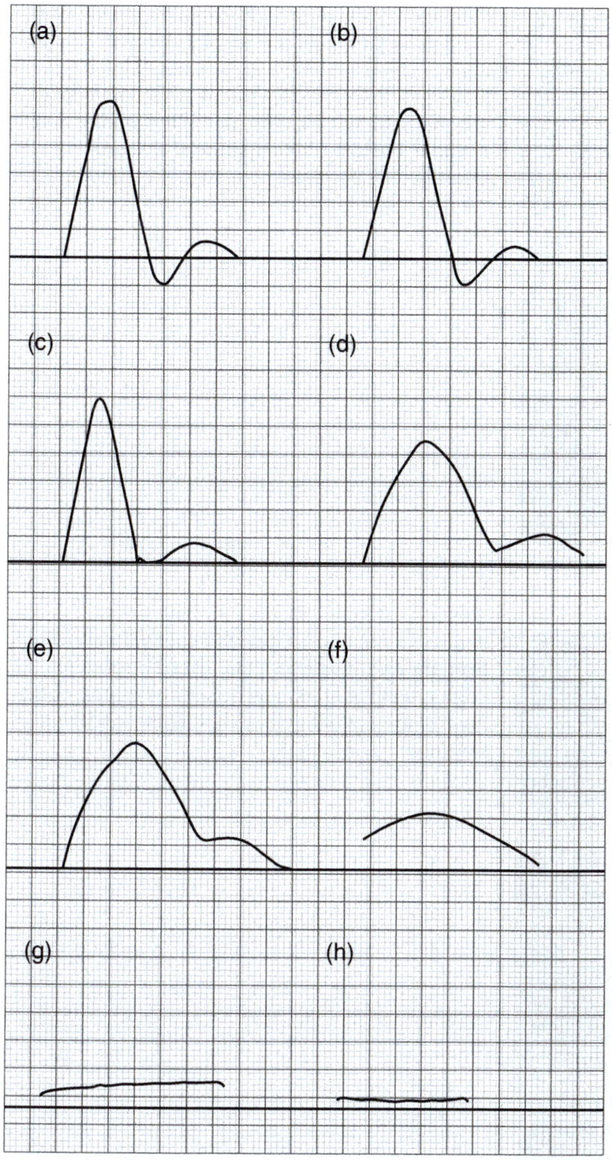

Figure 7.10 Qualitative analysis of spectral waveforms proximal to the site of the probe. (a) Normal. (b) Mild arterial stenosis causing turbulence during systole. (c, d) Loss of reverse flow due to more severe stenosis. (e, f) As the degree of stenosis increases, the rate of acceleration of the upstroke decreases, the peak becomes rounded (e) and the wave becomes continuous and less pulsatile (f–h). Completely damped waveforms (f–h) in the pedal arteries are compatible with multilevel vessel disease and indicate the presence of blood flow resulting from the development of a collateral circulation.

7.1.6.2 Quantitative Analysis of the Waveform

The most widely used criterion for the diagnosis of peripheral arterial stenosis is the peak systolic velocity ratio. This ratio expresses the relationship of the intrastenotic peak systolic velocity to the lowest post-stenotic or pre-stenotic peak systolic velocity. The peak systolic velocity ratio allows an estimation of the degree of a stenosis without distortion by a second stenosis located at a more distal or proximal site (Table 7.2). Other criteria used for the estimation of arterial stenosis are presented in Table 7.3.

Table 7.2 Peak systolic velocity (PSV) ratio in the determination of degree of stenosis.

PSV ratio	Reduction in cross-sectional area
<2.5	0–49%
>2.5	50–74%
>5.5	75–99%

Table 7.3 Criteria for lower limb arterial stenosis in spectral analysis.

Percent stenosis	Pre-stenotic spectrum	Intra-stenotic spectrum	Spectrum just past the stenosis
0–50%	Normal: Triphasic or biphasic Narrow frequency band Clear spectral window	Increase in PSV (by <100% and/ or < 180 cm s^{-1})	No significant turbulence Possible flow reversal
51–75%	Normal	Increase in PSV (by >100% and/ or > 180 cm s^{-1})	Flow reversal Possible slight turbulence
76–99%	Normal or slightly reduced velocity	Increase in PSV (by >250% and/ or > 180 cm s^{-1})	Significant turbulence Complete infill of the spectral window

PSV, peak systolic velocity.

Duplex ultrasonography has a sensitivity of 80% and specificity above 90% for detecting femoral and popliteal stenosis compared with angiography, but it is less reliable for the assessment of the severity of stenosis in the tibial and peroneal arteries. Normal and abnormal spectral waveform recordings are shown in Figures 7.11–7.18.

7.1.7 Other Non-Invasive Methods

Modern methods for the assessment of peripheral arteries include helical or spiral CTA and MRA.

Spiral CTA has the ability to generate three-dimensional images and is most useful in the evaluation of large arteries (e.g. thoracic or abdominal aorta) (Figure 7.19). Disadvantages include the intravascular administration of iodinated contrast (with its inherent allergic and nephrotoxic effects) and the inability to assess small-vessel disease. A number of recent reports of small

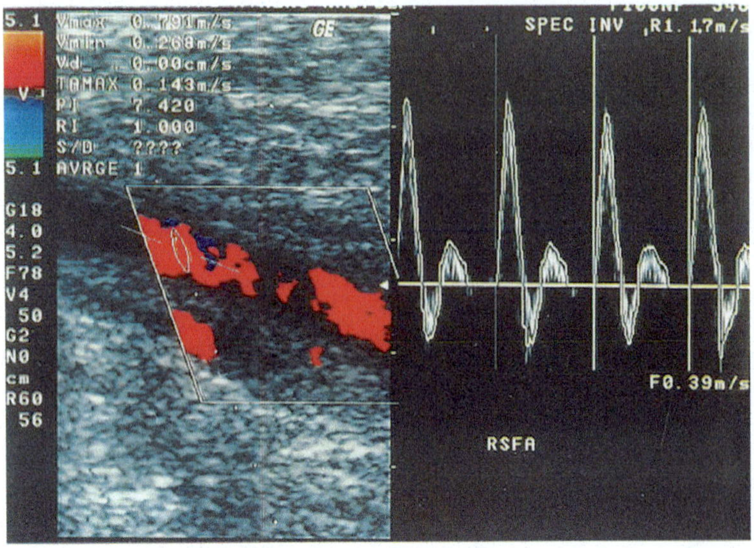

Figure 7.11 A normal triphasic spectral waveform from the right superficial femoral artery. Notice the narrow, steep increase and decrease of the waveform. Peak systolic velocity is 79.1cm second^{-1} (normal peak systolic velocities in the arteries above the knee being 50–100cm second^{-1}). *Source:* Courtesy of C. Revenas.

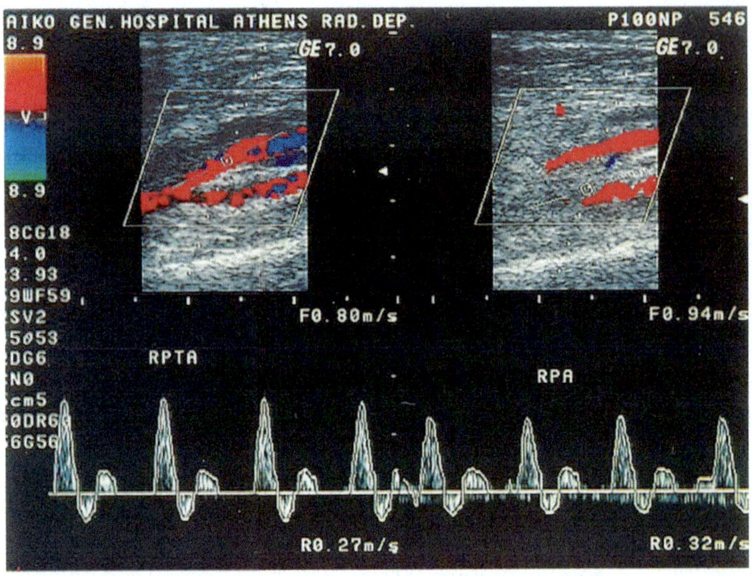

Figure 7.12 A normal triphasic spectral waveform from the right posterior tibial artery. Duplex scanning of the artery can be seen at the top of the figure. Peak systolic velocity is 49cm second. *Source:* Courtesy of C. Revenas.

series of patients have noted excellent correlation between CTA and digital subtraction angiography (DSA) in the detection of aortic and lower extremity arterial disease (Figure 7.20), but these findings have not been universal. In addition, the total burden of radiation is relatively high.

MRA has mainly been used for examining the cerebral vessels and carotid arteries. Recent data suggest that this method might replace angiography as a primary imaging examination for PVD. Angiography might be preserved only for percutaneous interventions and for cases with equivocal findings. In addition, MRA is a simple, non-toxic and relatively inexpensive method (Figure 7.21–7.23). A rare but serious complication in patients with severe renal failure requiring dialysis is nephrogenic systemic fibrosis and nephrogenic fibrosing dermopathy with use of gadolinium contrast material, so the technique should be used with caution in this population.

7.2 Invasive Vascular Testing: Arteriography

Arteriography remains the definitive diagnostic procedure before any form of surgical intervention. It should **not** be used as a diagnostic procedure to establish the presence of arterial disease. Contrast material may

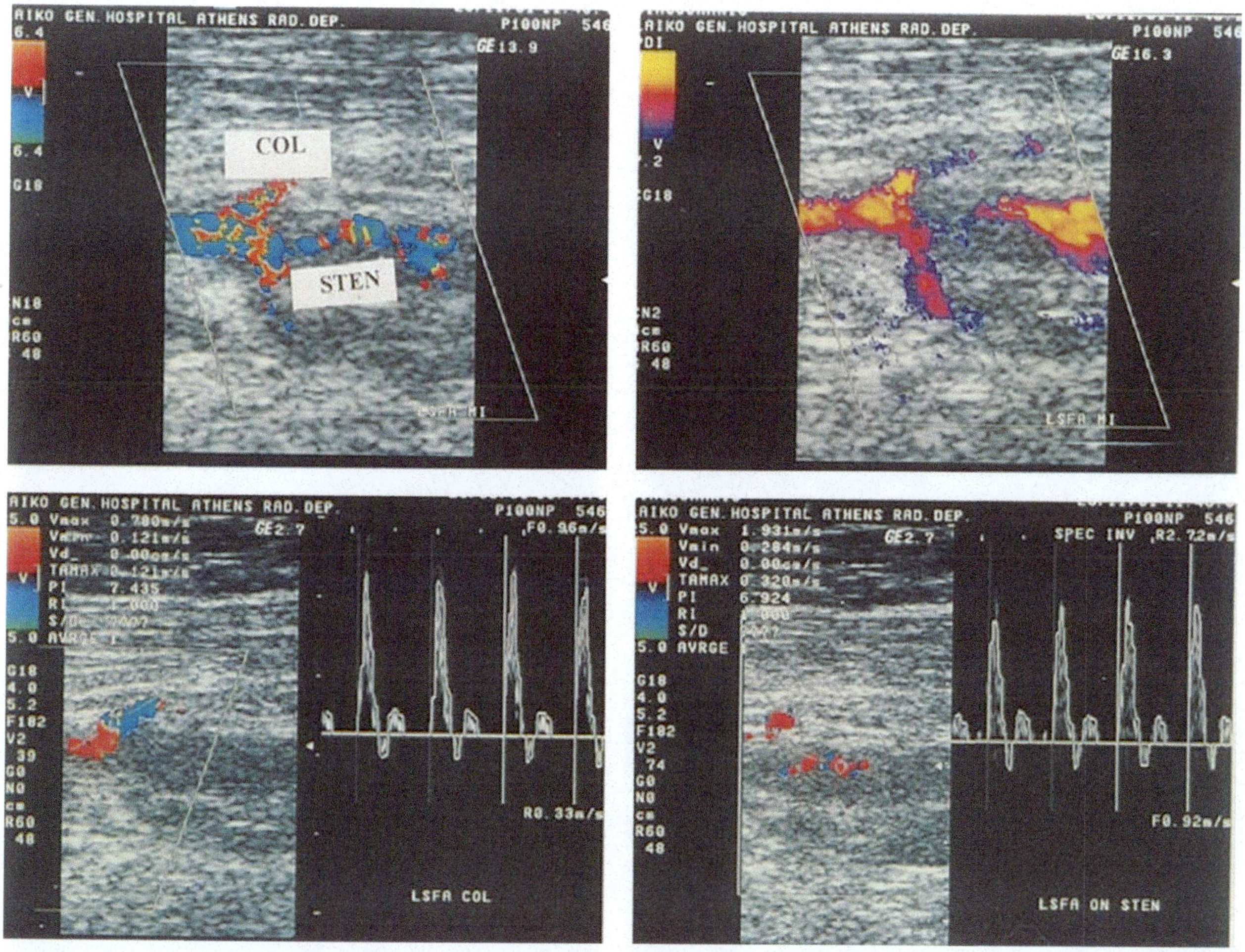

Figure 7.13 The upper left panel shows a significant stenosis (STEN) of the left superficial femoral artery with development of a collateral circulation (COL). Note (lower left panel) the triphasic spectral waveform of the collateral vessel, and that the peak systolic velocity is 78 cm $second^{-1}$, which is too high for such a vessel. In the area of the femoral artery stenosis, peak systolic velocity is high (193cm $second^{-1}$) and the waveform is triphasic, but blood flow during diastole is low, as seen from the short duration of the reverse flow (lower right panel). Next to the spectral waveform, the artery with the stenosis is seen in color duplex scanning. These findings suggest the presence of a stenosis of approximately 50–80%. The upper right panel shows a dynamic Doppler recording, which images the collateral vessels better. *Source:* Courtesy of C. Revenas.

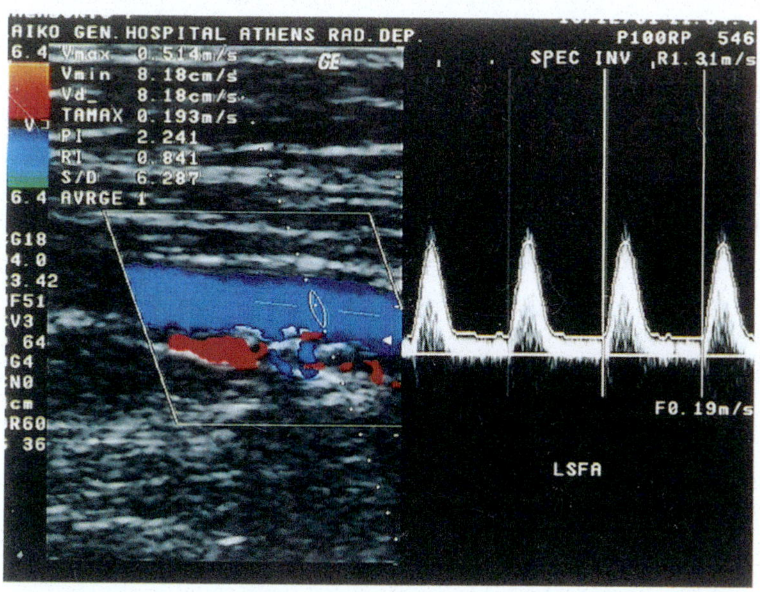

Figure 7.14 Biphasic spectral waveforms obtained from the left superficial femoral artery. The spectral window is widened and filled in, although not completely. Peak systolic velocity is low (51.4cm $second^{-1}$). These findings denote the presence of significant proximal stenosis at one or multiple levels. *Source:* Courtesy of C. Revenas.

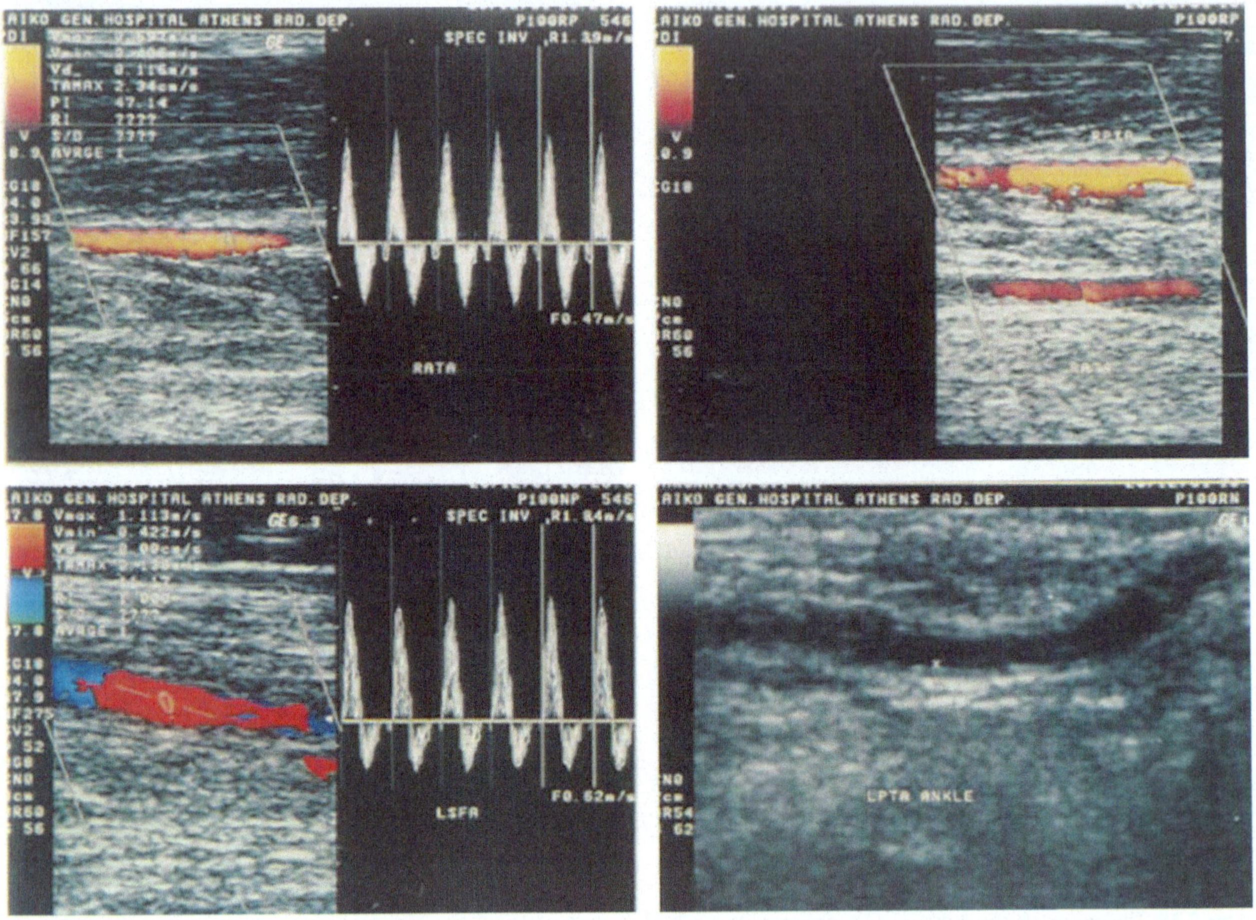

Figure 7.15 The spectral waveform from the right anterior tibial artery in an area of stenosis is seen in the upper left panel. Peak systolic velocity is high (69.7cm $second^{-1}$) – peak systolic velocities in the arteries below the knee are usually approximately 50cm $second^{-1}$ – and there is mild widening of the spectrum during both systole and diastole. This record corresponds to a stenosis of about 30%. The spectral waveform from the left superficial femoral artery is shown in the lower left panel. There is mild spectral widening and loss of presystolic flow. The right tibial arteries are shown in color duplex imaging in the upper right panel. A duplex scan of the left posterior tibial artery is seen in the lower right panel. *Source:* Courtesy of C. Revenas.

exaggerate any pre-existing renal disease, so, for this reason, the contrast material used must be limited as much as possible. In addition, the International Meeting on the Assessment of Peripheral Vascular Disease in Diabetes strongly recommends that arteriography should be performed before revascularization procedures and the decision to amputate is made in diabetic patients, in order to assess the exact status of the vascular tree, particularly when the ABI and toe systolic pressure indicate that arterial disease is present.

Nowadays, DSA, which improves visualization of the arteries by eliminating background soft tissue and bone, has nearly universally replaced conventional angiography in the evaluation of vessel disease (Figures 7.24–7.27).

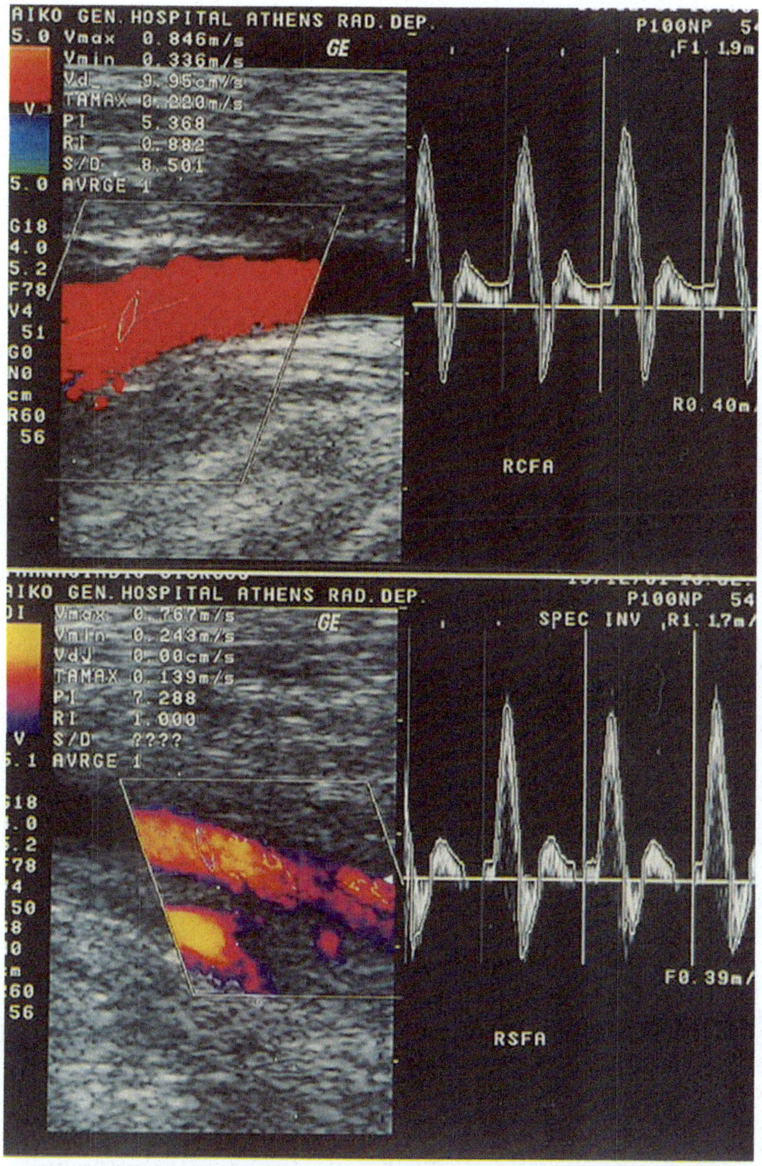

Figure 7.16 Near-normal spectral waveforms obtained from the right common (upper panel) and right superficial (lower panel) femoral arteries. The peak systolic velocity is reduced slightly, the waveform is triphasic, and there is minimal widening of the spectral window. These findings suggest the presence of a mild proximal stenosis. *Source:* Courtesy of C. Revenas.

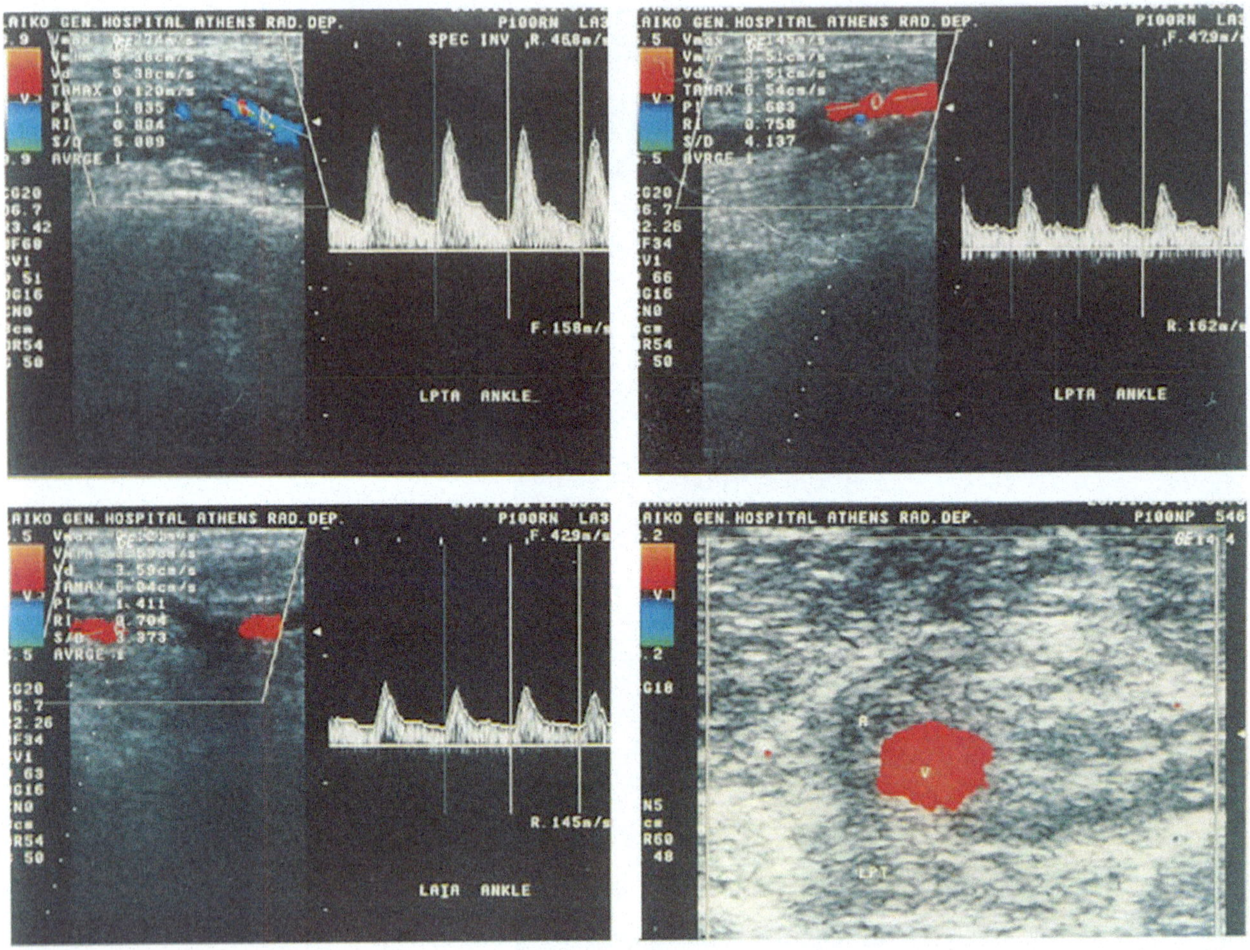

Figure 7.17 The upper left panel shows a biphasic waveform of the left posterior tibial artery at ankle level. Peak systolic velocity is reduced (27.4cm second^{-1}), there is a widening of the spectral window during systole, while velocity is high during diastole. The artery diameter is normal as seen in a color duplex image on the left of the spectral waveform. These findings suggest the presence of a proximal stenosis of about 40%. The upper right panel shows the same artery at another site after a stenosis. Notice the low peak systolic velocity (14.5cm second^{-1}), the biphasic waveform, and the spectral widening during systole, as well as the high velocity during diastole. These findings suggest the presence of a proximal stenosis of more than 50%. The lower left panel shows duplex scanning of the left anterior tibial artery from the same patient and the spectral waveform recorded. An even lower peak systolic velocity (12.1cm second^{-1}), significant widening of the systolic spectral window and a high diastolic velocity are seen. The diameter of the artery is normal (lower right panel). The above findings signify the presence of proximal stenosis of about 50–60%. *Source:* Courtesy of C. Revenas.

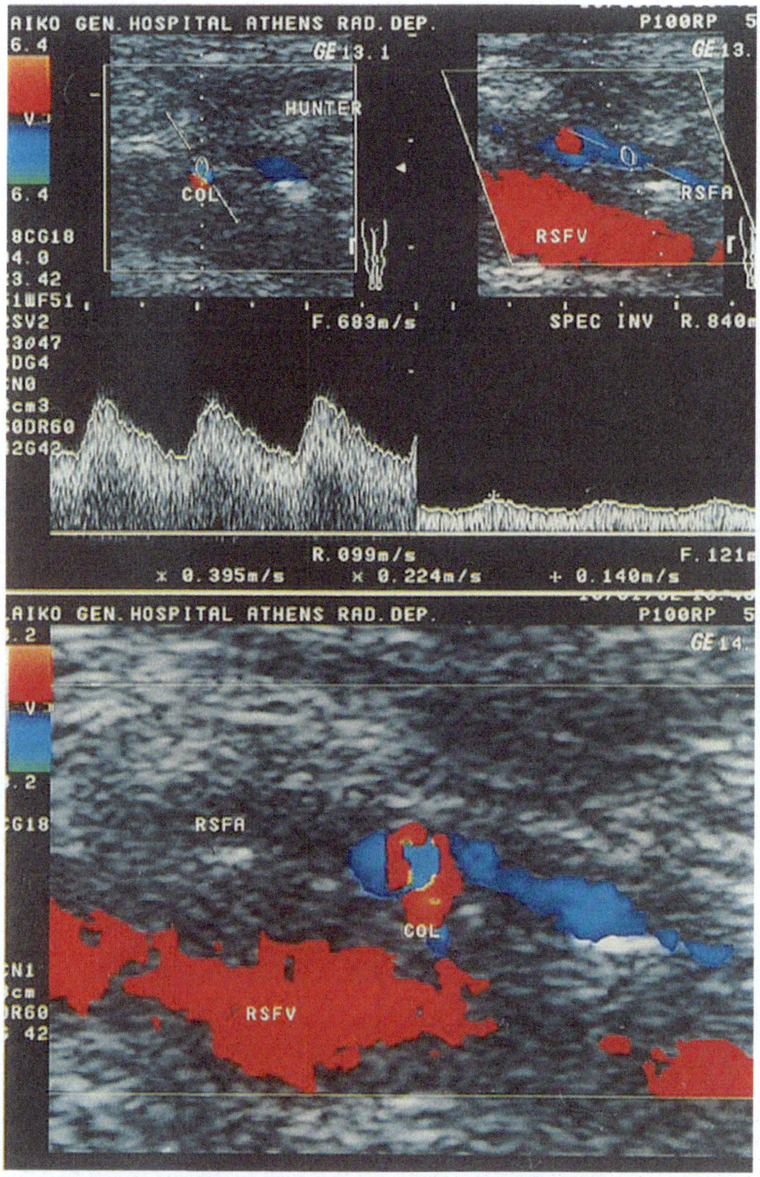

Figure 7.18 The lower panel shows complete obstruction of the right superficial femoral (RSFA) artery at the canal of Hunter. A collateral vessel (COL) is seen proximal to the stenosis. Distal to the site of the obstruction, there is blood flow in the superficial femoral artery from collateral vessels. The upper panel shows the spectral waveform obtained from the collateral vessel shown in the previous part of the figure. The waveform is biphasic, both peak systolic and diastolic velocities are high, and there is widening of the systolic spectral window. Following this, the waveform obtained from the right superficial femoral artery distal to the site of the complete obstruction is shown. Note the low peak systolic and high diastolic velocities. This waveform is called tardus pardus. This type of spectral waveform is similar to that obtained from the venous circulation; it signifies the presence of flow in an artery from the development of a collateral circulation. As more collateral vessels fill the artery, the spectral waveform may be triphasic, but the peak systolic velocity will be reduced. *Source:* Courtesy of C. Revenas.

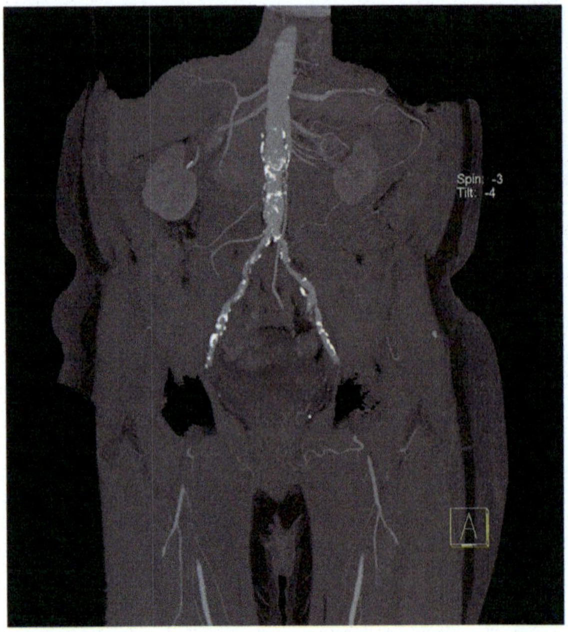

Figure 7.19 Computed tomography angiography. Three-dimensional reconstruction of the abdominal aorta and the iliac arteries. Notice the extensive calcification of the vessels. *Source:* Courtesy of R. Efthymiadou.

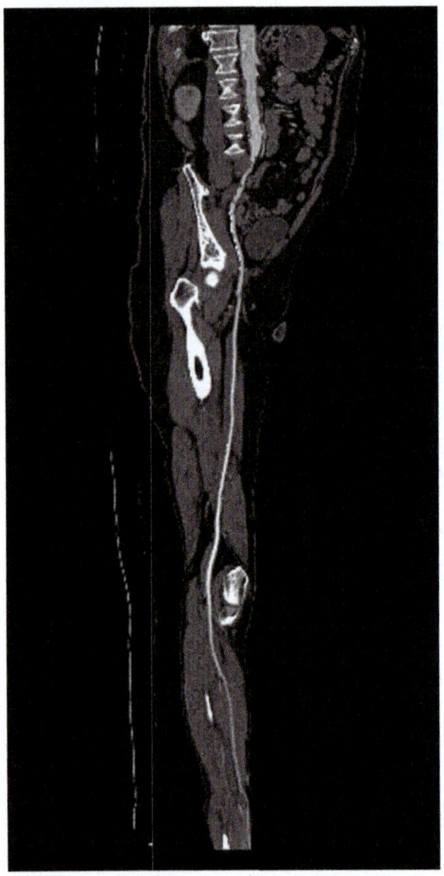

Figure 7.20 Computed tomography angiography. Three-dimensional reconstruction of the arterial system of the right leg. *Source:* Courtesy of R. Efthymiadou.

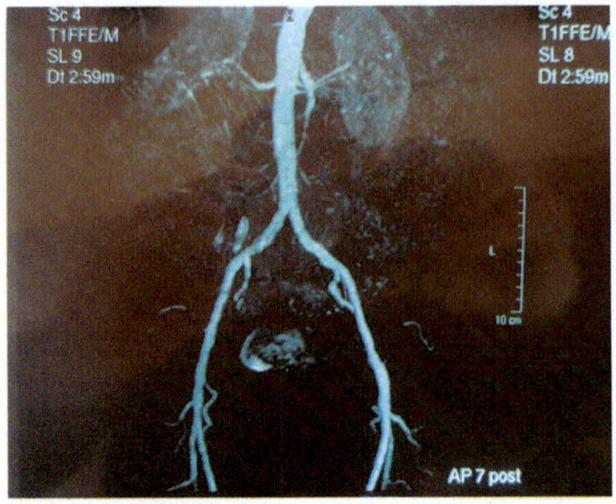

Figure 7.21 Magnetic resonance angiography of the abdominal aorta and iliac arteries. *Source:* Courtesy of R. Efthymiadou.

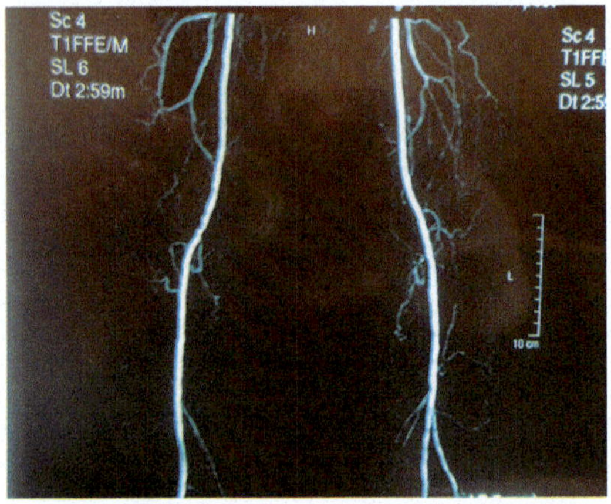

Figure 7.22 Magnetic resonance angiography of the femoral arteries of the same patient as in Figure 7.21. Notice the diffuse atherosclerotic disease in the right superficial femoral artery. *Source:* Courtesy of R. Efthymiadou.

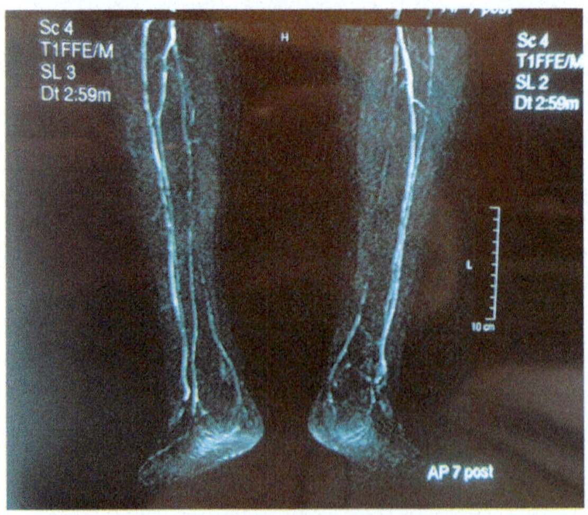

Figure 7.23 Magnetic resonance angiography of the tibial and peroneal arteries of the same patient as in Figure 7.21. Note that the posterior tibial arteries are completely occluded at their origin (seen especially on the left) and the vessels fill with blood retrogradely from the plantar arch. *Source:* Courtesy of R. Efthymiadou.

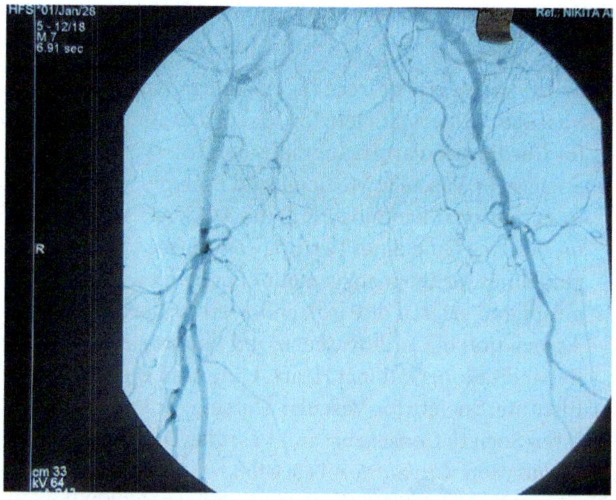

Figure 7.24 Digital subtraction angiography of a diabetic patient with significant peripheral vascular disease of the lower extremities. Both common iliac arteries are shown as having extensive atherosclerotic lesions, but they are patent.

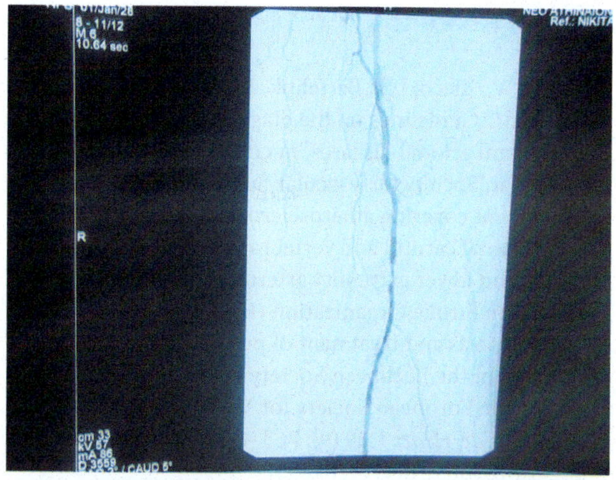

Figure 7.26 Digital subtraction angiography of the right superficial femoral artery of the same patient as in Figure 7.24, showing diffuse severe atherosclerotic stenoses.

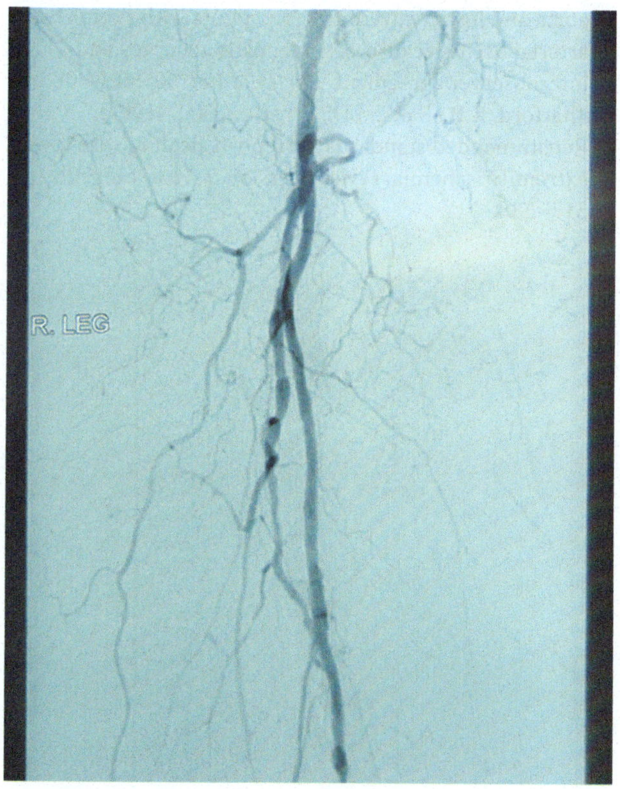

Figure 7.25 Digital subtraction angiography of the right common femoral artery of the same patient as in Figure 7.24, showing adequate patency.

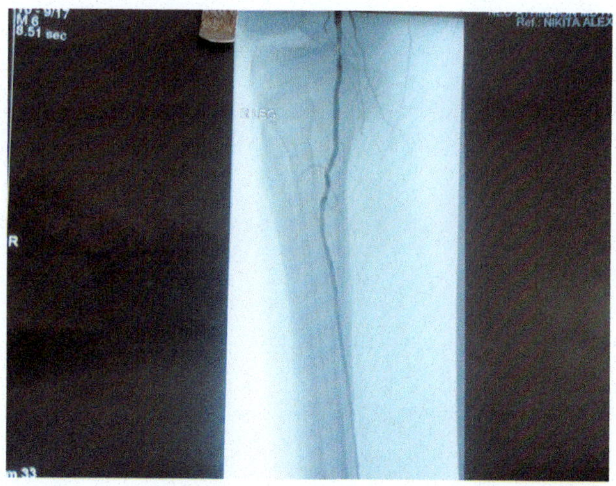

Figure 7.27 Digital subtraction angiography of the right popliteal and tibioperoneal arteries of the same patient as in Figures 7.24 and 7.25. Note the near-total occlusion of the right popliteal artery. In addition, distal to the trifurcation of the tibial arteries, only one main tibial artery is seen (the intraosseous artery), which provides perfusion to the lower foot.

Reference

Dormandy, J.A. and Rutherford, R.B. (2000). Management of peripheral arterial disease (PAD). TASC Working Group. TransAtlantic Inter-Society Consensus (TASC). *J Vasc Surg.* 31 (1 Pt 2): S1–S296.

Further Reading

Aboyans, V., Ricco, J.B., Bartelink, M.L.E.L. et al. (2018). 2017 ESC Guidelines on the diagnosis and treatment of peripheral arterial diseases, in collaboration with the European Society for Vascular Surgery (ESVS): Document covering atherosclerotic disease of extracranial carotid and vertebral, mesenteric, renal, upper and lower extremity arteries Endorsed by: the European Stroke Organization (ESO) The task force for the diagnosis and treatment of peripheral arterial diseases of the European Society of Cardiology (ESC) and of the European Society for Vascular Surgery (ESVS). *Eur. Heart J.* 39 (9): 763–816. https://doi.org/10.1093/eurheartj/ehx095.

Gerhard-Herman, M.D., Gornik, H.L. et al. (2017). 2016 AHA/ACC Guideline on the management of patients with lower extremity peripheral artery disease: A report of the american college of cardiology/American Heart Association task force on clinical practice guidelines. *Circulation* 135: e726–e779.

Heijenbrok-Kal, M.H., Kock, M.C., and Hunink, M.G. (2007). Lower extremity arterial disease: multidetector CT angiography meta-analysis. *Radiology* 245: 433–439.

Hirsch, A.T., Haskal, Z.J., Hertzer, N.R. et al. (2006). ACC/AHA 2005 Practice Guidelines for the management of patients with peripheral arterial disease (lower extremity, renal, mesenteric, and abdominal aortic): a collaborative report from the American Association for Vascular Surgery/Society for Vascular Surgery, Society for Cardiovascular Angiography and Interventions, Society for Vascular Medicine and Biology, Society of Interventional Radiology, and the ACC/AHA task force on Practice Guidelines (writing committee to develop guidelines for the management of patients with peripheral arterial disease): endorsed by the American Association of Cardiovascular and Pulmonary Rehabilitation; National Heart, Lung, and Blood Institute; Society for Vascular Nursing; TransAtlantic Inter-Society Consensus; and Vascular Disease Foundation. *Circulation* 113: e463.

Norgren, L., Hiatt, W.R., Dormandy, J.A. et al. (2007). Inter-Society Consensus for the management of peripheral arterial disease (TASC II). *J. Vasc. Surg.* 45 (Suppl): S5–S67.

Romano, M., Mainenti, P.P., Imbriaco, M. et al. (2004). Multidetector row CT angiography of the abdominal aorta and lower extremities in patients with peripheral arterial occlusive disease: diagnostic accuracy and interobserver agreement. *Eur. J. Radiol.* 50: 303–308.

Rutherford, R.B., Baker, J.D., Ernst, C. et al. (1997). Recommended standards for reports dealing with lower extremity ischemia: revised version. *J. Vasc. Surg.* 26: 517–538.

8

Ischemic and Neuro-Ischemic Ulcers and Gangrene

S. Liatis[1] *and P. Tsapogas*[2]

[1] First Department of Propaedeutic Internal Medicine, National and Kapodistrian University of Athens, Medical School, Laiko General Hospital, Athens, Greece
[2] Center for Diabetes and Metabolism, Henry Dunant Hospital Center, Athens, Greece

Although atherosclerotic lesions in the arteries of diabetic patients occur at sites similar to those of non-diabetic individuals (such as arterial bifurcations), advanced disease is more common in diabetic patients, affecting even collateral vessels. The pathology of the affected arteries is similar in both those with and those without diabetes.

Typical atherosclerotic lesions in diabetic patients with peripheral vascular disease include diffuse multifocal stenosis and a predilection for the tibioperoneal arteries. All tibial arteries may be occluded, with distal reconstitution of a dorsal pedal or common plantar artery. Diabetes has the greatest impact on the smaller vessels (diameter less than 5 mm) in the body.

The atherosclerotic procedure starts at a younger age and progresses more rapidly in those who have diabetes than those who do not. Although non-diabetic men are affected by peripheral vascular disease much more commonly than non-diabetic women (a male-to-female ratio of 30:1), diabetic women are affected half as often as diabetic men.

Gangrene is characterized by the presence of cyanotic, anesthetic tissue associated with or progressing to necrosis. It occurs when the arterial blood supply falls below minimal metabolic requirements. Gangrene can be described as dry or wet, wet gangrene being dry gangrene complicated by infection.

8.1 Blue toe Syndrome

An embolism of cholesterol crystals and other debris from friable atherosclerotic plaques in the aorta or arteries of the proximal lower extremities may lodge in the distal circulation and infarct the tissues ("blue toe syndrome"). Clinically, the syndrome is presented with sudden blue or violaceous discoloration of one or more toes. Another common cutaneous finding is livedo reticularis, consisting of macular reddish, blue, or purple-colored connecting rings that form a network.

Case 8.1

Blue toe syndrome developed in a 61-year-old patient with type 2 diabetes as manifested by rest pain for more than two weeks, a history of smoking and intermittent claudication, and ischemic purple patches on the toes (Figure 8.1) and forefoot (Figures 8.2 and 8.3). Digital subtraction angiography (DSA) revealed multiple stenotic lesions in the deep femoral arteries (Figure 8.4), significant occlusive lesions in the right anterior tibial artery, and total occlusion of the right posterior and left anterior tibial arteries (Figure 8.5).

8.2 Critical Limb Ischemia (CLI)

Critical leg ischemia is any condition where there is an overwhelming likelihood that the limb is at risk for amputation or significant tissue loss within six months. However, for most patients presenting with critical limb ischemia, the risk for limb loss is fairly immediate, and the need for revascularization is more urgent than for patients with claudication. Critical limb ischemia occurs when distal limb perfusion is impaired to the extent that oxygen delivery is insufficient to meet resting metabolic tissue demands, and it usually follows inadequate adaptation of the peripheral circulation to chronic ischemia (collateral recruitment and vasodilatation). As a result, CLI is associated with increased risk for amputation,

Atlas of the Diabetic Foot, Third Edition. Ioanna Eleftheriadou, Alexandros Kokkinos, Stavros Liatis, Konstantinos Makrilakis, Nicholas Tentolouris, Anastasios Tentolouris, and Panagiotis Tsapogas.

Companion website: www.wiley.com/go/tentolouris/atlas_diabetic_foot

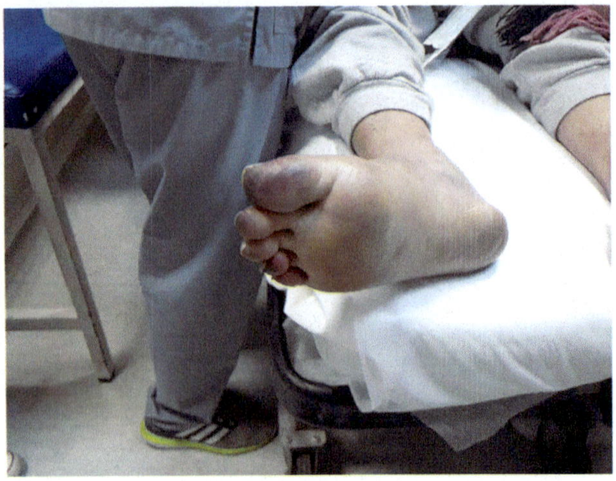

Figure 8.1 "Blue toe syndrome."

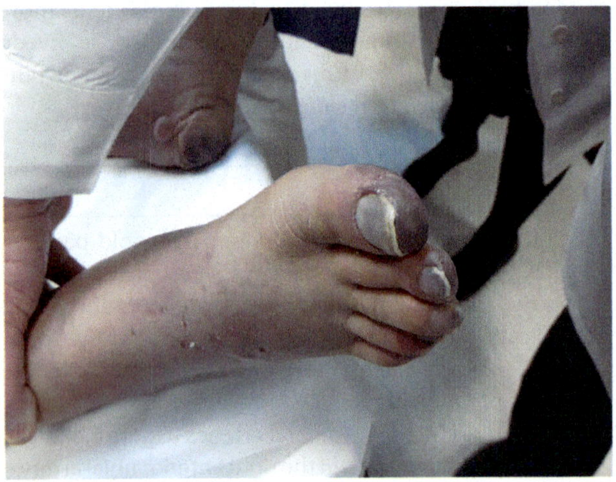

Figure 8.2 Case 8.1: "blue toe syndrome." Ischemic purple patches on the toes and the forefoot of a patient with peripheral artery disease.

decreased quality of life, and increased mortality. Amputation rates remain high at 25%, and long-term survival is poor.

According to the consensus statement on critical limb ischemia, critical leg ischemia is defined as either of the following two criteria:

1) *persistently recurring ischemic rest pain* requiring regular adequate analgesia for more than two weeks, with an ankle systolic pressure of 50mmHg or less and/or a toe pressure of 30mmHg or less;
2) *ulceration or gangrene* of the foot or toes, with an ankle systolic pressure of 50mmHg or below and/or a toe pressure of 30mmHg or less.

Similar ankle pressure parameters have been suggested by the European Society of Cardiology (ESC) guidelines. The Society for Vascular Surgery defines severe ischemia as an ABI less than 0.4, an ankle pressure less than 50mmHg, or a toe pressure less than 30mmHg.

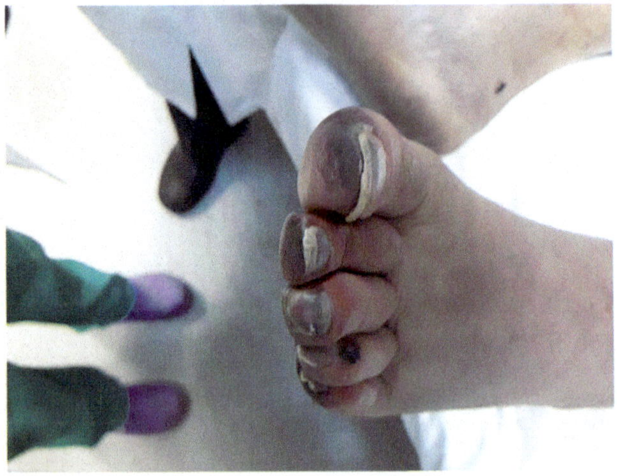

Figure 8.3 Case 8.1: "blue toe syndrome." Ischemic purple patches on the toes of a patient with critical limb ischemia.

Critical limb ischemia is manifested by rest pain (Rutherford classification category 4) or tissue loss. Critical leg ischemia is dominated by pedal pain, which may not be present in certain patients with diabetes and peripheral neuropathy. In such patients, the superficial pain sensation may be altered and they may experience only deep ischemic pain, such as calf claudication and ischemic rest pain). In most cases, the pedal pain is intolerably severe; it may respond to foot dependency, but otherwise responds only to opiates. In such patients, it is important to differentiate neuropathic pain from ischemic rest pain. Measurement of the ankle–brachial index or toe pressure can easily differentiate the two conditions.

8.3 Ischemic Ulcers

Ischemic ulcers are often located distally and on the dorsum of the foot or toes (Figures 8.6–8.9, and see Case 8.2). Arterial ulcers also occur commonly in the nail bed if the toenail cuts into the skin or if the patient has had recent aggressive toenail trimming or an ingrown toenail removed (see Case 8.3).

Initially, ischemic ulcers have irregular edges, but they may progress to have a better-defined appearance (Figure 8.7). On manipulation, such as debriding, these ulcers bleed very little or not at all. The patient may report characteristic pain, especially at night when supine, which is relieved by dependency of the extremity. Upon examination, characteristic findings of chronic ischemia, such as hairlessness, pale skin and absent pulses, are noted. Calcification of the metatarsal and digital arteries is often present (see Figure 8.14).

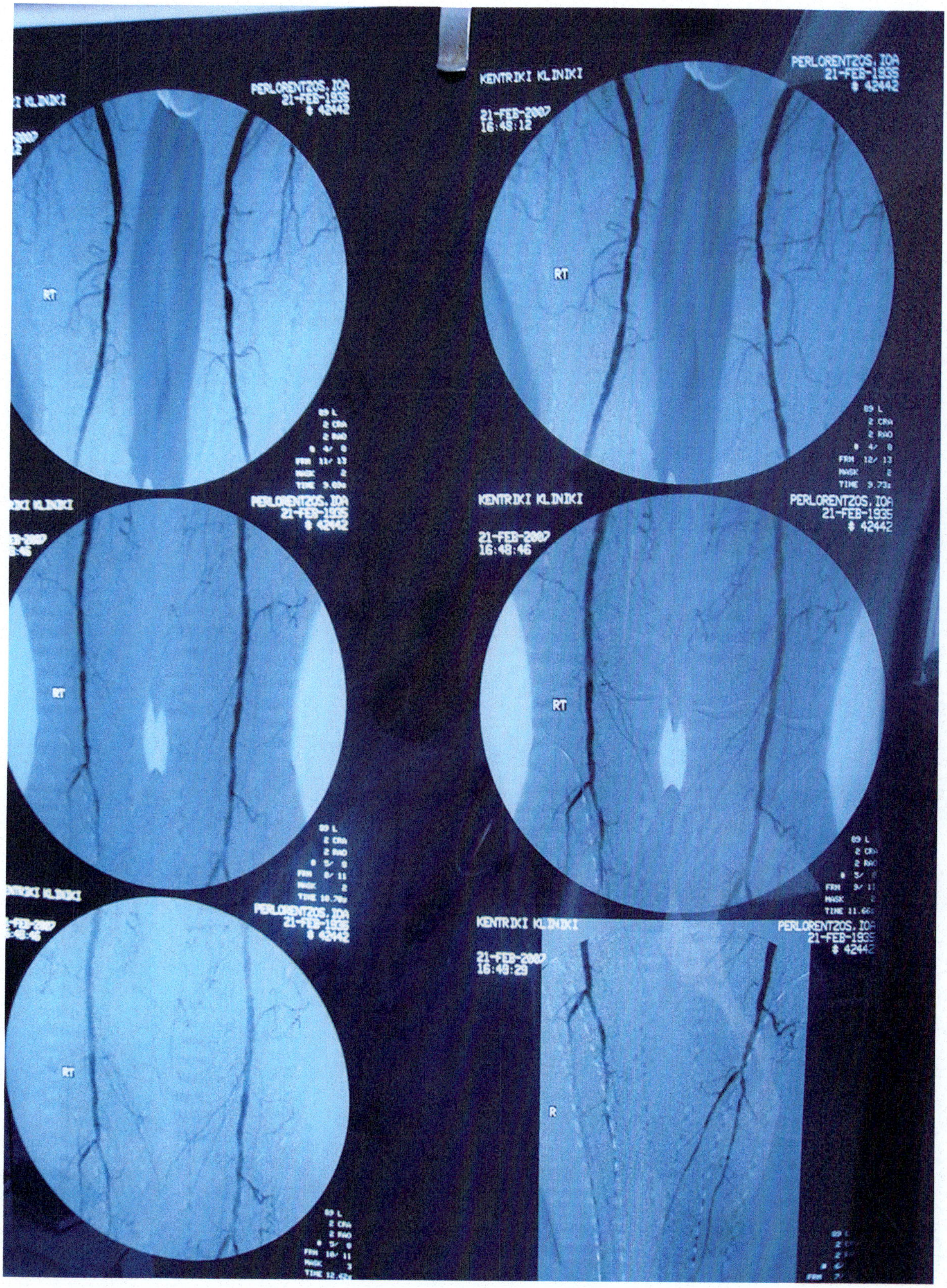

Figure 8.4 Case 8.1: Digital subtraction angiography showing multiple insignificant atheromatous lesions in the deep femoral arteries.

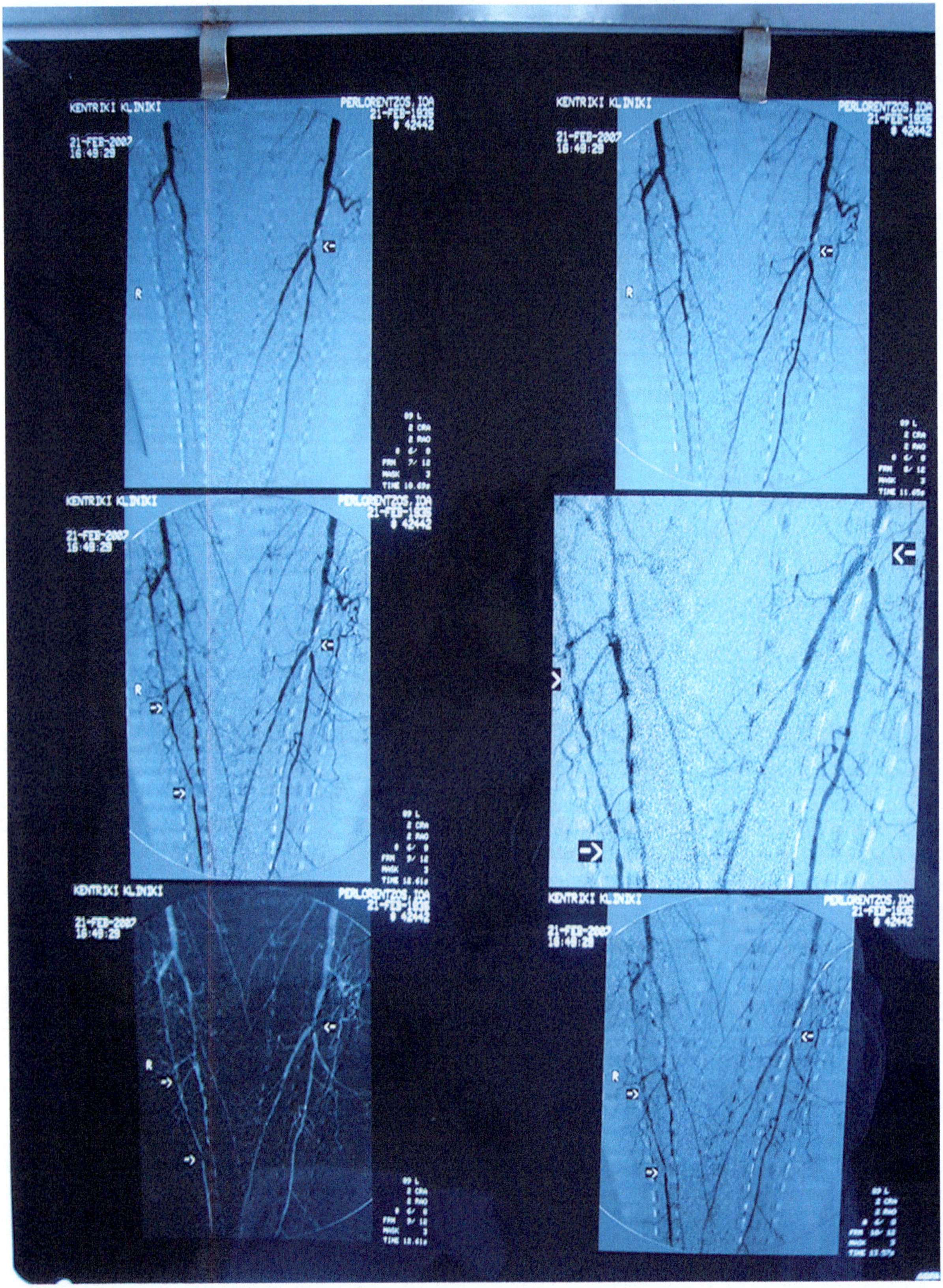

Figure 8.5 Case 8.1: Digital subtraction angiography. Note two significant occlusive lesions in the right anterior tibial artery (arrows), and total occlusion of the right posterior and left anterior tibial artery.

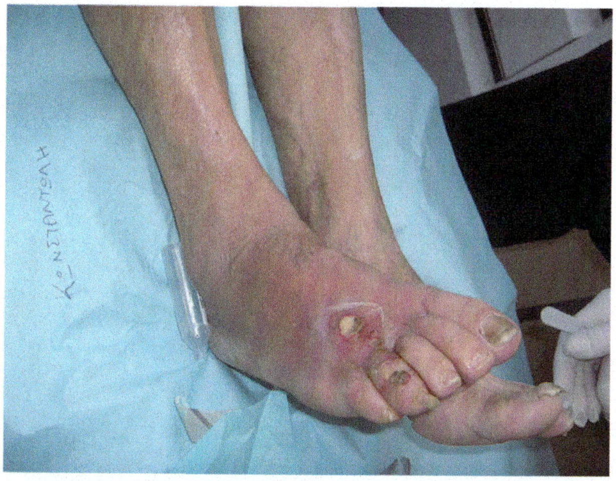

Figure 8.6 A painful infected ischemic ulcer over the fourth metatarsal head that appeared after minor trauma (from a protruding shoe seam). Note the absence of callosity and the yellowish base of the ulcer, as well as cellulitis (less than 2cm) around the ulcer.

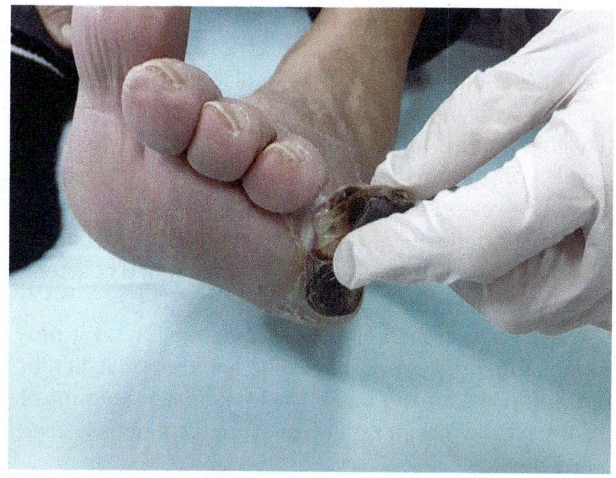

Figure 8.8 A painful ischemic ulcer involving the entire fifth toe and the interdigital space between the fourth and fifth toe. Concomitant dry gangrene of the fifth toe (expanding to the fifth metatarsal area) and wet gangrene of the interdigital space are noted.

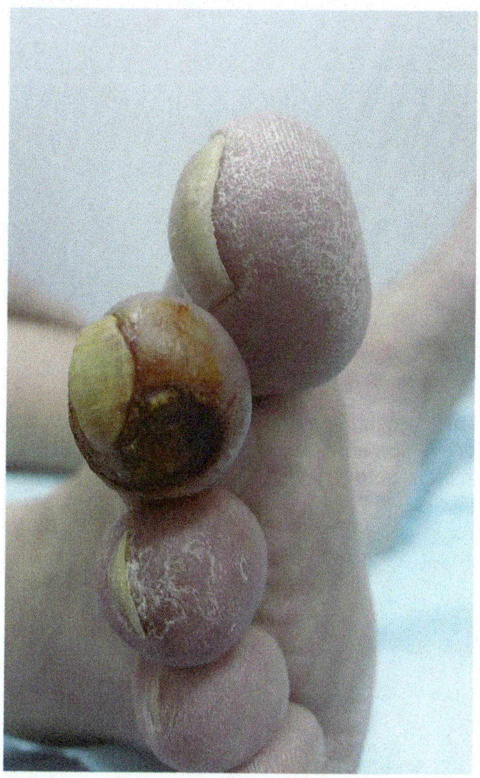

Figure 8.7 An ischemic ulcer with a necrotic lesion at the top right of the second toe.

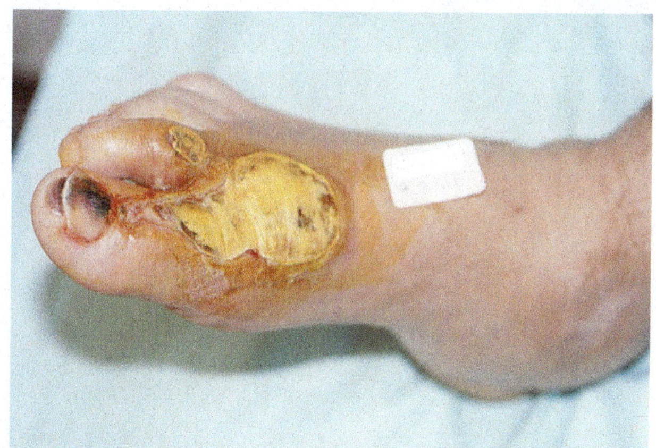

Figure 8.9 A large neuro-ischemic ulcer with exposed fascia on the dorsum of the forefoot. There is a subungual hematoma of the hallux and a healing neuro-ischemic ulcer on the second toe, in addition to significant ankle edema.

8.4 Superficial Neuro-Ischemic Ulcers of the Dorsum of the Foot

When a minor trauma occurs and local edema occludes a superficial branch of a small artery of the skin below it in the presence of neuropathy, a shallow neuro-ischemic

Case 8.2

Case 8.2 involves a painful, infected ischemic ulcer over the left fourth metatarsal head of an 85-year- old lady with longstanding type 2 diabetes (Figure 8.13). A minor trauma – a stumble over a table leg – had preceded this. Cellulitis (less than 2cm) is present around the ulcer. Calcification of the dorsal metatarsal arteries is evident in the X-ray of the foot (Figure 8.14). Aggressive antibiotic treatment on a home basis was started, and the ulcer was healing normally (Figure 8.15). This patient then had to be admitted due to acute respiratory distress, and two weeks after her initial visit to the diabetic foot clinic, she died in hospital.

Case 8.3

A 50-year-old lady with type 1 diabetes mellitus presented with an infected neuro-ischemic ulcer on her left hallux (Figure 8.16); this had started with an infected toenail. A phlegmon then spread over the base of the great toe. DSA revealed multiple stenotic lesions of both deep femoral arteries (Figure 8.17) and total obstruction of both popliteal arteries, as well as an extended collateral vasculature (Figure 8.18).

DSA has replaced film screen angiography as it provides superior contrast resolution and the capability for post-processing the data. It uses a smaller amount of contrast and maximizes the guidance for minimally invasive therapy.

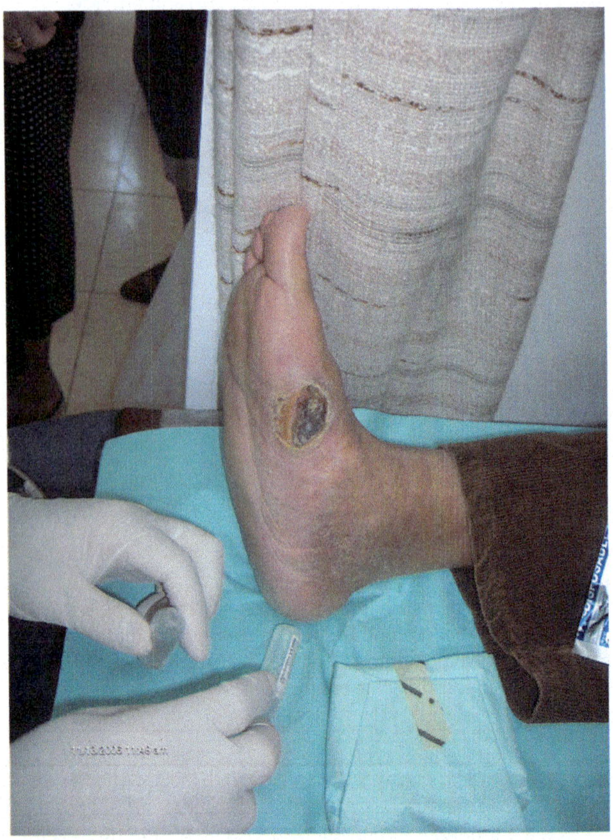

Figure 8.10 A painless superficial neuro-ischemic ulcer on the medial aspect of the foot of a patient with known diabetic neuropathy. Note the mixed features of ischemia and neuropathy. The patient described the development of this ulcer (and its expansion to this size) as spontaneous, and he did not bother reporting it.

ulcer may form over the ischemic area. This ulcer may be self-limiting and painless (Figures 8.10 and 8.11), or it may be complicated by infection, develop cellulitis (Figure 8.12) and become painful.

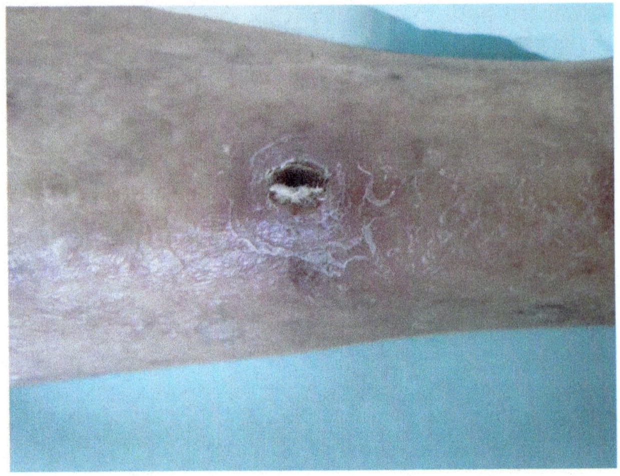

Figure 8.11 A relatively painless healing ischemic ulcer on the anterior lower leg.

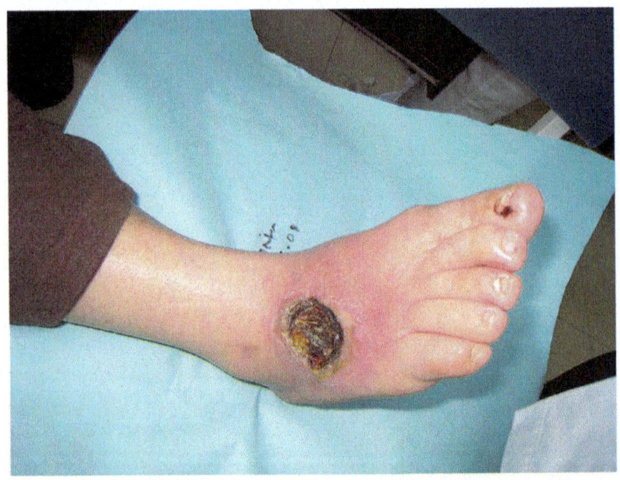

Figure 8.12 A shallow neuro-ischemic ulcer on the dorsum of the foot. The base of the ulcer is painless and necrotic, while cellulitis around the hard callus border of the ulcer is painful.

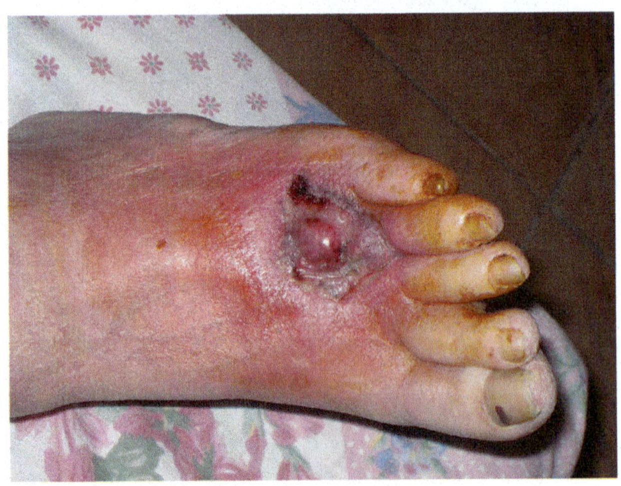

Figure 8.13 Case 8.2: A painful infected ischemic ulcer over the left fourth metatarsal head. Cellulitis is apparent over the ulcer.

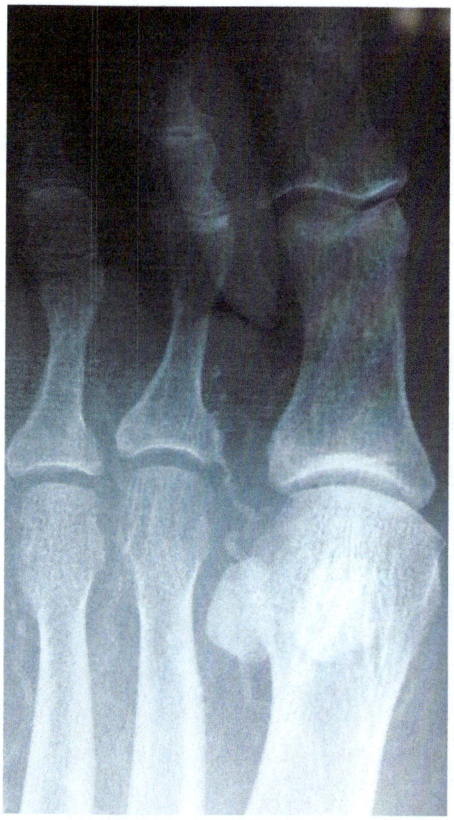

Figure 8.14 Case 8.2: Calcification of the first dorsal metatarsal artery in an 85-year-old lady with type 2 diabetes.

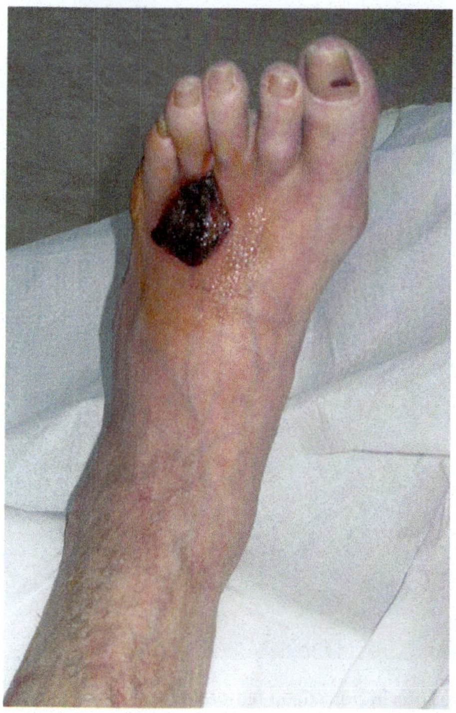

Figure 8.15 Case 8.2: A healing ulcer from the patient shown in Figure 8.13, six days after the patient's first visit.

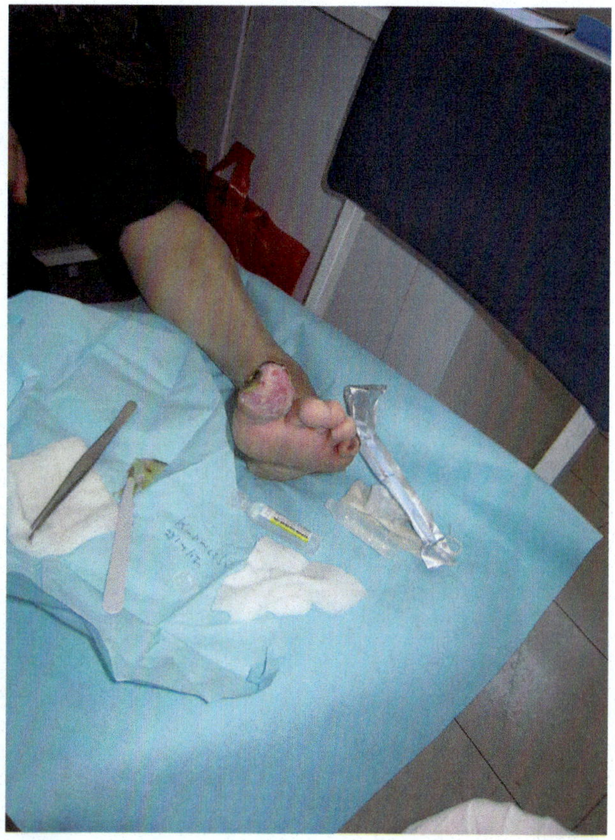

Figure 8.16 Case 8.3: An infected neuro-ischemic ulcer on the medial aspect of the tip of the left hallux revealed after the removal of phlegmon. There are necrotic borders to the lesion, and a small hemorrhage is seen on the fifth toe.

Clinically, a smooth, round, distinct border of callosity (a neuropathic feature) and the black sturdy necrotic base of the ulcer (an ischemic feature) are present. It may or may not need to be treated with aggressive antibiotic treatment. Off-loading is usually easy in this area of the foot.

8.5 Diabetic Gangrene ("End-artery" Disease)

"End-artery" disease, a term used for coronary heart disease or kidney artery disease, is sometimes applied to -the diabetic foot. In the normal foot, major injuries and operations are well tolerated by means of the arterial circulation distal to the ankle, since the plantar and the dorsal arches, their communications and the smaller arteries are patent.

In the diabetic foot, however, smaller unnamed arteries may function as "end-arteries" due to multiple complete blockade and/or partial constrictive atherosclerotic lesions. Therefore local edema and thrombosis due to

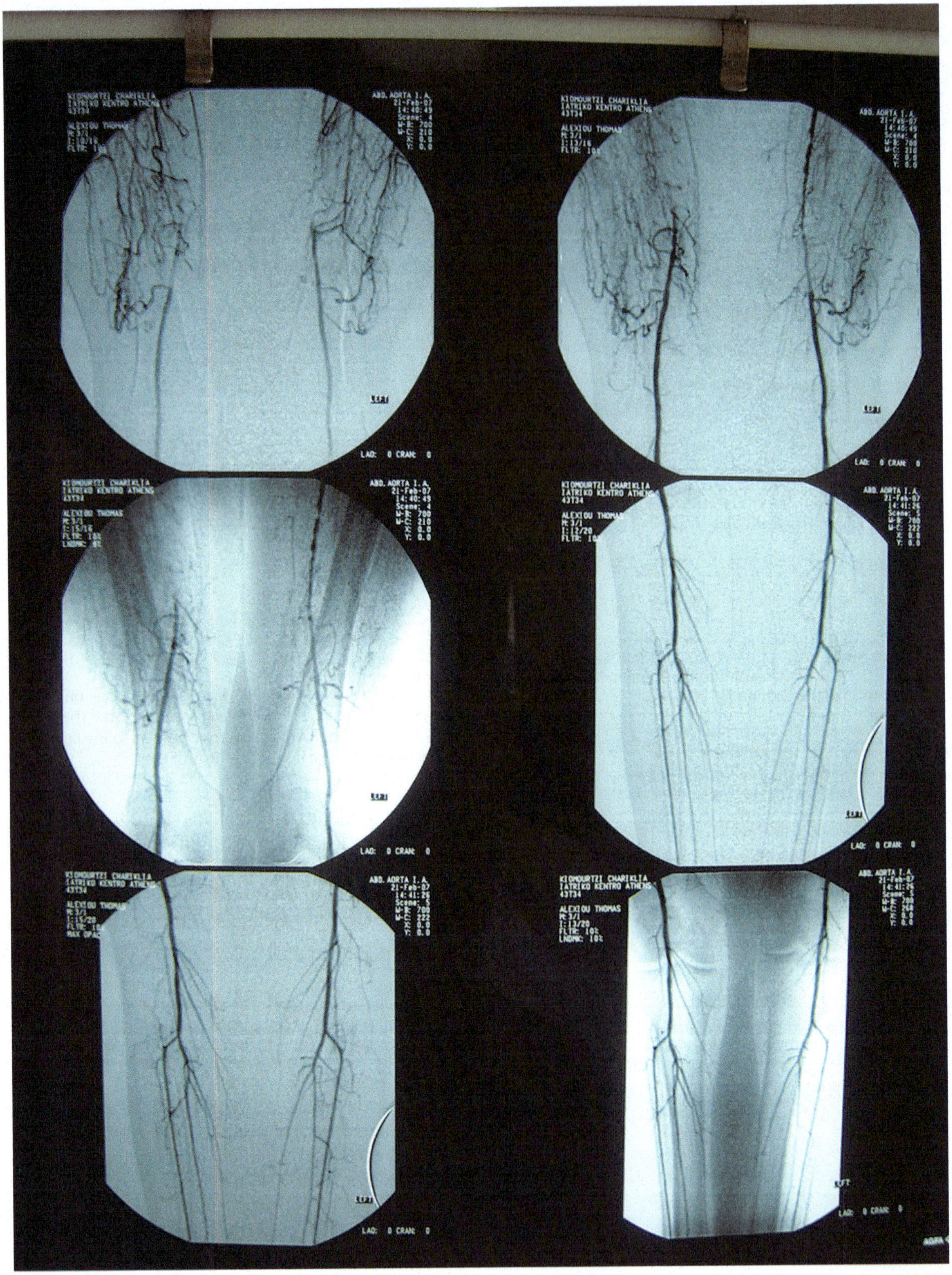

Figure 8.17 Case 8.3: Digital subtraction angiography showing multiple atherosclerotic lesions in both deep femoral arteries (lower panel).

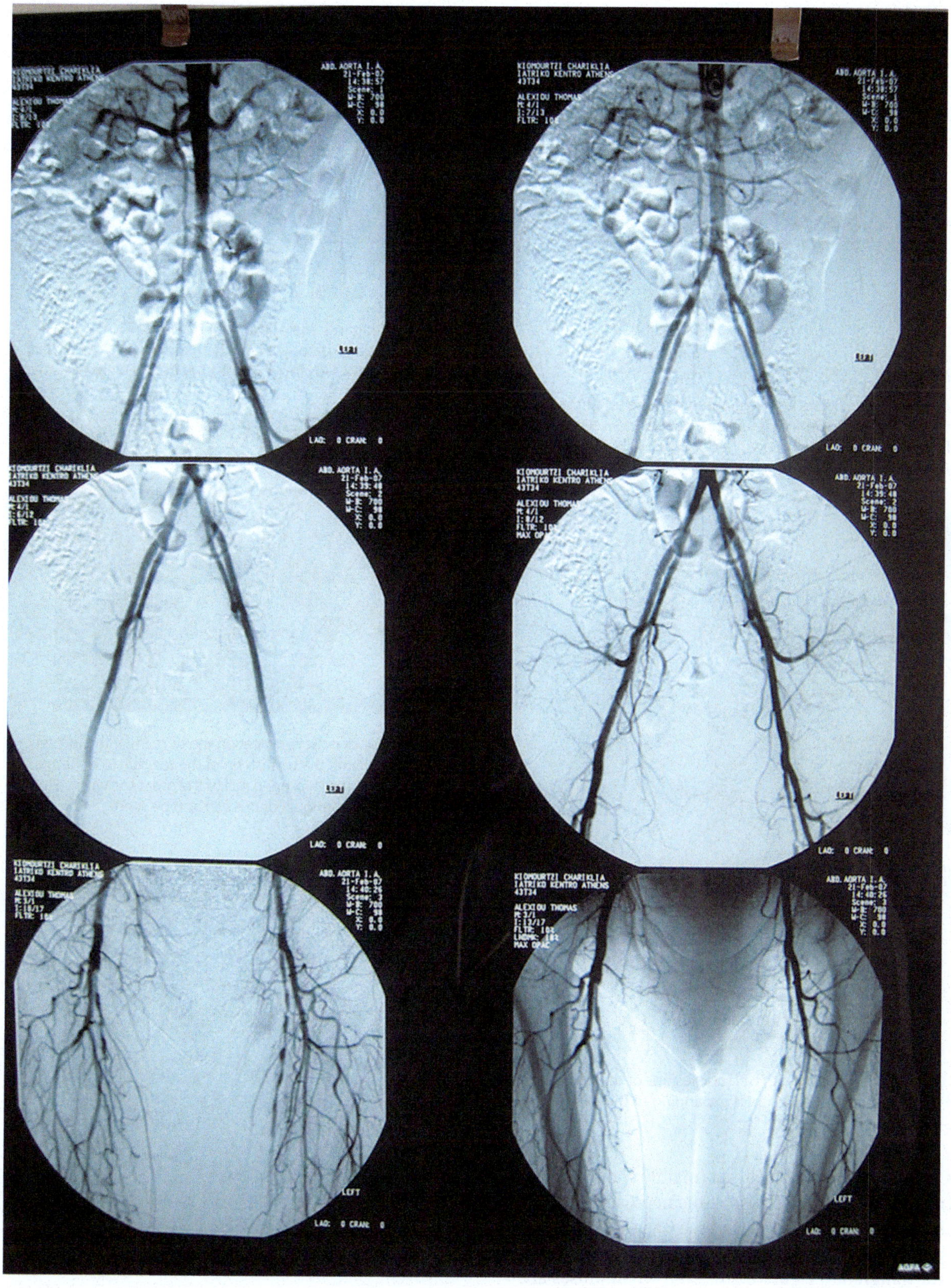

Figure 8.18 Case 8.3: Digital subtraction angiography showing total obstruction of both popliteal arteries with a significant collateral circulation (upper panel).

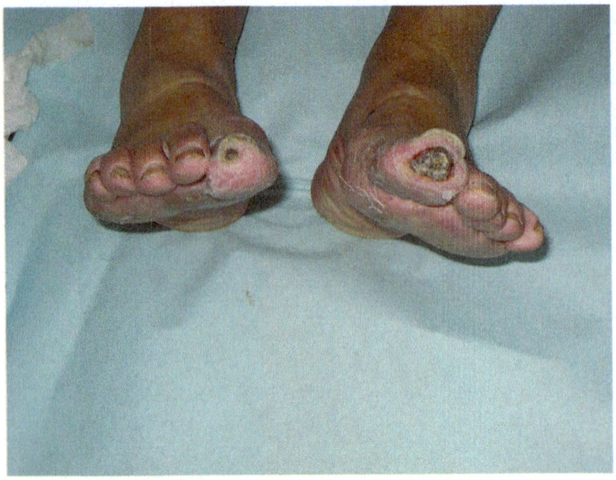

Figure 8.19 Ischemic necrosis (dry gangrene) of the tip of the halluxes, which started as pressure ulcers (the toe tips were pressed against by the patient's own bedding). Dry skin and claw toes are also apparent.

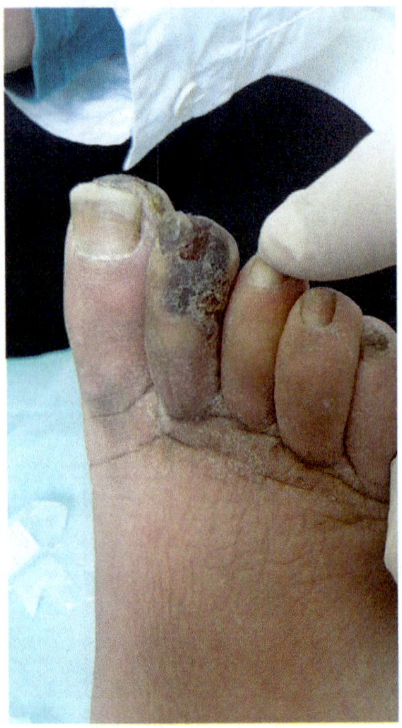

Figure 8.20 Ischemic ulcers with necrotic lesions of the first and second toe. The second toe's lesion is expanding to the exterior surface of the second phalange.

toxins produced by some bacteria (mainly staphylococci and streptococci) may cause ischemic necrosis of the tip of a toe (Figures 8.19 and 8.20, and see Case 8.4), of a part of its surface (Figures 8.21–8.22) or of one or more toes ("diabetic gangrene"; Figure 8.23), even when pulses are present in the foot arteries.

In the case of localized necrosis of the tip of a toe, removal of the gangrenous tissue, together with aggressive treatment of the infection, may lead to healing as long as the small arteries are still patent (see Case 8.4). Transluminal

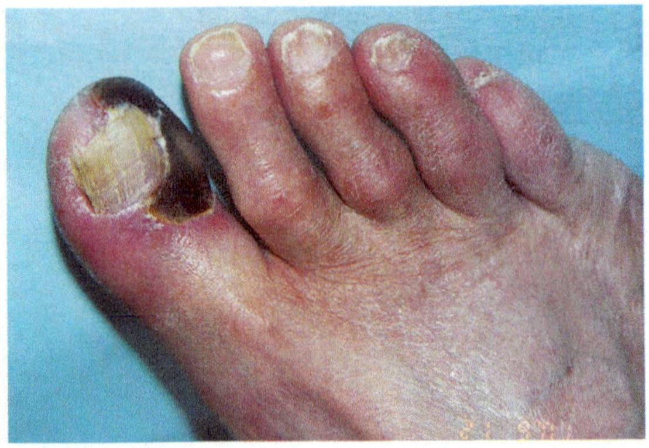

Figure 8.21 Wet gangrene of the right hallux due to onychocryptosis and paronychia. Ischemic changes (loss of hair, redness over the toes, dystrophic nail changes) can also be seen.

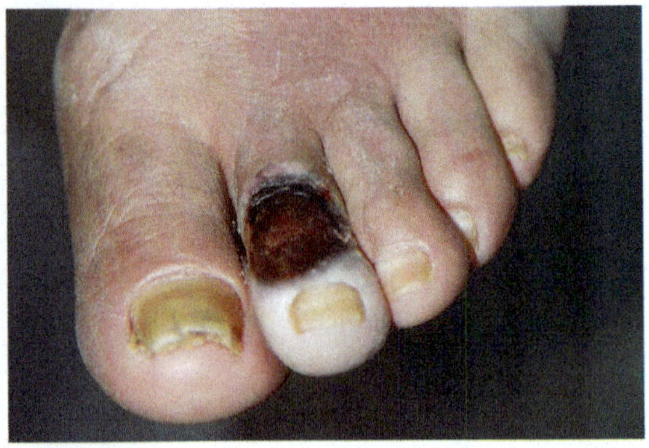

Figure 8.22 A black ischemic ulcer on the dorsum of the left second toe, with edema. Note the whitish tip of the toe due to ischemia. A fungal infection of the thickened nail of the great toe with yellowish discoloration and subungual debris can also be seen.

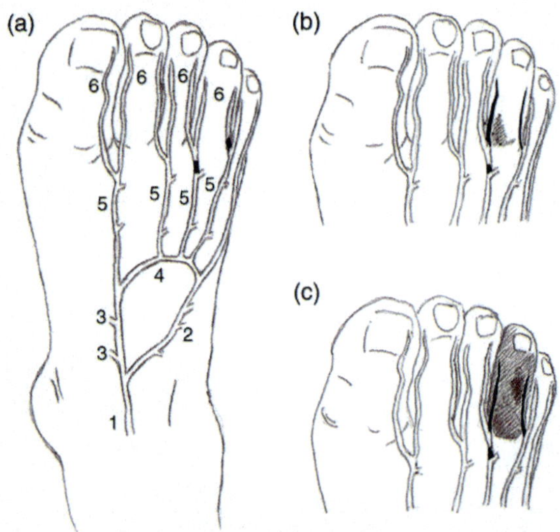

Figure 8.23 The mechanism underlying diabetic gangrene. Obliteration of the small arteries by atheromatosis (a), complicated by infection (b), results in gangrene (c). Arteries of the dorsum of the foot: (1) dorsal artery of the foot; (2) lateral tarsal artery; (3) medial tarsal arteries; (4) arcuate artery; (5) dorsal metatarsal arteries; (6) dorsal digital arteries.

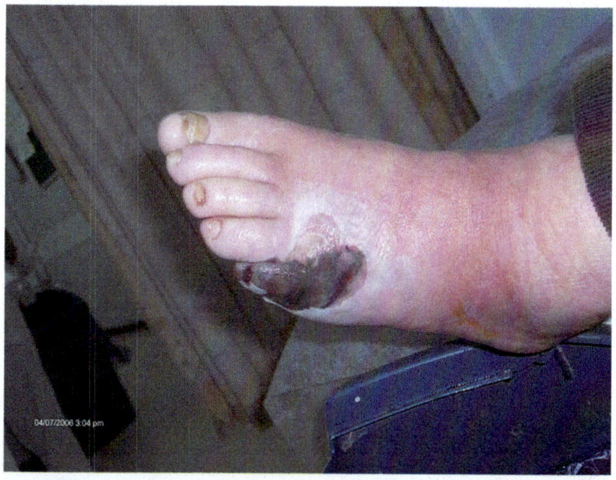

Figure 8.24 Wet gangrene of the fifth toe. Fontaine stage IV, Rutherford grade III, category 5.

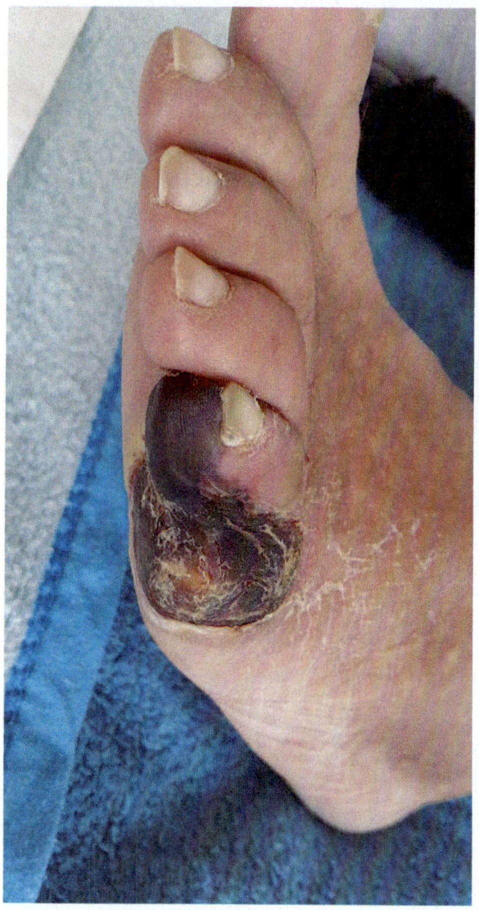

Figure 8.25 Dry gangrene covering the exterior surfaces of the fifth toe and fifth metatarsal area. Note the well-defined limits of the lesion.

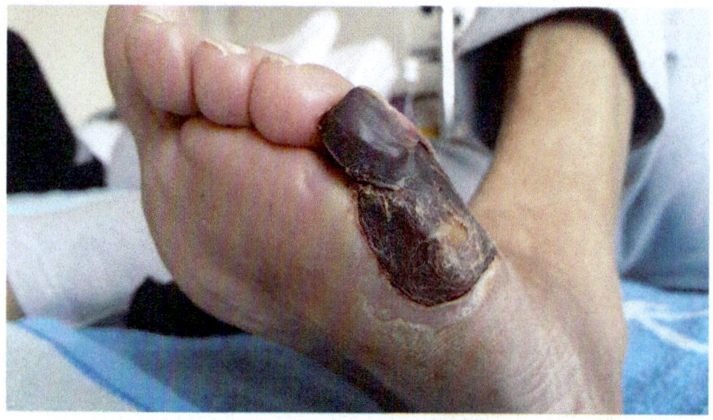

Figure 8.26 Dry gangrene covering the exterior surfaces of the fifth toe and fifth metatarsal area. Note the well-defined limits of the lesion.

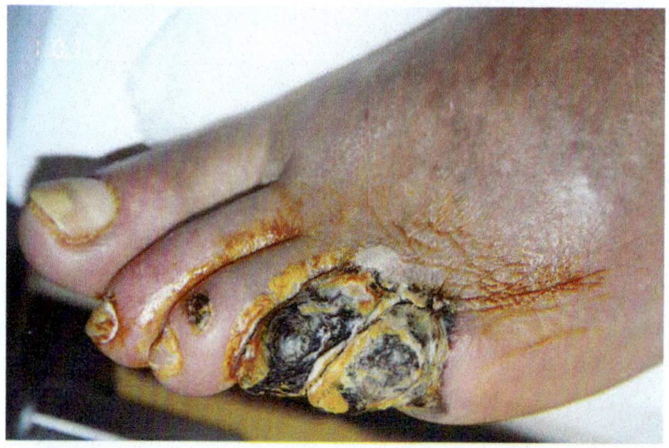

Figure 8.27 Dry gangrene of the fourth and fifth toes. Injury to the fifth toe preceded the situation, and gangrene of the fourth toe followed. An ischemic ulcer is seen on the dorsum of the third toe. *Source:* Courtesy of E. Bastounis.

angioplasty or stenting of the occluded arteries will allow proper antibiotic treatment and salvage of the foot, while a gangrenous toe will be isolated by mummification (dry gangrene) without major consequences (see Case 8.5). Gangrene of the fifth toe (Figures 8.24–8.27) or the hallux (Figures 8.28 and 8.29–8.31) is due to more extended atherosclerotic disease and will probably lead to toe amputation or disarticulation (Figure 8.31).

Case 8.4

Infected neuro-ischemic ulcers were seen on the tips of the big toes of a 60-year-old lady with type 2 diabetes (Figure 8.32) who had undergone right second ray amputation (Figure 8.33). The patient refused right hallux amputation, so was given aggressive treatment for the osteomyelitis, together with alcohol treatment of the gangrenous lesions of the tips of the great toes, which led to a successful result (Figure 8.34). This disease was Fontaine stage IV, Rutherford grade III (minor tissue loss), category 5.

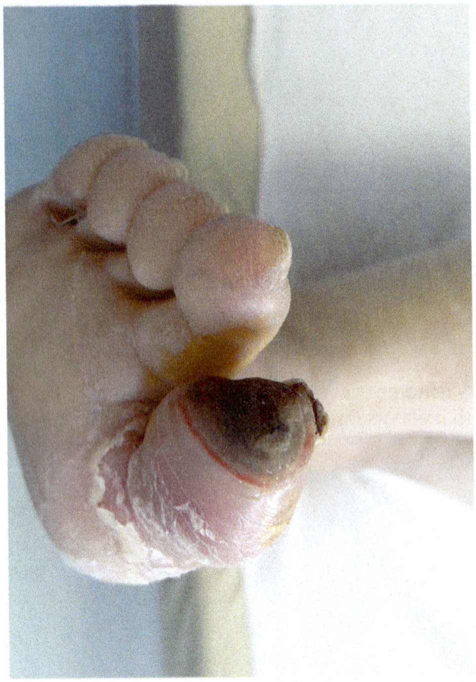

Figure 8.28 Necrotic lesion on the tip of the hallux in a patient with known peripheral artery disease. The necrotic area is well-defined but there is a small amount of apparent exudate production (wet gangrene).

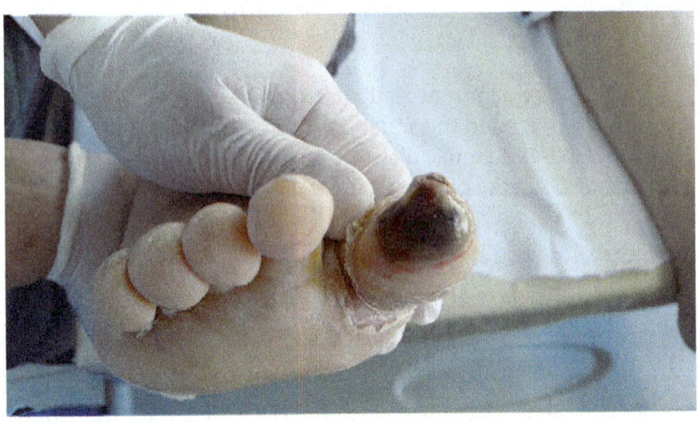

Figure 8.29 Necrotic lesion on the tip of the hallux in a patient with known peripheral artery disease. The necrotic area is well-defined but there is a small amount of apparent exudate production (wet gangrene).

A superficial skin hematoma may sometimes be misdiagnosed as ischemic necrosis of the skin, due to deep dark tissue discoloration. Careful physical examination, a history of trauma and duplex ultrasonography are usually adequate means to successfully differentiate these conditions (Case 8.6).

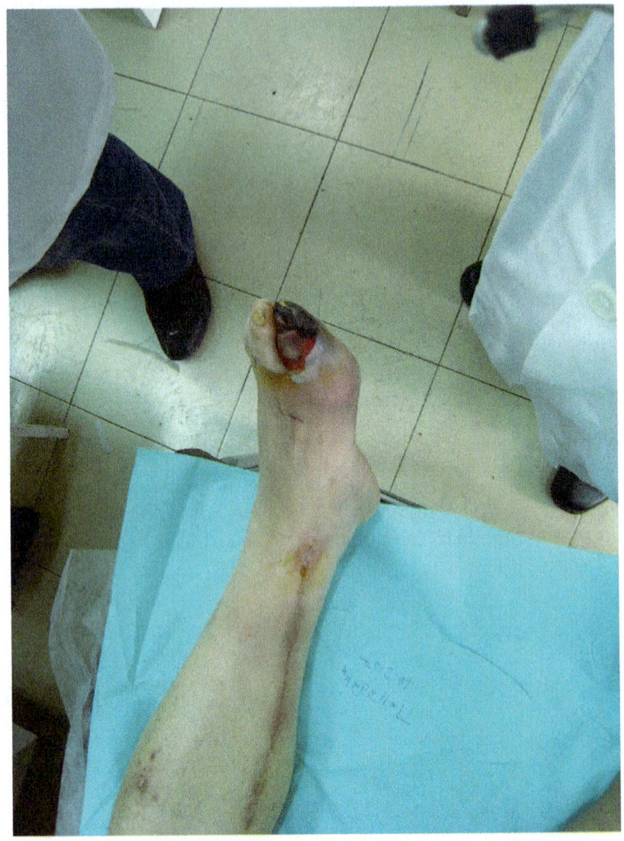

Figure 8.30 Diabetic gangrene (wet gangrene) of the left hallux. Note the below-knee femoropopliteal bypass scar. Fontaine stage IV, Rutherford grade III (minor tissue loss), category 5.

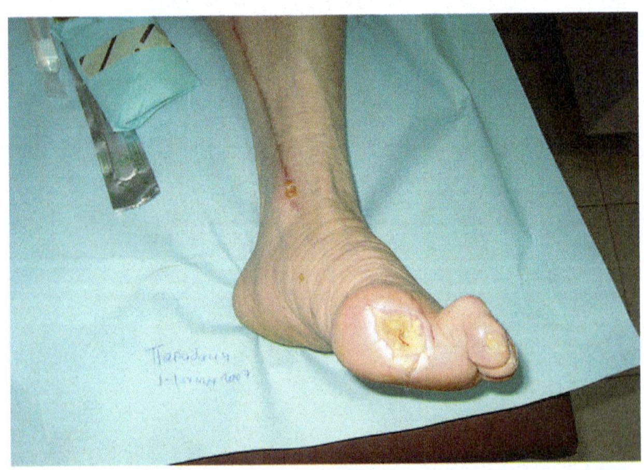

Figure 8.31 Hallux disarticulation and claw toes on the same foot as in Figure 8.37, one month after the procedure.

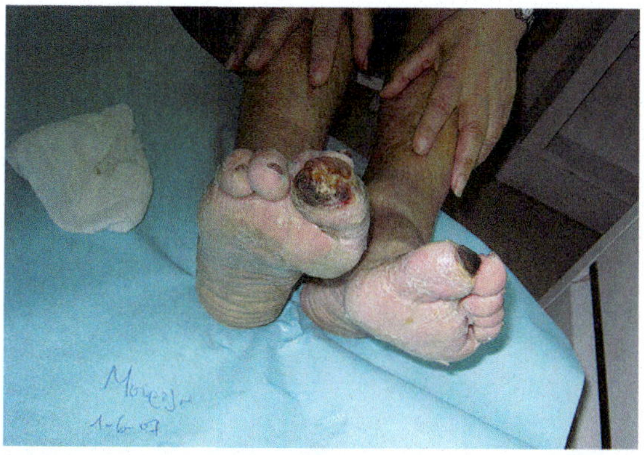

Figure 8.32 Case 8.4: Bilateral ischemic ulcers of the hallux, with osteomyelitis of the right hallux.

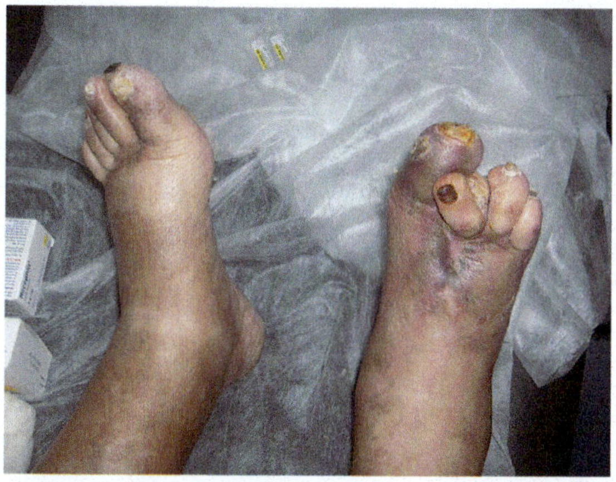

Figure 8.33 Case 8.4: A right second ray amputation with a second overriding toe. There is osteomyelitis of the right hallux and also an infected neuro-ischemic ulcer.

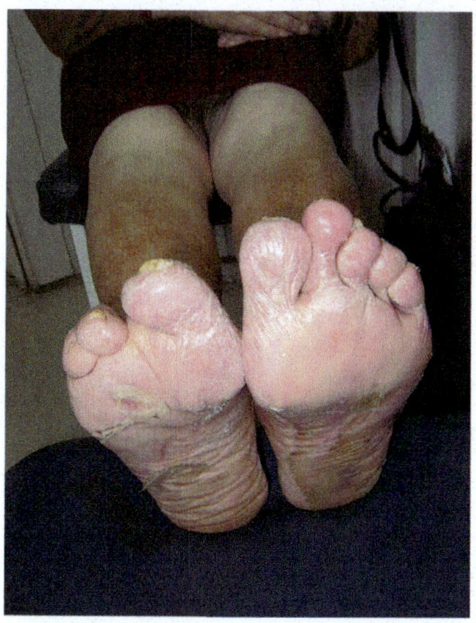

Figure 8.34 Case 8.4: Healed bilateral ischemic ulcers of the great toes. The plantar scaling arose due to alcohol dressings.

Case 8.5

Gangrene of the right fourth toe occurred in a 71-year-old gentleman with type 2 diabetes. This man was admitted due to an infected neuro-ischemic ulcer under his fourth metatarsal head, and wet gangrene of his fourth toe. A stress fracture of the proximal phalanx of the fifth toe was present on a plain radiograph (Figure 8.35), while osteomyelitis of the head of the fourth metatarsal could not be excluded. DSA was carried out, which disclosed multiple sites of stenosis in both the iliac and superficial femoral arteries (Figure 8.36). A suboptimal angioplasty was carried out on both arteries, and stents were inserted (Figure 8.37). The infection was treated successfully and the fourth toe was mummified (dry gangrene; Figure 8.38).

During percutaneous transluminal angioplasty, a balloon catheter is used to increase the diameter of the lumen of the arteriosclerotic artery. This is a relatively safe and minimally invasive technique (compared with surgery); it preserves the saphenous veins and reduces the length of hospital stay. However, this procedure fails more often in diabetic than in non-diabetic patients, due to intimal hyperplasia.

Stents are used to treat suboptimal angioplasty, lesions with severe dissections and significant residual stenosis after angioplasty. The first endovascular stent approved for use in the iliac arteries was the Palmaz stent, a single stainless steel tube, deployed by balloon expansion. The Wallstent, a flexible self-expanding stent that is available in several different diameters, is also in use. New covered stents are being evaluated, with the hope that they may mimic surgical grafts and resist re-stenosis.

Case 8.6

A 68- year old man was referred to the diabetes foot clinic as having possible ischemic necrosis of the lateral aspects of the left hallux, presenting 24 hours after total onychectomy. The patient noticed the development of "black colored spots" on the nail bed a few hours after the procedure (Figures 8.39 and 8.40). He had mild pain. The patient had type 2 diabetes since the age of 50 and he had been previously diagnosed with diabetic neuropathy and peripheral arterial disease. A careful close-up examination revealed as most probable explanation for the skin discoloration the formation of a hematoma, produced due to tissue injury during the onychectomy. Note that the lesions are located on both lateral aspects of the nail bed (a common place for a hematoma to occur) and not on the tip of the toe (the most probable site for ischemic necrosis). In addition, the irregular shape of the lesions are more compatible with a skin hematoma. Finally, the lesion was soft and "elastic" in palpation, not resembling to a firm and well-defined necrotic injury. The hematoma was then carefully removed (Figure 8.41).

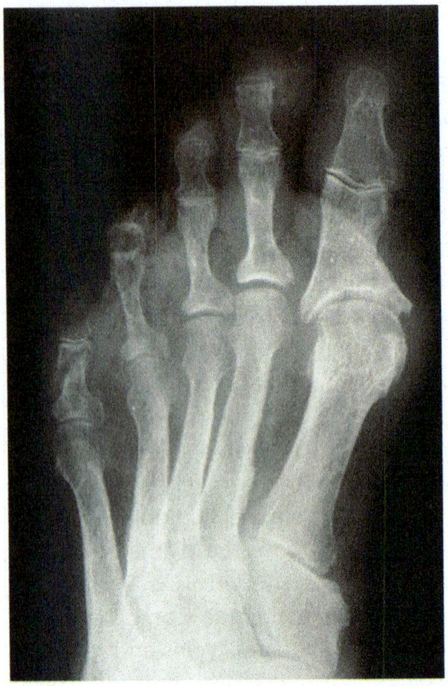

Figure 8.35 Case 8.5: A plain radiograph of the patient shown in Figures 8.44–8.46. There is a stress fracture of the proximal phalanx of the fifth toe, and osteoarthritis of the first and fourth metatarsophalangeal joints.

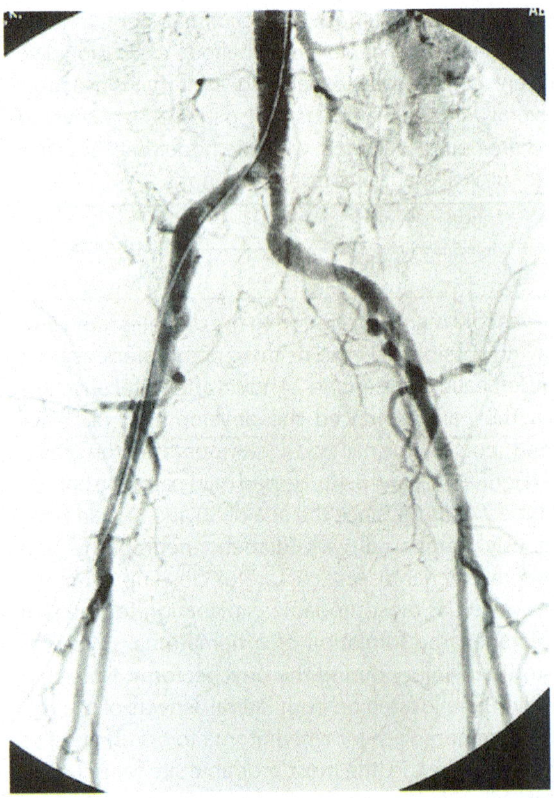

Figure 8.36 Case 8.5: Digital subtraction angiography showing severe stenosis after the bifurcation of the celiac aorta. *Source:* Courtesy of C. Liapis.

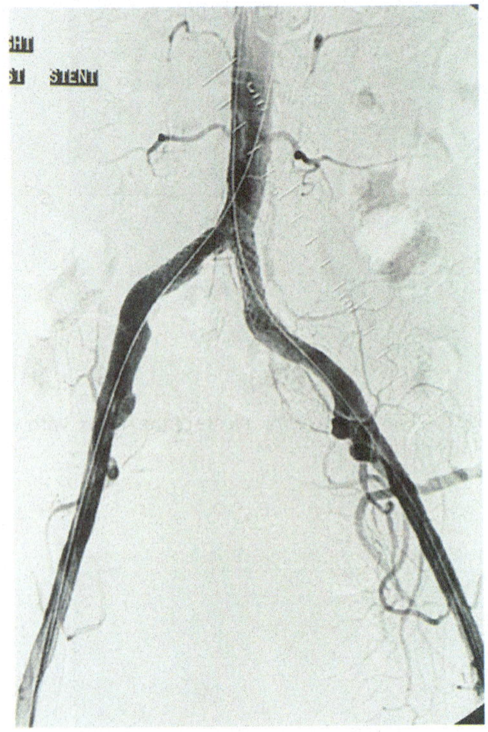

Figure 8.37 Case 8.5: Post-stenting digital subtraction angiography. *Source:* Courtesy of C. Liapis.

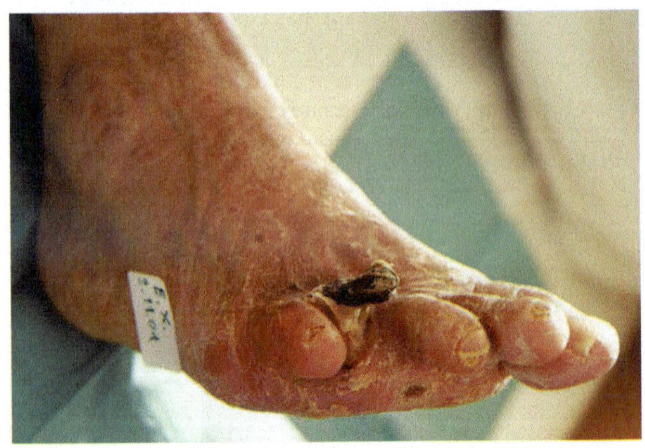

Figure 8.38 Case 8.5: Dry gangrene of the right fourth toe. A neuro-ischemic ulcer is present under the third metatarsal head.

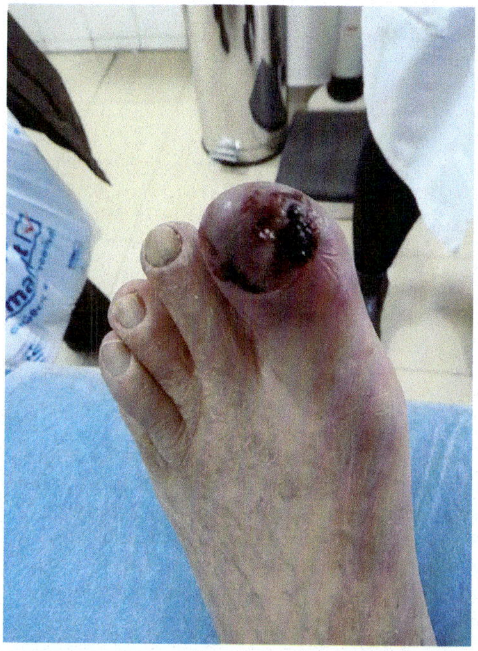

Figure 8.39 Case 8.6: A hematoma of the bed nail of the hallux after total onychectomy. Note the location (lateral) and the irregular shape of the lesion, (together with the patient history) differentiates it from gangrene.

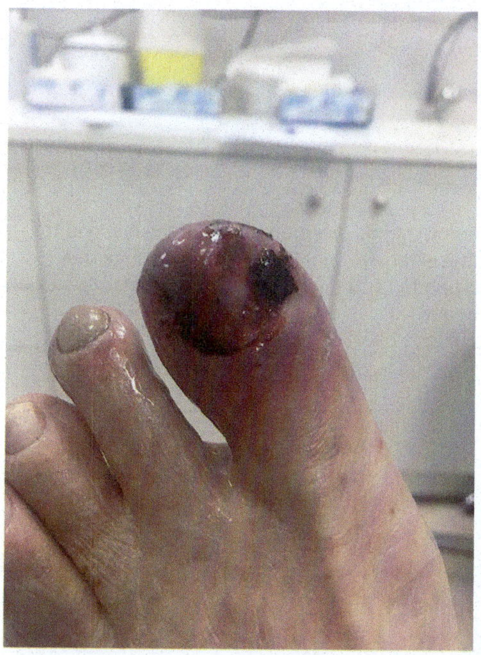

Figure 8.40 Case 8.6 : a hematoma of the bed nail of the hallux after total onychectomy. Note the location (lateral) and the irregular shape of the lesion, (together with the patient history) differentiates it from gangrene.

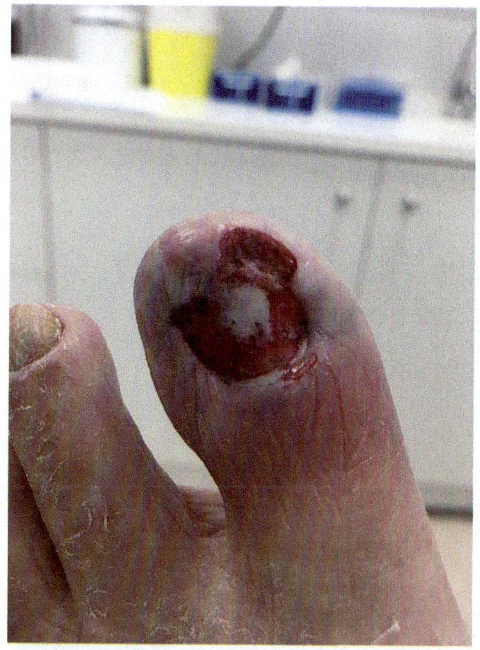

Figure 8.41 The same foot as in Figures 8.38 and 8.39 after removal of the hematoma.

8.6 Neuro-Ischemic Ulcers of the Toes or Forefoot

The neuro-ischemic ulcer combines features both of a neuropathic ulcer (location over a bony prominence, some callus formation – but not as extended as for a typical neuropathic ulcer – and the presence of diabetic neuropathy) and of an ischemic ulcer (irregular borders, necrotic tissue – when collateral circulation is absolutely inadequate – and the presence of peripheral artery disease) (Figures 8.42–8.46).

The site of neuro-ischemic ulcers is somewhat different from the site of the typical neuropathic ulcer, since they tend to develop on less loaded points of the toes; on the dorsum (Figure 8.47) and the lateral or medial aspects of the toes (Figures 8.48 and 8.49); on the medial aspect of the head of the first metatarsal (Figure 8.50) or the lateral aspect of the head of the fifth metatarsal (Figures 8.51); or on the dorsum of the foot (Figures 8.51 and 8.52). However, any typical painless neuropathic ulcer (located under a metatarsal head, for example) is often diagnosed with ischemia, particularly when it resists healing; it is then considered to be neuro-ischemic (Figure 8.53). Any infected neuro-ischemic ulcer may progress to osteomyelitis (Figure 8.54).

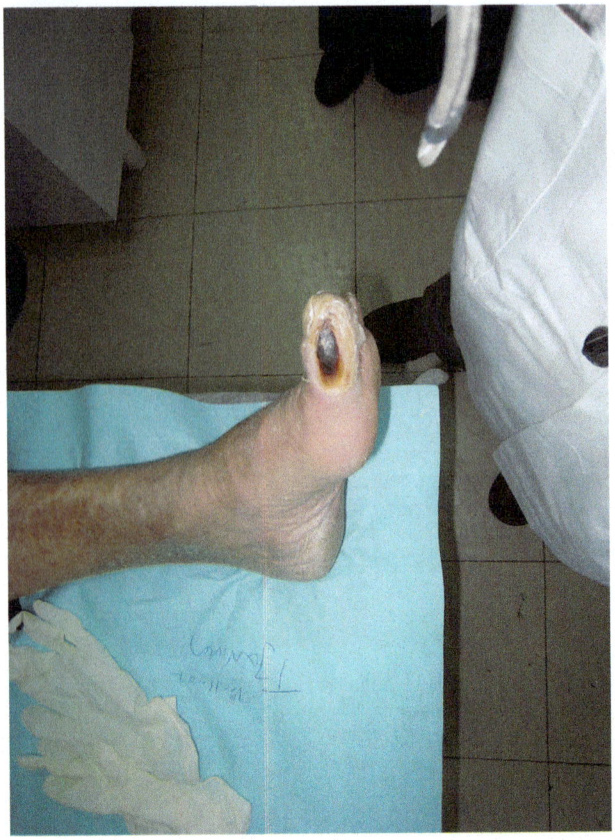

Figure 8.42 A neuro-ischemic ulcer on the medial surface of the hallux.

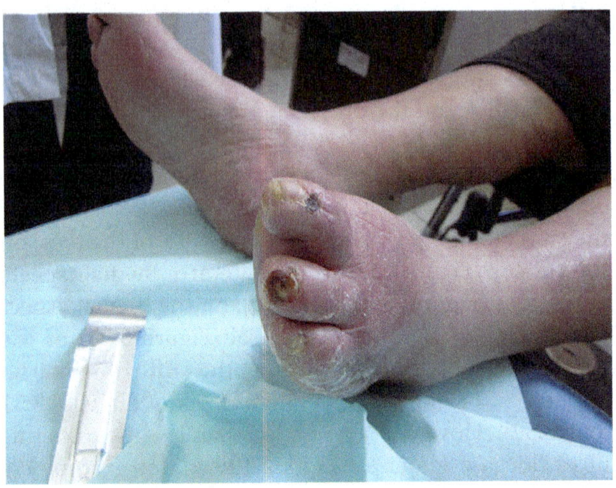

Figure 8.43 Neuroischemic ulcers on the top of the fourth toe and the dorsum of the third toe. This diabetic patient's first and second toes have been previously amputated.

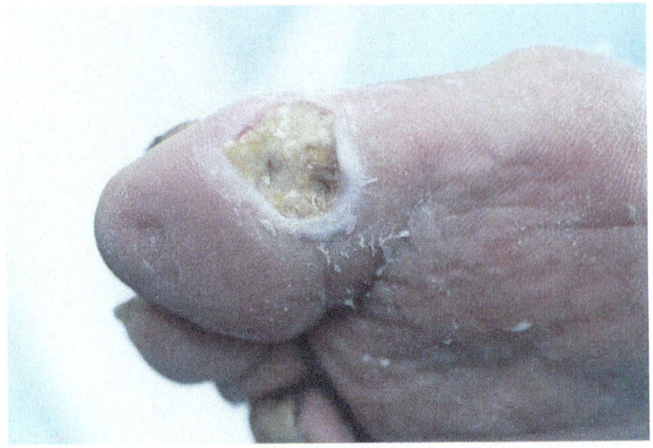

Figure 8.44 A neuro-ischemic ulcer on the tip of a hallux valgus caused by friction from a shoe seam. Off-loading and dextranomer beadlets (Debrisan; Johnson & Johnson Corp., New Brunswick, NJ, USA) were used, after a short course of antibiotics. Surgical debridement was not possible due to the hard tissue of the base of the ulcer, and the pain, which the patient could not tolerate.

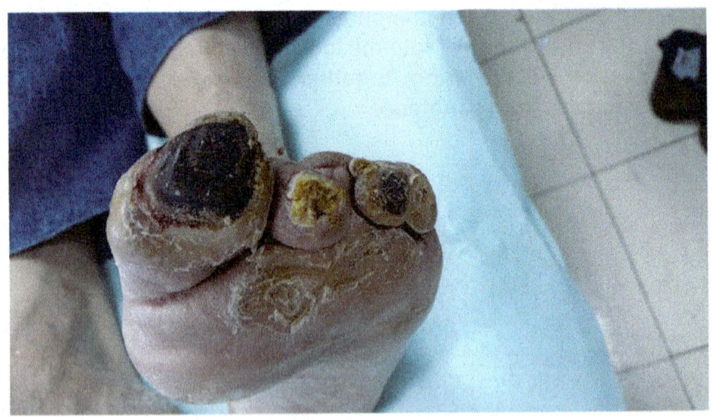

Figure 8.45 Neuroischemic ulcers on the tip of the first and the third toe. Note the extensive, in this case, callus formation (a hallmark of neuropathy) and the necrotic areas (dry gangrene), a hallmark of ischemia.

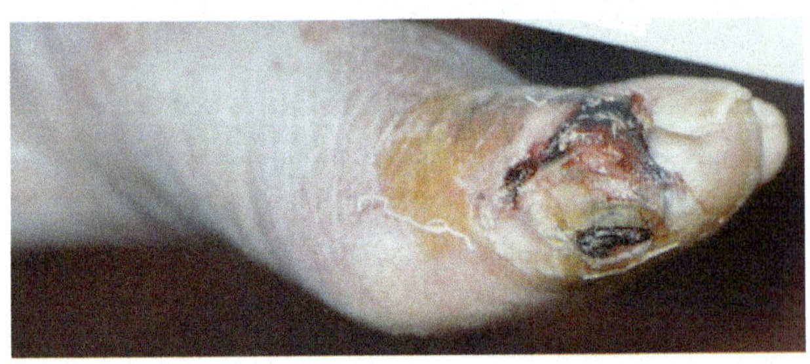

Figure 8.46 A neuro-ischemic ulcer on the medial aspect of the hallux. Note the irregular shape of the ulcer and the necrotic tissue.

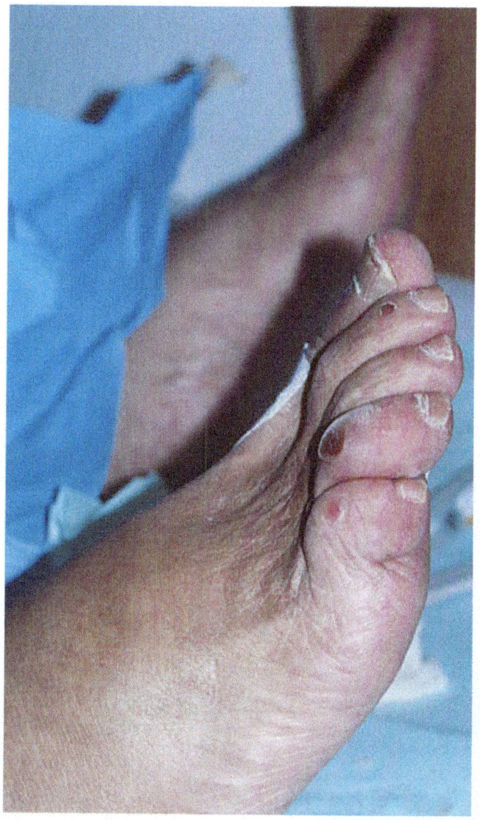

Figure 8.47 Neuro-ischemic ulcers on the dorsum of claw toes.

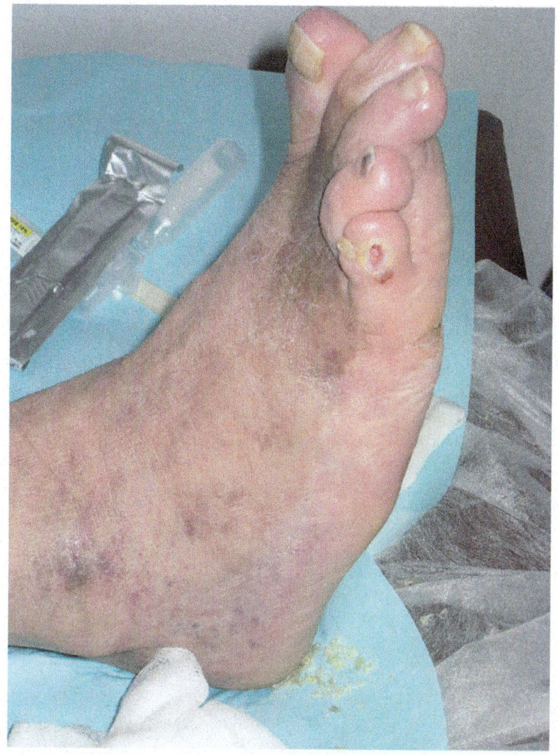

Figure 8.49 A neuro-ischemic ulcer of the fifth toe.

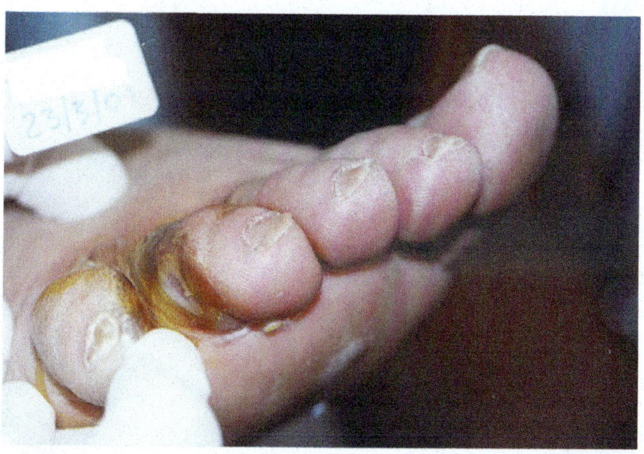

Figure 8.48 Painless interdigital neuro-ischemic ulceration caused by tight shoes.

Friction in the shoes is probably the most common cause of neuro-ischemic ulcers, and off-loading is fundamental for their cure. Revascularization is the cornerstone of treatment of these ulcers, yet in some areas of the foot and in simple cases, proper local treatment (off-loading, debridement, wet gauze) may suffice, especially when no aggressive infection is present (Figures 8.55–8.57).

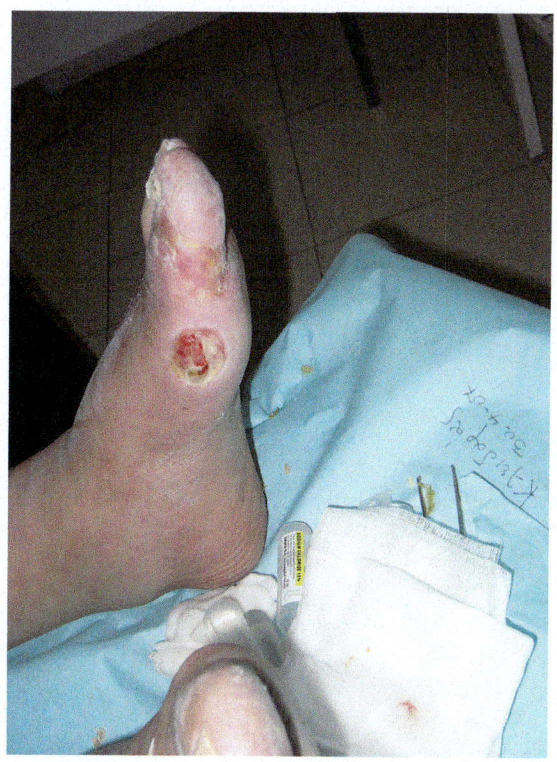

Figure 8.50 A neuro-ischemic ulcer on the medial aspect of the first metatarsal head. Scaling of the hallux is due to previous cellulitis and edema.

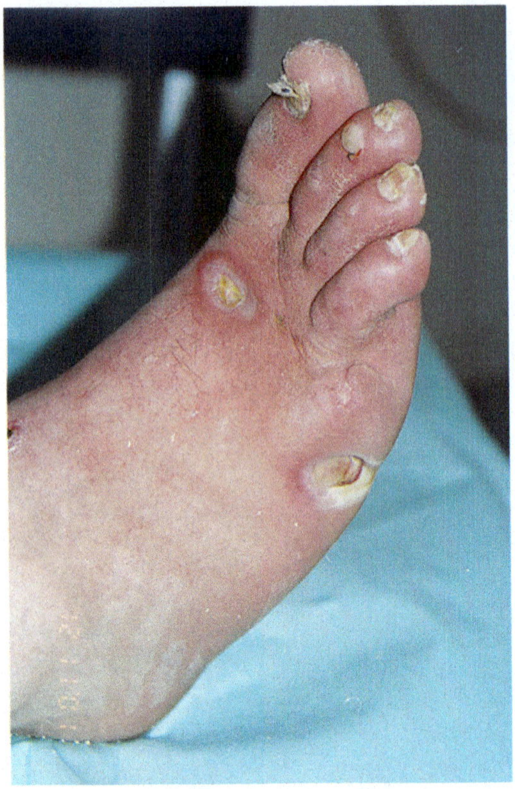

Figure 8.51 Neuro-ischemic ulcers over the first and fifth metatarsal heads. Fifth toe disarticulation can be seen. A superficial ulcer is present on the second toe, as well as onychodystrophy.

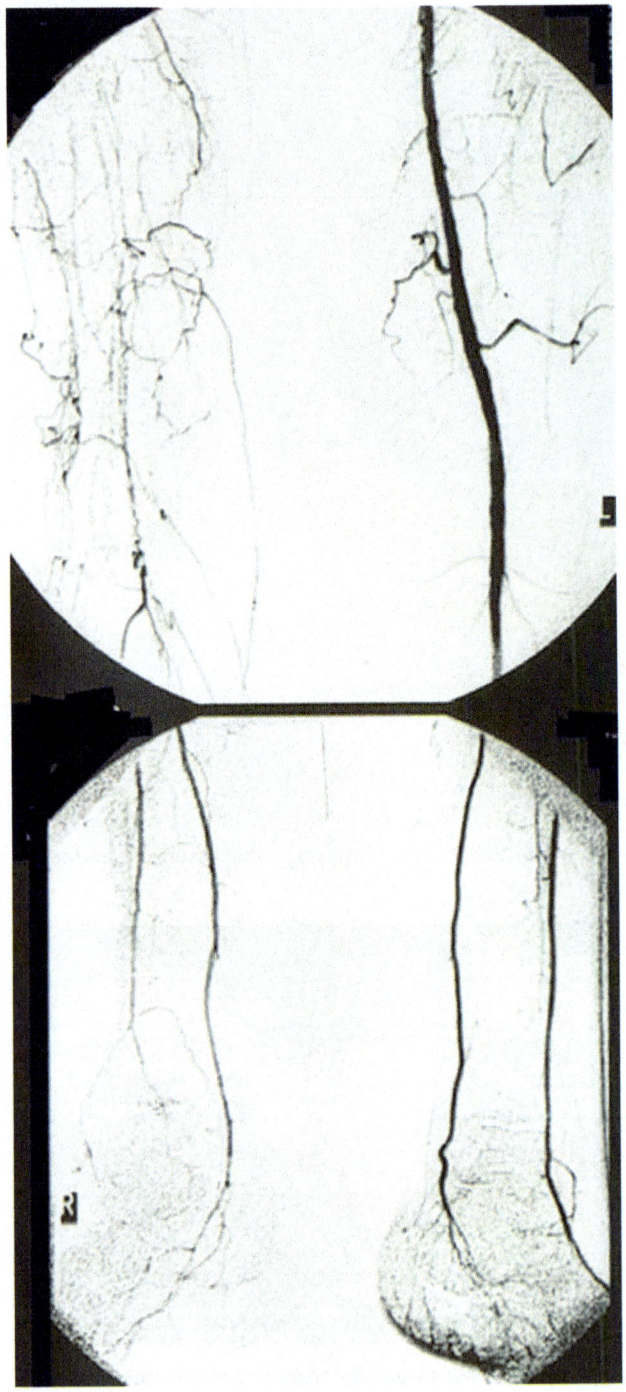

Figure 8.52 Arteriography of the patient whose foot is shown in Figure 8.60. There is severe obstruction of the distal part of the right femoral and popliteal arteries; the pedal arteries are patent and filled by a collateral circulation.

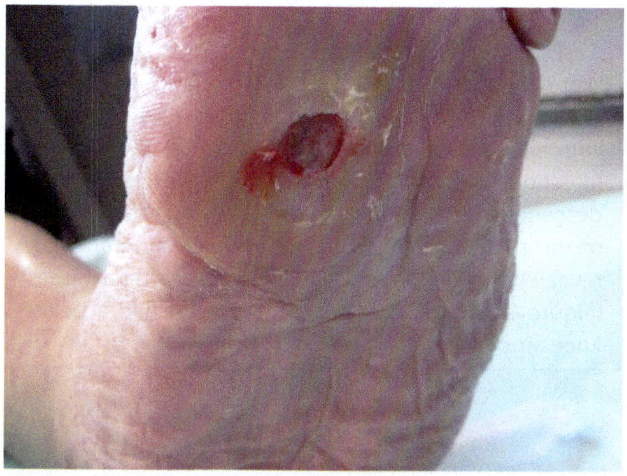

Figure 8.53 A persisting neuro-ischemic ulcer under an osteolytic lesion of the first metatarsal (osteomyelitis). The left femoral artery of this patient was totally obstructed due to peripheral artery disease.

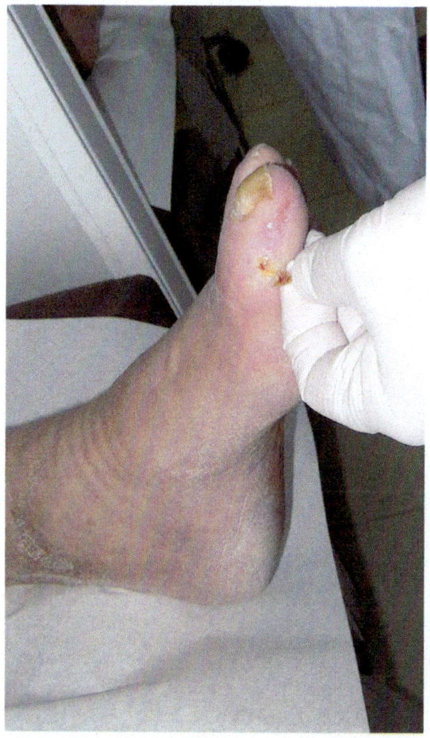

Figure 8.55 A healing neuro-ischemic ulcer on the medial surface of the hallux, four months after the first presentation of the patient in Figure 8.43 above.

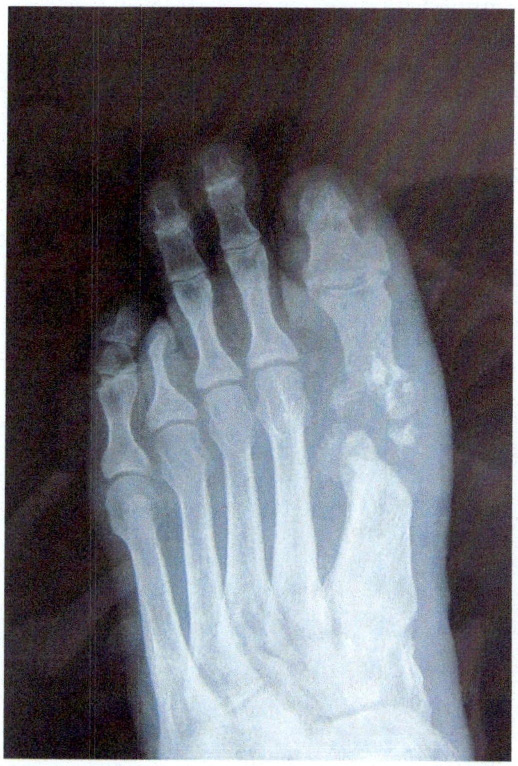

Figure 8.54 Osteomyelitis of the first metatarsal on the foot seen in Figure 8.54.

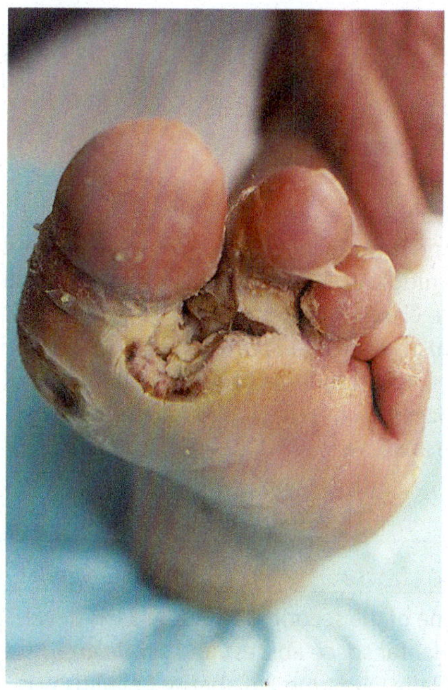

Figure 8.56 An infected neuro-ischemic ulcer soaked in profound discharge, on the plantar area between the first and second left metatarsal heads and extending into the second web space. A second ulcer surrounded by callus is also seen under the first metatarsal head.

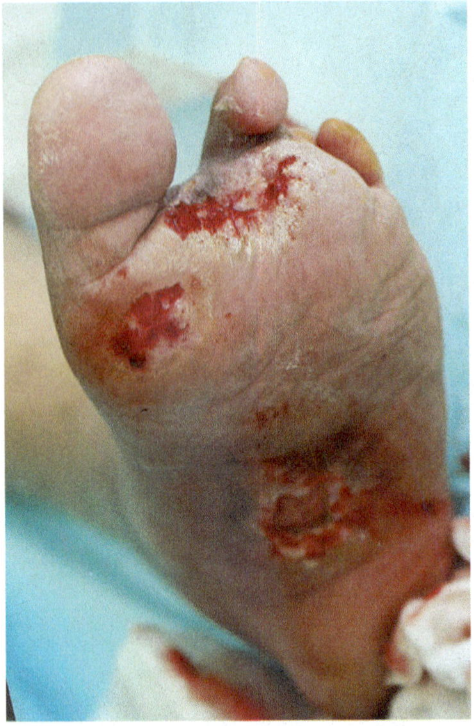

Figure 8.57 The same patient whose foot is illustrated in Figure 8.56, two years after second toe disarticulation. A neuro-ischemic ulcer caused by a worn-out insole is seen in the mid-sole area. A recurrent neuro-ischemic ulcer is present under the first metatarsal head, and a callus has formed below the disarticulated second toe.

8.7 Gangrene due to Abscess of the Plantar Space

In a plantar space abscess, edema can obliterate the plantar arterial arch and its branches, leading to ischemia and necrosis of the middle toes, together with the central plantar space (see Cases 8.7 and 8.8 below; Figures 8.58 and 8.59; mechanism shown in Figure 8.60). The fifth toe and the hallux receive branches through the lateral and medial plantar spaces, respectively, and may survive central plantar space abscesses.

Case 8.7

Diabetic gangrene of the second toe (Figure 8.61) developed due to a plantar space abscess and septic arteritis in a 63-year-old lady with type 2 diabetes. Cellulitis was seen on the dorsum and the plantar aspect of the foot (Figures 8.62 and 8.63). This patient eventually underwent Lisfranc disarticulation. The lesion was Fontaine stage IV, Rutherford grade III, category 5.

Case 8.8

Wet gangrene of the sole of the forefoot and the third toe (Figure 8.64) was seen in a 70-year-old gentleman with a fourth toe disarticulation that had never healed. Infection of the disarticulation site (Figure 8.65) descended into the plantar space, causing septic arteritis of the plantar arch and eventually wet gangrene. DSA revealed inoperable extended peripheral arterial disease (Figure 8.66), and eventually the patient had a below-knee amputation.

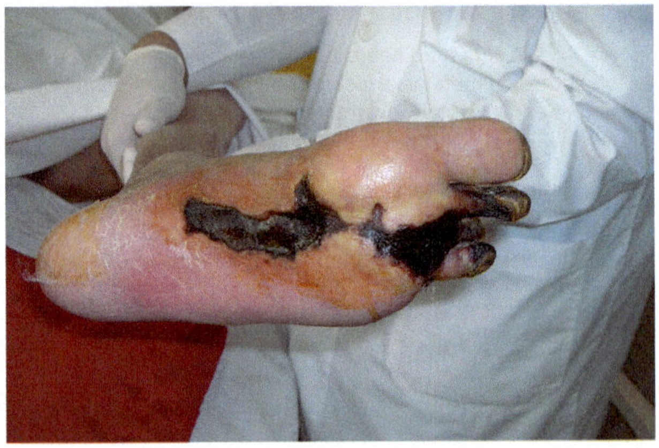

Figure 8.58 Wet gangrene of the plantar space and dry gangrene of the second, third and fourth toes. Note the cellulitis on the lateral aspect of the sole. Pus from an infection of the long-standing gangrenous toes descended into the plantar space forming an abscess there, which eventually produced a septic arteritis of the plantar arch and gangrene. See Figure 8.61 below for the underlying mechanism.

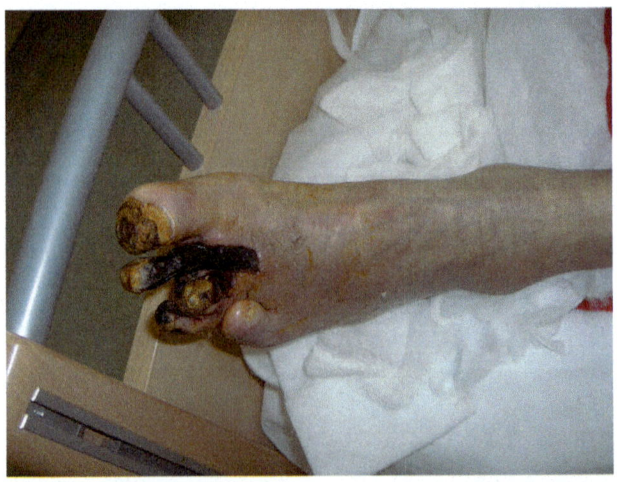

Figure 8.59 Dry gangrene of the tip of the hallux and the second, third and fourth toes. There is also a congenitally overriding fifth toe. This is the dorsal aspect of the foot shown in Figure 8.59.

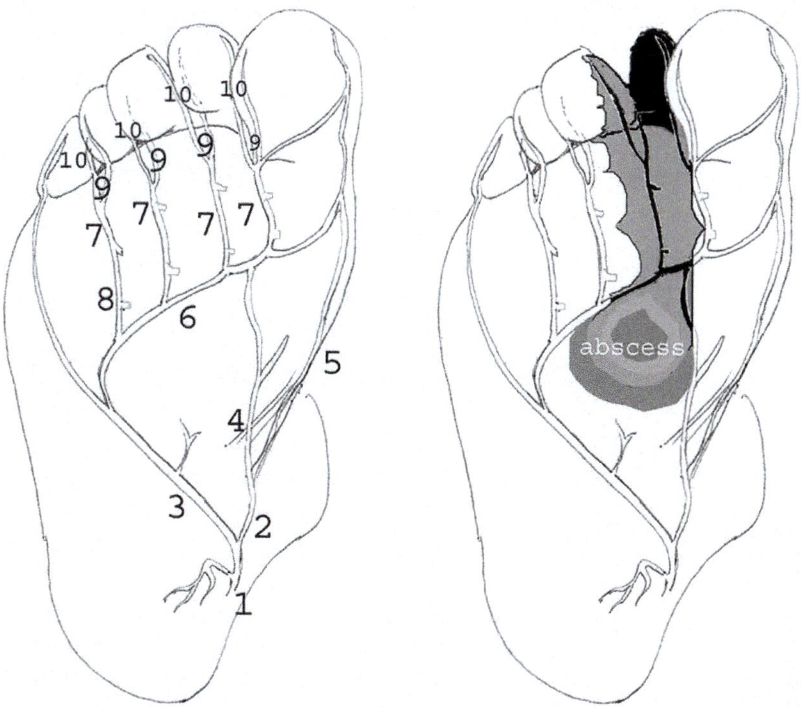

Figure 8.60 The normal plantar arch receives contributions from the medial and lateral branches of the posterior tibial artery and from the dorsalis pedis artery via a perforating artery (A). Gangrene of one or more of the middle toes will result when a central plantar space abscess occludes the plantar arch (B). Arteries of the plantar surface of the foot: (1) posterior tibial artery; (2) medial plantar artery; (3) lateral plantar artery; (4) arcuate artery; (5) superficial branch; (6) plantar arch; (7) common plantar digital arteries; (8) perforating arteries (usually two in each interosseous space, passing to dorsum of the foot); (9) plantar metatarsal arteries; (10) proper plantar digital arteries.

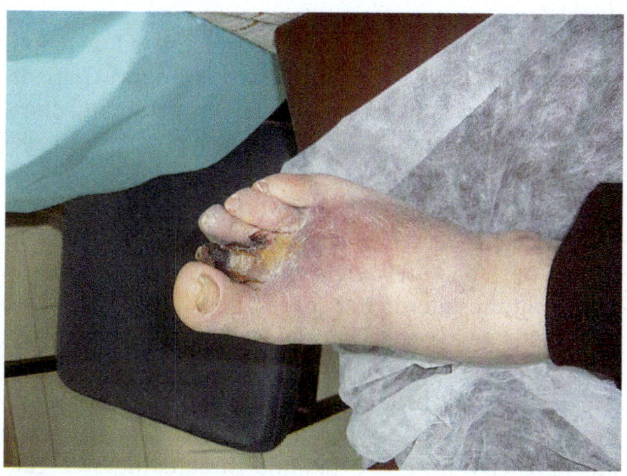

Figure 8.61 Case 8.7: Gangrene of the second toe and cellulitis of the dorsum of the foot.

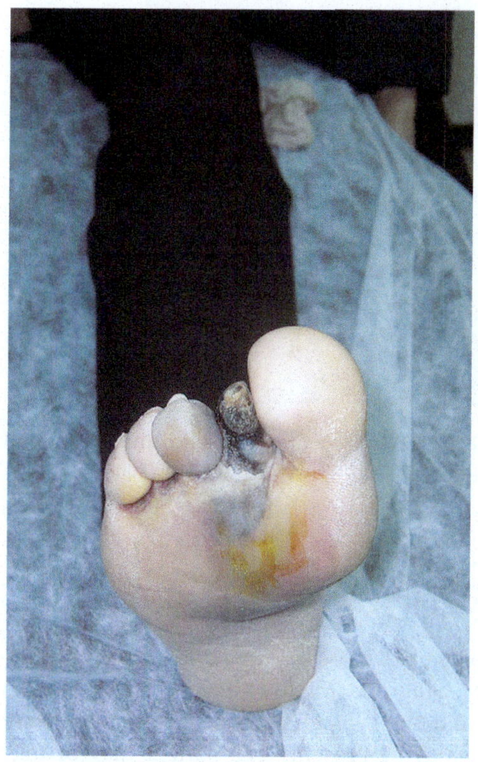

Figure 8.62 Case 8.7: Wet gangrene of the second toe due to a plantar space abscess.

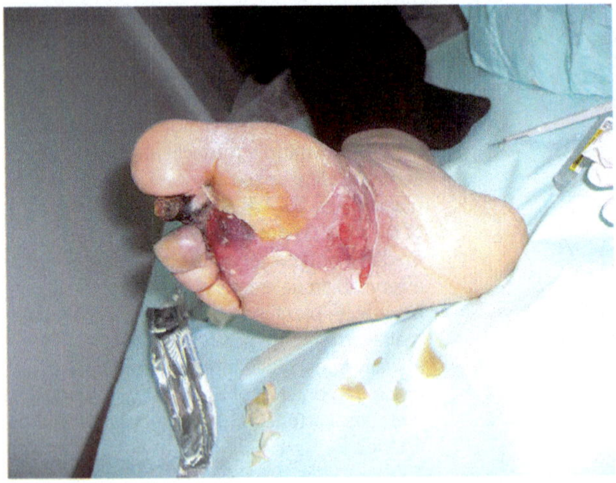

Figure 8.63 Case 8.7: Wet gangrene of the second toe due to a plantar space abscess, after removal of the loose dead skin over the infected ischemic tissue.

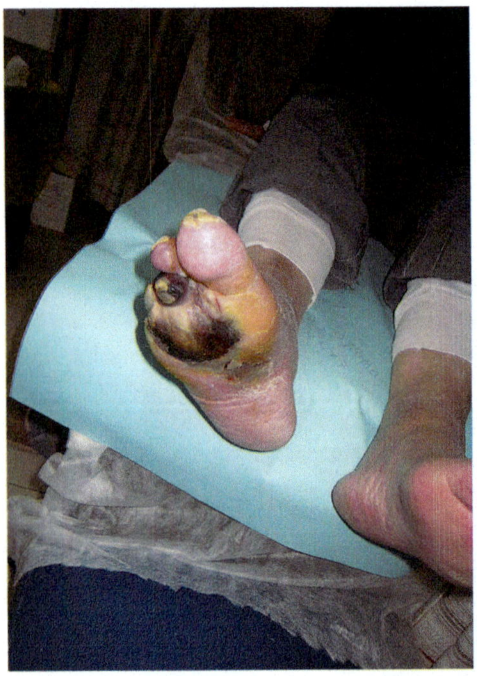

Figure 8.64 Case 8.8: Wet gangrene of the sole of the forefoot and the fourth toe. See Figure 8.60 above for the underlying mechanism.

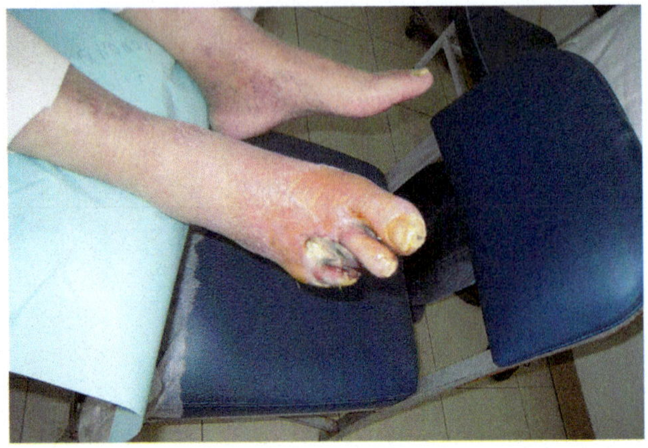

Figure 8.65 Case 8.8: Wet gangrene of the lateral aspect of the right forefoot. The initial lesion was located on the site of the previously disarticulated fourth toe.

8.8 Wet Gangrene

A moist appearance, gross swelling and blistering characterize wet gangrene (Figures 8.67–8.71). Cellulitis (erythema) and the typical signs of inflammation are evident. Pus may be present. The patient may or may not be febrile, and pain is present unless there is loss of pain sensation due to diabetic neuropathy. Small vesicles or yellow, bluish or black bullae may form, and eventually a black eschar covers the infected necrotic area (Figures 8.72 and 8.73, and see Figures 8.30, 8.58, 8.59, 8.63 and 8.64).

This is an emergency occurring in patients with severe ischemia who sustain an unrecognized trauma to their toe or foot. Urgent debridement of all affected tissues and the use of antibiotics often results in healing if sufficient viable tissue is present to maintain a functional foot, together with adequate circulation.

If wet gangrene involves an extensive part of the foot, urgent guillotine amputation at a level proximal enough to encompass the necrosis and gross infection may be life-saving. At the same time, bypass surgery or a percutaneous transluminal angioplasty needs to be performed, if feasible. Saline gauge dressings, changed every eight hours, work well for open amputations. Revision to a below-knee amputation may be considered three to five days later.

Wet gangrene is the most common cause of foot amputation in persons with diabetes. It often occurs in patients with severe peripheral vascular disease after infection. Dry gangrene may be infected and progress to wet gangrene.

Patients with dry gangrene who are awaiting a surgical procedure need education about meticulous foot care. They must be taught to inspect their feet daily, including the interdigital spaces, and wash them twice daily with gentle soap and lukewarm water; their feet should be dried thoroughly, particular the web spaces. It is extremely important for patients to avoid wet dressings and debriding agents, as their use may convert a localized dry gangrene to limb-threatening wet gangrene. Proper footwear is crucial to avoid further injury to the ischemic tissue.

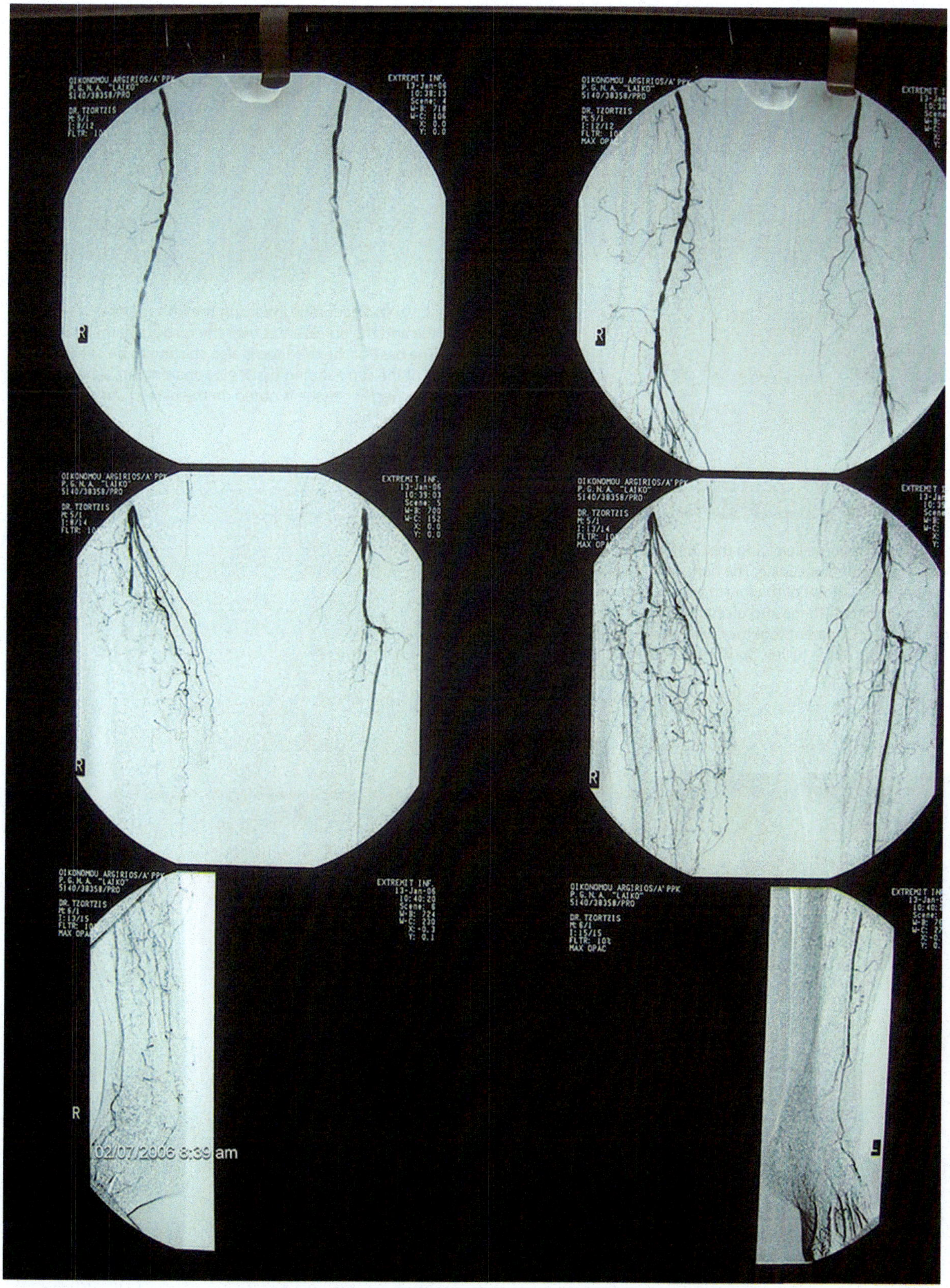

Figure 8.66 Case 8.8: Digital subtraction angiography showing obstruction of the right popliteal artery and a significant collateral circulation. Multiple atherosclerotic lesions are apparent on both femoral arteries and on the left tibial artery.

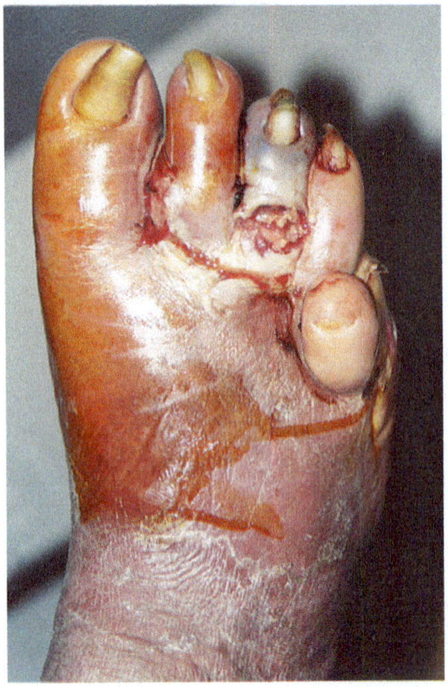

Figure 8.67 Wet gangrene involving the forefoot, with cellulitis extending as far as the right ankle. The bone and articular surfaces of the interphalangeal joint of the fourth toe are exposed. Congenital overriding fifth toe and ulceration under the fifth metatarsal head are apparent together, with onychodystrophy and an ingrown nail of the hallux. *Source:* Courtesy of E. Bastounis.

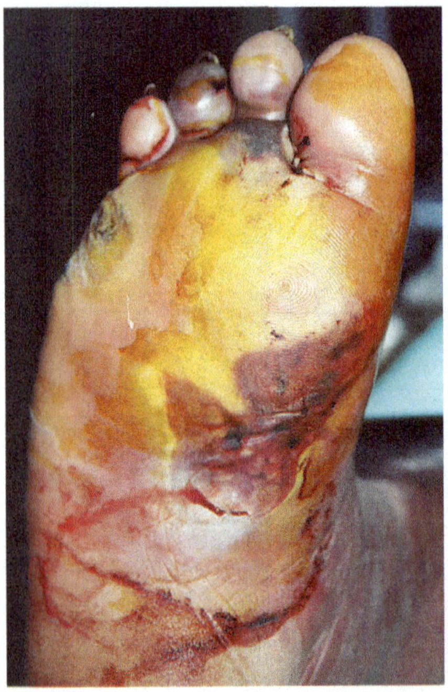

Figure 8.68 The sole of the foot shown in Figure 8.67 with wet gangrene of the forefoot, ulceration under the fifth metatarsal head, and ruptured blisters. *Source:* Courtesy of E. Bastounis.

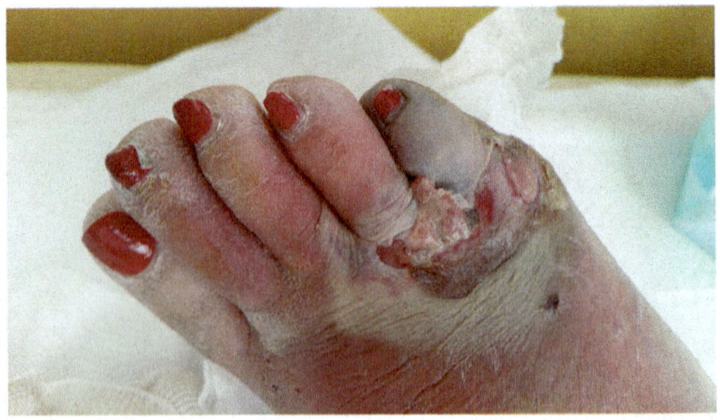

Figure 8.69 Wet gangrene involving the fifth toe, the base of the fourth toe and the dorsal areas over the respective metatarsal heads. The base of the third toe is also starting to be affected. Cellulitis of the surrounding tissues is apparent. An ischemic ulcer covered by necrotic tissue is noted on the plantar surface over the fifth metatarsal head.

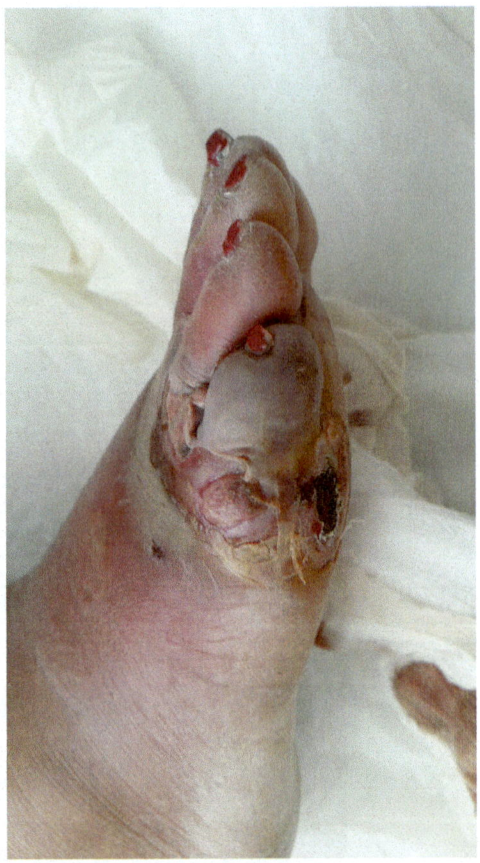

Figure 8.70 Wet gangrene involving the fifth toe, the base of the fourth toe and the dorsal areas over the respective metatarsal heads. The base of the third toe is also starting to be affected. Cellulitis of the surrounding tissues is apparent. An ischemic ulcer covered by necrotic tissue is noted on the plantar surface over the fifth metatarsal head.

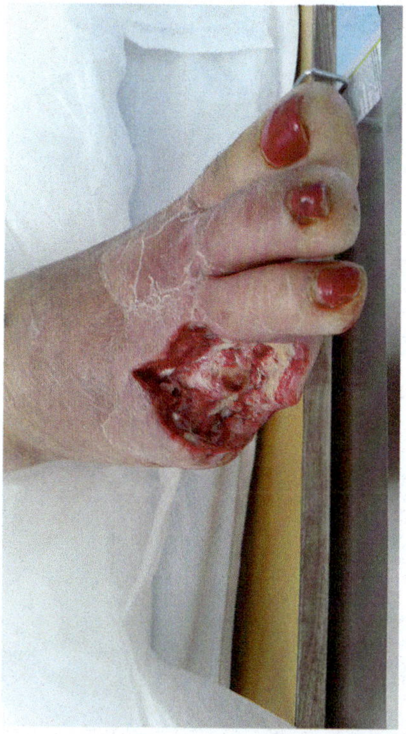

Figure 8.71 The same foot as in Figures 8.69 and 8.70, three days after disarticulation of the fourth and fifth digits, debridement of necrotic tissue and administration of broad-range antibiotics. Note the absence of inflammation signs in contrast to the situation before the amputation.

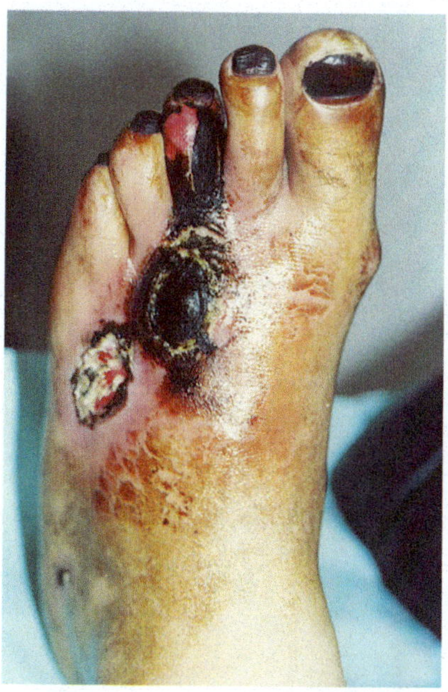

Figure 8.72 Wet gangrene of the midfoot and an infected necrotic (ischemic) ulcer over the fifth metatarsal head. The black color of the toenails is due to a long immersion of the foot in povidone-iodine solution. See Figure 8.61 above for the underlying mechanism.

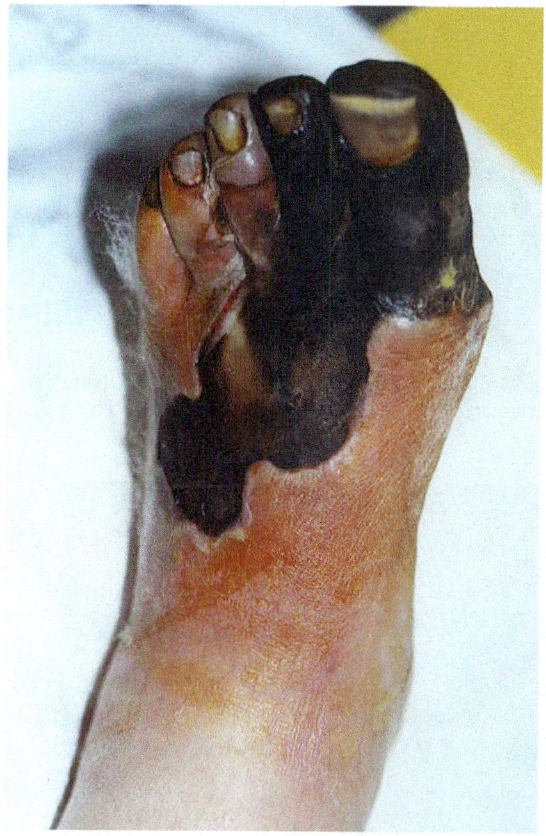

Figure 8.73 Wet gangrene of the right foot. Redness and edema, due to infection, extend as far as the lower third of the tibia. *Source:* Courtesy of E. Bastounis.

Case 8.9

Dry gangrene occurred on the right hallux of 57-year-old gentleman with type 1 diabetes and end-stage renal disease, who showed bounding pulses (Figure 8.74). The patient refused hallux disarticulation. An ischemic ulcer on the medial aspect of the first metatarsal head communicated with the base of the gangrene (Figure 8.75). Osteomyelitis of the head of the first and second metatarsals was evident on plain radiographs (Figure 8.76).

The lesion was stabilized for a few weeks (Figures 8.77 and 8.78) with the use of aggressive antibiotic treatment, and some evidence of control over the bone infection was present (Figure 8.79). A new ulcer formed under the base of the third toe (Figure 8.80), which was also treated. Two months later, a fulminant infection and wet gangrene of the forefoot developed (Figure 8.81), and a below-knee amputation was performed, even though the dorsal artery of the foot and the posterior tibial artery were patent.

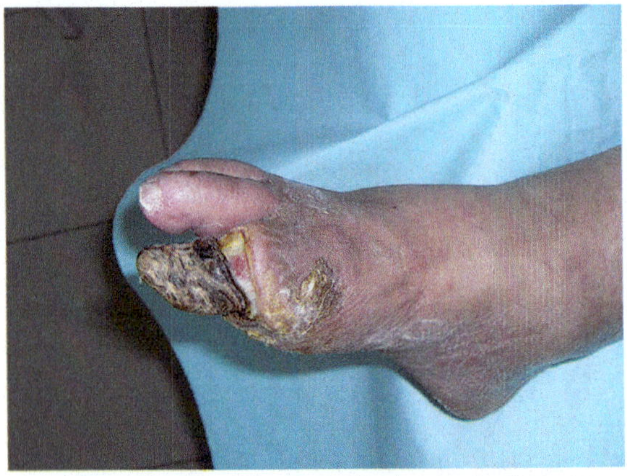

Figure 8.74 Case 8.9: dry gangrene of the right hallux. Note the distinct demarcation line between the viable and dead tissue.

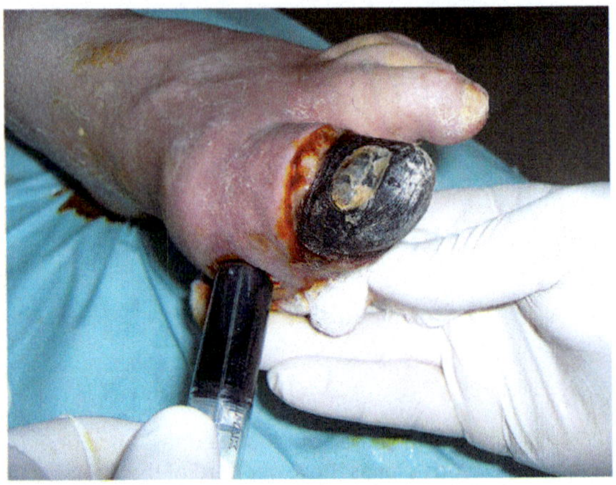

Figure 8.75 Case 8.9: dry gangrene of the great toe. An infusion of povidone-iodine through a medial ulcer revealed the communication of the ulcer with the base of the gangrene.

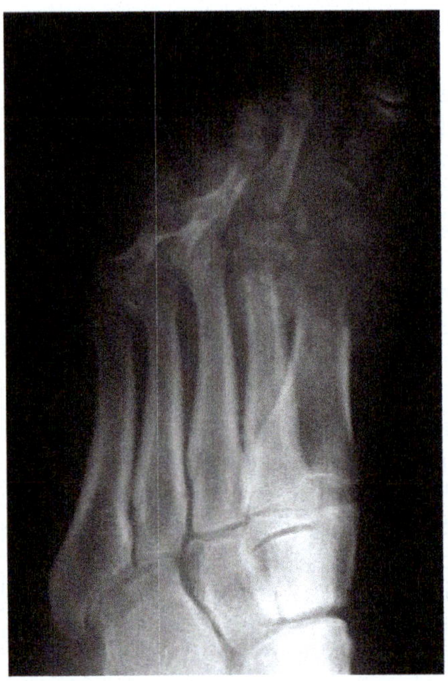

Figure 8.76 Case 8.9: A plain radiograph of osteomyelitis of the first and second metatarsal heads.

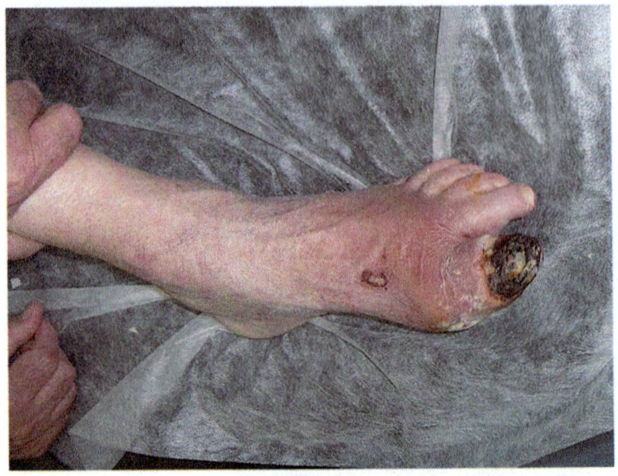

Figure 8.77 Case 8.9: Dry gangrene of the great toe.

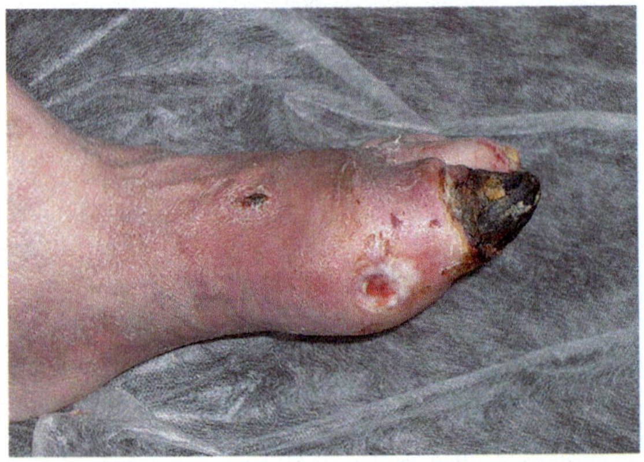

Figure 8.78 Case 8.9: Dry gangrene of the great toe. An ischemic ulcer is present over osteomyelitis of the head of the first metatarsal.

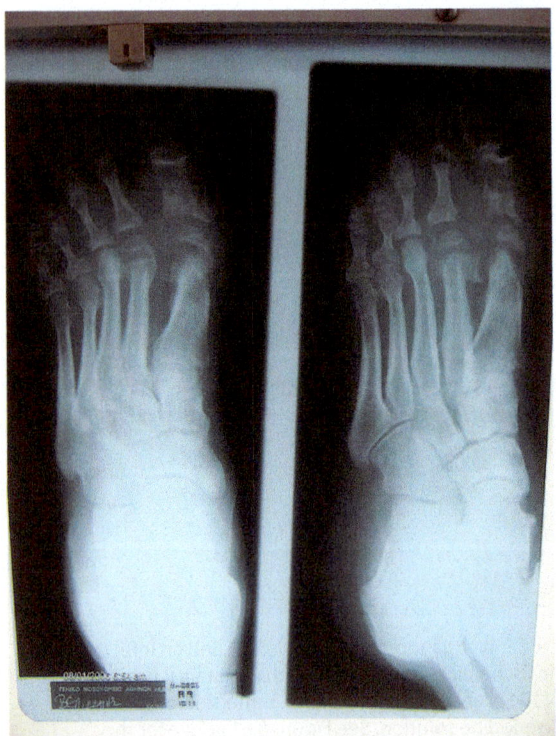

Figure 8.79 Case 8.9: A plain radiograph of osteomyelitis of the first and second metatarsal heads.

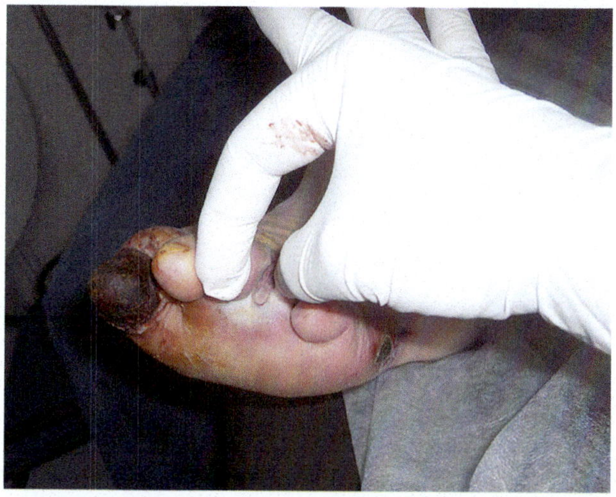

Figure 8.80 Case 8.9: Dry gangrene of the great toe. An ischemic ulcer is present at the base of the third toe, surrounded by whitish infiltrated tissue.

8.9 Dry Gangrene

Dry gangrene is characterized by its hard, dry and wrinkled dark brown or black texture; it usually occurs on the distal aspects of the toes (Figure 8.82 and 8.83), often with a clear demarcation between viable and necrotic tissue. Once demarcation has occurs the involved toes may be allowed to autoamputate. However, this process is long (several months) and disturbing. In addition, many patients do not have an adequate circulation to heal a distal amputation. For these reasons, it is common practice to evaluate the arteries angiographically and perform a bypass or a percutaneous transluminal angioplasty with concomitant limited distal amputation, in order to improve the chance of wound healing. In the case of extended gangrene (Figure 8.84), amputation at a higher level is unavoidable.

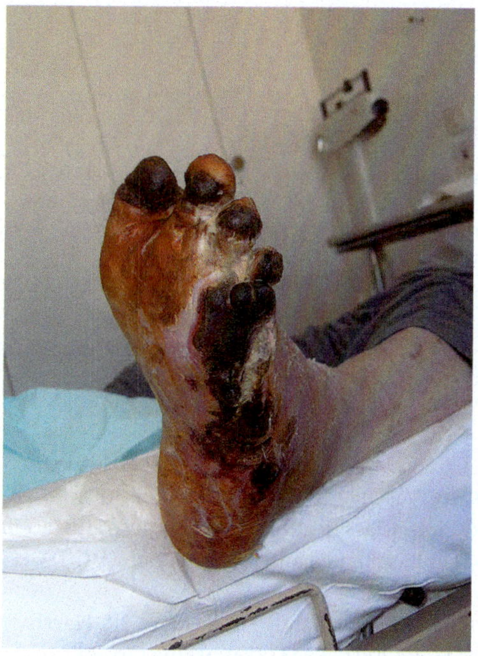

Figure 8.81 Case 8.9: Wet gangrene of the plantar aspect of the foot after a fulminant infection. Pus is coming out of the bases of the lateral toes and a gash under the fourth toe extending to the lateral mid-sole. Dry gangrene of the hallux and the top of the ischemic areas can also be seen.

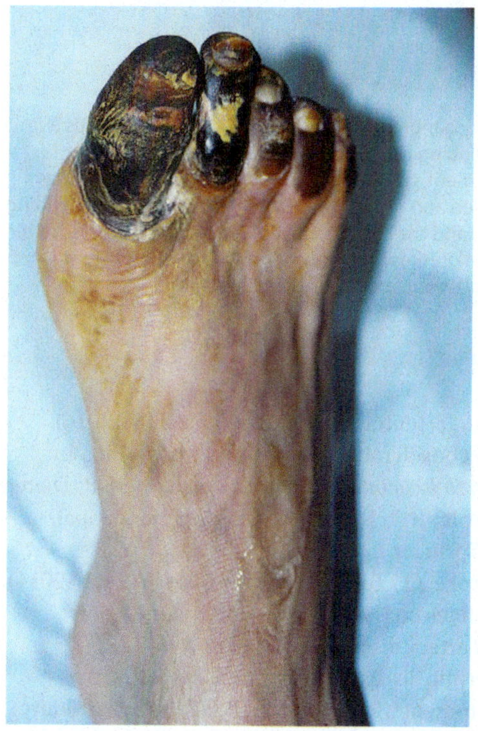

Figure 8.82 Dry gangrene of the toes. Note the black, hard and wrinkled wood-like texture of the dead tissue, and the distinct demarcation line between dead and viable tissue.

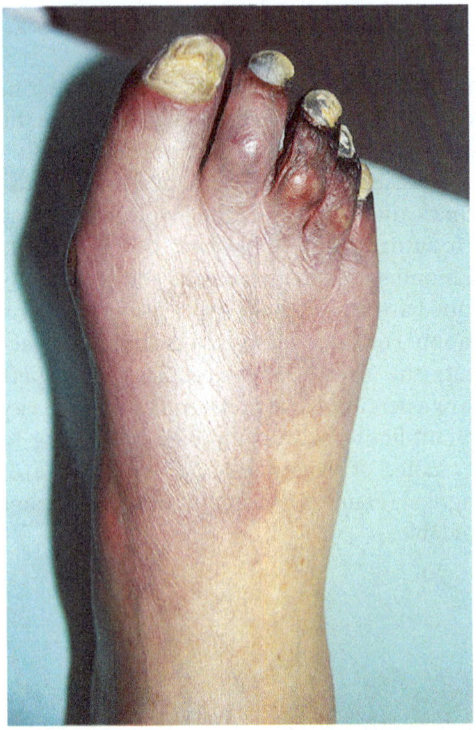

Figure 8.83 Dry gangrene of the tips of all the toes. Cellulitis (wet gangrene) extending all over the dorsum of the foot is under antibiotic treatment, the edema is diminishing, and the skin has become wrinkled and dry. The well-demarcated red area extending up to the ankle and the lateral aspect of the foot indicates ischemic necrosis of the skin. Onychogryphosis of the toenails is a feature of chronic ischemia. *Source:* Courtesy of E. Bastounis.

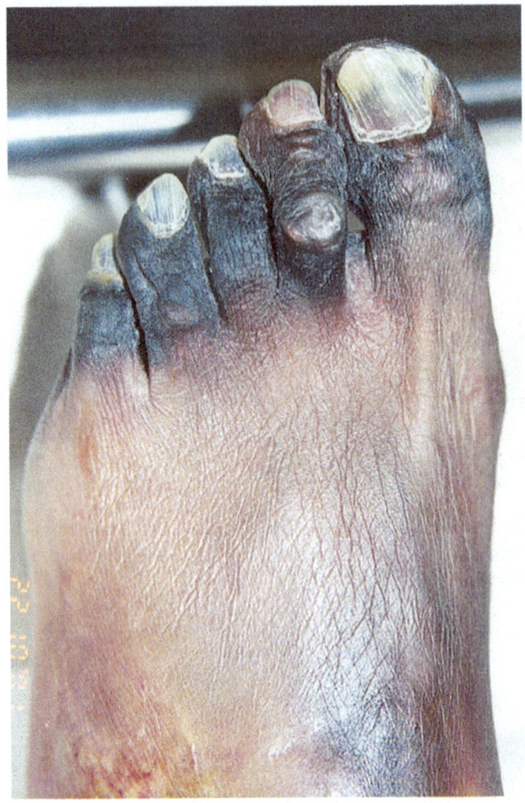

Figure 8.84 Dry gangrene involving all the toes of the left foot with a necrotic area over the mid-dorsum. The condition of the dorsum renders salvation of the foot questionable. *Source:* Courtesy of E. Bastounis.

Further Reading

Eleftheriadou, I., Tentolouris, N., and Jude, E.B. (2016). Endocrine considerations in critical leg ischemia. In: *Critical Limb Ischemia, Acute and Chronic* (ed. R. Dieter, R.A. Dieter Jr., R.A. Dieter III and A. Nanjundappa), 543–560. Springer.

European Stroke, O., Tendera, M., Aboyans, V. et al. (2011). ESC guidelines on the diagnosis and treatment of peripheral artery diseases: document covering atherosclerotic disease of extracranial carotid and vertebral, mesenteric, renal, upper and lower extremity arteries: the task force on the diagnosis and treatment of peripheral artery diseases of the European Society of Cardiology (ESC). *Eur. Heart J.* 32 (22): 2851–2906.

Gabriel A, Camp MC, Paletta C, Massey B. Vascular ulcers. Available at: http://emedicine.medscape.com/article/1298345-overview (accessed February 2009).

Hirschmann, J.V. and Raugi, G.J. (2009). Blue (or purple) toe syndrome. *J. Am. Acad. Dermatol.* 60: 1–20.

Mills, J.R. Sr. (2008.). Open bypass and endoluminal therapy: complementary techniques for revascularization in diabetic patients with critical limb ischaemia. *Diabetes Metab. Res. Rev.* 24 (Suppl. 1): S34–S39.

Mills, J.L. Sr., Conte, M.S., Armstrong, D.G. et al. (2014). The Society for Vascular Surgery Lower Extremity Threatened Limb Classification System: risk stratification based on wound, ischemia, and foot infection (WIfI). *J. Vasc. Surg.* 59 (1): 220–234. e221–222.

Norgren L, Hiatt WR, Dormandy JA, Nehler MR, Harris KA, Fowkes FGR. 2007. TASC II Working Group. "Inter-Society Consensus for the management of peripheral arterial disease (TASC II)." *J. Vasc. Surg.* 45(Suppl. 1): S5–S67.

O'Neal, L.W. (2001). Surgical pathology of the foot and clinicopathologic correlations. In: *Levin and O'Neal's The Diabetic Foot*, 6e (ed. J.H. Bowker and M.A. Pfeifer), 483–512. St Louis: Mosby.

Swischuk, J.L., Smouse, H.B., and Vargo, C. (2001). Lower extremity arterial revascularizations. In: *Peripheral Vascular Interventions* (ed. K. Kandarpa), 315–328. Philadelphia: Wolter Kluwer/Lippincott Williams & Wilkins.

9

Heel Ulcers

A. Kokkinos[1] *and P. Tsapogas*[2]

[1] *First Department of Propaedeutic Internal Medicine, National and Kapodistrian University of Athens, Medical School, Laiko General Hospital, Athens, Greece*
[2] *Center for Diabetes and Metabolism, Henry Dunant Hospital Center, Athens, Greece*

9.1 Heel Cracks and Common Diabetic Heel Ulcers

Thick callosity formation is not unusual in the heel region, but usually it is evenly distributed, so pure neuropathic full-thickness ulcers are not often seen on the heel. In the case of preceding operations or healed ulcers, a callus may form over scar tissue, and a new ulcer may develop (Figures 9.1–9.4). Corns may be found on the heel even when clinical neuropathic findings are absent (Figure 9.5).

Cracked heels (heel fissures) are common and are caused by dry skin (Figures 9.6 and 9.7). When the cracks are deep, they are painful to stand on and the skin can bleed; in severe cases, they can become infected (Figures 9.8 and 9.9, and see Figure 9.6). A black necrotic eschar is formed at the base of the ulcer, which may be too hard to remove manually (Figures 9.9–9.14) and will remain after the infection has been treated (Figure 9.10).

Ulcers on the heels of diabetic patients are mainly of ischemic etiology, and pressure or friction ulcers will resist healing owing to peripheral arterial disease. Other findings of ischemia may also be present (Figures 9.15 and 9.16). Most of these ulcers are painful, especially when the patient has no diabetic neuropathy. The presence of ischemia further exacerbates pain, and can make the ulcers tender to even the lightest touch; the loss of pain sensation may allow the diabetic patient to tolerate a heel ulcer.

Infection of a heel ulcer may be present in the form of cellulitis, a phlegmon, an abscess or osteomyelitis (see Case 9.1). Infection demands prompt diagnosis, and sometimes an ultrasound scan will reveal an abscess or a cavity. Debridement of the ulcer, cultures of discharge, aggressive antibiotic treatment, and off-loading should all be employed, as for other foot ulcers.

9.2 Pressure Ulcers

Advanced age, peripheral neuropathy, deformity, ischemia, edema, limited joint mobility, trauma and lower limb immobility lead to a gradual thinning of the heel pad and reduce its capacity to absorb shock during walking. These predisposing factors are present in people with diabetes mellitus who develop heel ulcers, either due to friction of the shoes or from the shearing forces encountered during walking (repetitive trauma) or standing, or because of gravity pressure on the heels, as is the case of bed-ridden patients during hospitalization. Inactivity, incontinence (both fecal and urinary), poor nutritional status and an altered mental status are additional risk factors.

Comatose patients, patients with coronary heart disease, and patients who have suffered a cerebrovascular accident are also at risk for the development of pressure ulcers. Patients undergoing hip surgery, as well as burn patients, are at high risk for heel ulcers due to the combination of increased external pressure from immobility, friction, shear forces and decreased blood flow as a result of vasoconstriction (caused by catecholamine excess due to hypovolemia, epinephrine infusions, pain, cigarette smoking and changes in temperature). Pressure ulcers are also possible over the spine, sacrum, coccyx, ischial tuberosities, trochanters, malleoli and elbows, in side-lying positions, and on the occiput or behind the ears.

A hard, unyielding mattress under an immobilized patient may lead to heel ulceration as a direct result of gravity pressure, and reduced heel blood flow with soft tissue necrosis, even after a few hours of immobility. Lying supine in a hospital bed generates a heel-to-bed pressure of 50–94mmHg, which exceeds the normal

Atlas of the Diabetic Foot, Third Edition. Ioanna Eleftheriadou, Alexandros Kokkinos, Stavros Liatis, Konstantinos Makrilakis, Nicholas Tentolouris, Anastasios Tentolouris, and Panagiotis Tsapogas.

Companion website: www.wiley.com/go/tentolouris/atlas_diabetic_foot

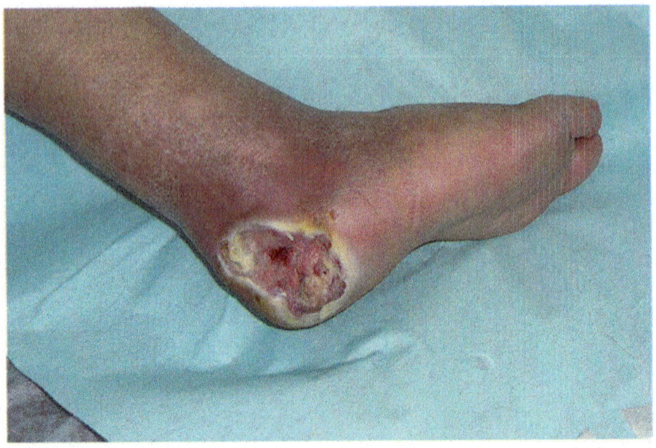

Figure 9.1 A stage 4 infected pressure ulcer of the heel extending to the muscle over the base of (but not exposing) the Achilles tendon.

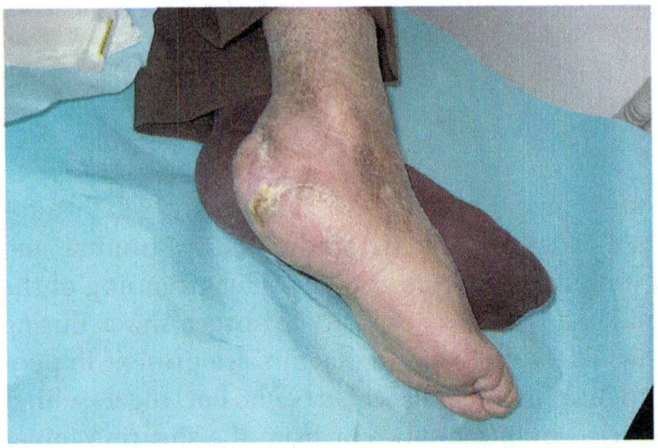

Figure 9.2 A healed ulcer of the heel. Callus formation is evident over the scar and is a concern for future ulceration. This is the foot of the patient shown in Figure 9.1.

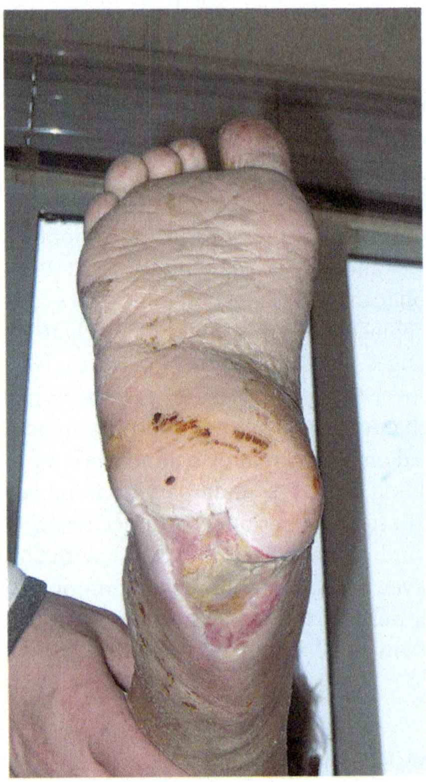

Figure 9.3 A healing stage 3 pressure ulcer that developed on the scar of a previous ulcer at the same location. This is the foot of the patient shown in Figures 9.1 and 9.2.

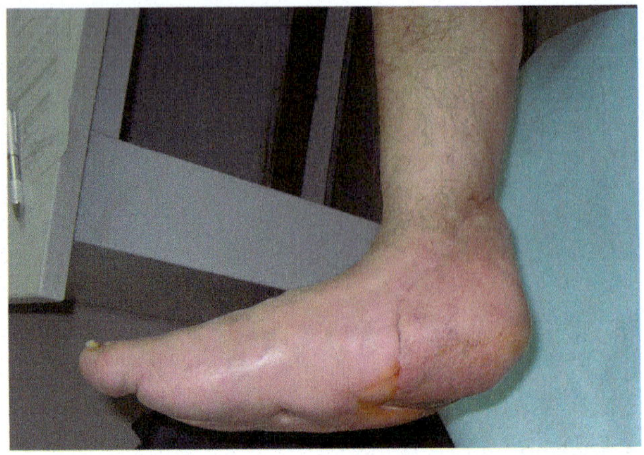

Figure 9.4 Plastic reconstruction of the heel after removal of a melanoma. Proper footwear prevents callosity and ulceration.

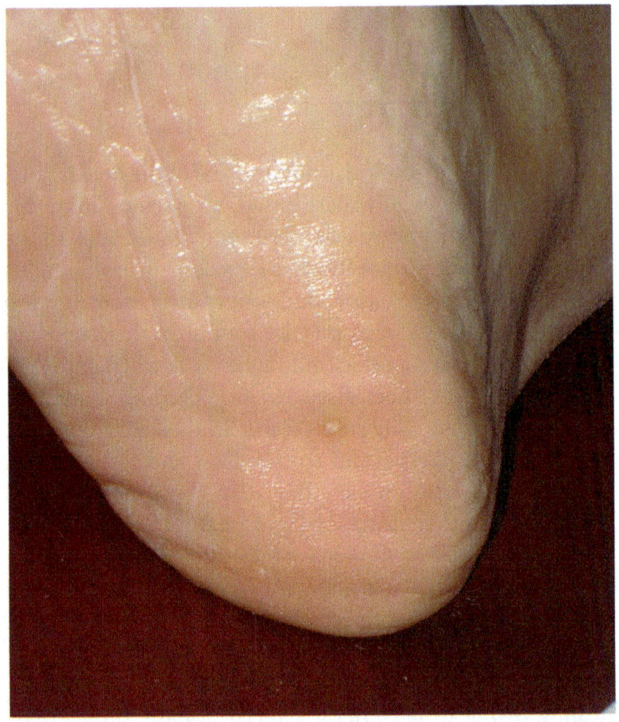

Figure 9.5 A painful corn under the heel of an obese 70-year-old lady with long-standing type 2 diabetes. Peripheral artery disease was found on a triplex scan (both posterior tibial arteries being occluded), yet neither claudication nor any neuropathic signs were present.

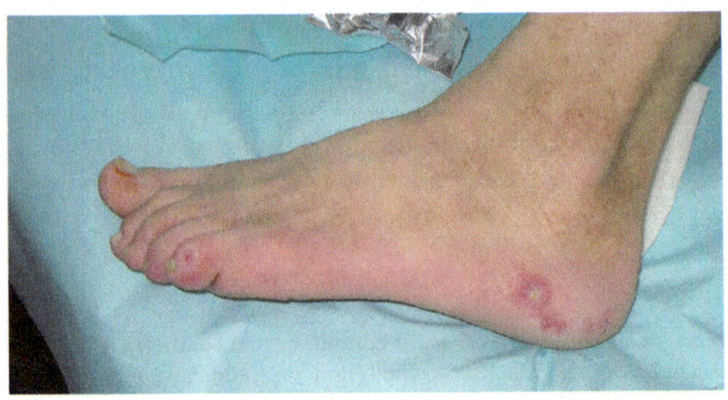

Figure 9.6 Painful superficial skin cracks on the lateral aspect of the heel. A neuro-ischemic ulcer is seen on the fifth toe.

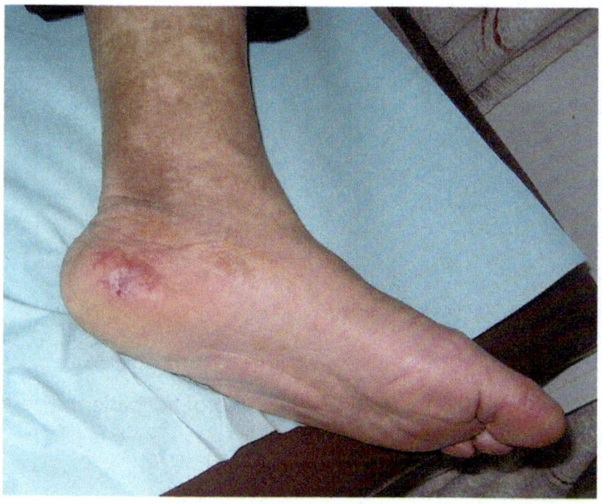

Figure 9.7 A painful skin crack is seen on the medial aspect of the heel. Erythema and edema around the tear denote the presence of an infection.

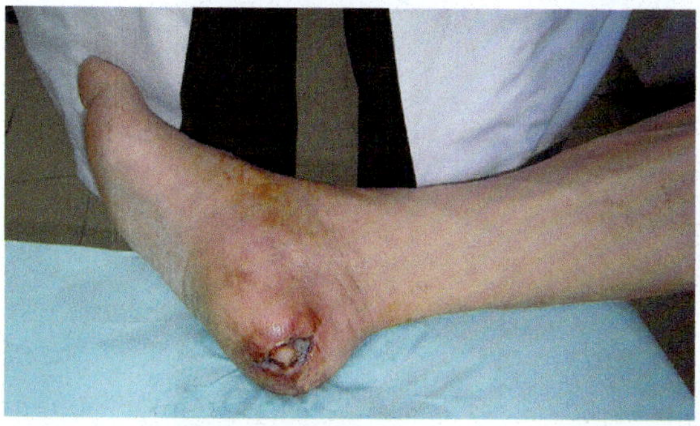

Figure 9.8 A painless, infected neuro-ischemic heel ulcer that had been preceded by a heel crack.

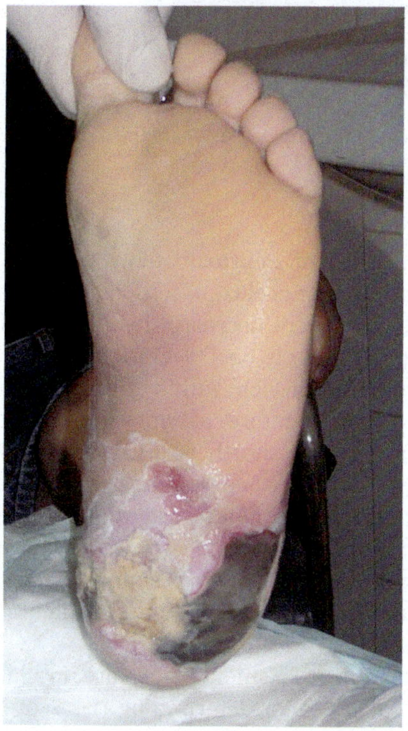

Figure 9.9 A painless, infected (neuro-ischemic) heel ulcer with superficial wet gangrene, formed after minor trauma to the sole of this ischemic patient. No abscess was found on an ultrasound scan. Healing was slow but successful.

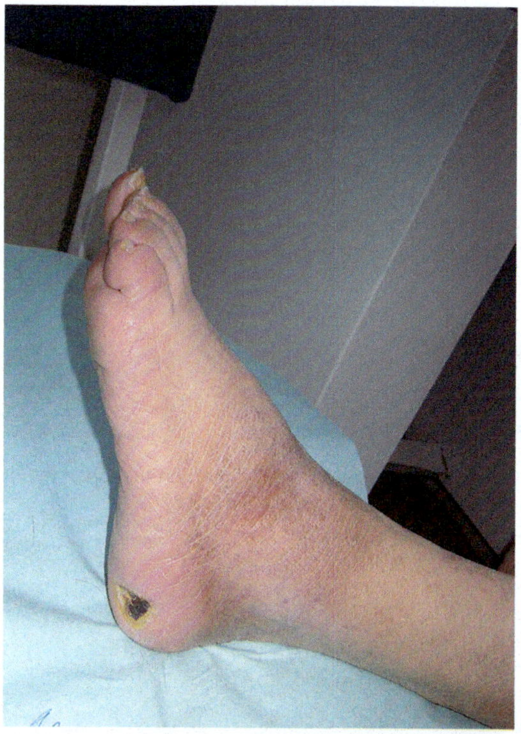

Figure 9.10 A heel ulcer with a black eschar is seen on the lateral aspect of the heel. Infection of the ulcer has been treated successfully.

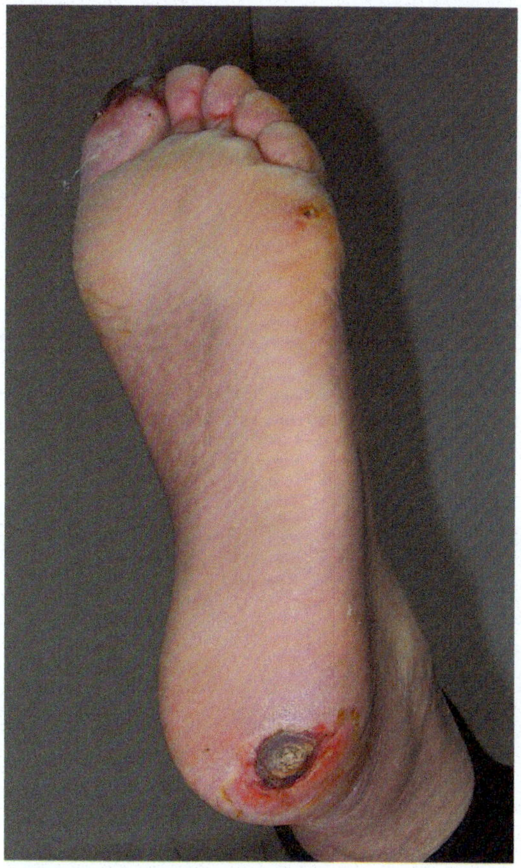

Figure 9.11 An unstageable skin ulcer on the lateral aspect of the heel. After removal of the eschar, this was found to be a shallow ulcer. A triplex scan revealed biphasic flow in both anterior tibial arteries (80% obstruction), and complete obstruction of the left posterior tibial artery.

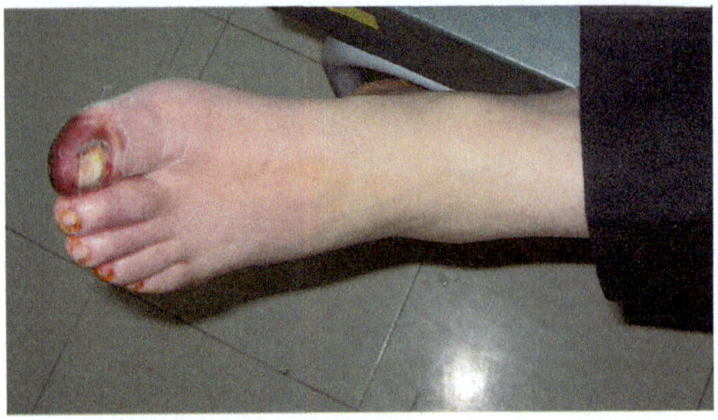

Figure 9.12 An infected neuro-ischemic ulcer on the top of the hallux on the foot of the patient shown in Figure 9.11.

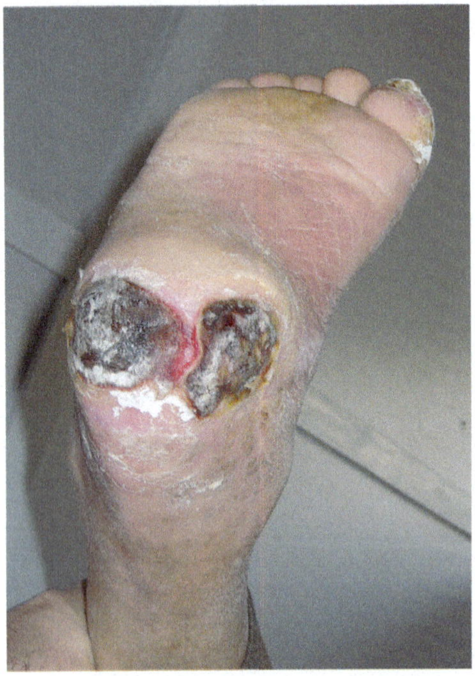

Figure 9.13 Painless neuro-ischemic heel ulcers in a heavy-smoking diabetic patient with severe atherosclerosis in his right leg.

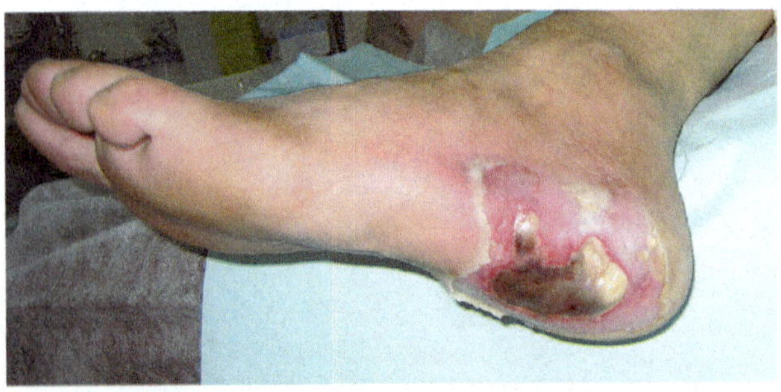

Figure 9.14 Wet gangrene of a heel ulcer. Sharp debridement determines the depth of the ulcer. An ultrasound may be helpful in determining an underlying abscess.

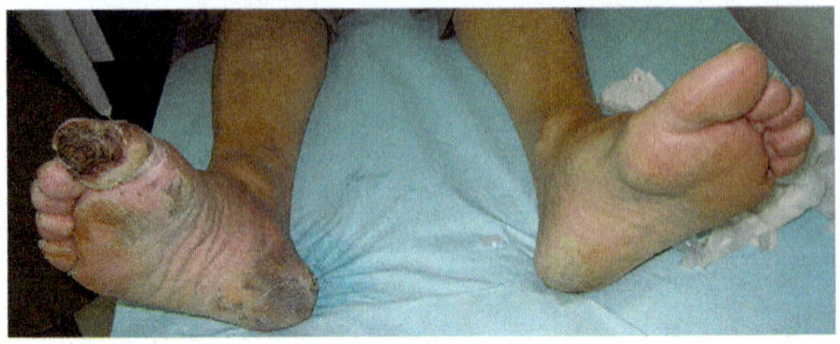

Figure 9.15 Dry gangrene of the right hallux of the patient whose foot is seen in Figure 9.13.

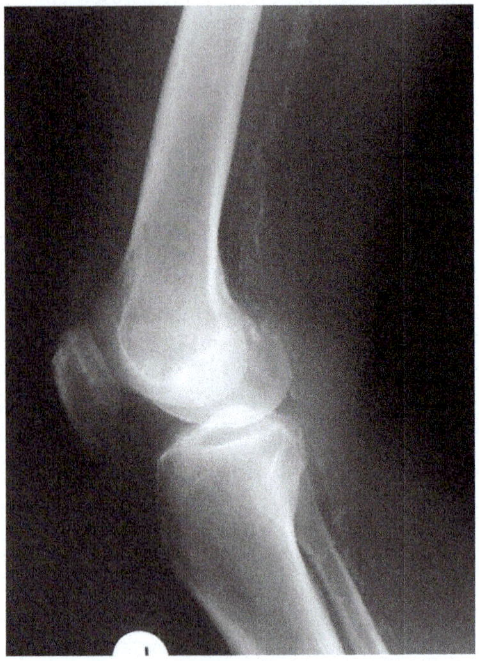

Figure 9.16 Calcification of the popliteal artery of the patient whose foot is shown in Figure 9.13.

capillary filling pressure of approximately 32mmHg. This can cause local vascular occlusion sufficient to produce ischemia and subsequent necrosis of the skin and subcutaneous tissues, leading to heel ulceration.

Pressure ulcers usually develop within the first two weeks of hospitalization; therefore, patients who are at risk should be identified both shortly after admission to a healthcare setting, as well as when there is a significant change in the individual's condition (transfer to intensive care, system or organ failure, sepsis, chronic intensive care status with prolonged ventilatory support, fever, hemodynamic instability, urinary tract infection in nursing home residents, etc.).

Several risk-screening assessment tools are available that consist of subscales for determining risk score. The Braden scale (which encompasses six parameters:

Case 9.1

A 69-year-old lady with recently diagnosed type 2 diabetes and a body mass index of $45 kg/m^2$ was referred to the foot clinic by her local health center. She had sepsis due to a large irregular wound under her right heel with extremely macerated borders and a massive production of pus (Figure 9.17). This ulcer had formed after minor trauma caused by a pin in her shoe, and the ulcer had extended to the bone within a few days.

Complete bed rest and aggressive antibiotic treatment were recommended. A multi-antibiotic-susceptible strain of *Pseudomonas aeruginosa* was isolated in all cultures. The infection was treated successfully and the ulcer granulated normally (Figures 9.18–9.20), yet a tunnel was formed, which reached to the bone (as shown in a plain radiograph after the infusion of lipiodol; Figure 9.21), resisting all debridement.

The strain of *P. aeruginosa* became more and more resistant to antibiotics in serial isolations, yet no clinical infection was present three months after the initial visit (see Figure 9.20), and all inflammation indexes were negative. Antibiotics were stopped in the fourth month of treatment, and the presence of the bacterium was considered to be colonization rather than infection. A chronic neuropathic ulcer was present 10 months after the initial visit (Figure 9.22), and debridement was performed on a two to three-weekly schedule.

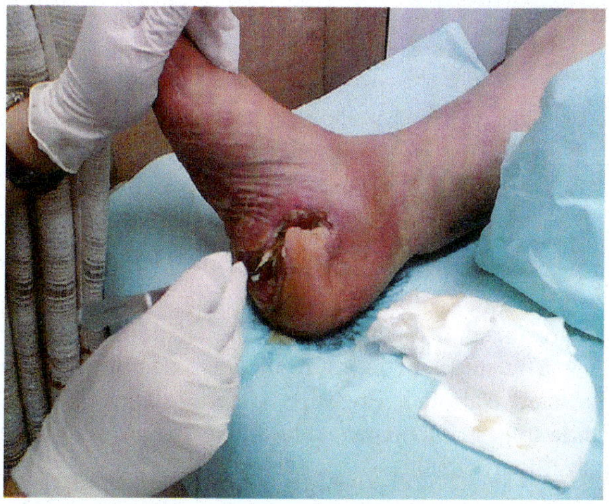

Figure 9.17 Case 9.1: A deep irregular cut with macerated borders and massive production of pus has formed after a wound caused by a pin in the patient's shoe under her right heel.

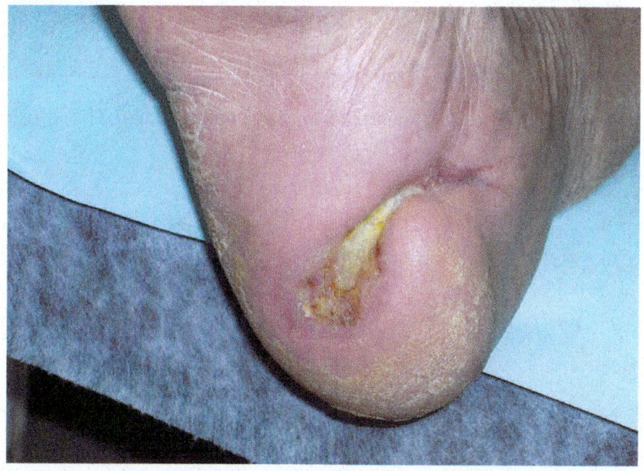

Figure 9.19 Case 9.1: A neuropathic ulcer of the heel one month after the initiation of aggressive antibiotic treatment. Note the formation of yellow fibrin at the base of the ulcer.

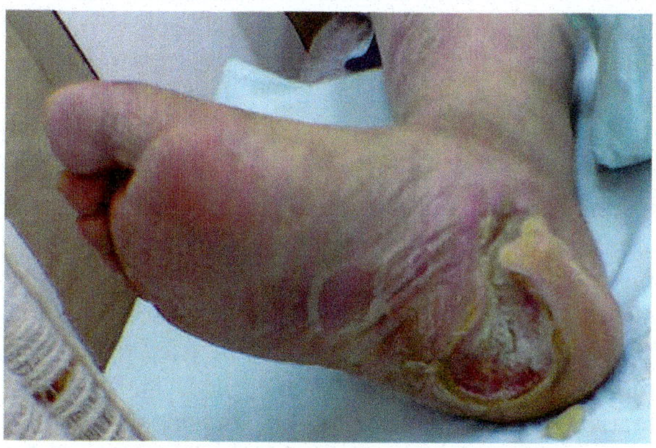

Figure 9.18 Case 9.1: A neuropathic ulcer of the heel one month after the initiation of aggressive antibiotic treatment. Note the presence of granulating tissue and fibrin formation in the base of the ulcer. Callosity at the borders of the ulcer denotes incomplete bed rest.

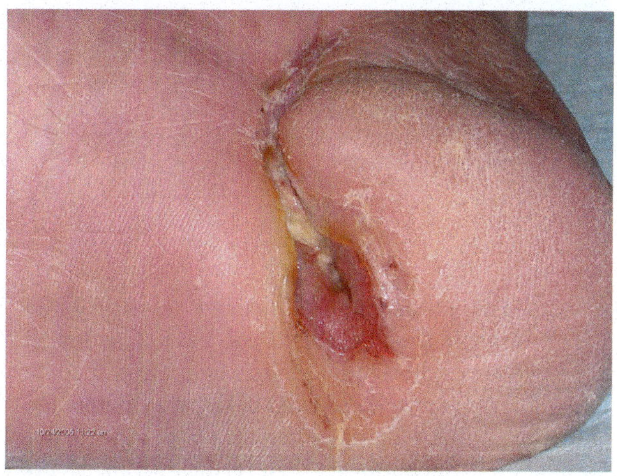

Figure 9.20 Case 9.1: A chronic neuropathic ulcer of the heel is actually the entrance to a 4cm tunnel to the fascia.

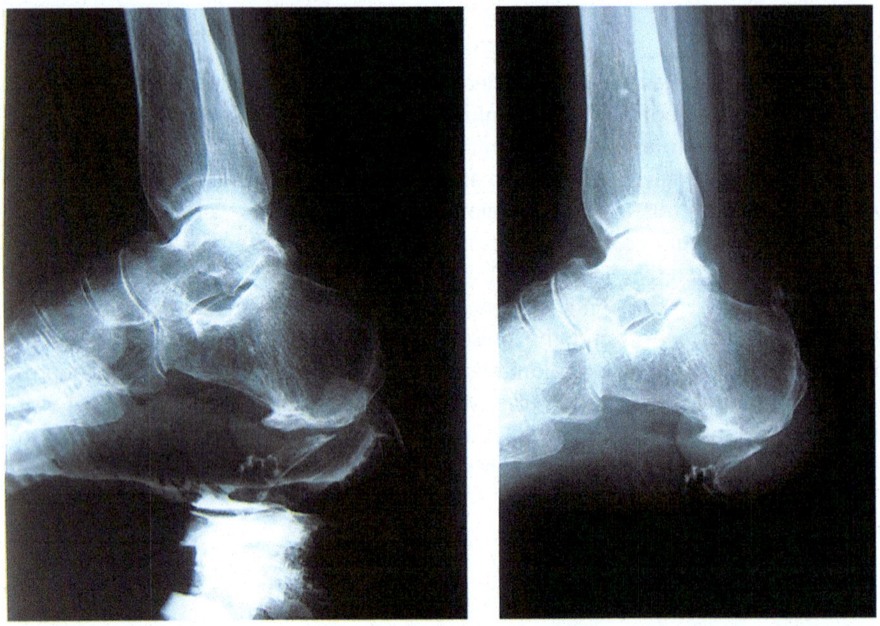

Figure 9.21 Case 9.1: A plain radiograph of a heel ulcer. The infusion of lipiodol revealed a tunnel extending to the fascia.

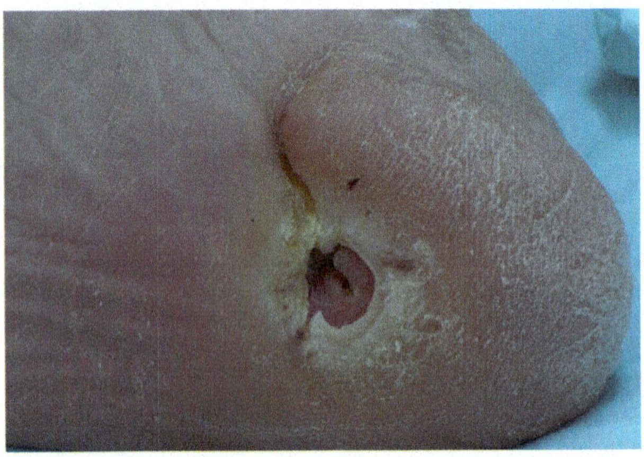

Figure 9.22 Case 9.1: A chronic neuropathic ulcer of the heel that was actually the entrance of a 4cm tunnel to the bone surface. Callosity is present around the ulcer due to walking. Special heel-off-loading shoes were not tolerated by the patient, who refused surgical intervention.

sensory perception, mobility, activity, moisture, nutrition, and friction and shear) is the only scale that has been extensively tested in adults across healthcare settings. The Norton scale consists of five parameters (general physical condition, mental condition, activity, mobility, and incontinence). Nevertheless, an accurate predictive ability of pressure ulcer risk scales has not yet been determined.

9.3 Staging of Pressure Ulcers

Pressure ulcers are staged to define the level of tissue injury. The stages of pressure ulcers, as defined by the American National Pressure Ulcer Advisory Panel, include stages 1–4, unstageable, and deep tissue pressure injury (Figure 9.23):

- *Stage 1* is a localized area of intact skin with non-blanchable erythema, which may appear differently in the case of darkly pigmented skin. The ulcer may differ from the surrounding healthy tissue in terms of texture (firm or soft), temperature, and sensation, and these changes may precede visual changes. Purple or maroon discoloration indicate deep tissue pressure injury, not a stage 1 ulcer.
- *Stage 2* refers to partial-thickness loss of skin with exposed dermis (see Figure 9.28). The bed of the wound is viable, pink or red in color, and moist. It may also initially present as a blister filled with serum (ruptured or intact). Subcutaneous fat and deeper tissues are not visible. There are no granulation tissue, slough and eschar. This stage should not be used to describe moisture associated skin damage (MASD), or traumatic wounds (skin tears, burns, abrasions).
- *Stage 3* refers to an ulcer with full-thickness loss of skin and visible adipose tissue. Granulation tissue and epibole (rolled wound edges) are often present, as well as slough and/or eschar. Undermining and tunneling may occur. Deeper tissues, such as fascia, muscle, tendon,

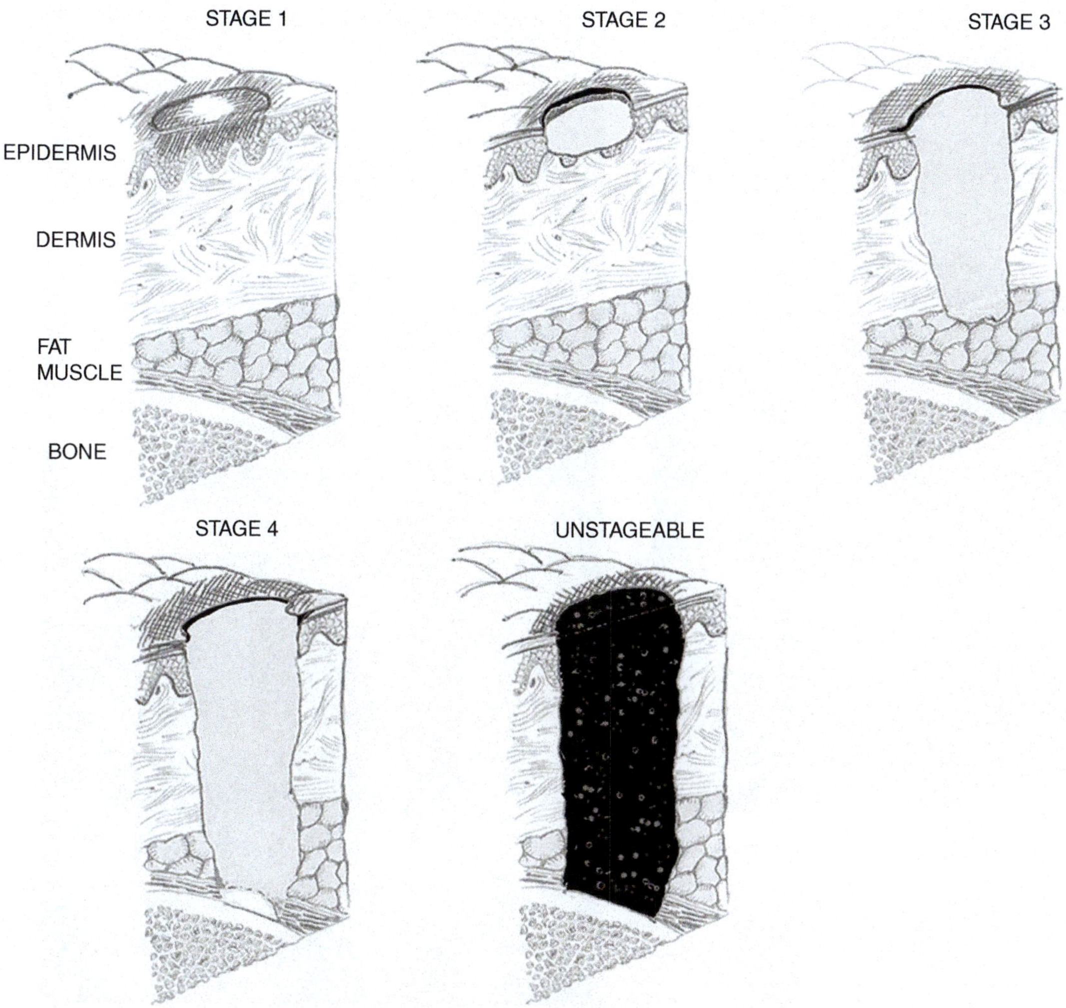

Figure 9.23 Stages of pressure ulcers (*Source:* Adapted from the National Pressure Ulcer Advisory Panel: http://www.npuap.org/pr2.htm). See text for details.

ligament, cartilage and bone are not visible. In the case that slough or eschar obscures the extent of tissue loss, this should be classified as an Unstageable Pressure Injury.

- *Stage 4* is a full-thickness ulcer with skin and tissue loss extending into fascia, muscle, tendon, ligament, cartilage or bone (see Figure 9.1). Osteomyelitis may complicate this ulcer. Epibole (rolled edges), undermining and tunneling may also be associated with stage 4 pressure ulcers. Slough or eschar can be present, but these do not obscure depth estimation. If they do, then this is an Unstageable Pressure Injury.
- *Unstageable* pressure ulcers have full-thickness tissue loss with the base of the ulcer covered by slough or eschar. Thus, the extent of tissue damage cannot be assessed (Figures 9.24–9.27). These ulcers must be debrided to allow depth identification and staging, in which case, once slough or eschar is removed, a Stage 3 or Stage 4 pressure injury will usually be revealed. Stable eschar (i.e. dry, adherent, intact without erythema or fluctuance) on the heel or ischemic limb should not be softened or removed.
- *Deep tissue pressure injury* refers to lesions where there is intact or non-intact skin with a localized area of persistent non-blanchable deep red, maroon, purple discoloration or epidermal separation which reveals a dark wound bed or a blister filled with blood. Skin changes may follow pain or temperature change, and may appear differently in darkly pigmented skin. This type of injury is usually the result of intense and/or prolonged pressure and shear forces at the bone-muscle interface. It may evolve (usually rapidly) and reveal the extent of tissue injury, or it may resolve without tissue loss.

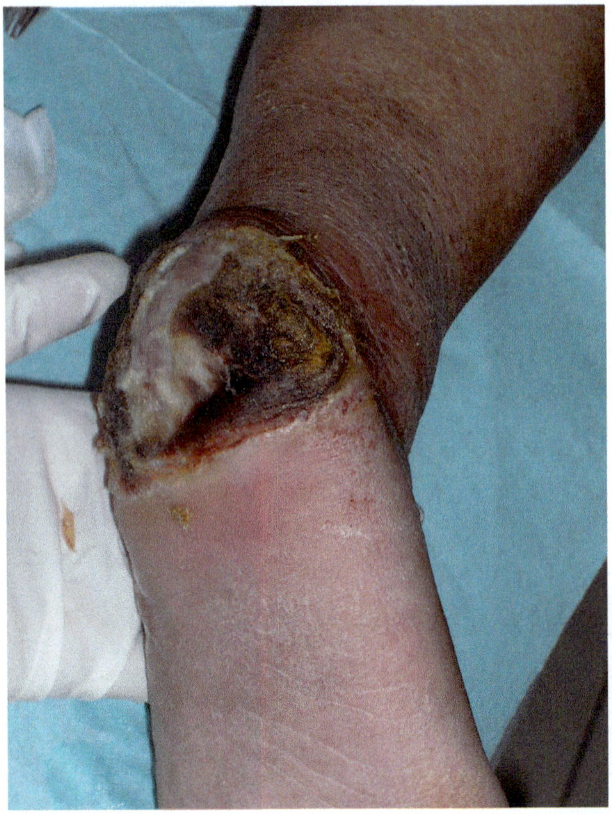

Figure 9.24 An unstageable pressure ulcer. Removal of the eschar revealed a stage 3 ulcer.

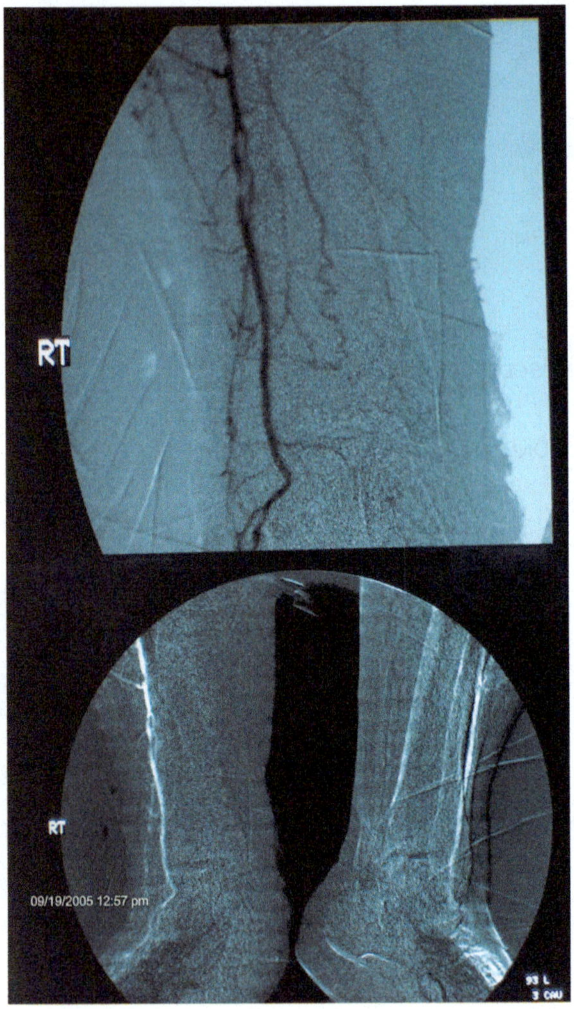

Figure 9.25 Digital subtraction angiography of the patient whose foot is seen in Figure 9.20. Note the atherosclerotic lesions of the right popliteal artery (upper panel), and the occlusion of the posterior tibial arteries (lower panel).

Case 9.2

A 79-year old lady with recently diagnosed type 2 diabetes mellitus developed pressure heel ulcers (Figure 9.28) during a long stay in intensive care because of a myocardial infarction. Diffuse atherosclerotic lesions were present on digital subtraction angiography. No neuropathic signs were present. The ulcers were categorized as stage 2 after removal of the slough, which was done with great difficulty since the ulcers were extremely painful, to the point that this patient was unable to sleep at night. Enzymatic debridement was applied to avoid any manipulations (Figure 9.29).

After a second hospitalization because of cardiac insufficiency, the ulcers were categorized as stage 3, since they were full-thickness ulcers and tunneling, but bone, tendon and muscle were not exposed (Figure 9.30). The same approach as before was chosen, with minimal results. In her last visit after a third admission, the ulcers were extending over the Achilles tendon and were unstageable (Figure 9.31), but still very painful. A new, fatal myocardial infarction prevented any further follow-up.

Case 9.3

An 88-year old man with type 2 diabetes mellitus since his early fifties presented to the clinic with a round pressure ulcer on his left heel, after having been hospitalized for 10 days for a myocardial infarction. The ulcer was covered with a dry eschar, the removal of which was very difficult, because the patient experienced excruciating pain, and concurrent symptoms of angina during the procedure. In fact, topical anesthesia was needed in order to debride the ulcer; a stage 3 lesion was exposed, with full-thickness skin loss and visibility of the subcutaneous adipose tissue (Figure 9.32). He was treated with oral antibiotics and the ulcer was covered with a silver containing foam dressing. Fifteen days later, there was moderate improvement, but the patient was lost to follow up thereafter.

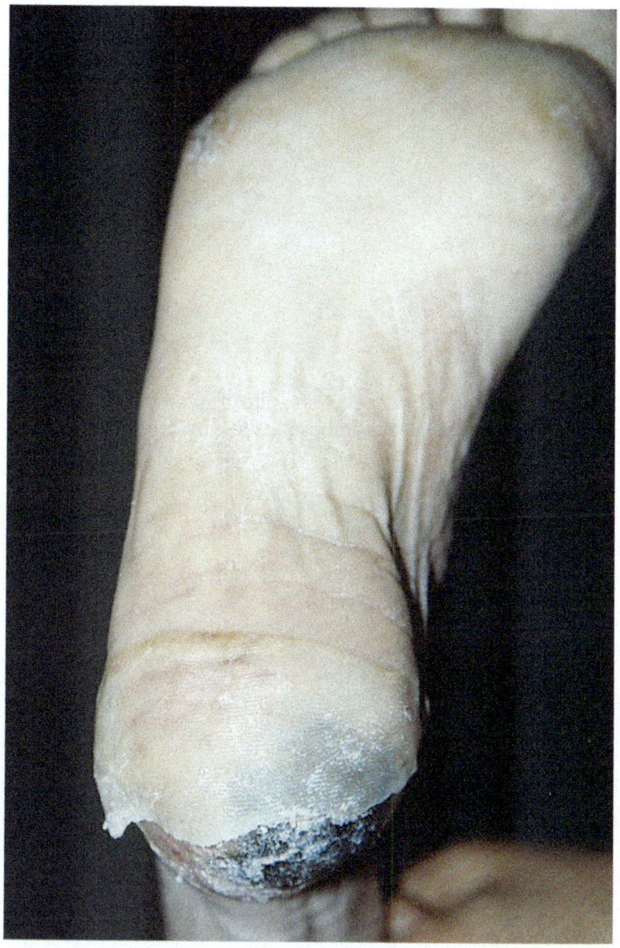

Figure 9.26 An unstageable heel pressure ulcer. Removal of the loose skin and the eschar revealed a stage 3 ulcer.

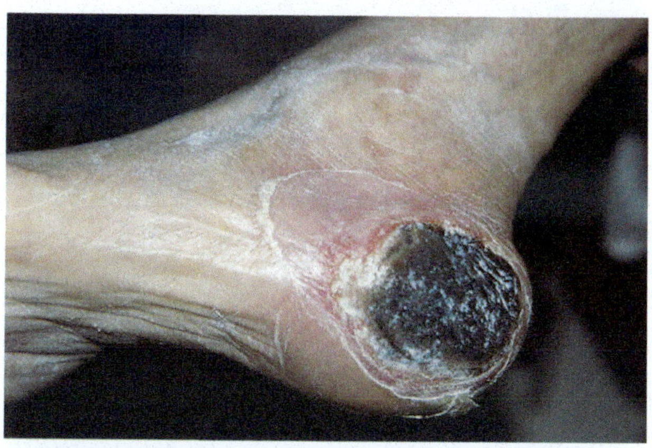

Figure 9.27 An unstageable heel pressure ulcer. Removal of the eschar revealed a stage 3 ulcer.

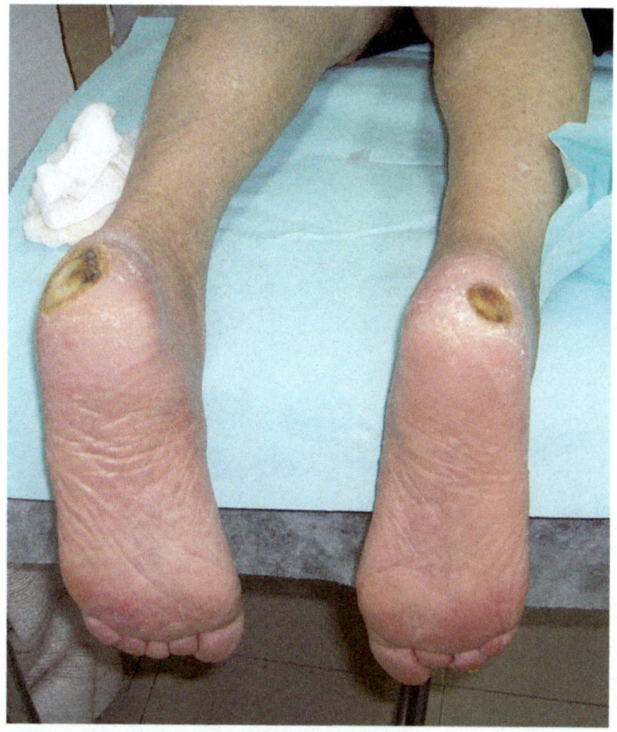

Figure 9.28 Case 9.2: Stage 2 pressure ulcers.

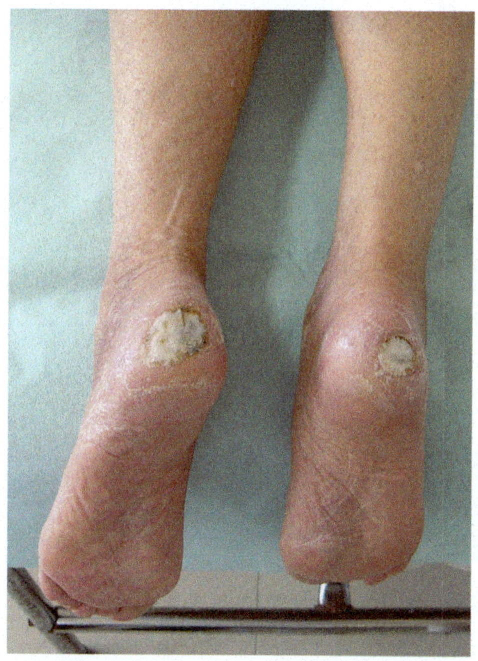

Figure 9.29 Case 9.2: Stage 2 pressure ulcers covered with Debrisan beadlets to allow enzymatic debridement as the patient had experienced extreme pain during manipulations.

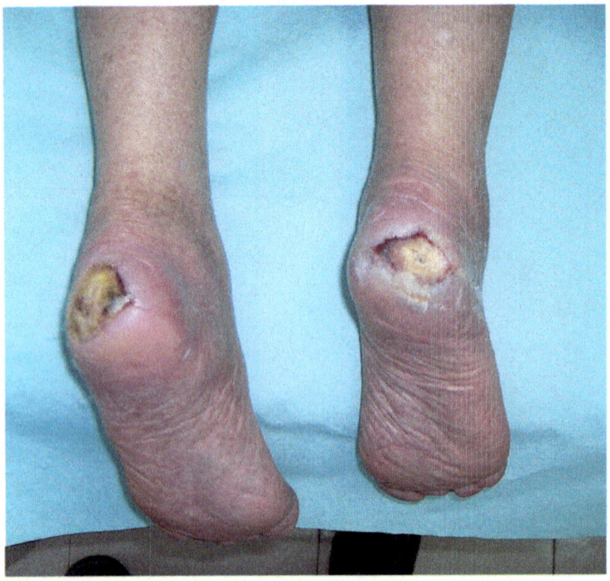

Figure 9.30 Case 9.2: Stage 3 pressure ulcers. A fissure to the adipose tissue, without muscle exposure, is seen on the right heel.

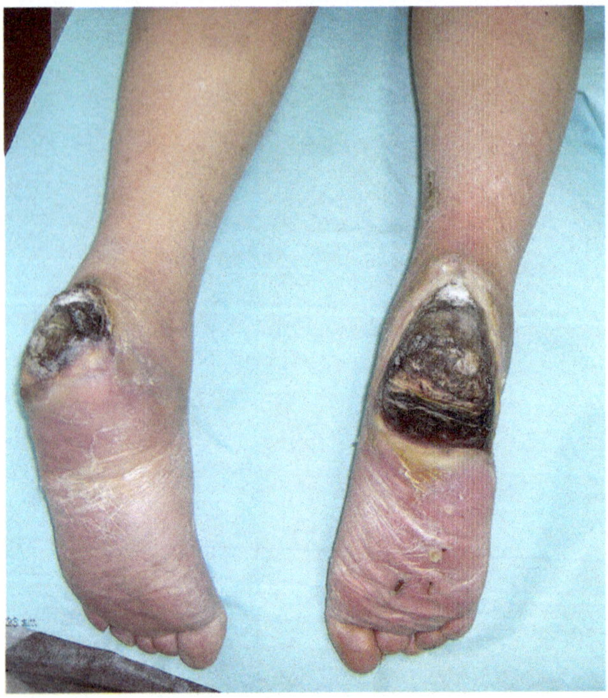

Figure 9.31 Case 9.2: Unstageable pressure ulcers.

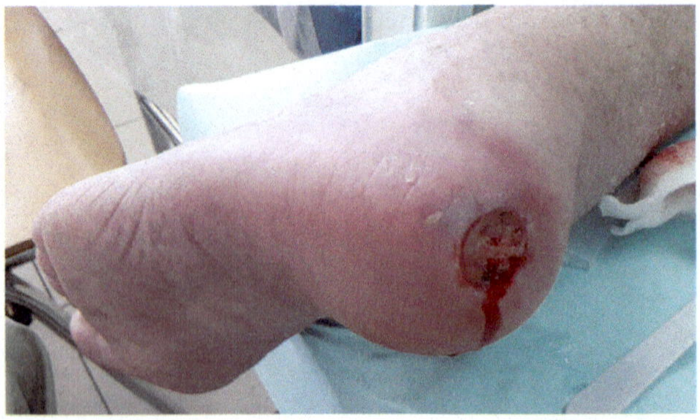

Figure 9.32 Case 9.3: A stage 3 pressure ulcer on the left heel. Exposure of subcutaneous adipose tissue is evident.

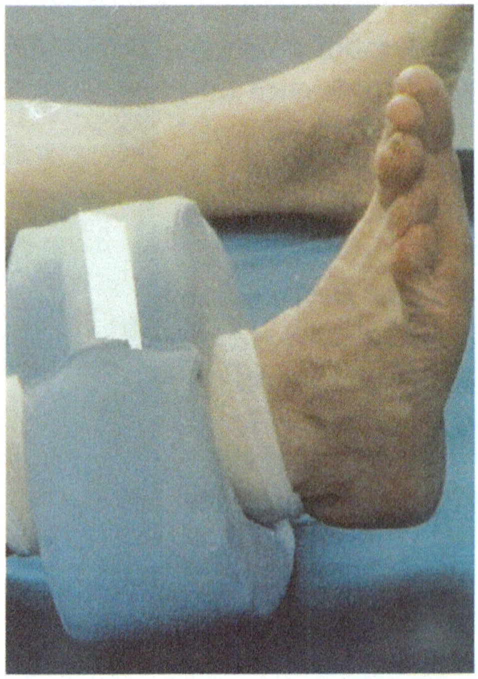

Figure 9.33 A heel protector ring, which keeps the heel suspended and completely off the mattress.

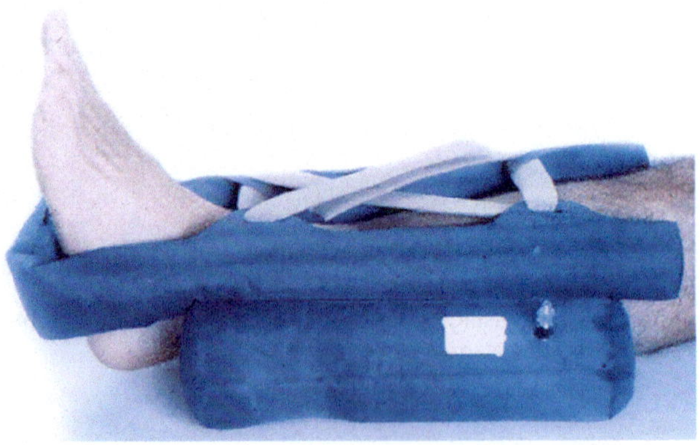

Figure 9.34 A calf support device, which provides a larger resting surface, thus off-loading pressure from the heel.

9.4 Prevention of Pressure Ulcers

These ulcers may account for extended hospitalization, and they are recognized as detrimental to an individual's quality of life, and a financial burden to the healthcare system. Pressure ulcers of the heel may be preventable using a heel protector ring (Figure 9.33) or other calf support devices (Figure 9.34). The calf has a larger resting surface, so the pressure over bony prominences is redistributed. Again, some ring cushions or doughnut devices have been shown to increase edema and venous congestion. In addition, revascularization should urgently be performed in patients with gangrene of the heel, since such ulcers heal slowly and may be infected. Even in the case of healed or healing ulcers, the best approach in terms of offloading for patients who are able to walk remains a matter of controversy.

Further Reading

Braden scale. Available at: www.bradenscale.com (accessed September 2009). This page also carries a link to the Copyright Permission Form.

D'Ambrogi, E., Giacomozzi, C., Macellari, V., and Uccioli, L. (2005). Abnormal foot function in diabetic patients: the altered onset of Windlass mechanism. *Diabet. Med.* 22: 1713–1719.

Healy, A., Naemi, R., and Chockalingam, N. (2014). The effectiveness of footwear and other removable off-loading devices in the treatment of diabetic foot ulcers: a systematic review. *Curr. Diabetes Rev.* 10: 215–230.

National Pressure Ulcer Advisory Panel. Updated pressure ulcer stages. Available at: http://www.npuap.org/resources/educational-and-clinical-resources/npuap-pressure-injury-stages (accessed February 2018).

Stechmiller, J.K., Cowan, L., Whitney, J.A.D. et al. (2008). Guidelines for the prevention of pressure ulcers. *Wound Repair Regen.* 16: 151–168.

Wong, V.K., Stotts, N.A., Hopf, H.W. et al. (2007). How heel oxygenation changes under pressure. *Wound Repair Regen.* 15: 786–794.

10

Charcot Foot

K. Makrilakis

First Department of Propaedeutic Internal Medicine, National and Kapodistrian University of Athens, Medical School, Laiko General Hospital, Athens, Greece

In 1703, William Musgrave first described a neuropathic joint as an arthralgia caused by venereal disease. In 1868, Jean-Martin Charcot gave the first detailed description of the disease, which was therefore named after him. Charcot noted this disease process as a complication of syphilis, but nowadays diabetes is the commonest etiology of Charcot arthropathy.

Also called Charcot neuro-osteoarthropathy (CNO), Charcot osteoarthropathy, neuropathic joint or Charcot joint, CNO is a progressive condition of the musculoskeletal system characterized by joint dislocations, pathologic fractures and debilitating deformities. It results in a progressive destruction of bone and soft tissues at weight-bearing joints; in its most severe form, it may cause significant disruption of the bony architecture. Charcot arthropathy can occur at any joint. However, it occurs most commonly in the lower extremities, at foot and ankle level. The most frequently involved joints are the tarsus and tarso-metatarsal (TMT) joints, followed by the metatarsophalangeal joints and the ankle. Although unusual, involvement of upper limb joints can occur.

CNO represents one of the most serious complications of diabetes (both type 1 and type 2). Its prevalence ranges between 0.3 and 7.5% (its true prevalence may actually be underestimated because of frequent misdiagnosis by untrained clinicians). A high prevalence of Charcot neuroarthropathy (12%) has been reported in patients following simultaneous pancreatic and kidney transplantation, a group characterized by severe and longstanding diabetes. It is usually unilateral, but bilateral involvement has been reported to occur in 6–40% in several series. In approximately 20% of cases the contralateral limb is affected later, usually within a couple of years. The development of this complication depends on peripheral somatic and autonomic neuropathy, together with an adequate blood supply to the foot. A minor trauma, often unrecognized by the patient, may initiate the process of joint and bone destruction. Some cases of CNO have been reported after infection of the foot, surgery to the ipsilateral or contralateral foot, or restoration of foot circulation. The mean age of presentation is approximately the 60th year, and the majority of the patients have diabetes for duration of more than 15 years. Men and women are affected equally. A majority of patients with Charcot foot will also have nephropathy and around 80–90% will develop medial calcifications of the arteries as well.

Two major theories exist regarding the pathophysiology of this condition:

- The *neurotraumatic theory* states that Charcot arthropathy is caused by an unperceived trauma or injury to an insensate foot. The sensory neuropathy renders the patient unaware of the osseous destruction that occurs with ambulation. This microtrauma leads to progressive destruction and damage to bone and joints.
- The *neurovascular theory* suggests that the underlying condition leads to the development of autonomic neuropathy, causing the extremity to receive an increased blood flow. This in turn results in a mismatch in bone destruction and synthesis, leading to osteopenia.

The general consensus is that CNO most likely results from a combination of these processes. The loss of proprioception and deep sensation leads to recurrent trauma, which ultimately leads to progressive destruction, degeneration and disorganization of the joint. In addition, a neurally mediated vascular reflex results in hyperemia, which can cause osteoclastic

Atlas of the Diabetic Foot, Third Edition. Ioanna Eleftheriadou, Alexandros Kokkinos, Stavros Liatis, Konstantinos Makrilakis, Nicholas Tentolouris, Anastasios Tentolouris, and Panagiotis Tsapogas.

Companion website: www.wiley.com/go/tentolouris/atlas_diabetic_foot

bone resorption. However, since the classic neurotraumatic and neurovascular theories fail to explain all the features of CNO, especially the common asymmetrical damage and self-limiting process, other hypotheses have recently been put forward. The signaling pathway of the receptor activator of nuclear factor-kB (RANK), RANK ligand (RANKL), and its decoy receptor osteoprotegerin (OPG) has been suggested as the link between vascular and bone metabolism. In fact, RANKL has been shown to mediate osteolysis in CNO by stimulating osteoclastic differentiation of monocytes/macrophages, an effect that is attenuated by OPG, the decoy receptor. This has led to nascent theories implicating RANKL/OPG signaling as the potential pathogenetic basis for Charcot arthropathy and has stimulated interest for new therapies.

10.1 Classification of Neuro-Osteoarthropathy Based on Characteristic Anatomic Patterns of Bone and Joint Destruction

Numerous classification systems based on clinical, radiographic and anatomic pathology describe Charcot arthropathy. Anatomic classification systems are the most commonly used and have the added benefit of predicting outcome and prognosis.

The classification proposed by **Sanders and Frykberg** (1991) is as follows:

- *Pattern I:* forefoot (involvement of the interphalangeal joints, phalanges, metatarsophalangeal joints and distal metatarsal bones). The frequency of this pattern is 26–67%, and it is often associated with ulceration over the metatarsal heads.
- *Pattern II:* tarsometatarsal joints. The frequency of this pattern is 15–48%. It often causes collapse of the midfoot and inversion of the plantar arch, the so-called rocker-bottom foot deformity.
- *Pattern III:* naviculocuneiform, talonavicular and calcaneocuboid joints. The frequency of this pattern is 32%. It often causes collapse of the midfoot and a rocker-bottom foot deformity, particularly when it is combined with pattern II.
- *Pattern IV:* ankle and subtalar joints. Although this pattern accounts for only 3–10% of CNO, it invariably causes severe structural deformity and functional instability of the ankle.
- *Pattern V:* calcaneus. Avulsion fracture of the posterior tubercle of the calcaneus. This pattern is not in fact neuro-osteoarthropathy, since no joint involvement occurs. This pattern is rare.

A simpler anatomical classification distinguishes between three types, the forefoot type, involving the interphalangeal (IP) and metatarsophalangeal (MTP) joints, the midfoot type, involving the TMT and tarsal joints, and the hindfoot variation, in which the ankle joint and calcaneum are involved.

Other classification systems have also been described (Harris & Brand 1966; Lennox 1974; Horibe et al. 1988; Saunders & Mrdjencovich 1991; Barjon 1993; Brodsky & Rouse 1993; Johnson 1995; Schon et al. 1998). A detailed description of these classification systems can be found in the literature.

10.2 Clinical Presentation and Laboratory Findings

The clinical presentation of CNO can vary widely depending on the stage of the disease. Thus, symptoms can range from mild swelling and no deformity to moderate deformity with significant swelling, and to severe deformity.

Acute Charcot arthropathy almost always presents with signs of inflammation. Profound unilateral swelling, an increase in local skin temperature (generally, 3–7°C above the skin temperature of the unaffected foot), erythema, joint effusion and bone resorption in an insensate foot are present. These characteristics, in the presence of intact skin and a loss of protective sensation, are often pathognomonic of acute Charcot arthropathy. The diagnosis is, however, very often missed by the treating clinician, because symptoms may be attributed to infection (cellulitis, osteomyelitis), gout, deep venous thrombosis, or sprain (especially if a minor trauma is preceded). It is also not unusual that an infectious process co-exists with CNO. Standard radiographs may usually show no abnormalities at this stage, contributing to delays in diagnosis.

Pain can occur in more than 75% of patients; however, the severity of the pain is significantly less than would be expected based on the severity of the clinical and/or radiographic findings. Instability and loss of joint function also may be present. Approximately 40% of patients with acute Charcot arthropathy have concomitant ulceration, which complicates the diagnosis and raises concerns that osteomyelitis is present.

A typical clinical presentation is a patient with a swollen, warm, and red foot, with mild pain or discomfort. Usually, there is a difference in skin temperature of more than 2°C compared with the unaffected foot (this can be best measured with a special skin thermometer; Figure 10.1). Most patients do not mention any trauma; some may, however, recall a minor one, such as a mild ankle sprain. On examination, pedal

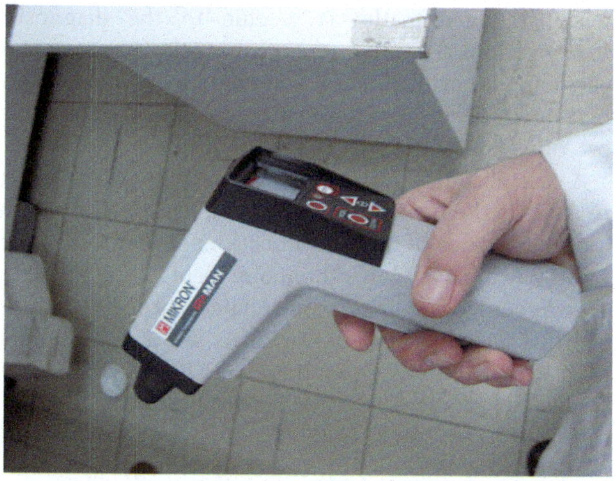

Figure 10.1 A thermometer for measuring skin temperature using infrared radiation, without touching the skin.

pulses are bounding, and findings of peripheral neuropathy are constantly present.

Charcot fractures that are not identified and treated properly may progress to marked joint deformity and to skin ulceration over a bony prominence. The ulceration can result in a severe infection, which may lead to osteomyelitis and a need for amputation of the extremity. Another complication of Charcot arthropathy is foot collapse, leading to the formation of a clubfoot, or a rocker-bottom foot, in which collapse and inversion of the plantar arch occurs. These deformities may, in turn, predispose to skin ulceration, an established risk factor for amputation. Other complications include ossification of the ligamentous structures, or the formation of intra-articular and extra-articular exostoses.

The white blood cell (WBC) count is usually normal, the erythrocyte sedimentation rate (ESR) may be slightly increased (20–40 mm $hour^{-1}$ – as opposed to usually >70 mm $hour^{-1}$ in osteomyelitis) and the C-reactive protein (CRP) level is often normal.

Recurrent acute attacks may occur, or there can be a slowly progressing arthropathy with insidious swelling over months or years.

10.3 Radiologic Findings

These depend on the stage of the disease. Eichenholtz (1966) described three clinico-radiologically distinct stages:

1) The stage of *development*, characterized by soft tissue swelling, hydrarthrosis, subluxations, cartilage debris (detritus), erosion of the cartilage and subchondral bone, diffuse osteopenia, thinning of the joint space and bone fragmentation (Figure 10.2).

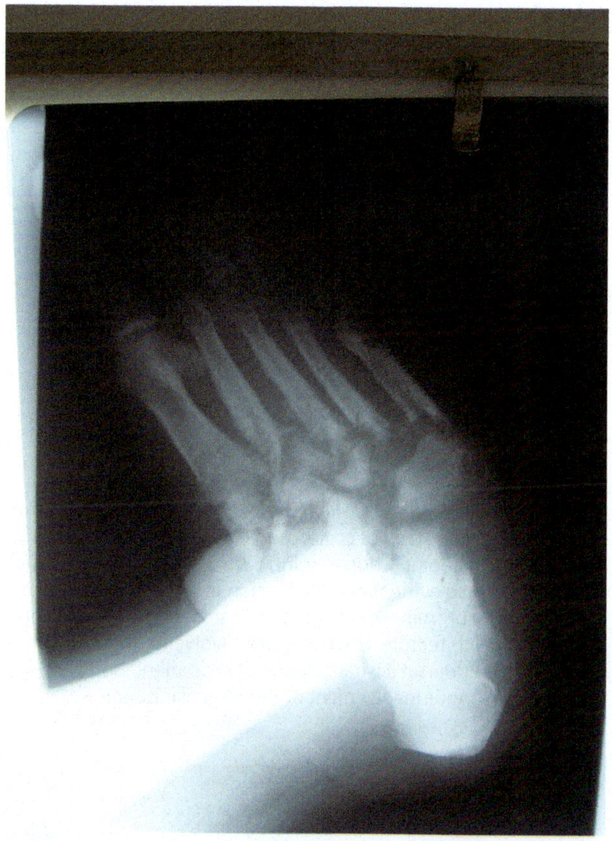

Figure 10.2 A patient with acute Charcot arthropathy of the midfoot, with hyperfragmentation of the midfoot bones. Also evident is old osteomyelitis of the head of the fifth metatarsal bone and amputation of the second toe.

2) The stage of *coalescence*, characterized by an attempt at restoration of the tissue damage. The inflammation subsides, fine debris is absorbed, periosteal bone is formed, bone fragments fuse to the adjacent bones and the affected joints are stabilized (Figure 10.3).
3) The *reconstructive* stage, characterized by subchondral osteosclerosis, periarticular spurring, exuberant intra-articular and marginal osteophytes, and ossification of the ligaments and joint cartilage. Joint mobility is reduced. Fusion and rounding of large bone fragments may be seen (Figure 10.4).

Exclusion of osteomyelitis in such patients is not always easy. Bone scintigraphy studies and magnetic resonance imaging (MRI) or computed tomography may not easily distinguish neuro-osteoarthropathy from osteomyelitis. In patients in whom MRI is unable to distinguish between infection and Charcot neuroarthropathy, labeled WBC scanning can be more specific, but should always be correlated with clinical findings. Patients with contraindications to MRI (e.g. a pacemaker) may be assessed using positron emission tomography (PET) scan or PET/CT, if available (at the moment, further study of PET scanning

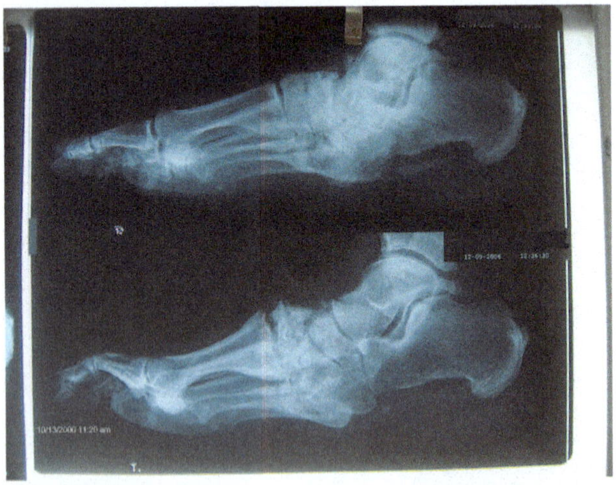

Figure 10.3 Upper picture: The right foot of a patient with Charcot arthropathy at the stage of coalescence. There is involvement of the talonavicular joint (Chopart joint) with distortion of its normal architecture. Also evident are calcification of the plantar fascia and a plantar bony prominence due to the Charcot foot distortion of the midfoot architecture. Lower picture: Involvement of the cuneiform–metatarsal (Lisfranc) joints of the patient's left foot. There is less serious involvement of the navicular bone.

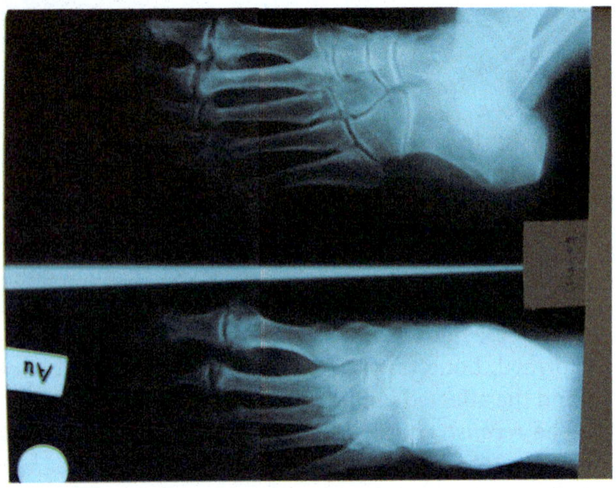

Figure 10.4 Involvement of the first, second and third metatarsophalangeal joints of a patient with a chronic Charcot forefoot arthropathy at the reconstructive stage, showing severe inflammatory changes of these joints.

is needed to determine the sensitivity and specificity of this imaging modality as a test to distinguish neuropathic arthropathy from osteomyelitis).

10.4 Differential Diagnosis

The diagnosis of acute CNO requires a high level of alertness for the disease. The acute development of foot swelling in a patient with long-standing diabetes and peripheral neuropathy is a clue to the diagnosis. Investigations are aimed at confirming the diagnosis and excluding other conditions that could be confused with neuropathic arthropathy, the most important of which is osteomyelitis/septic arthritis.

A careful clinical history and examination are essential to confirm the presence of peripheral neuropathy and to look for portals of entry of infection. Diabetes mellitus may be complicated by other coincidental joint diseases such as gout, calcium pyrophosphate arthropathy, osteoarthritis and inflammatory arthritis. As a result, joints with effusion should be aspirated and the fluid obtained evaluated for organisms and crystals. Exclusion of osteomyelitis is always a problem. Inflammatory indices (WBC count, ESR, CRP), radiologic images (plain X-rays, MRI, bone scintigraphy), and local cultures may sometimes help.

10.5 Treatment

A high index of suspicion, early diagnosis, and timely treatment are the keys to arrest progression of the disease. The treatment of Charcot arthropathy is primarily non-operative. Treatment consists of two phases: an acute and a post-acute phase. The management of the acute phase includes immobilization and a reduction of stress to the affected limb.

Immobilization usually is accomplished by casting. Total-contact casts have been shown to allow patients to ambulate, while preventing the progression of deformity. These can be worn permanently (Figure 10.5) or can be custom-made for the patient (Figure 10.6), who can take it off for bathing, sleeping, etc. (Figures 10.7 and 10.8).

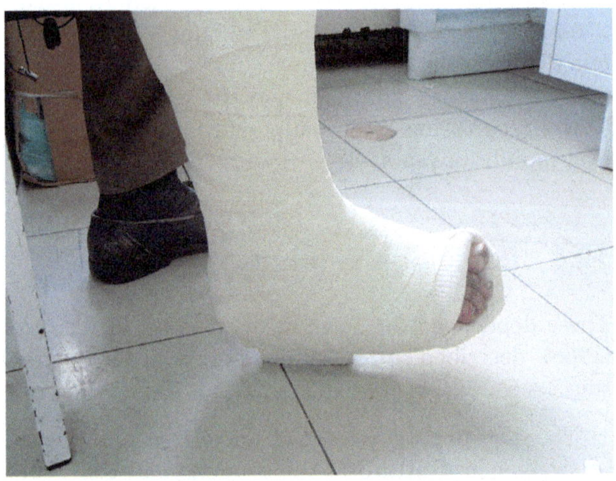

Figure 10.5 A total-contact cast placed on a patient with acute Charcot neuro-osteoarthropathy, to allow for some ambulation while at the same time off-loading the foot.

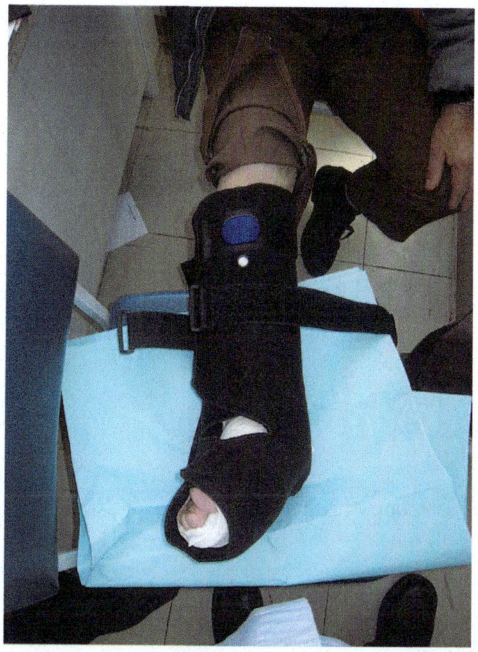

Figure 10.6 A special custom-made total-contact cast for a patient with Charcot arthropathy.

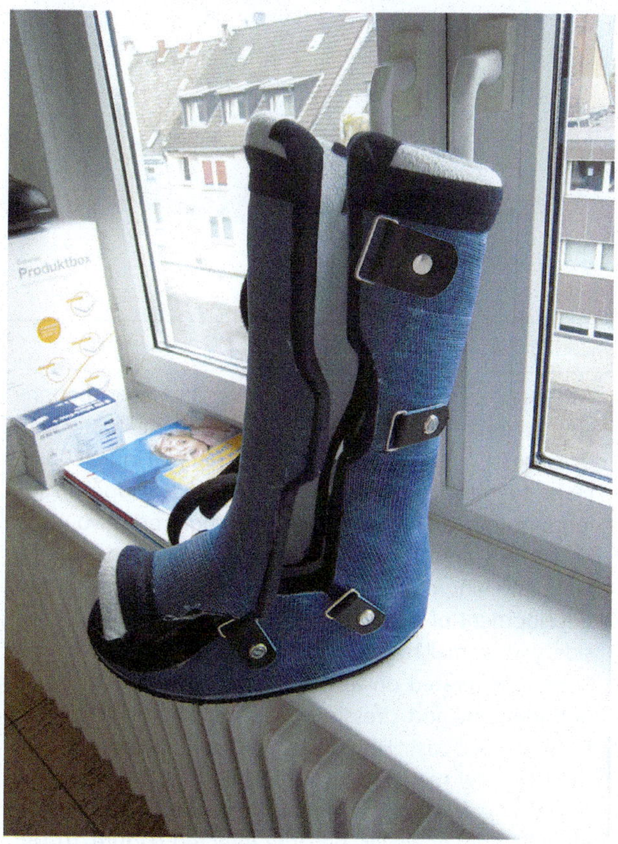

Figure 10.7 Another special custom-made total-contact cast for a patient with Charcot arthropathy.

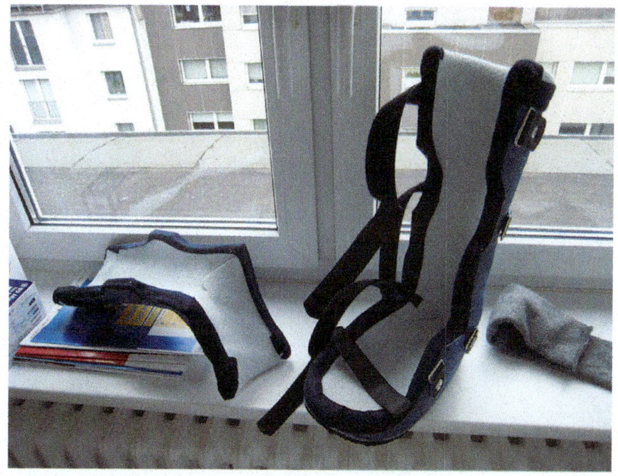

Figure 10.8 The special custom-made total-contact cast for Charcot arthropathy shown in Figure 10.8, showing details of its interior. The patient can take it off for sleeping, bathing, etc.

The cast is well molded with minimal padding, allowing total contact with the lower leg and foot. By molding casting material to the foot and leg, weight-bearing forces are spread out along the entire surface of contact, thus substantially reducing the vertical force per unit area and allowing an even distribution of pressures to the sole of the foot.

Casts must be checked weekly to evaluate for proper fit, and they should be replaced every one to two weeks as edema of the foot improves. Patients with concomitant ulceration must have their casts changed weekly for ulcer evaluation and debridement. Serial plain radiographs should be taken approximately every month during the acute phase to evaluate progress.

Casting usually is necessary for three to six months and is discontinued based on clinical, radiographic and dermal thermometric signs of quiescence. A minimum of eight weeks without weight-bearing has been recommended for disease of the midfoot, progressing through partial weight-bearing in a cast brace to full weight-bearing in about four to five months. Other methods of immobilization include special braces (Figure 10.9) and ankle–foot orthoses (Figure 10.10), but these may prolong healing times.

Reduction of stress is accomplished by decreasing the amount of weight-bearing on the affected extremity. While total non-weight-bearing is ideal for treatment, patients are often not compliant with this treatment. Studies have shown that partial weight-bearing with assistive devices (e.g. crutches [Figures 10.11 and 10.12] or walkers [Figure 10.13]) also is acceptable, without compromising healing time. However, full weight-bearing in the acute phase tends to lengthen the total time in the cast.

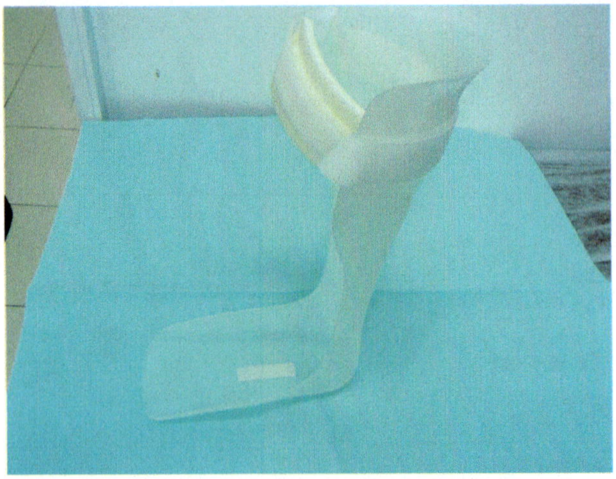

Figure 10.9 A special brace for ankle–foot joints.

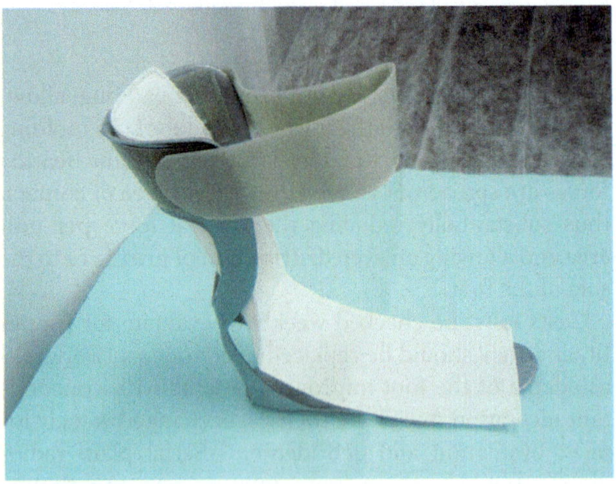

Figure 10.10 Special ankle–foot orthoses.

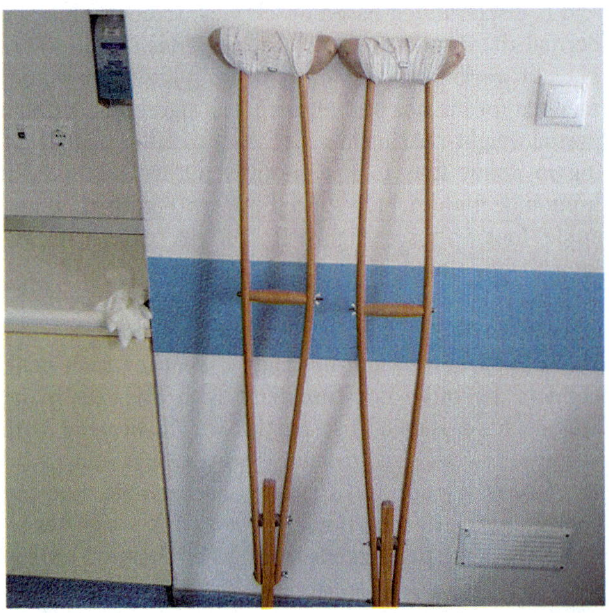

Figure 10.11 Armpit support crutches.

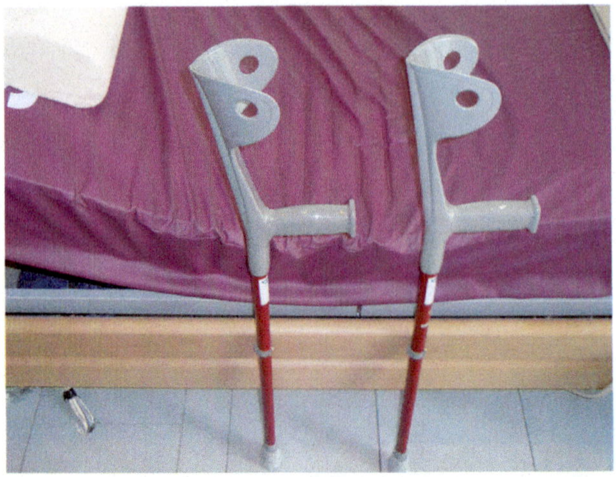

Figure 10.12 Elbow support crutches.

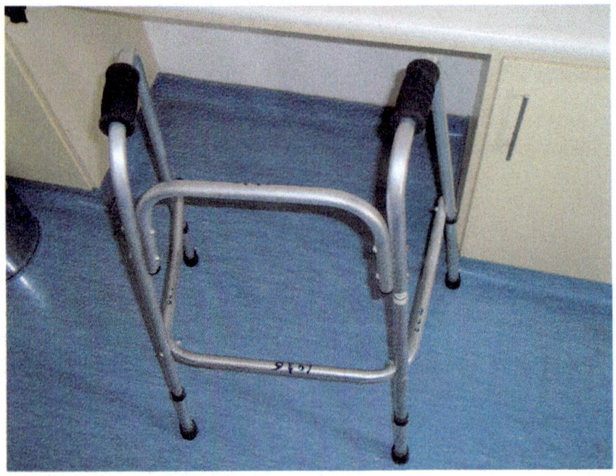

Figure 10.13 A walker.

Case 10.1

A 69-year-old man with type 2 diabetes and severe peripheral neuropathy presented to the diabetic foot clinic because of ulcers on the soles of both feet (Figure 10.14). He had a history of bilateral CNO that had developed in the left foot four years earlier and in the right one two years before. His right foot had a more prominent deformity, with flattening of the arch, widening of the foot and the development of a bony prominence on the inner lateral side, with a small hyperkeratosis over it (Figure 10.15).

He was treated on a weekly basis with local wound debridement and dressing changes, but he refused a total-contact cast. His ulcers gradually improved over the next few months (Figure 10.16), and the right one actually healed completely one year later (Figure 10.17). The left one, however, became infected (Figure 10.18), with a purulent discharge and the development of various microorganisms from local cultures, and had to be treated with systemic antibiotics.

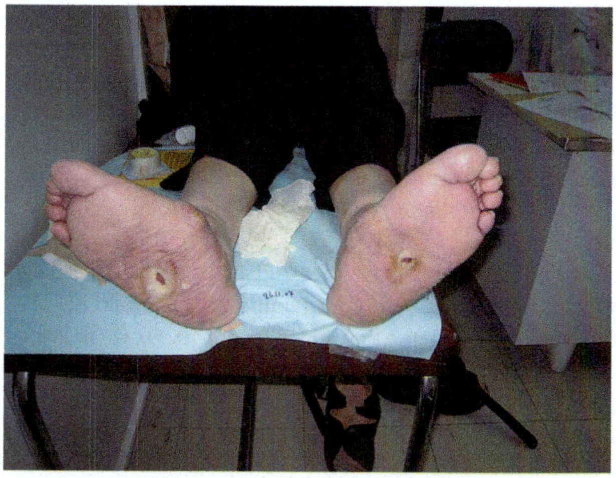

Figure 10.14 The feet of a patient with bilateral Charcot neuro-osteoarthropathy and ulcers on the soles. The right foot has a more prominent deformity, with flattening of the arch, widening of the foot and the development of a bony prominence on the inner lateral side, with a small hyperkeratosis over it.

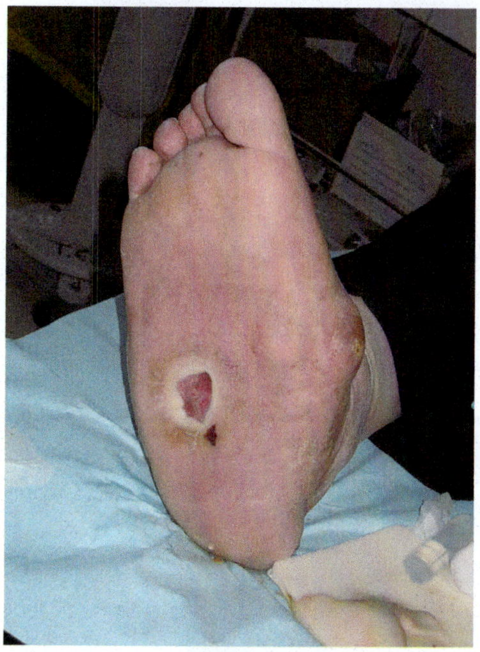

Figure 10.15 The right foot of the patient in Figure 10.14.

Management following removal of the cast includes a lifelong protection of the involved extremity. Patient education and professional foot care on a regular basis are integral aspects of lifelong foot protection. After cast removal, patients should wear a brace to protect the foot. Custom footwear includes extra-depth shoes with rigid soles and a plastic or metal shank (see Chapter 12). If ulcers are present, a rocker-bottom sole can be used. In addition, Plastazote inserts can be used for insensate feet.

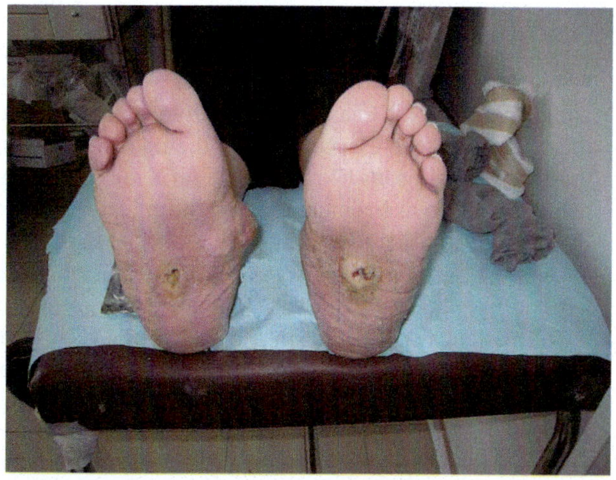

Figure 10.16 The feet of the patient with bilateral Charcot neuro-osteoarthropathy and ulcers on the soles shown in Figure 10.15, 2.5 months later. The ulcers have considerably improved with local wound care.

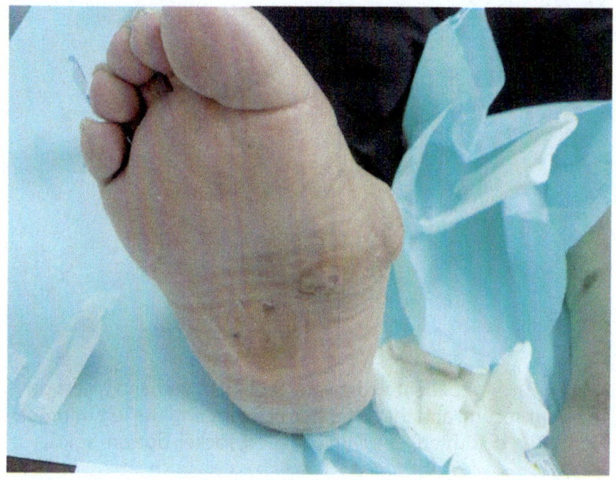

Figure 10.17 One year later, the right foot of the patient shown in Figure 10.15, with the ulcer on the sole nearly completely healed.

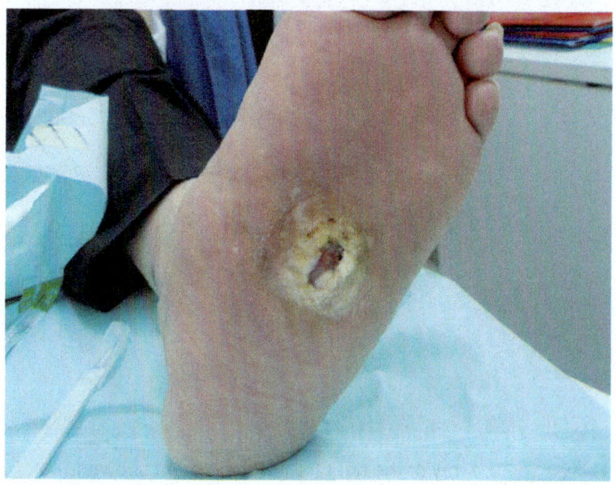

Figure 10.18 The left foot of the patient shown in Figure 10.15, with a persistent ulcer on the sole of the midfoot, which became infected.

Case 10.2

A 56-year-old man with type 2 diabetes of 11 years' duration and bilateral chronic Charcot feet presented with ulcers on the soles of his feet, especially under the right second and third metatarsal heads (Figure 10.19). An X-ray of the feet revealed extensive fragmentation of the metatarsals and the metatarsophalangeal joints, with a pencil-like appearance of the right foot metatarsals (Figure 10.20), while the left side was not particularly badly damaged (Figure 10.21).

The patient was treated on a weekly basis with local wound debridement and dressing changes for several months. He was advised on foot off-loading with a special boot for total non-weight-bearing, but was not compliant. Because of concerns of osteomyelitis, he was treated with systemic antibiotics and hyperbaric oxygen, and a half-foot cast was placed on his right foot to help with off-loading of the ulcer (Figure 10.22). Unfortunately, his condition did not improve. Local cultures grew different microbes (*Staphylococcus aureus*, *Proteus mirabilis*, *Escherichia coli*, *Morganella morgagni*), and systemic antibiotics had to be given.

The ulcer on his right foot did not heal and actually looked worse one year later (Figure 10.23), while his left foot developed a large new ulcer (Figure 10.24). On moving the foot, the right looked like "a loose bag of bones." The patient was advised on foot amputation but refused. He continued to require close medical attention with repeated admission to the hospital for antibiotic-resistant soft tissue infections of the foot.

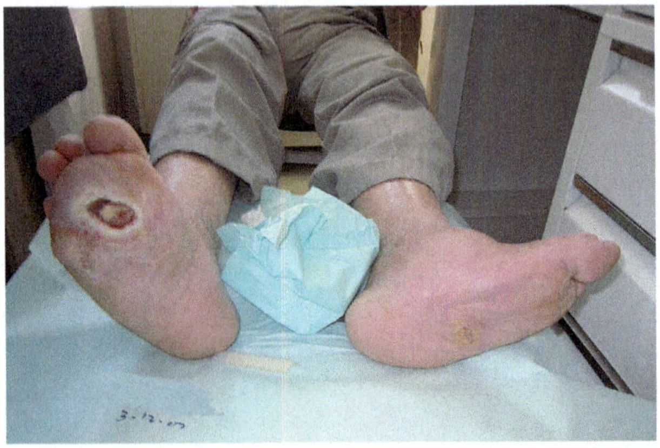

Figure 10.19 A patient with bilateral Charcot feet and ulcers on the right second and third metatarsal heads and the left midfoot. Notice the deformed feet, with widened, rocker-bottom soles.

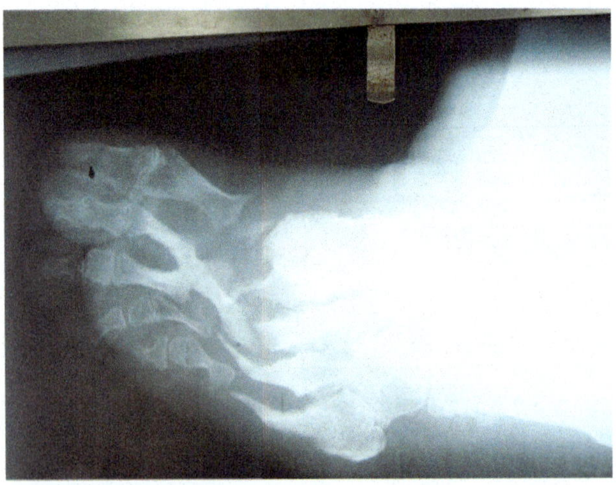

Figure 10.20 X-ray of the right foot of the patient shown in Figure 10.19, with extensive fragmentation of the metatarsals and the metatarsophalangeal joints, and a pencil-like appearance of the metatarsals.

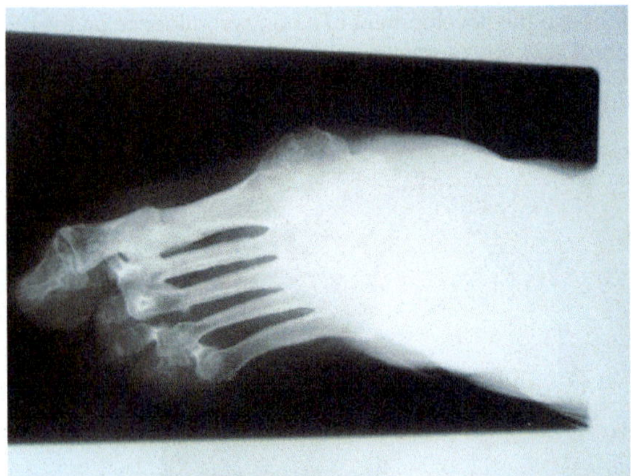

Figure 10.21 X-ray of the left foot of the patient shown in Figure 10.19, showing much less severe involvement than on the right.

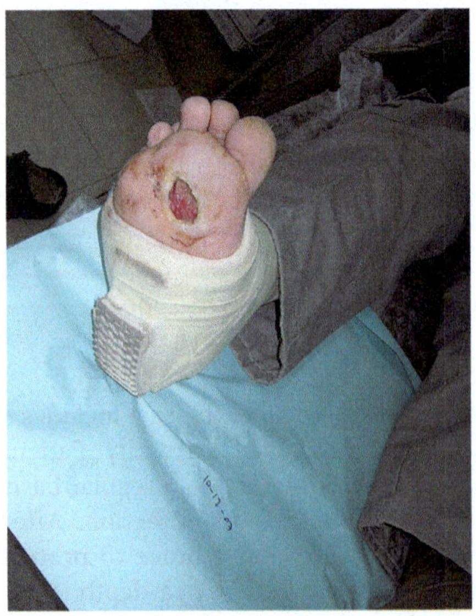

Figure 10.22 A half-shoe ambulatory cast has been placed on the right foot of the patient shown in Figure 10.19 to off-load the forefoot and help with ulcer healing.

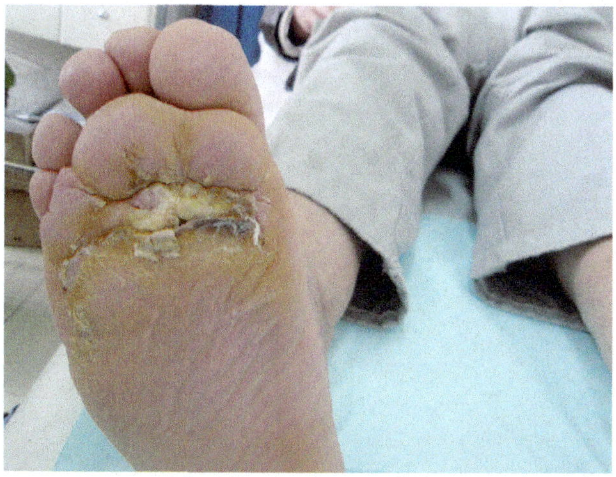

Figure 10.23 The right foot of the patient shown in Figure 10.19 one year later. Note the deformed chronic ulcer under the second and third metatarsals.

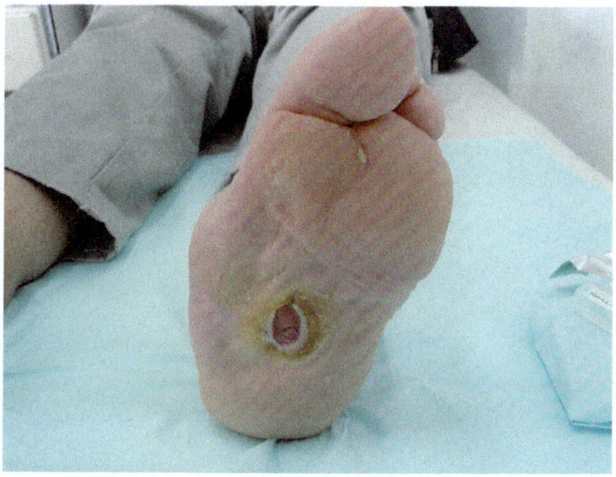

Figure 10.24 The left foot of the patient shown in Figure 10.19 one year later. The ulcer on the midfoot has re-emerged.

This regimen may be eliminated after 6–24 months, based on clinical, radiographic and dermal thermographic findings. The continued use of custom footwear in the post-acute phase for foot protection and support is essential. The total healing process typically takes one to two years. Preventing further injury, noting temperature changes, checking the feet every day, reporting trauma and receiving professional foot care also are important principles of treatment.

Surgical procedures and techniques vary based on the location of the disease and on the surgeon's preference and experience with Charcot arthropathy. Surgery has generally been advised for resecting infected bone (osteomyelitis), removing bony prominences that could not be accommodated with therapeutic footwear or custom orthoses, or correcting deformities that could not be successfully accommodated with therapeutic footwear or custom ankle-foot orthoses. Surgical procedures

Case 10.3

A 62 year-old man, with history of type 2 diabetes for 12 years, working as a civil servant with a physically very light office job, developed a swollen, red, warm right foot, causing minimal discomfort on walking, without any apparent trauma. Evaluation by his primary care physician allegedly revealed a fracture on X-ray of his right mid-foot. He was referred to an orthopedic physician, who advised rest for a while and anti-inflammatory medications. The patient over the next few months continued to walk on the foot, which gradually got disfigured, remained swollen, with flattening of the arch, widening of the sole and development of a bony prominence on the inner lateral side (Figure 10.25), together with a large, purulent ulceration of the sole at the level of the arch (Figure 10.26). An X-ray of the foot showed disarticulation of the TMT joints, fractures of the third and fourth metatarsal bones, osteopenia and calcification of a mid-foot artery between the first and second metatarsals (Figure 10.27). Clinical examination showed loss of protective sensation of light touch, temperature and vibration on the feet. WBC count, CRP, and ESR were elevated. A diagnosis of CNO together with possible osteomyelitis was made. He was started on antibiotic treatment together with advice on complete off-loading of the right foot. He was prescribed a removable air-cast boot to start using after a couple of months. The ulcer was completely healed over the following six months (Figure 10.28) and he was able to return to work, but with a permanent deformity of the right foot (Figure 10.29), needing special custom-made shoes to accommodate it. An orthopedic surgical consultation was planned for the future in case the ulcer would recur.

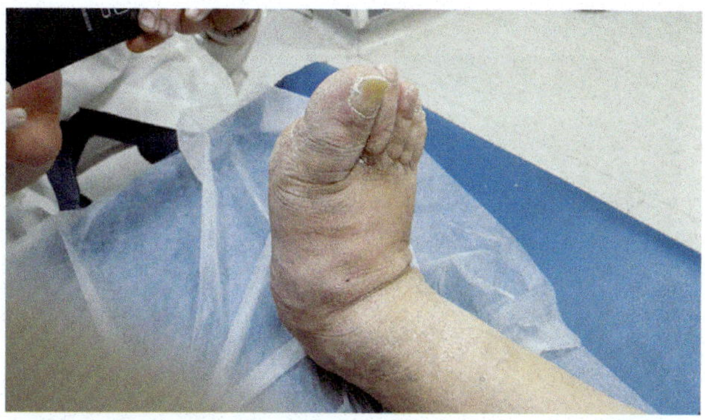

Figure 10.25 Dorsal aspect of the right foot of a 62-year old male depicting swelling and disfiguration of the foot.

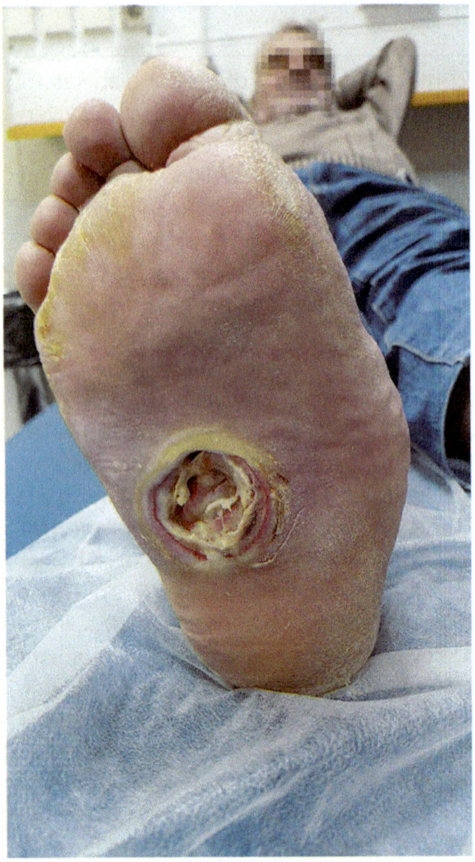

Figure 10.26 Plantar aspect of the right foot of the patient showing flattening of the arch, widening of the sole and development of a bony prominence on the inner lateral side, together with a large, purulent ulceration of the sole at the level of the arch.

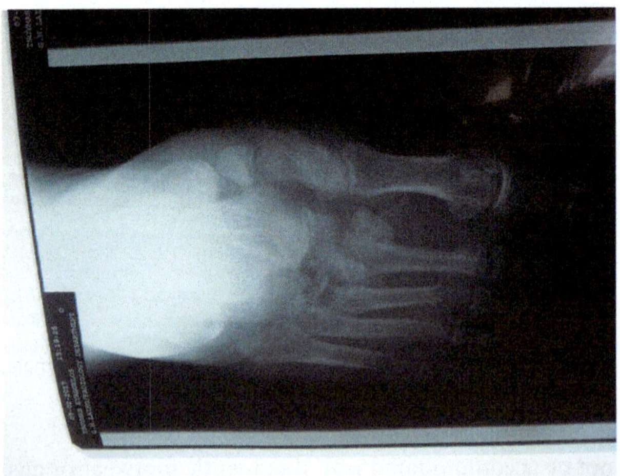

Figure 10.27 X-ray of the right foot of the patient shown in Figures 10.25 and 10.26, revealing disarticulation of the tarso-metatarsal joints, fractures of the third and fourth metatarsal bones, osteopenia and calcification of a mid-foot artery between the first and second metatarsals.

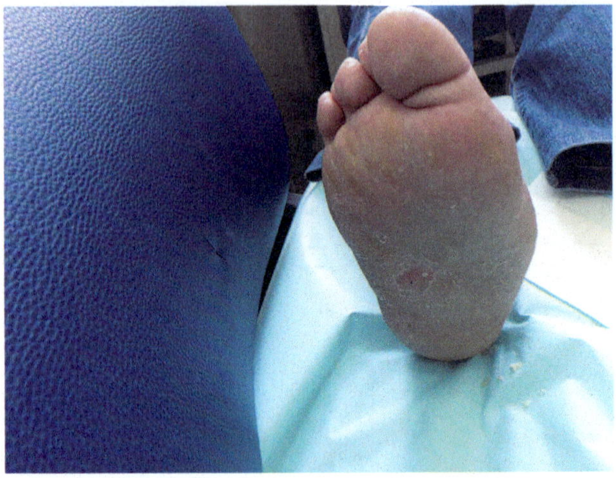

Figure 10.28 Plantar aspect of the right foot of the patient shown in Figure 10.26, depicting healing of the ulcer, but with persistent flattening of the arch, widening of the sole and development of a bony prominence on the inner lateral side.

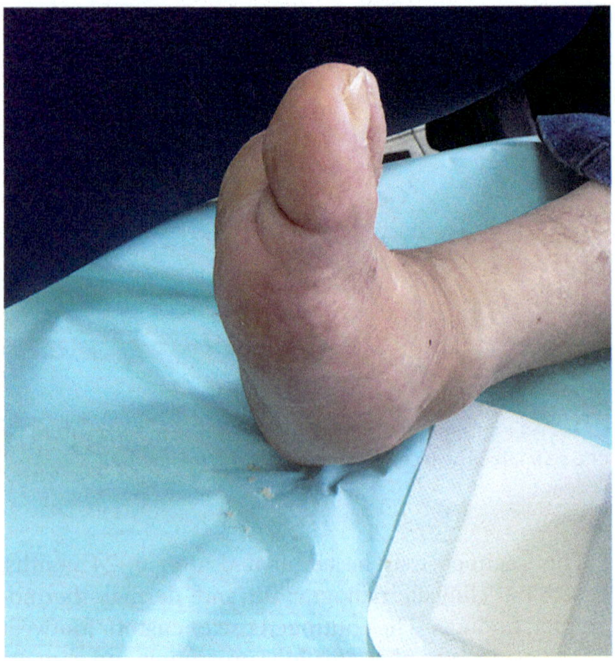

Figure 10.29 Lateral view of the foot showing the persistent deformity with formation of a bony prominence on the inner side of the sole.

include exostosectomy of bony prominences, osteotomy, arthrodesis, screw and plate fixation, open reduction and internal fixation, reconstructive surgery, fusion with Achilles tendon lengthening, autologous bone grafting and amputation. Patients treated with surgery have longer healing times.

Case 10.4

An 82-year old man with history of Type 2 diabetes for 40 years and venous insufficiency of his lower extremities bilaterally, developed ulcers of his medial malleoli, which got infected and required hospitalization and i.v. antibiotic treatment. The ulcers healed and the patient was discharged home in stable condition. A few months later, during a routine clinic visit, he was noted to have a swollen left ankle, warm to touch but non-tender, with mild external rotation (Figure 10.30). An X-ray revealed osteopenia and bone resorption of the posterior edge of the tibia in the left medial malleolus, with narrowing of joint space (Figure 10.31). Soft tissue edema and ostyeophytes of the talus bone were also noted. A scintigram with Tc99m (Figure 10.32) showed increased uptake of radiation in the left tarsal bones, consistent with an active inflammatory process (an MRI could not be performed because the patient had an unknown type of pacemaker since 20 years earlier). WBC count, ESR and CRP were normal.

The patient was considered to have acute Charcot arthropathy of the left ankle and was advised on immediate immobilization with a total contact cast. He refused casting and opted for an air-cast removable boot because he wanted to retain some mobility. A few days later he presented with recurrent inflammation of the left medial malleolus ulcer, with was apparently injured by the boot (Figure 10.33). and worsening of the external rotation of the ankle (Figure 10.34). A new X-ray (Figure 10.35) revealed deterioration of the bone resorption of the posterior edge of the tibia in the left medial malleolus with formation of some osseous cysts and sclerosis and disorganization of the subtalar joint. ESR was still within normal limits for the patient's age (35 mm $hour^{-1}$), together with WBC count and CRP. The patient was admitted to the hospital for intravenous antibiotic treatment. He now accepted total contact casting of the left foot, after the ulcer would be healed.

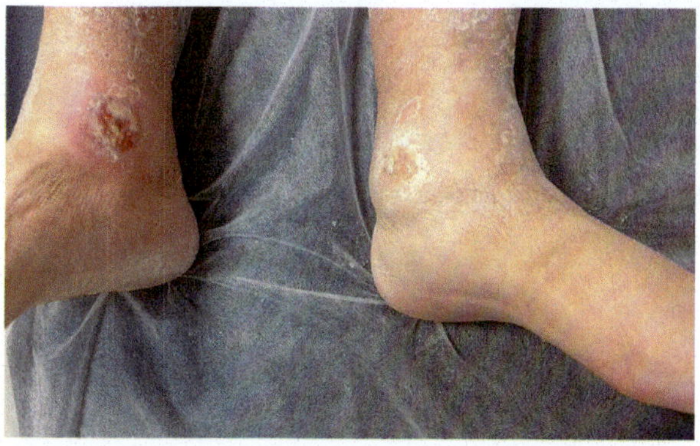

Figure 10.30 Photograph of both ankles of an 82-year old male with diabetes of long duration. Notice the healed ulcers of bilateral medial malleoli and the external rotation of the left ankle. The left ankle was actually more swollen and warmer than the right one, although the ulcer on the right side seemed more erythematous.

Other treatment options that have been tested include the use of bisphosphonates, which are potent inhibitors of bone resorption and have minimal effect on bone formation. This action stops the osteoclastic activity of bone breakdown, promotes healing, and decreases local inflammation. However, this treatment appears rather ineffective and even deleterious for the resolution time of the acute stage and, moreover, data on long-term outcomes are not available. There is, therefore, currently little evidence to support the use of bisphosphonates as part of the routine management of patients with diabetes complicated by acute CNO. Given the involvement of the RANKL pathway in the pathogenesis of CNO, anti-RANKL agents (e.g. denosumab) is another treatment option currently being tested.

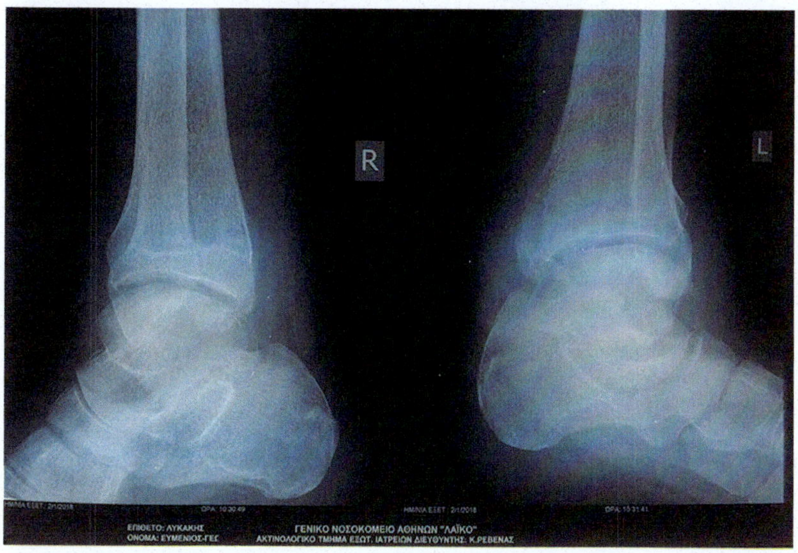

Figure 10.31 X-ray of both ankle joints of the patient in Figure 10.30. Notice the bone resorption of the posterior edge of the tibia in the left medial malleolus, with narrowing of joint space.

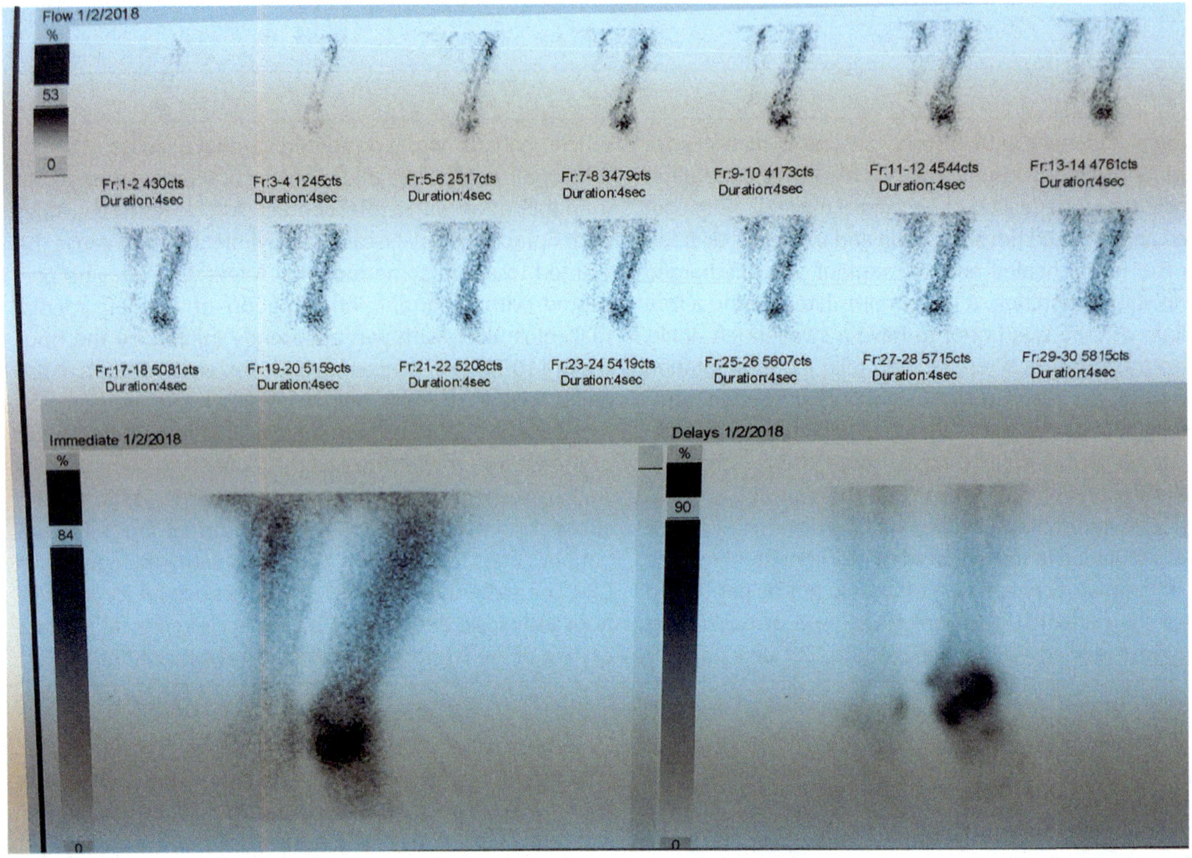

Figure 10.32 Three-phase scintigram with Tc99m of the patient shown in Figure 10.30, depicting increased uptake of radiation in the left tarsal bones.

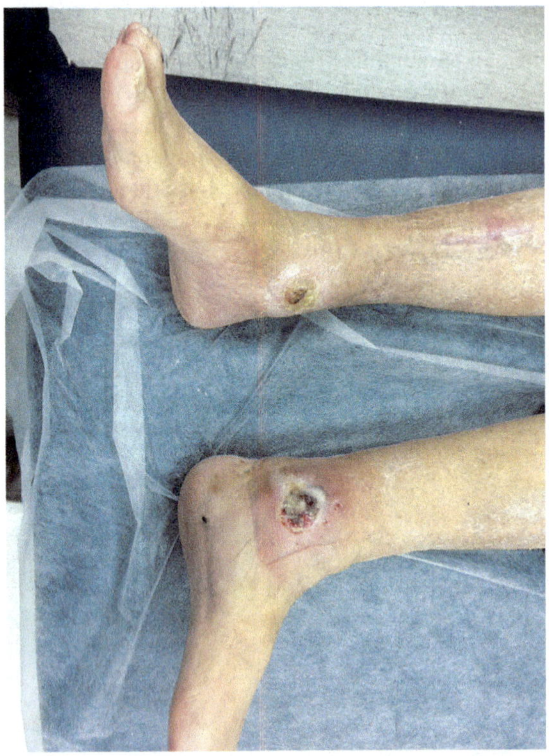

Figure 10.33 Photograph of the left ankle of the patient in Figure 10.30, showing a recurrent inflamed ulcer of the left medial malleolus.

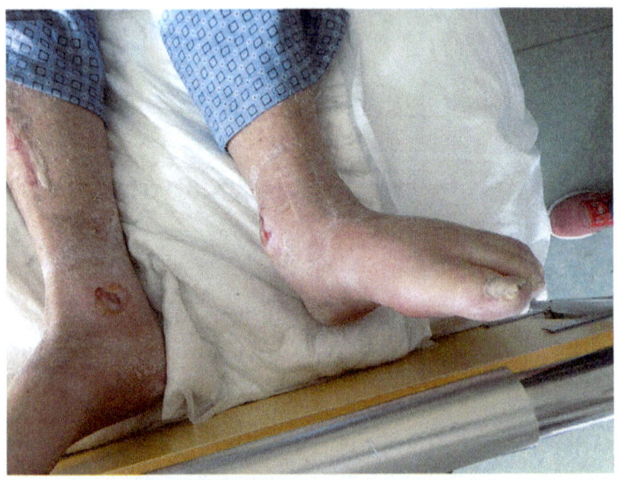

Figure 10.34 Photograph of the left ankle of the patient in Figure 10.30, showing more prominent external rotation of the foot.

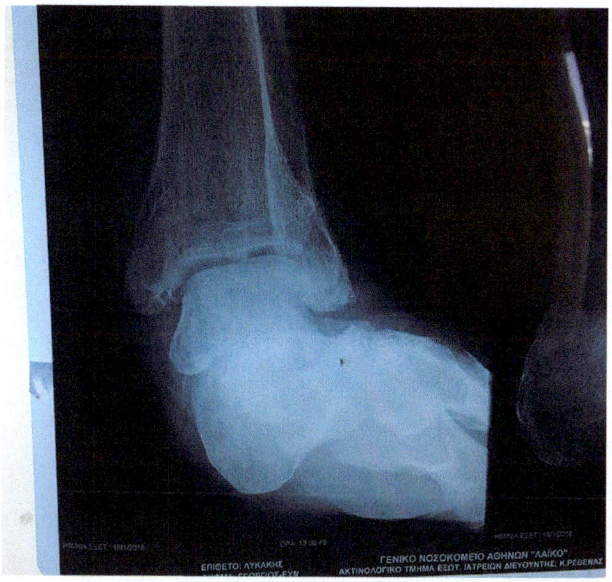

Figure 10.35 X-ray of the left ankle joint of the patient shown in Figure 10.33 with bone resorption of the posterior edge of the tibia in the left medial malleolus and formation of some osseous cysts as well as sclerosis and disorganization of the subtalar joint.

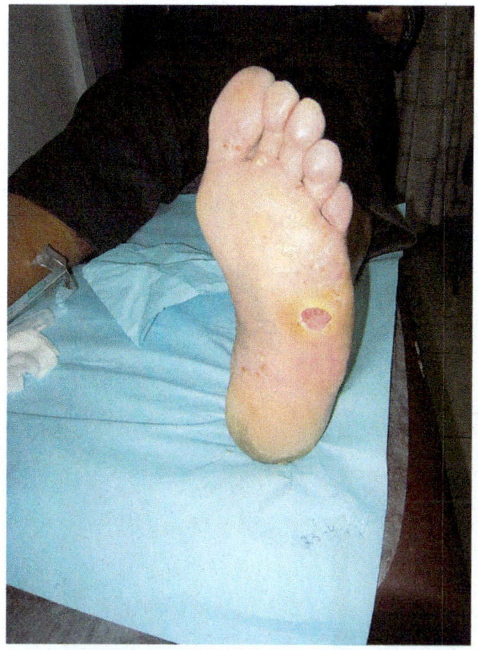

Figure 10.36 The left foot of a diabetic patient with a neuropathic ulcer under the fifth metatarsal.

Case 10.5

A 60-year-old man with long-standing diabetes was referred to the diabetic foot clinic by his primary care physician because of an ulcer under his left fifth metatarsal (Figure 10.36) and a Charcot foot on the right side (Figure 10.37). A plain X-ray of the right foot revealed a midfoot Charcot arthropathy with a navicular fracture (Figure 10.38), while the left foot showed a fracture of the fifth metatarsal (Figure 10.39).

The temperature of his right foot was 2°C higher than that of his left. He had increased ESR and CRP levels, and a culture of the ulcer bed on the left foot after debridement grew *E. coli* and *S. aureus*. Because of the consideration of osteomyelitis of the left foot, the patient was admitted to the hospital for a few days for intravenous antibiotic treatment and intravenous bisphosphonate (he received intravenous zoledronic acid).

One month later, he returned with a new ulcer on the sole of the right foot, with purulent discharge (Figure 10.40). He was again treated with antibiotics and alendronate by mouth. Despite aggressive antibiotic therapy, his condition did not improve (Figure 10.41), and he developed an abscess on his right foot (Figure 10.42) with a fistula on his right sole communicating with the lateral side of the foot (Figure 10.43).

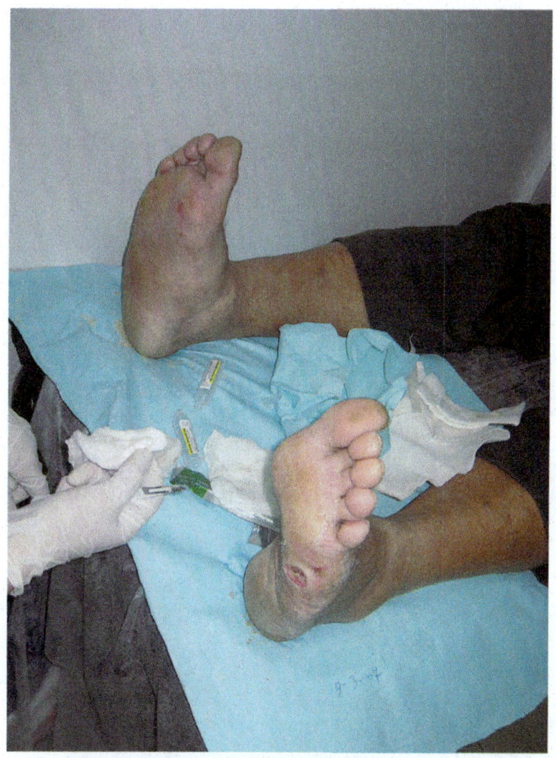

Figure 10.37 Both feet of the patient in Figure 10.35 showing Charcot foot on the right side (note the deformed, widened right foot) and a neuropathic ulcer under the left fifth metatarsal.

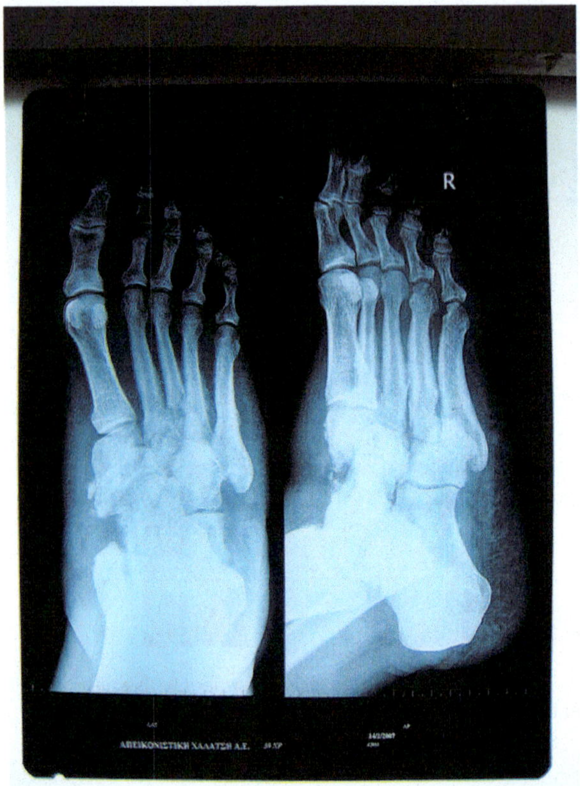

Figure 10.38 X-ray of the right foot of the patient shown in Figure 10.36, revealing a midfoot Charcot arthropathy with a navicular fracture.

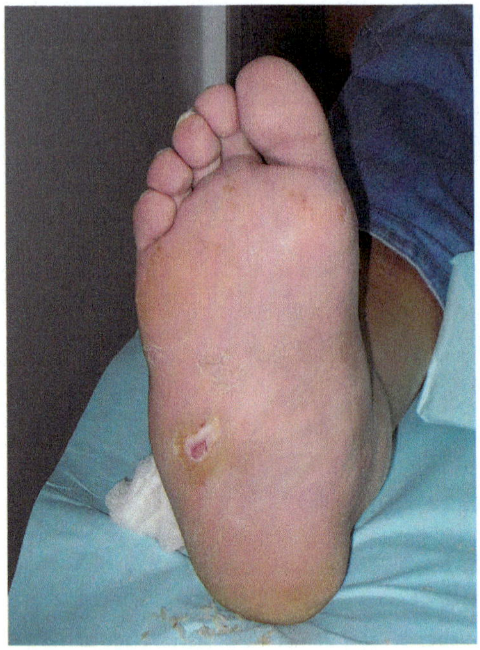

Figure 10.40 The right foot of the patient shown in Figure 10.36, one month later, showing a new ulcer on the sole, under the base of the fifth metatarsal, with purulent discharge.

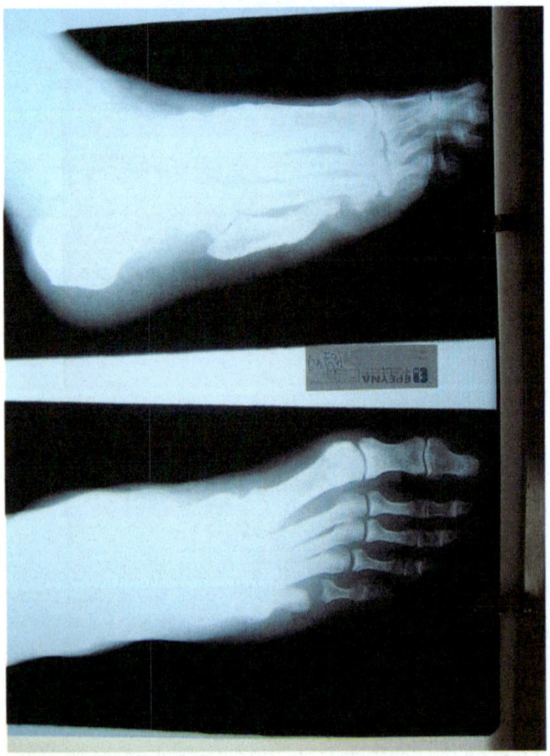

Figure 10.39 X-ray of the left foot of the patient shown in Figure 10.36, revealing a fracture of the fifth metatarsal.

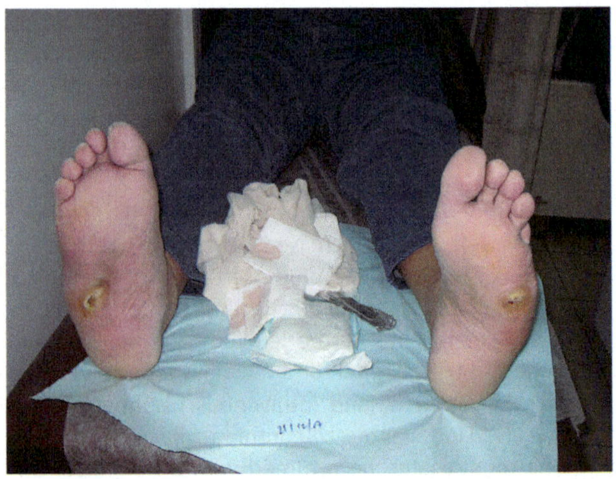

Figure 10.41 The feet of the patient shown in Figure 10.36, nine months later, showing bilateral fifth metatarsal ulcers.

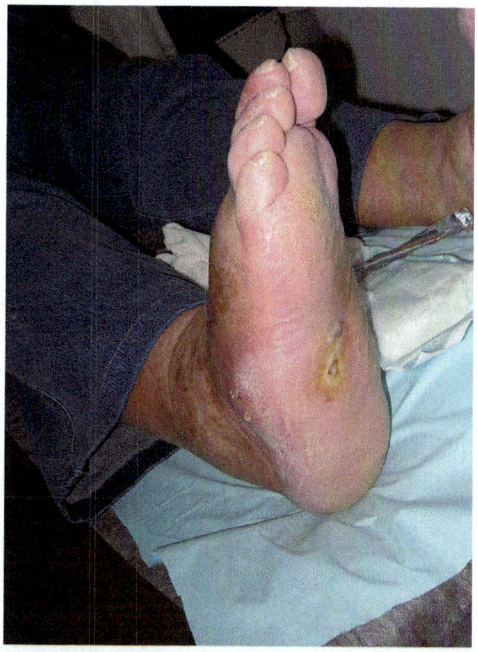

Figure 10.42 The right foot of a patient with an ulcer at the base of the fifth metatarsal and an abscess on the dorsum of the foot.

Case 10.6

A 45-year-old man with type 2 diabetes was referred to the diabetic foot clinic for evaluation and treatment of a swollen, warm, mildly painful foot. He had a history of nephrotic syndrome, and had had a right second toe amputation 2 years earlier because of thrombosis of the digit. His right foot was widened, with a rocker-bottom deformity (Figure 10.44). A plain X-ray showed hyper-fragmentation of the midfoot bones and evidence of osteomyelitis of the head of the fifth metatarsal bone and amputation of the second toe (see Figure 10.2). His foot was swollen and painful (Figure 10.45).

Acute Charcot arthropathy was diagnosed, and the patient received intravenous bisphosphonate treatment. He was advised on proper footwear and bed rest for foot off-loading. A few months later, a repeat X-ray showed the disease had entered a quiescent phase (Figure 10.46).

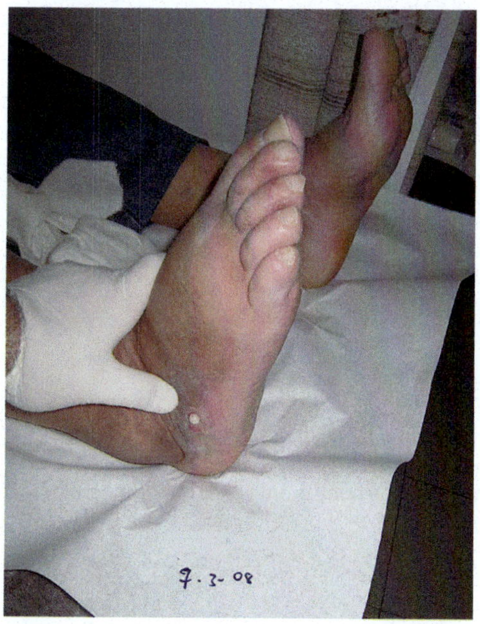

Figure 10.43 The right foot of the patient shown in Figure 10.36, two months later, with a fistula communicating between the ulcer on the sole and the lateral side of the dorsum of the foot.

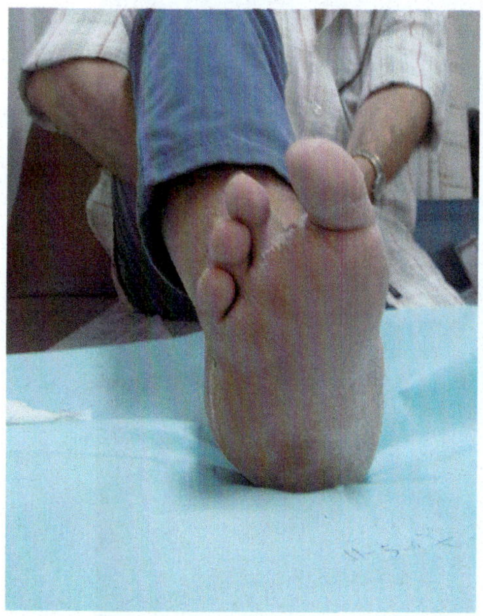

Figure 10.44 A diabetic patient with a widened right foot with a rocker-bottom deformity. An amputation of the second toe is evident.

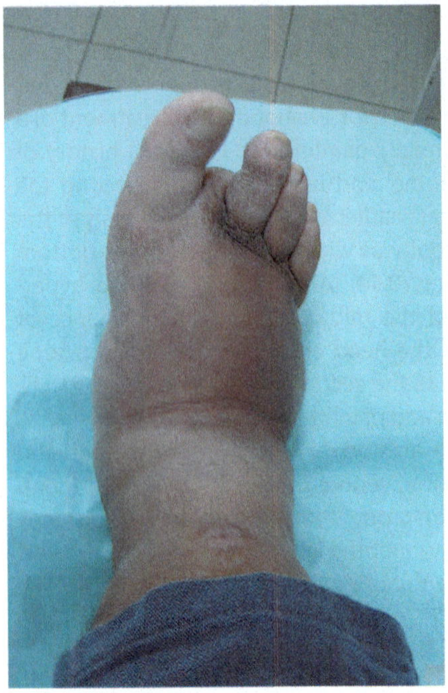

Figure 10.45 The right foot of the patient shown in Figure 10.41 viewed from above. Notice the wide, edematous foot, and the second toe amputation.

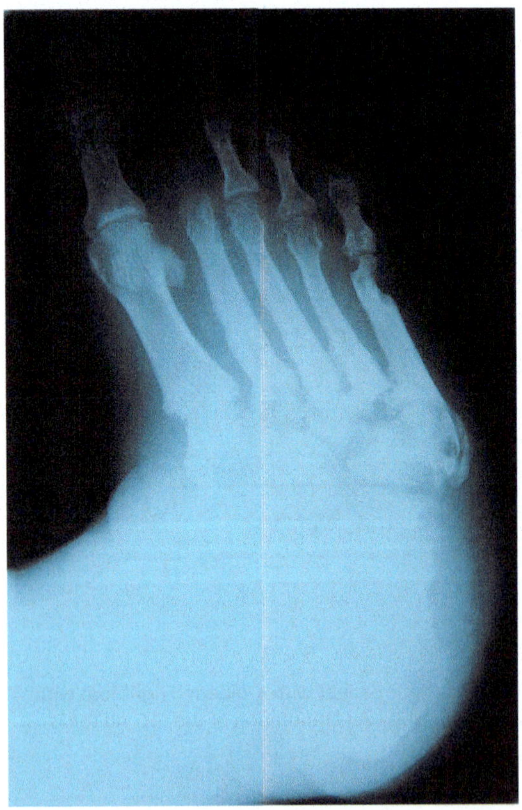

Figure 10.46 X-ray of the right foot of the patient shown in Figure 10.41, six months later, showing marginal osteophytosis of the cuboid bone, and fusion and rounding of the large bone fragments of the midfoot, indicative of the reconstructive stage of the disease. Again, the osteomyelitis of the fifth metatarsal and the amputated second toe can be noted.

Case 10.7

A 62-year-old woman with history of a right Charcot foot and an ulcer on her right sole (Figure 10.47) was seen in the diabetic foot clinic. She had repeated sessions of debridement of the ulcer. Her foot had a permanent rocker-bottom deformity (Figure 10.48). The deformity and the ulcer were still present seven months (Figure 10.49) and eight months (Figure 10.50) after her first visit, when the patient was seen in the clinic.

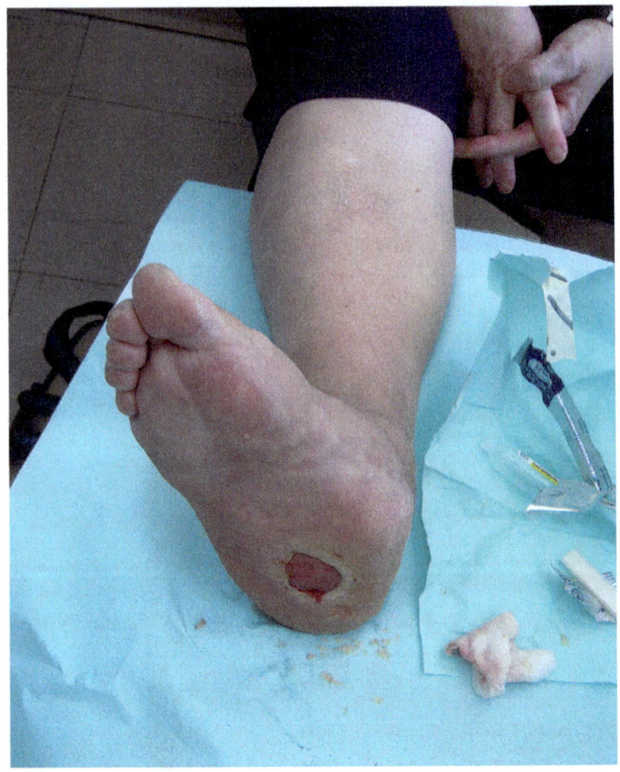

Figure 10.47 The right foot of a female diabetic patient with Charcot foot and a large ulcer at the base. Notice the rocker-bottom deformity and the bony prominence on the inner side.

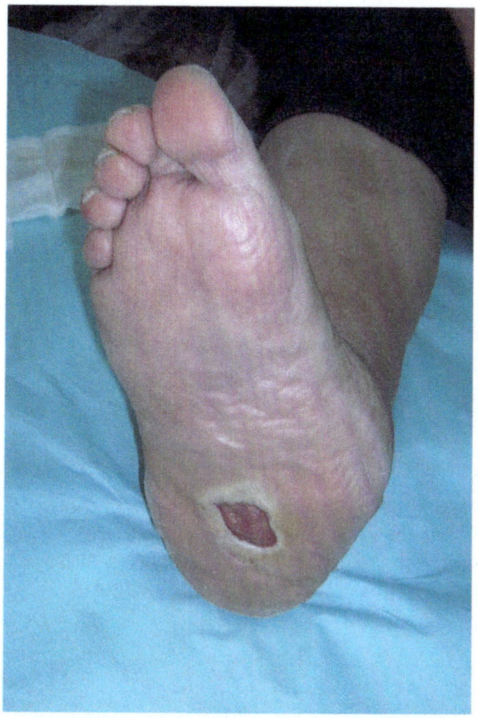

Figure 10.48 The right foot of the patient shown in Figure 10.44, four months later, with the Charcot foot and the large ulcer at the base. Notice the rocker-bottom deformity and the bony prominence on the inner side.

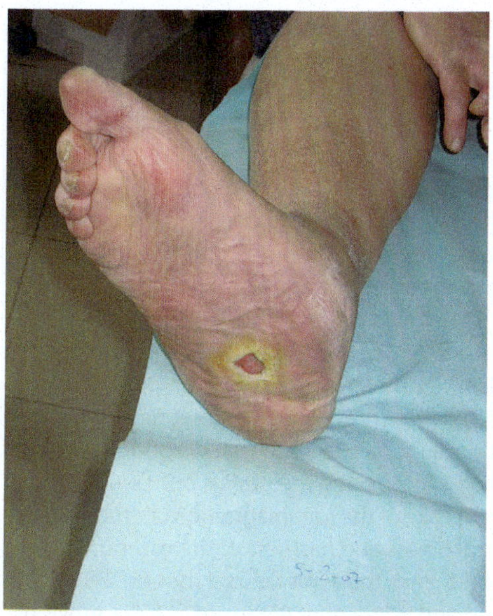

Figure 10.49 The foot of the patient shown in Figure 10.44, seven months later, with persistence of the deformity.

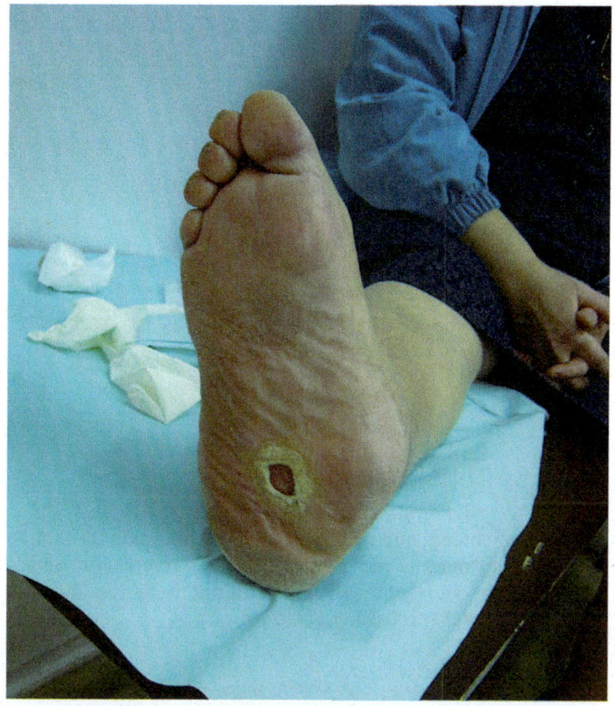

Figure 10.50 The foot of the patient shown in Figure 10.44, eight months later, with persistence of the deformity.

Case 10.8

A 61-year-old woman with type 2 diabetes for 22 years and chronic renal insufficiency had developed a chronic Charcot foot after a fracture of her right leg six years earlier. She presented to the diabetic foot clinic with a large (5 × 6cm) non-healing ulcer on her right sole, together with a smaller one (1 × 1cm) on the outer surface of her sole (Figure 10.51). She was seen nearly twice a month in the clinic, with local debridement of the ulcers, and was advised on off-loading of the foot with appropriate footwear, which she was not compliant with. Because of concerns of infection of the ulcers, she was not a candidate for a total-contact cast.

Around 10 months later, the ulcers were still persisting (Figure 10.52), and one month after that the large ulcer started showing signs of infection with a purulent discharge (Figure 10.53). A plain X-ray of her foot (Figure 10.54) showed evidence of CNO of the rear foot, but osteomyelitis could not definitely be ruled out.

The patient was treated with repeated sessions of antibiotics, but unfortunately, she developed a very aggressive infection with the development of necrotizing fasciitis of the tibia, for which she required repeated surgical interventions and finally needed amputation of the leg below the knee.

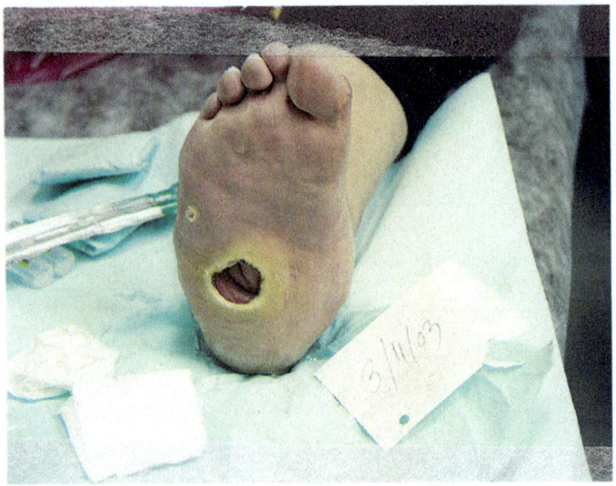

Figure 10.51 The right foot of a 61-year-old woman with a chronic Charcot foot and a large (5 × 6cm) non-healing ulcer of the right sole, together with a smaller one (1 × 1cm) on the outer surface of the sole. Note the hyperkeratosis at the rims of the ulcers and the widened rocker-bottom foot.

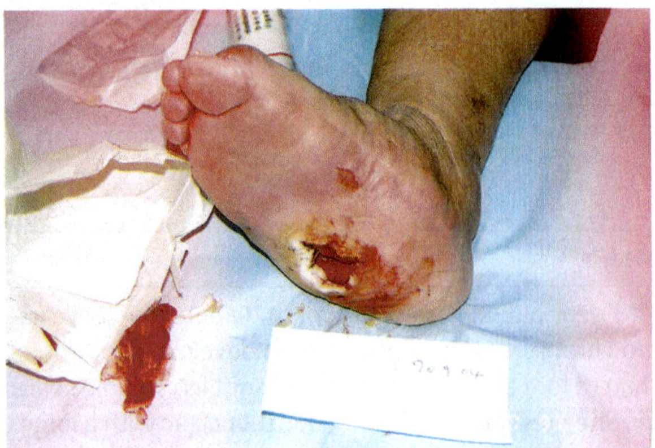

Figure 10.52 Persistence of the ulcers of the patient shown in Figure 10.48, 10 months later.

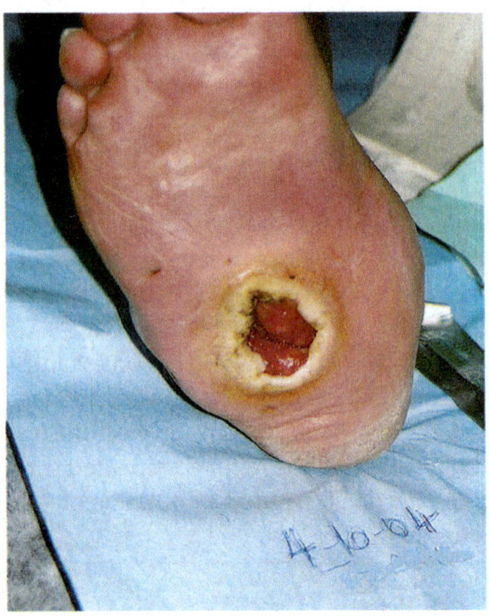

Figure 10.53 One month later, the ulcer shown in Figure 10.51 is still persisting, with signs of infection (purulent discharge).

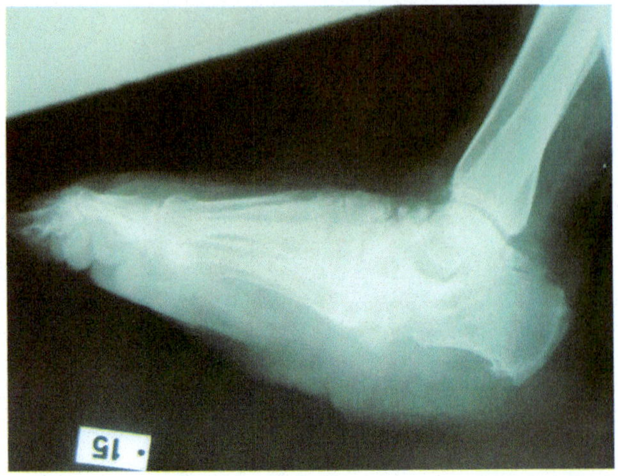

Figure 10.54 Plain X-ray of the right foot of the patient shown in Figure 10.50. Note the involvement of the talus and the talonavicular joint, with the possibility of osteomyelitis. Also evident is excessive edema of the soft tissues of the sole of the foot.

Case 10.9

A 55 year-old man developed a callus on the plantar surface of his right big toe from an ill-fitted new shoe at work, which he scratched and an ulcer developed. Over the following couple of weeks, the whole foot got swollen and warm, but without tenderness (Figure 10.55). At the same time, he developed symptoms of increased thirst and polyuria, which prompted laboratory examinations and the diagnosis of new onset diabetes (HbA1c 10.2%). The patient was treated with antibiotics by mouth by his primary care physician for four weeks. X-ray examination revealed extensive bony destruction of the mid-foot with osseous fragmentation, sclerosis, subluxation of TMT joints and new bone formation (bony debris) adjacent to the cuboid and second metatarsal (Figure 10.56). An MRI examination of the foot (Figure 10.57), with intravenous paramagnetic contrast administration (Figure 10.58), revealed abnormal magnetic signal on all tarsal and metatarsal bones with inhomogeneous uptake of the paramagnetic material around the metatarsal bones and haziness of the osseous cortex of the second and third metatarsal bones. ESR was 75 mm $hour^{-1}$ and WBC count 8600 mm^{-3}. A diagnosis of acute CNO of the midfoot together with possible osteomyelitis was made. He was advised on complete foot off-loading and continuation of the antibiotic treatment. One month later there was mild improvement of the leg edema (Figure 10.59 and Figure 10.60), with periosteal bone formation around the metatarsals, fusion of bony fragments to the adjacent bones and stabilization of the affected joints (Figure 10.61). Antibiotic treatment and foot off-loading were continued.

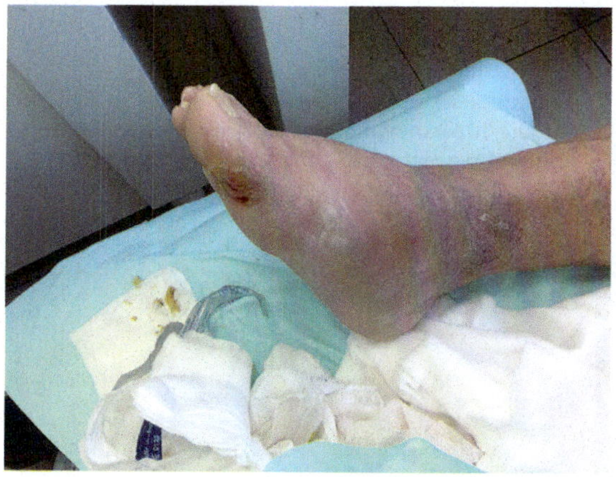

Figure 10.55 Photograph of the right foot of a 55-year old male. Notice the extreme edema of the whole foot and an ulcer on the plantar surface of the big toe. The foot was warm but not tender.

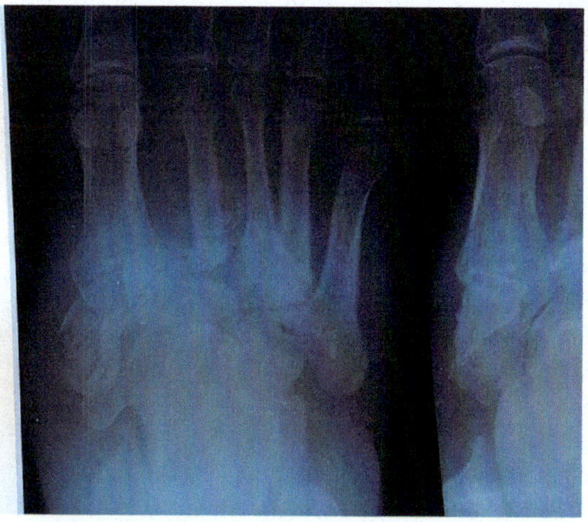

Figure 10.56 X-ray of the right foot of the patient in Figure 10.54 showing extensive bony destruction of the mid-foot with osseous fragmentation, sclerosis, subluxation of tarso-metatarsal joints and new bone formation (bony debris) adjacent to the cuboid and second metatarsal.

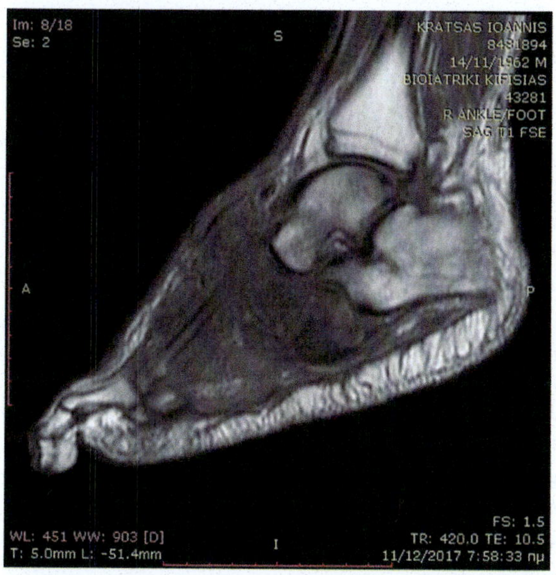

Figure 10.57 MRI examination of the right foot of the patient shown in Figure 10.54 revealing abnormal magnetic signal on all tarsal and metatarsal bones.

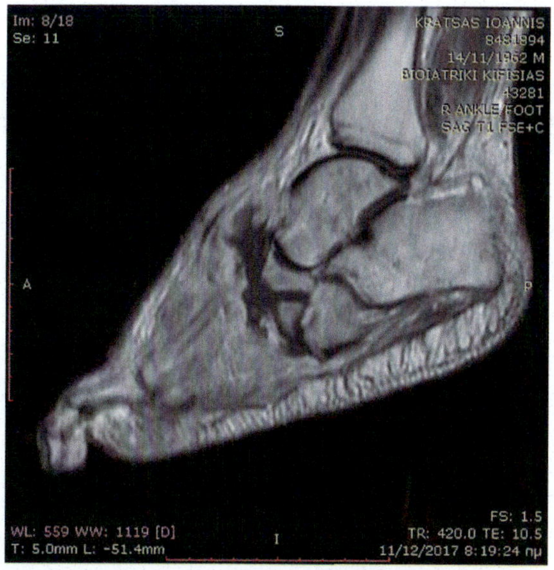

Figure 10.58 MRI examination of the right foot of the same patient after intravenous paramagnetic contrast administration showing inhomogeneous uptake of the paramagnetic material around the metatarsal bones.

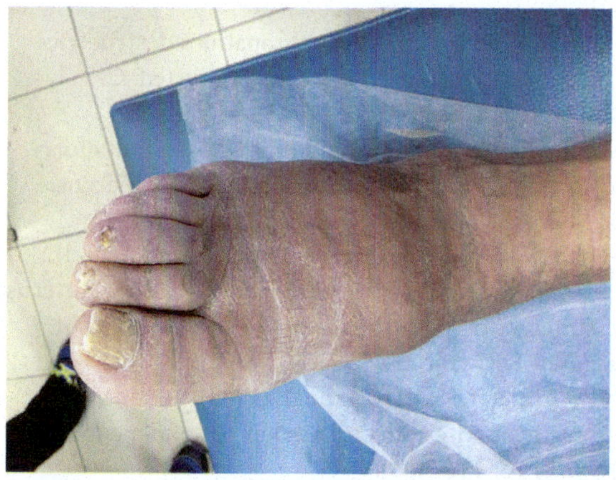

Figure 10.59 Dorsal aspect of the right foot of the patient shown in Figure 10.54, one month later. The edema has subsided a bit.

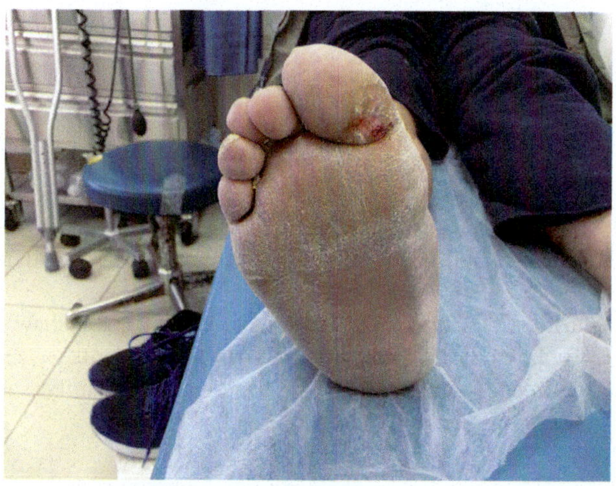

Figure 10.60 Plantar aspect of the right foot of the patient shown in Figure 10.54, one month later.

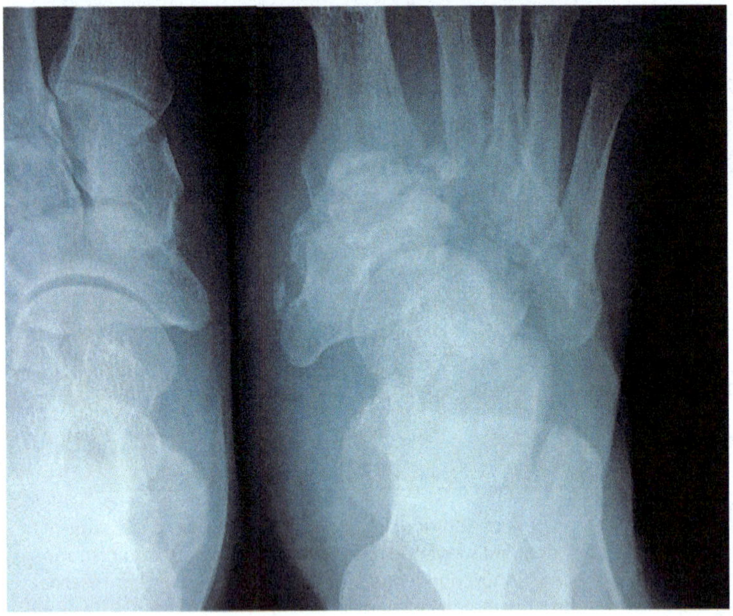

Figure 10.61 X-ray of the right foot of the patient in Figure 10.58 showing periosteal bone formation around the metatarsals, fusion of bony fragments to the adjacent bones and stabilization of the affected joints.

References

Barjon, M.C. (1993). Les ostéoarthropathies destructrices du pied diabétique. In: *Le pied diabétique* (ed. C. Hérisson and L. Simon), 77–91. Paris: Masson.

Brodsky, J.W. and Rouse, A.M. (1993). Exostectomy for symptomatic bony prominences in diabetic Charcot foot. *Clin. Orthop. Relat. Res.* 296: 21–26.

Eichenholtz, S.N. (1966). Charcot Joints. Springfield, IL: Charles C. Thomas. Harris JR, Brand PW. 1966. Patterns of disintegration of the tarsus in the anaesthetic foot. *J Bone Joint Surg (Br.)* 5: 95–97.

Horibe, S., Tada, K., and Nagano, J. (1988). Neuroarthropathy of the foot in leprosy. *J. Bone Joint Surg. (Br.)* 70: 481–485.

Johnson JE. 1995. Neuropathic (Charcot) arthropathy of the foot and ankle. Handout for American Academy of Orthopedic Surgeons Instructional Course 349.

Lennox, W.M. (1974). Surgical treatment of chronic deformities of the anaesthetic foot. In: *Surgical Rehabilitation in Leprosy, and in Other Peripheral Nerve Disorders* (ed. F. McDowell and C.D. Enna), 350–372. Baltimore: Williams & Wilkins.

Sanders, L.J. and Frykberg, R.G. (1991). Diabetic neuropathic osteoarthropathy: the Charcot foot. In: *The High Risk Foot in Diabetes Mellitus* (ed. R.G. Frykberg), 297–338. New York: Churchill Livingstone.

Saunders, L.J. and Mrdjencovich, D. (1991). Anatomical patterns of bone and joint destruction in neuropathic diabetics. *Diabetes* 40: 529A.

Schon, L.C., Easley, M.E., and Weinfeld, S.B. (1998). Charcot neuroarthropathy of the foot and ankle. *Clin. Orthop.* 349: 116–131.

Further Reading

Charcot, J.M. (1868). Sur quelques arthropathies qui paraissent depender d'une lesion du cerveau ou de la moele epiniere. *Arch. Des. Physiol. Norm. Path.* 1: 161–171.

Ertugrul, B.M., Lipsky, B.A., and Savk, O. (2013 Nov). Osteomyelitis or Charcot neuro-osteoarthropathy? Differentiating these disorders in diabetic patients with a foot problem. *Diabet Foot Ankle.* 5: 4.

Giurini, J.M., Chrzan, J.S., Gibbons, G.W., and Habershaw, G.M. (1991). Charcot's disease in diabetic patients. Correct diagnosis can prevent progressive deformity. *Postgrad. Med.* 89: 163–169.

Gnanasegaran, G., Vijayanathan, S., and Fogelman, I. (2012). Diagnosis of infection in the diabetic foot using (18)F-FDG PET/CT: a sweet alternative? *Eur. J. Nucl. Med. Mol. Imaging* 9 (10): 1525–1527.

Kelly, M. (1963). William Musgrave's De Arthritide Symptomatica (1703): his description of neuropathic arthritis. *Bull. Hist. Med.* 37: 372–376.

Matricali, G.A., Bammens, B., Kuypers, D. et al. (2007). High rate of Charcot foot attacks early after simultaneous pancreas-kidney transplantation. *Transplantation* 83 (2): 245–246.

Papanas, N. and Maltezos, E. (2013 May 21). Etiology, pathophysiology and classifications of the diabetic Charcot foot. *Diabet Foot Ankle.* 4: https://doi.org/10.3402/dfa.v4i0.20872.

Richard JL, Almasri M, Schuldiner S. 2012. "Treatment of acute Charcot foot with bisphosphonates: a systematic review of the literature." *Diabetologia*. 55(5): 1258–1264.

Rogers, L.C., Frykberg, R.G., Armstrong, D.G. et al. (2011). The Charcot foot in diabetes. *Diabetes Care* 34: 2123–2129.

Rosenbaum, A.J. and DiPreta, J.A. (2015). Classifications in brief: Eichenholtz classification of Charcot arthropathy. *Clin. Orthop. Relat. Res.* 473: 1168–1171.

Wukich, D.K. and Sung, W. (2009). Charcot arthropathy of the foot and ankle: modern concepts and management review. *J. Diabetes Complicat.* 23 (6): 409–426.

11

Infections

P. Tsapogas

Center for Diabetes and Metabolism, Henry Dunant Hospital Center, Athens, Greece

Invasion of the foot tissues by microorganisms, usually accompanied by an inflammatory response, may follow colonization of the skin by initially harmless bacteria, or may occur as a primary event.

Diagnosing a foot ulcer infection must be based on clinical criteria. A superficial or a full-thickness ulcer, treated inadequately, predisposes to infection, although cellulitis or osteomyelitis can occur without a break in the skin. Infected ulcers are often asymptomatic, especially if the patient feels no pain due to diabetic polyneuropathy. Alternatively, they may cause mild discomfort and produce some drainage, which eventually may become purulent and odorous. A disturbance of blood glucose control may be early evidence of a local infection.

The clinical assessment of any ulcer includes a description of its location, appearance, extent, depth, temperature and odor:

- *Appearance* includes color, type and condition of the tissue, presence of drainage, and any eschar, necrosis or surrounding callus. Infected wounds may be purple or red, or even brown or black, depending on the pathogen and its etiology, and their drainage may be serous, hemorrhagic or purulent. Induration of the skin and swelling usually denote infection.
- *Extent* is measured either directly on a clear film or by defining the length and width of the ulcer.
- *Depth* is estimated with a sterile blunt probe, which also determines underlying sinus tracts, abscesses or penetration to a bone.
- *Temperature* is estimated using the examiner's hand or measured by a dermal thermometer. Underlying infections raise the skin temperature.
- The foul *odor* of an ulcer may denote infection by a specific pathogen (such as *Proteus, Pseudomonas,* anaerobes, a mixed infection or fungi) or simply a necrotic process.

Pain may be a warning symptom of an infection, although patients with diabetic neuropathy may not feel more than some discomfort. Therefore, early signs of any foot infection, or an infection complicating a chronic ulcer, should be looked for by clinicians, patients, and those who provide foot care for patients at home. These signs include an unpleasant smell, an increased amount or change in the quality of the exudate, or any change in the appearance, depth or extent of a chronic ulcer, and signs of inflammation of the surrounding skin (induration, temperature, redness). It is very important to diagnose and treat an early foot infection, and it should be treated as a medical emergency.

11.1 Classifications for Diabetic Foot Infections

Wound infections are categorized as mild, moderate or severe:

- *Mild* infections are superficial infections confined to the skin and subcutaneous fat, with minimal or no purulence or cellulitis.
- *Moderate* infections are deep and may involve the fascia, muscles, tendons, joints, or bones. They may present as cellulitis of 0–2cm in diameter or as a plantar abscess, and they may cause systemic symptoms; they impose a certain risk for amputation.
- *Severe* infection of a foot ulcer is a deep infection with more than 2cm of cellulitis, lymphangitis, gangrene and/or necrotizing fasciitis, threatening limb loss and causing systemic toxicity. The absence of symptoms or signs of systemic illness does not exclude a limb-threatening infection.

A research classification system has been developed by the International Working Group on the Diabetic Foot to

Atlas of the Diabetic Foot, Third Edition. Ioanna Eleftheriadou, Alexandros Kokkinos, Stavros Liatis, Konstantinos Makrilakis, Nicholas Tentolouris, Anastasios Tentolouris, and Panagiotis Tsapogas.

Companion website: www.wiley.com/go/tentolouris/atlas_diabetic_foot

facilitate communication in the field of research. The acronym PEDIS is used: P = perfusion; E = extent or size; D = depth or tissue loss; I = infection; and S = sensation or neuropathy.

Infection has the following grades:

- grade 1: no signs or symptoms of infection;
- grade 2: in the subcutaneous tissue only;
- grade 3: extensive erythema and infection of deeper tissue;
- grade 4: a systemic inflammatory response indicating severe infection.

These grades of infection correlate exactly with the Infectious Diseases Society of America categories (i.e. no infection, mild, moderate, severe). Any diabetic foot infection should be assessed for its severity using the Infectious Diseases Society of America (IDSA)/IWGDF classification. Several prospective studies have shown that the PEDIS system or the IDSA/IWGDF diabetic foot infection classification predict the need for hospitalization or lower extremity amputation.

11.1.1 Management of the Infected Diabetic Foot

Cultures for aerobic and anaerobic pathogens and fungi assist in the management of infection. Curettage of the base of the debrided ulcer (Figure 11.1 and 11.2), culture of material collected by surgical biopsy of deep tissue or bone, or aspiration of drainage fluid is preferred. Before culturing a wound, however, any overlying necrotic tissue should be removed by vigorous scrubbing with saline-moistened sterile gauze.

Bacteria that colonize normal skin are coagulase-negative staphylococci, α-hemolytic streptococci and other Gram-positive aerobes, as well as corynebacteria.

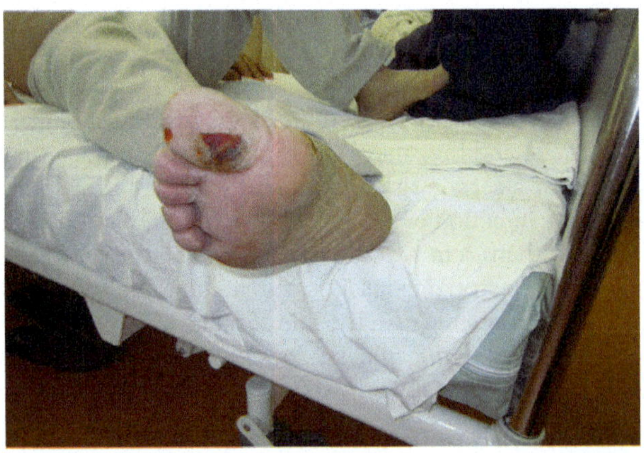

Figure 11.1 A clinically diagnosed infection of the big toe, should alert for an underlying cause and prompt for surgical debridement.

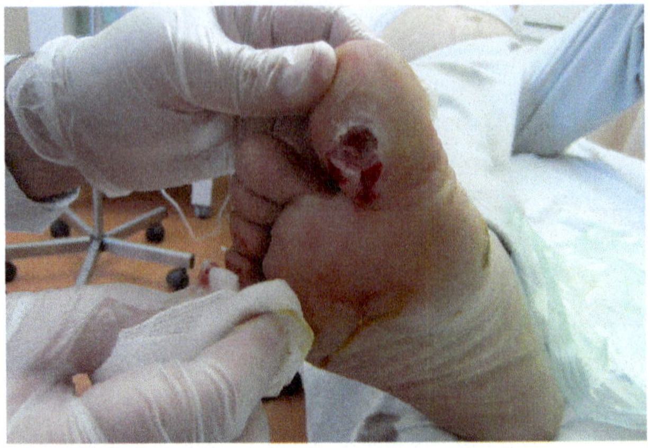

Figure 11.2 Surgical debridement of the ulcer of Figure 11.1 revealed a deep ulcer penetrating to the bone of the big toe. A PEDIS 3 (moderate) infection was diagnosed.

Staphylococcus aureus or β-hemolytic streptococci, pathogens that colonize the skin of diabetic patients, are the causative agents of acute infections in antibiotic-naive patients, and are nearly always the cause of cellulitis in non-ulcerated skin; *S. aureus* is the most commonly recovered pathogen in most infections in which a single agent is isolated.

Polymicrobial cultures, with an average of five or six organisms, are often obtained from patients with chronic lesions, especially when they have been treated with antibiotics for some time. Anaerobes, mostly *Bacteroides* species and various anaerobic Gram-positive cocci, are often isolated from deep necroses. *Proteus* species and *Escherichia coli* predominate among the Gram-negative bacilli, and *Pseudomonas* is often isolated from indurated, wet wounds.

In severe infections, Gram-negative pathogens and anaerobes predominate, versus Gram-positive pathogens and enterobacteriaceae, which are usually isolated from mild infections. The severity of infection does not, however, predict the causative microorganism.

Mild or moderate cellulitis may be treated with dicloxacillin, first-generation cephalosporins or clindamycin. Co-trimoxazole is an alternative for treating a proven staphylococcal infection, as well as for enterobacteriaceae. When the infection is mild and the causative pathogens and their susceptibility to antibiotics are predictable, empirical antibiotic therapy is justified. A narrower-spectrum agent may be chosen, such as a first-generation cephalosporin and/or clindamycin.

One to three weeks of therapy may suffice for soft tissue infections. The more severe the infection and the higher the prevalence of antibiotic resistance, the greater the need for microbiologic information. Second-generation oral cephalosporins, amoxicillin–clavulanic acid or fluoroquinolones, and clindamycin or metronidazole may be effective oral treatment against moderate infections, for patients who do not need hospitalization, when a mixed infection is suspected or before microbiologic data are available.

Patients with severe infections, and those in a systemic toxic condition, should be hospitalized and treated with intravenous antibiotics, since they may be unable to swallow or tolerate oral therapy. In addition, more predictable levels of antibiotics in infected tissues can be achieved with intravenous administration. Such patients are usually treated with broad-spectrum antibiotics, before cultures, and antibiograms are available. Imipenem–cilastin, ampicillin–sulbactam, piperacillin–tazobactam, third-generation cephalosporins or fluoroquinolones are usually effective; clindamycin or metronidazole may be added, and an agent with a narrower spectrum may be chosen later based on the antibiograms.

Urgent surgical drainage or removal of dead tissues may also be needed. Arterial insufficiency may compromise therapy as it prevents the antibiotics from reaching the site of infection. In this case, surgical revascularization of the limb is carried out. Radiographic evaluation is necessary when osteomyelitis is suspected or for wounds of long duration. Subcutaneous gas, foreign bodies, fractures, cortical erosions or neuro-osteoarthropathy may be seen on plain radiographs.

11.2 Methods of Appropriate Microbiologic Sampling

Soft tissue specimens from an infected diabetic foot have to be taken after the lesion is cleansed and debrided. Tissue specimens from an open wound should be obtained from the debrided base of the ulcer, by means of biopsy or curettage (scraping with a scalpel blade or a dermal curette). Material from a closed cavity is appropriate for microbiologic sampling as long as cleansing is adequate before opening (Figure 11.3). Purulent collections may be obtained by needle aspiration.

Deep soft tissue purulent collections may require imaging studies to be diagnosed; magnetic resonance imaging (MRI) seems to be most sensitive and specific. A culture of a bone sequestrum taken from an osteomyelitic lesion may provide useful microbiologic information, although an open wound penetrating to the bone may be colonized with incidental flora (Figures 11.4–11.7).

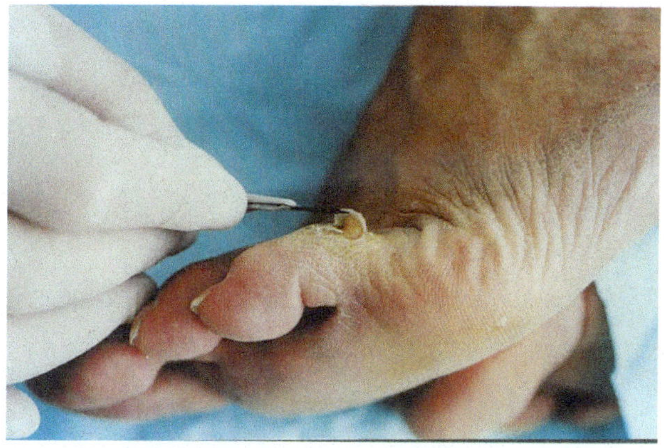

Figure 11.3 Accumulation of pus is revealed under a callus. Infectious material from a closed cavity is appropriate for microbiological sampling. A callus may seal off a purulent exudate, and this may cause the rapid spread of an infection. PEDIS 2 (mild) infection.

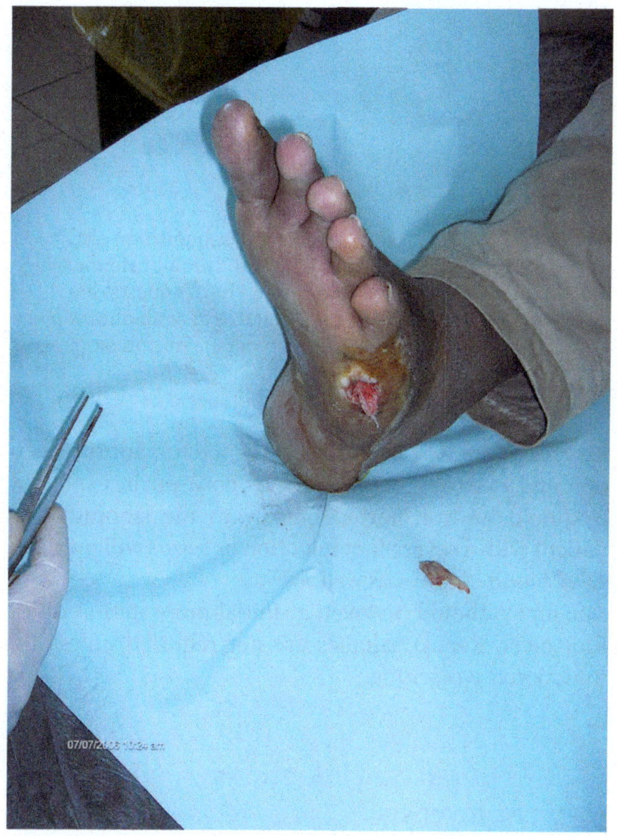

Figure 11.4 A neuropathic ulcer penetrating to the fifth metatarsal and causing osteomyelitis. PEDIS 3 (moderate) infection.

Superficial swabbing of undebrided ulcers or wound drainage is not recommended and should be avoided, due to the risk for contamination. Superficial swab cultures are not usually helpful, since they often produce different results from cultures of deep tissues, and colonization of the skin with any bacterium without concomitant infection does not need treatment. They are also difficult to interpret because of the number of pathogens found on the surface of a wound, and the technique is unsuitable

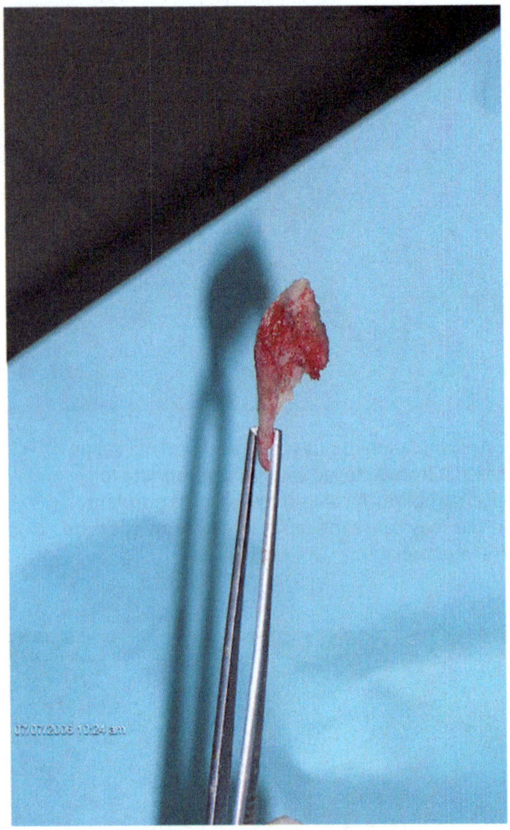

Figure 11.5 A devitalized infected bone (sequestrum) obtained from a neuropathic ulcer of a patient with chronic osteomyelitis of the fifth metatarsal bone (see Figure 11.4). Sequestra are avascular; therefore, they are impenetrable to antibiotics. A piece of surgically obtained tissue is an appropriate microbiological sample.

for anaerobes. A special swab designed for culturing aerobic and anaerobic organisms may, however, be exploited; it should be transported quickly to the laboratory. A patient with a severe foot infection or sepsis will probably need blood cultures as well.

Samples should be taken at initial presentation of the foot ulcer. Repeat samples are not required unless the infection is worsening.

11.3 Fungal Nail Infections (Onychomycosis)

Chronic onychomycosis is classified into three clinical types:

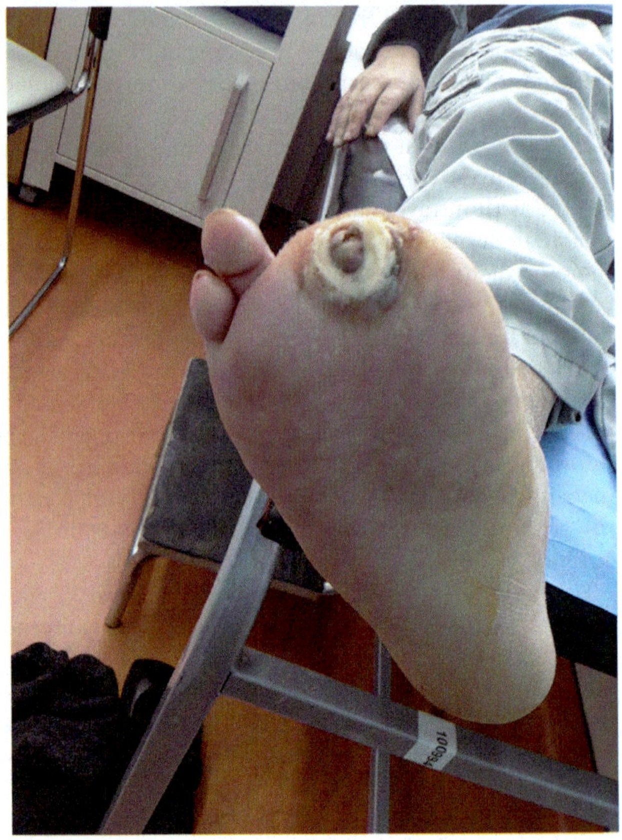

Figure 11.6 An infected neuropathic ulcer over the first metatarsal head two years after a big toe amputation. After removal of the calus a loose bone was palpated. PEDIS 3 infection.

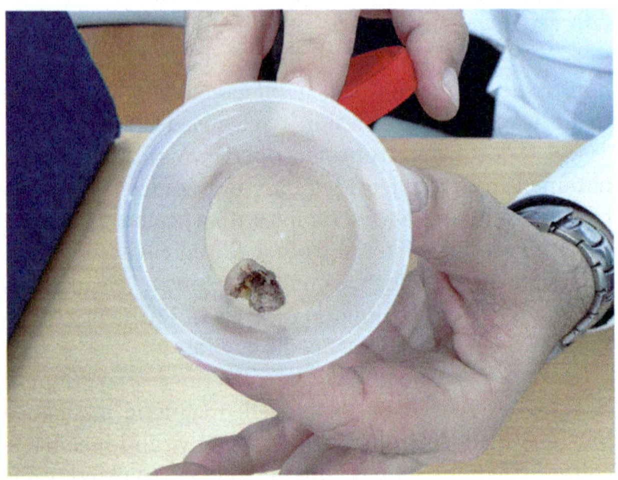

Figure 11.7 A sequestrum obtained from a neuropathic ulcer of a patient with chronic osteomyelitis of the first metatarsal bone (see Figure 11.6).

- In *distal subungual onychomycosis*, the distal edge of the nail becomes infected and a yellow discoloration, onycholysis and subungual debris develop (Figure 11.8). In *proximal subungual fungal infection*, *Trichophyton rubrum* accumulates hyperkeratotic debris under the nail plate and loosens the nail, eventually separating it from its bed (Figures 11.9–11.13).
- *Superficial white onychomycosis* (leuconychia mycotica), caused by *Trichophyton mentagrophytes*, infects the nail

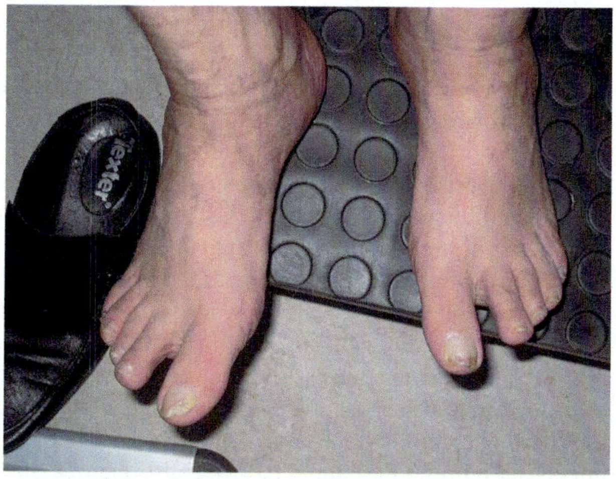

Figure 11.8 Distal onychomycosis of the nails of the great toes.

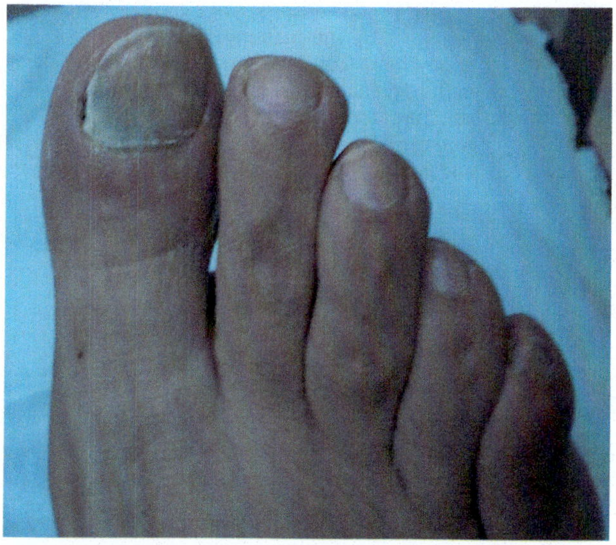

Figure 11.9 Onychomycosis of the nail of the great toe. Fungal invasion occurs from the proximal underside of the nail (proximal subungual fungal infection).

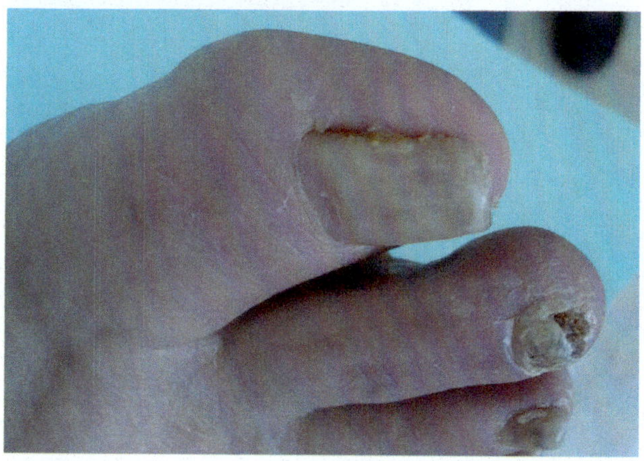

Figure 11.10 Subungual onychomycosis of the first two toes.

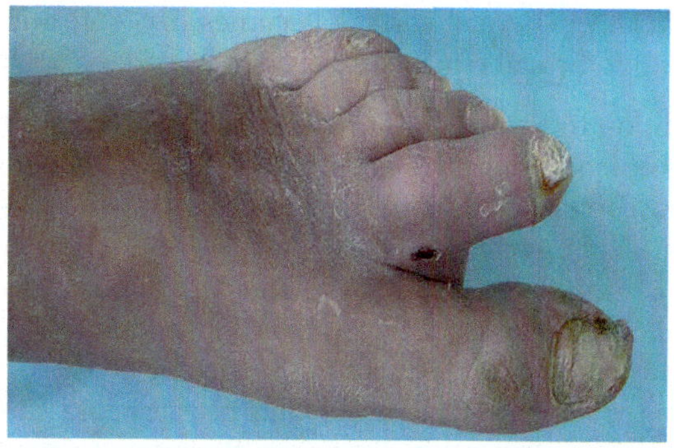

Figure 11.11 Onychomycosis of the nails of the first two toes. A neuropathic ulcer is present at the base of the second toe.

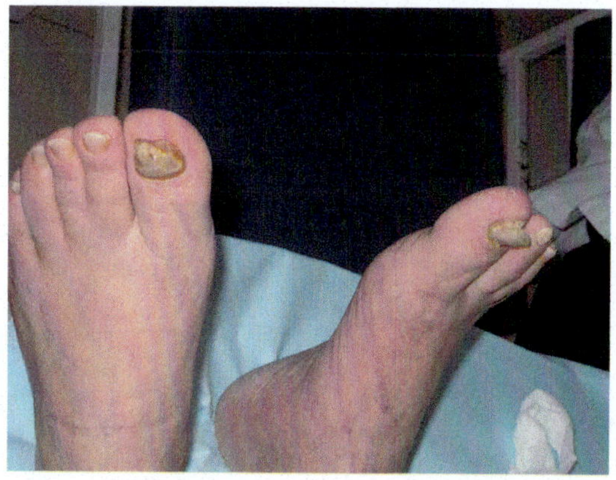

Figure 11.12 Onychomycosis of the nails of both great toes. The infection originates from the underside of the nail plate, separating it from its bed.

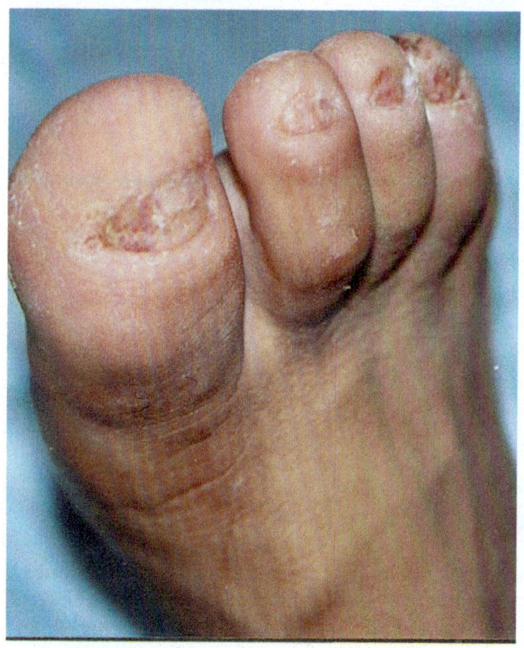

Figure 11.13 Apoptosis of the nails of all toes due to onychomycosis.

superficially. The nail surface becomes dry, soft and friable, but the nail remains attached to its bed.

In addition to these fungi, *Epidermophyton floccosum* may also be isolated from infected areas. A positive result on microscopical examination and culture of nail clippings with subungual debris, or from surface debris in superficial onychomycosis, is the standard method to diagnose onychomycosis. Tinea pedis and discoloration of the nails are sensitive criteria for the diagnosis.

Chronic trauma, lichen planus and psoriasis are the most common alternative diagnoses. Periungual squamous cell carcinoma (characterized by a single nail lesion and often pain) and yellow nail syndrome may also result in misdiagnosis.

Itraconazole and fluconazole are also effective in the treatment of chronic onychomycosis.

11.4 Paronychia

Acute or chronic paronychia (or perionychia) is an inflammatory reaction involving the folds of tissue surrounding a fingernail or toenail (Figure 11.14). It is the result of the breakdown of the protective barrier between the nail and the nail fold.

Direct or indirect trauma to the nail fold (cuticle) is the commonest cause of acute paronychia. Pedicure procedures (trimming or pushing back the cuticles; Figure 11.15), an injury from a splinter or thorn, or an ingrown nail may produce such a trauma. Friction in an unfit shoe may also cause the development of a blister at the perionychium, which may rupture and become infected (Figures 11.16 and 11.17; see also Figures 3.70 and 8.22).

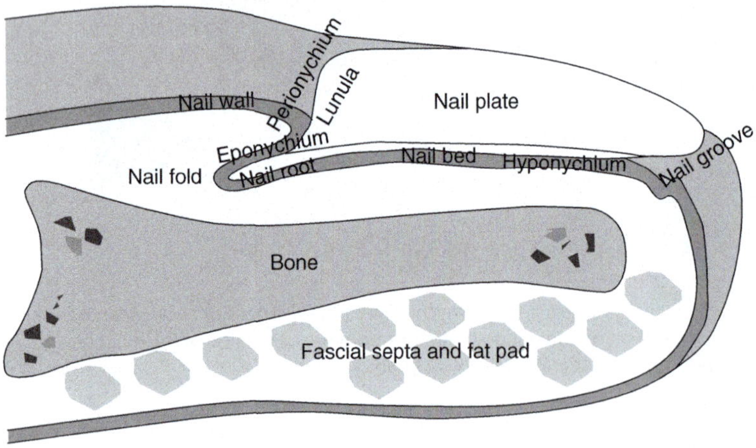

Figure 11.14 The anatomy of a nail. The eponychium (cuticle) is situated between the skin of the digit and the nail plate, fusing these structures together. This configuration provides a waterproof seal from external irritants, allergens and pathogens.

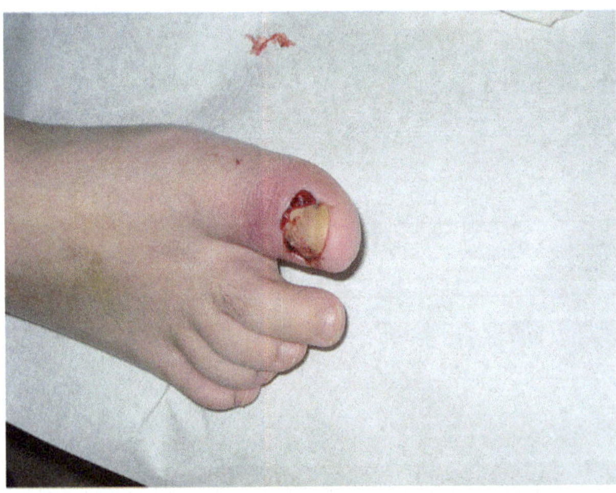

Figure 11.15 Acute painful paronychia after minor trauma due to a pedicure. Cellulitis and edema of the hallux are evident. The nail is loose and discolored, with pronounced transverse ridges such as Beau's lines (resulting from inflammation of the nail matrix). Gentle pressure on the nail plate exacerbates the pain arising from the infection under the nail.

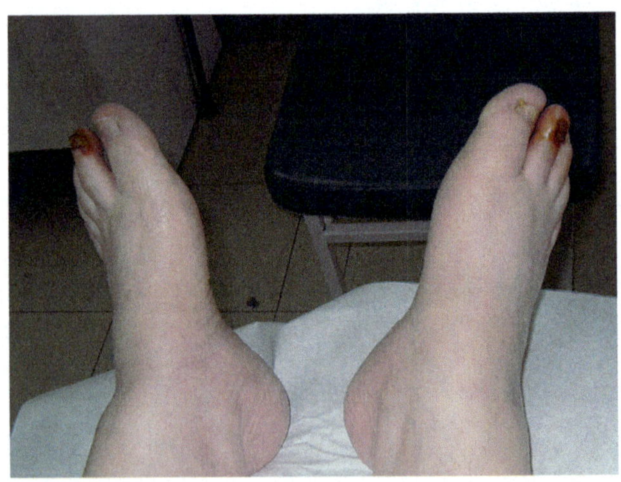

Figure 11.16 Acute paronychia due to friction from unfit shoes.

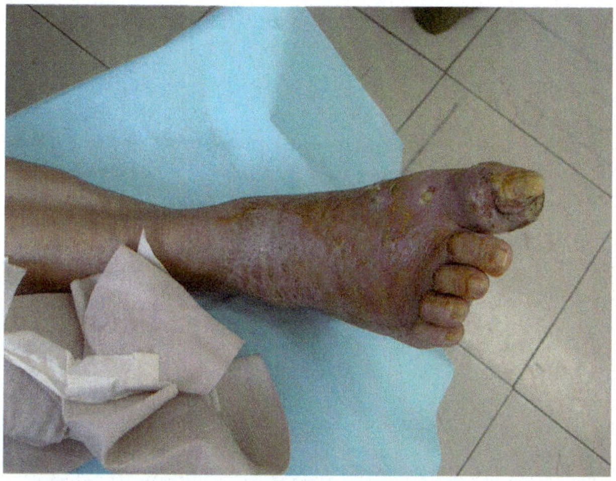

Figure 11.17 Untreated chronic paronychia of the hallux, complicated by an acute infection of the forefoot (arising from an infected neuro-ischemic ulcer at the base of the great toe). Edema of the forefoot is evident. Acute paronychia can also develop as a complication of chronic paronychia.

Erythema, edema, discomfort or tenderness, and pus accumulation under the nail folds characterize acute paronychia, which is typically restricted to one toe. If untreated, a subungual abscess may evolve, and the nail may become detached from the nail bed. Transient or permanent dystrophy of the nail plate may occur, while recurrent acute paronychia may evolve into chronic paronychia.

Eczema, psoriasis, Reiter syndrome and diseases affecting the fingertip may involve the nail folds. Squamous cell carcinomas, malignant melanomas and metastases from malignant tumors should be considered when chronic paronychia is unresponsive to treatment, and biopsies should be taken.

Rare inherited conditions like yellow-nail syndrome or nail-patella syndrome mimic paronychia (and resist treatment). A carefully taken family history may reveal an interesting hereditary pattern (Figures 11.18–11.20).

Surgical intervention for paronychia is generally recommended when an abscess is present, although there is no evidence that treatment with oral antibiotics is any better or worse than incision and drainage for acute paronychia.

11.5 Superficial Bacterial Foot Infections

Case 11.1 A Painless Foot Infection Due to an Ill-Fitting Shoe (Figure 11.21)

A 59-year old man with type 2 diabetes of a five-year duration, and a history of an amputation of his fifth left toe due to osteomyelitis, appeared in the diabetic foot clinic because of his foot wounds. On the previous day he had a lengthy walk in a new pair of shoes, and he noticed his wounds after he removed his shoes. He did not smoke or drink alcohol, and he was on alogliptin, metformin, atorvastatin, valsartan and amplodipine. He was not febrile and his blood pressure was 128/89 mmHg. On clinical examination he had superficial ulcers on both sides of his first toe and under the first metatarsal bone; and smaller lesions on his second and third toe. His big toe was red, warm, and slightly swollen; and a small pus collection was present under a callus. He felt no pain, and he could not feel light touch, pressure, vibrations, or temperature differences on either foot. His white blood count was 6390 Kμl^{-1} with a 74.2% PMN, an ESR of 57, and a CRP of 1.18 mg dl^{-1} (normal values <0.5). Blood glucose was 125 mg dl^{-1} nut other biochemistry was normal. A simple radiograph showed no bone lesion. A PEDIS 3 (moderate) infection was diagnosed. A color doppler of his leg arteries was normal. After washing his foot with normal saline, his callus was remover and a culture of a purulent liquid underneath was obtained with a sterile swab. Oral trimethoprime/sulfamethoxazole and clindamycin was started empirically and he was released with the advice of bed rest; and a simple saline gauze dressing in a half shoe. He visited the clinic daily. On the third day a multisensitive strain of *S. aureus* and an *Enterobacted cloacae* were isolated, both sensitive to his regimen; and his foot improved significantly. He continued this treatment for two weeks. A proper diabetic insole was made with the use of a pedobarograph after a month's time.

11.6 Fungal Soft Tissue Infections

Fungal infections develop as a result of poor foot hygiene, hyperhidrosis, or the accumulation of moist detritus in the webs. *Interdigital tinea pedis* (Figure 11.22) is the most common form of chronic fungal foot infection. Itching, redness, scaling, erosion, and soaking of the skin with fluid usually occur, while in the late phase the redness subsides. *T. mentagrophytes*, *T. rubrum*, or *E. floccosum* may be found. Topical terbinafine cream cures most infections caused by dermatophyta, and should be continued for two weeks after symptoms subside.

Superficial bacterial infections in the interdigital spaces may spread to deeper structures through the lumbrical tendons (Figure 11.23), or they may cause thrombosis of the adjacent digital arteries. Furthermore, edema impedes foot circulation, especially in the presence of peripheral vascular disease. Adequate foot hygiene and

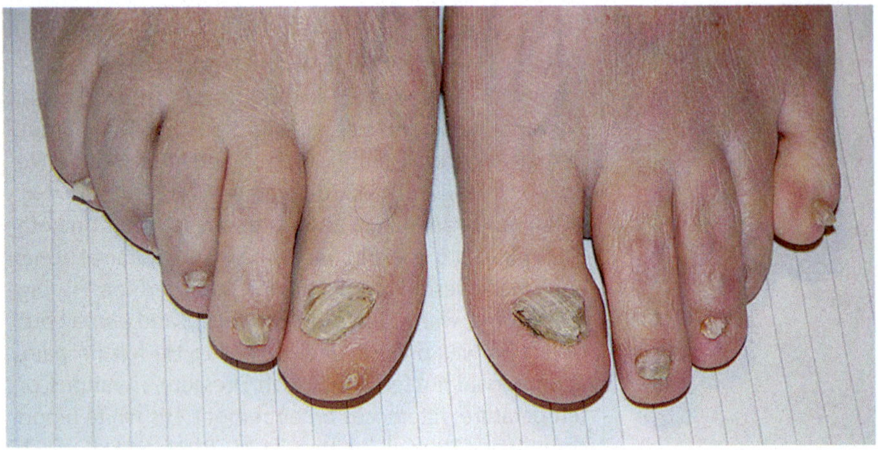

Figure 11.18 Nail-patella syndrome. Underdeveloped and discolored, split, ridged, or pitted nails. Skeletal abnormalities involving the knees, elbows, and hips are also common. Courtesy of Dr. Nikolaos Tsigaridas.

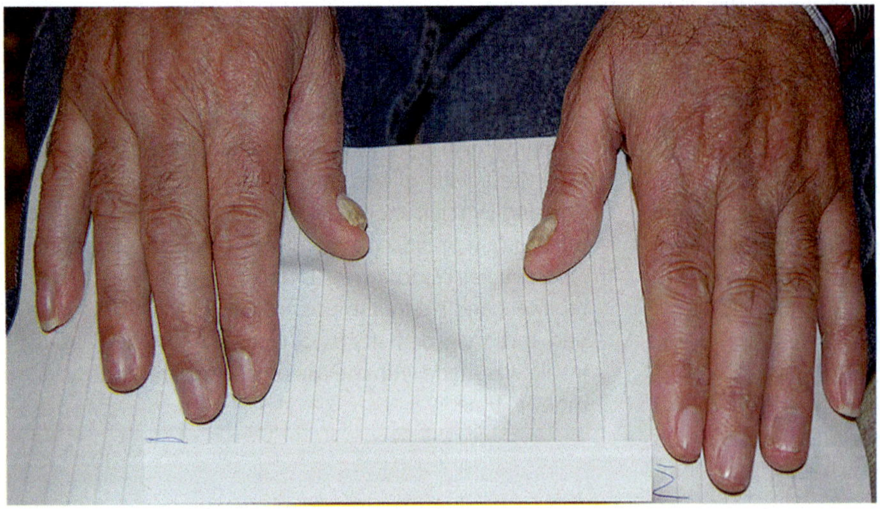

Figure 11.19 Nail-patella syndrome. Discolored and thick thumbnails of the gentleman of Figure 11.18. The fingernails in this hereditary condition are more likely to be affected than the toenails. Courtesy of Dr. Nikolaos Tsigaridas.

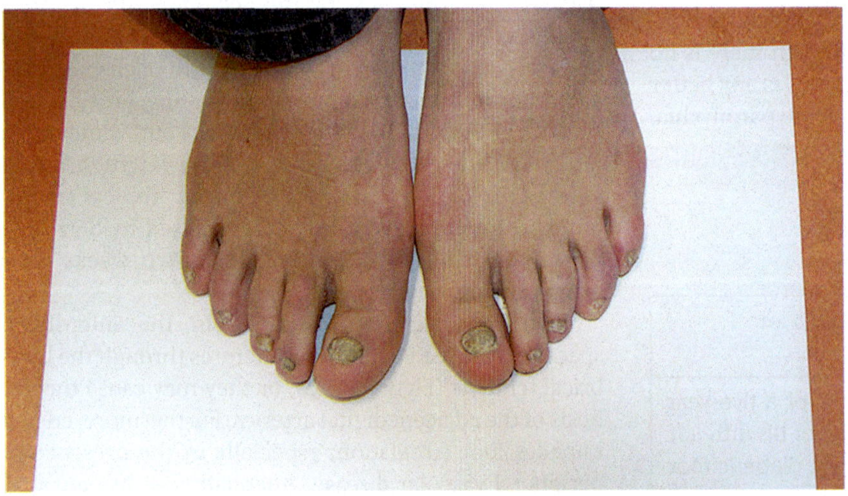

Figure 11.20 Nail-patella syndrome. Toenails of a cousin of the gentleman of Figure 11.18. A total of 11 members of both genders of an extended family of 19 examined had the traits of the syndrome on the toenails or fingernails or both. Courtesy of Dr. Nikolaos Tsigaridas.

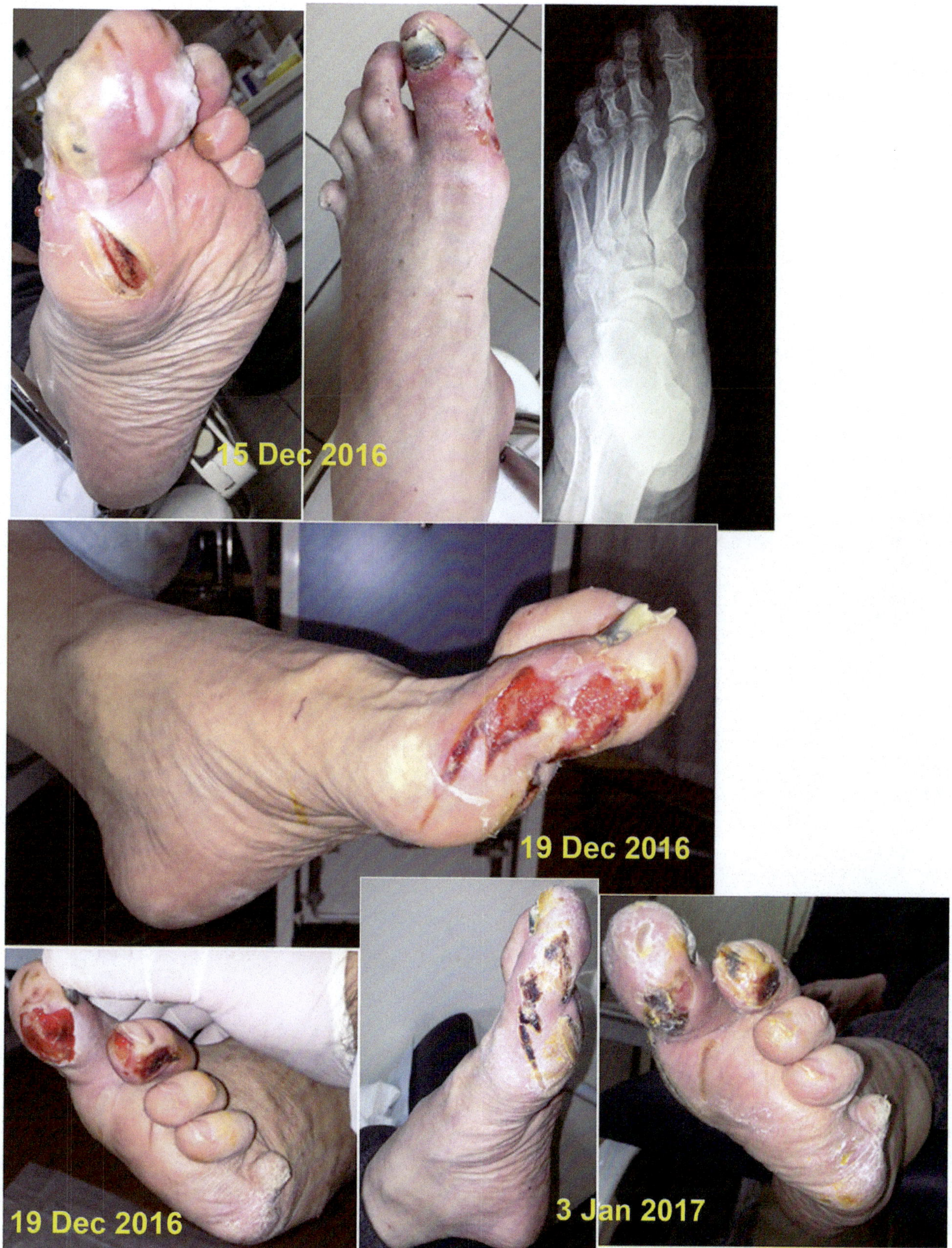

Figure 11.21 Superficial forefoot ulcers due to an ill-fitting shoe. PEDIS 2.

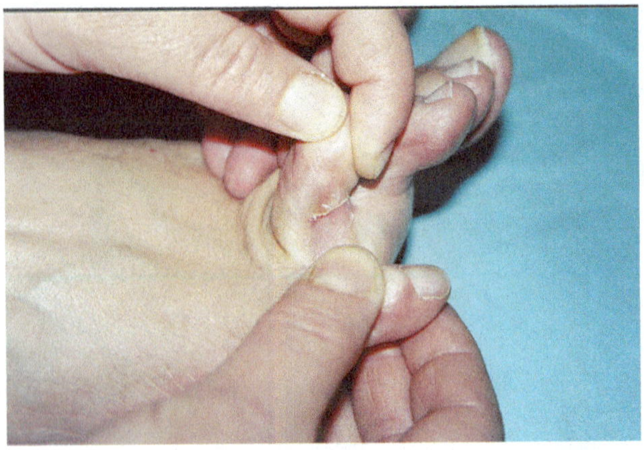

Figure 11.22 Tinea pedis. PEDIS 2.

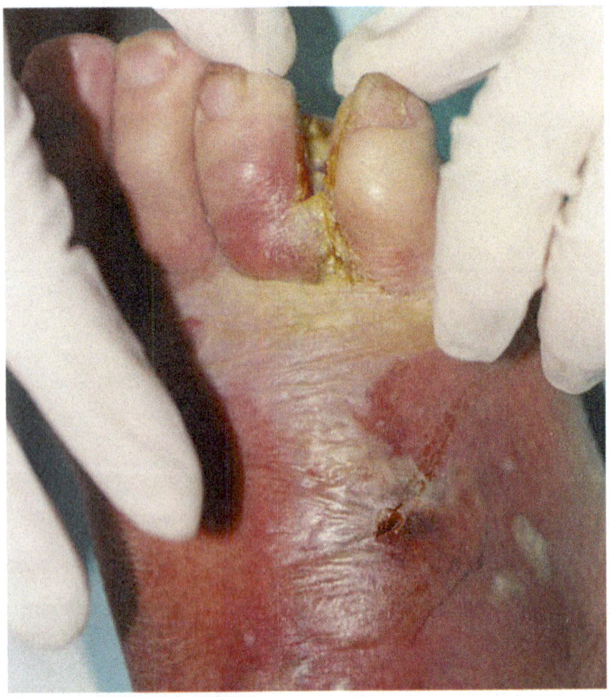

Figure 11.23 An interdigital fungal infection complicated by a combination of a staphylococcal and a streptococcal infection caused rapid generalized phlegmon of the foot. PEDIS 4.

treatment of the fungal infection could prevent this complication.

Fungal infections may also complicate improperly treated ulcers (Figure 11.24) and cases when changes of dressings are late and fluid production in the ulcer is significant (Figure 11.25). Sometimes the fungal infection may spread to the bone under the ulcer, causing fungal osteomyelitis (Figure 11.26).

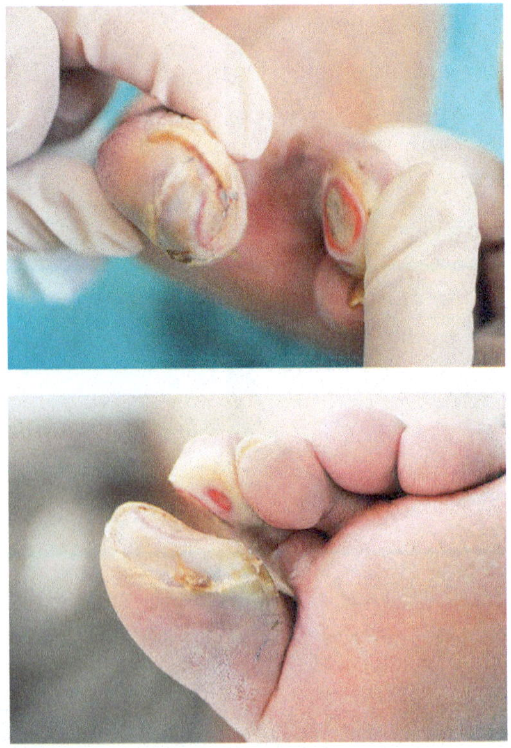

Figure 11.24 A fungal infection complicating kissing ulcers of the first and second toes. PEDIS 3.

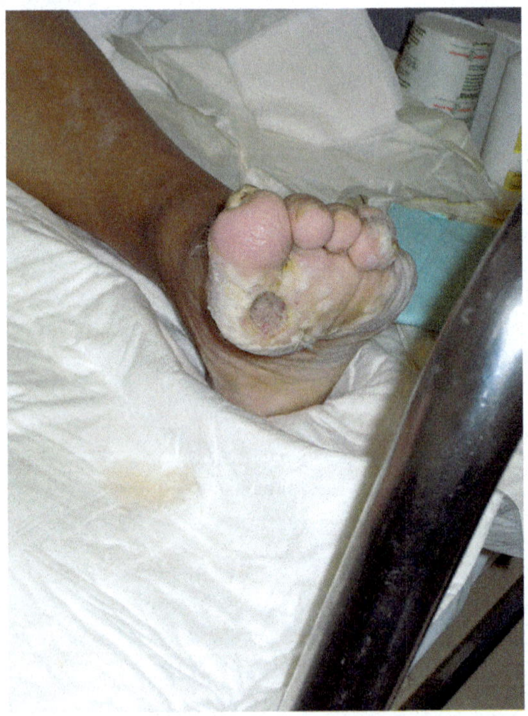

Figure 11.25 Maceration of the forefoot due to improper dressing of and significant fluid production from a neuropathic ulcer under the first metatarsal head. *Candida albicans* was isolated from both the base of the ulcer and the bone underneath.

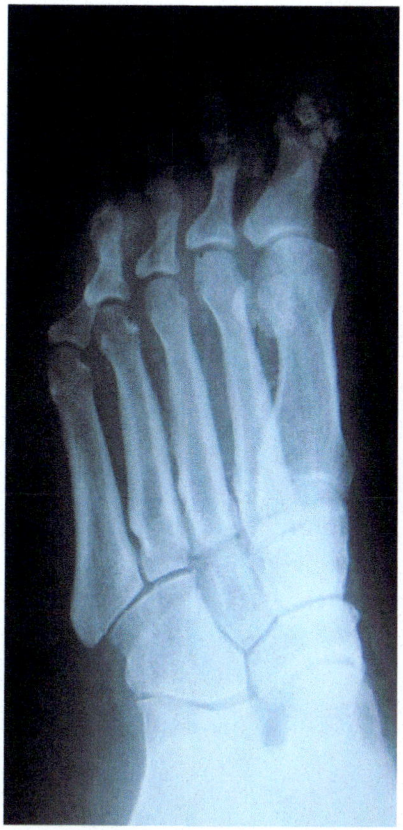

Figure 11.26 Osteomyelitis of the first metatarsal head, complicated by fungal infection as proved by bone culture. The last two phalanges show osteolysis from a past bacterial osteomyelitis. This is a radiograph of the foot shown in Figure 11.25. PEDIS 3.

11.7 Phlegmon

A phlegmon is a diffuse acute suppurative inflammation of the soft or connective tissue caused by infection. Clinically, it is a hard swelling with edema and cellulitis but without gross suppuration, as is seen with an abscess (Figure 11.27). A phlegmon may develop within hours or a few days, after an infection spreads from an infected ulcer to the adjacent soft tissues (Figure 11.28). Aggressive antibiotic treatment of the cellulitis, together with surgical decompression through debridement of the necrotic tissues, is the treatment of choice (Figures 11.29 and 11.30).

A septic abscess is an enclosed collection of pus. It is accompanied by cellulitis, by disappearing or bulging of the plantar arch (Figure 11.31) and, before drainage, by fluctuance on palpation.

11.8 Abscess

An abscess may be found in one of the four fascial compartments of the foot (Figure 11.32):

- the *medial compartment* – bordered by the inferior surface of the first metatarsal dorsally, an extension of the plantar aponeurosis medially, and the intermuscular septum laterally;
- the *central compartment* – bordered by the plantar aponeurosis inferiorly, the intermuscular septa medially and laterally, and the tarsometatarsal structures dorsally;

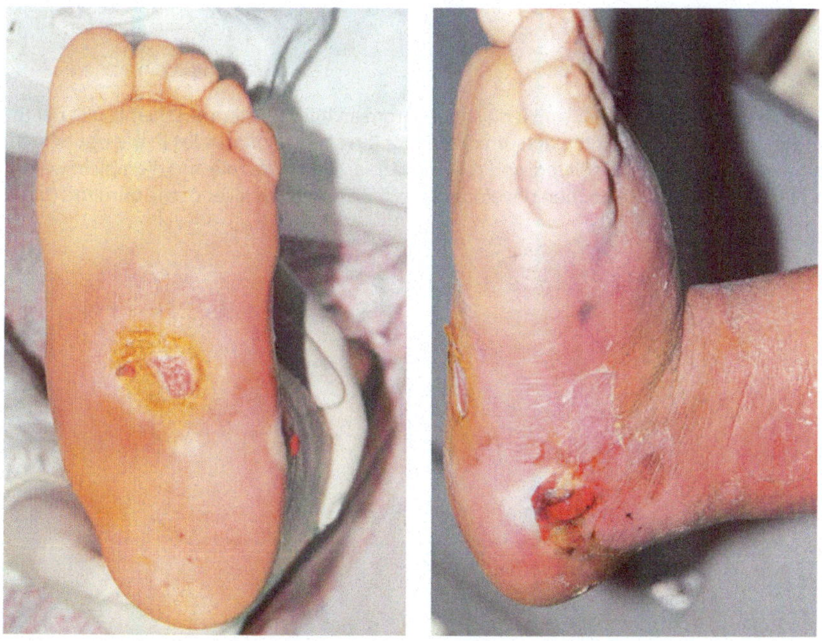

Figure 11.27 A phlegmon of a Charcot foot, caused by a spread of infection from a neuropathic ulcer of the midfoot. *Pseudomonas aeruginosa*, a strain susceptible only to colistin, was isolated. Generalized sepsis led to urgent amputation within two days of presentation of this patient and saved her life. PEDIS 4.

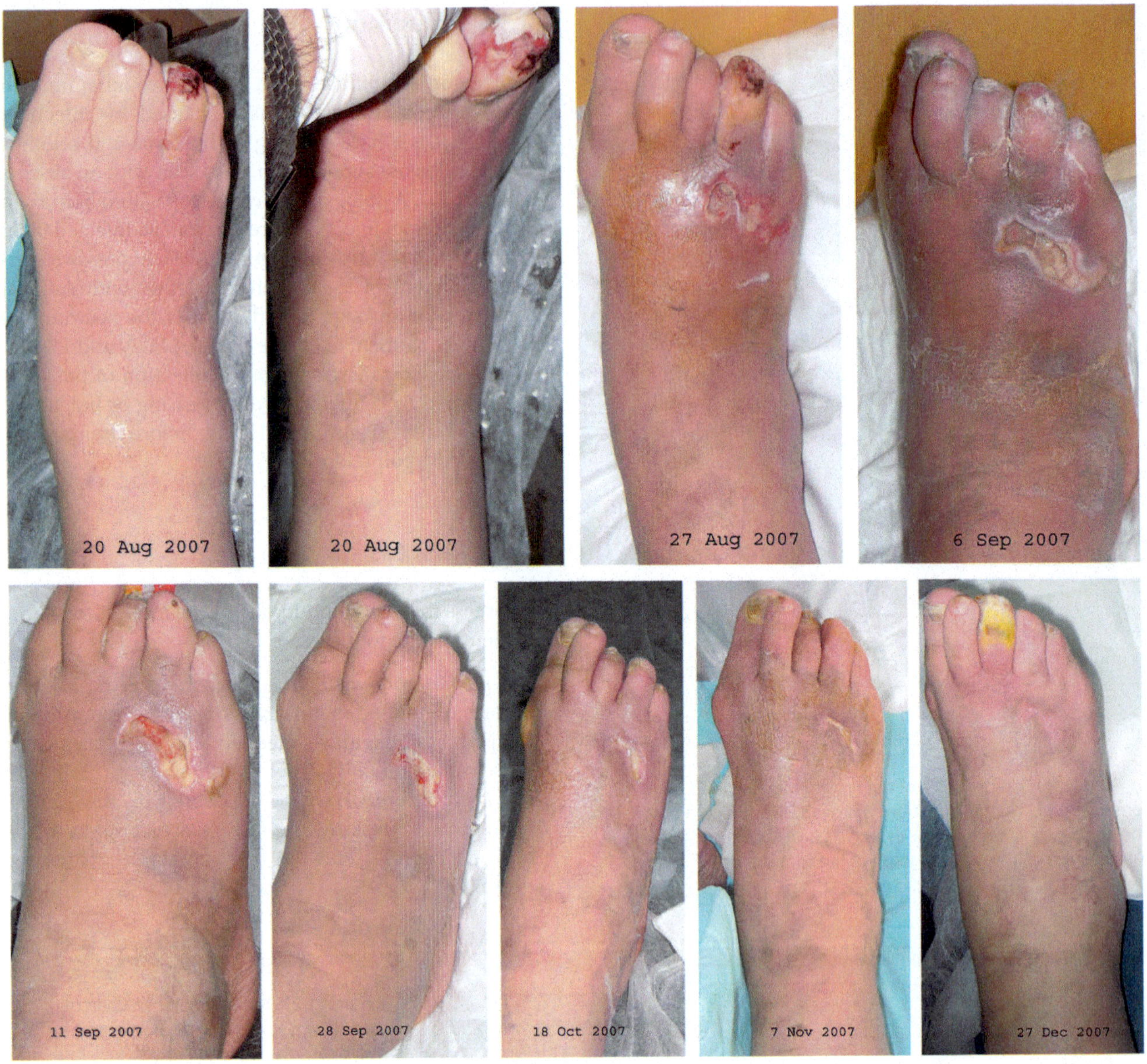

Figure 11.28 Progression of a treated phlegmon of the dorsum of the foot, which developed from an infected neuro-ischemic ulcer of the fourth toe. Cellulitis (induration, redness, high temperature) is present on the dorsum of the foot (first two photographs in the upper row), but there was no pain, owing to neuropathy. *Staphylococcus aureus* was isolated, and cotrimoxazole, metronidazole and rifampicin were given intravenously. One month after completion of treatment, a new infection developed, this time due to an ulcer of the third toe (far right photograph on the lower row). PEDIS 4.

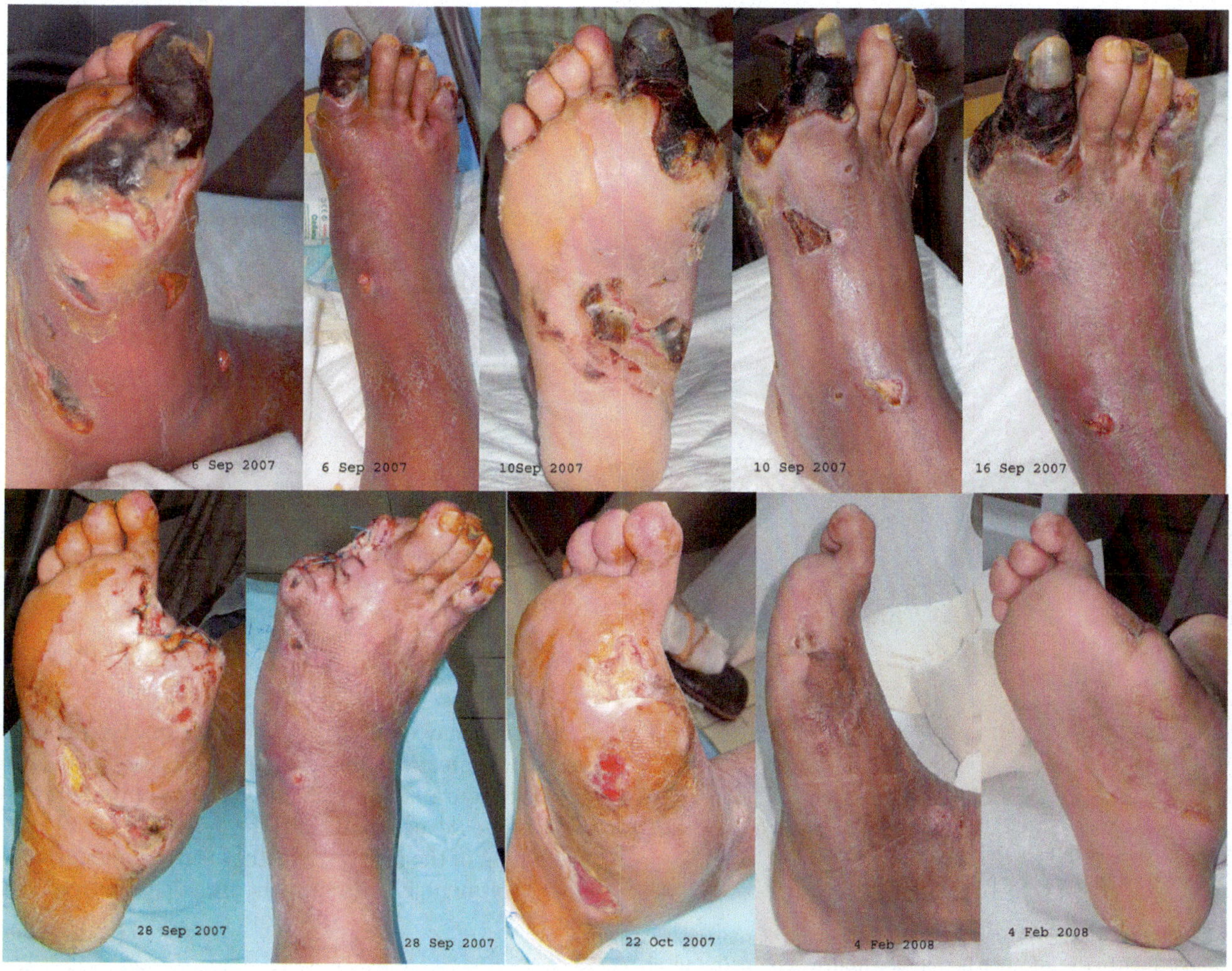

Figure 11.29 Treatment of a phlegmon of the foot, PEDIS 4 with first ray amputation, aggressive antibiotic treatment, and hyperbaric oxygen. This is the right foot of a 67-year-old gentleman with type 2 diabetes who was admitted because of a phlegmon of his right foot. A neuropathic ulcer at the base of his hallux had caused wet gangrene of the great toe two weeks before this presentation, while hospitalization in another hospital had failed to prevent further spread of the infection. A below-knee amputation was suggested. An amputation of this man's left leg had been performed two years before this event for osteomyelitis, and the patient was using a prosthesis for walking. On presentation to our hospital, dry gangrene of the hallux was present, and the infection at the base of the ulcer had spread to the medial and central compartments. New ulcers on the dorsum and sole of the foot had developed due to gravity. Cellulitis and edema of the foot were evident. All cultures were negative due to previous antibiotic treatment, while no previous culture results were available. The patient was afebrile, and his general condition was stable. Empirical intravenous treatment with amoxicillin–clavulanic acid and sulfamethoxazole–trimethoprim was started. Two weeks after the man's admission, the infection was controlled and hallux disarticulation was performed. Treatment with hyperbaric oxygen was recommended, and healing was smooth and successful.

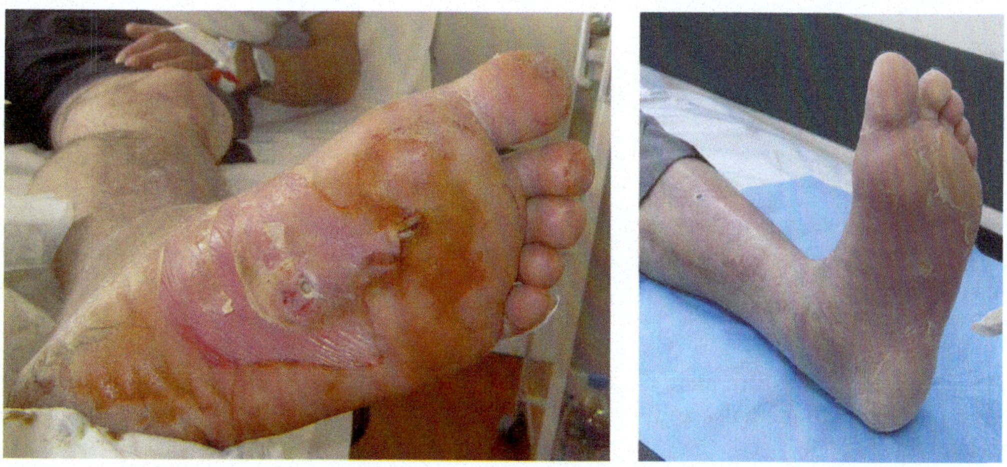

Figure 11.30 A phlegmon of the midfoot before and after intensive treatment with antibiotics. The lesion was painless and it was caused by a piece of broken glass. PEDIS 4.

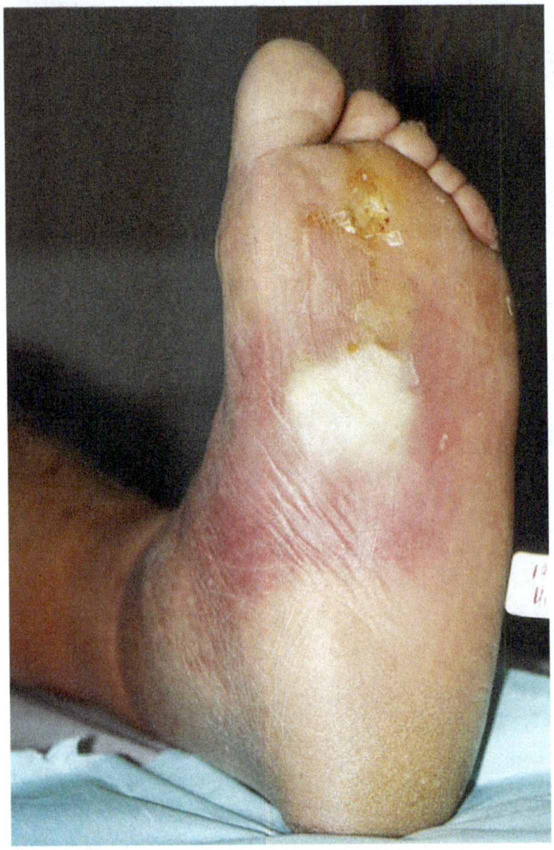

Figure 11.31 An abscess of the medial and central plantar compartments. The infection had spread from a neuropathic ulcer under the second metatarsal head. PEDIS 4.

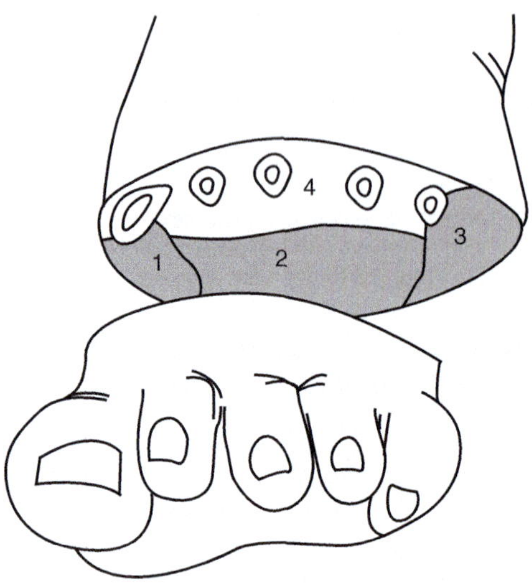

Figure 11.32 The four fascial compartments of the foot: (a) medial compartment; (b) central compartment; (c) lateral compartment; and (d) interosseous compartment.

- the *lateral compartment* – bordered by the fifth metatarsal dorsally, an intermuscular septum medially, and the plantar aponeurosis laterally;

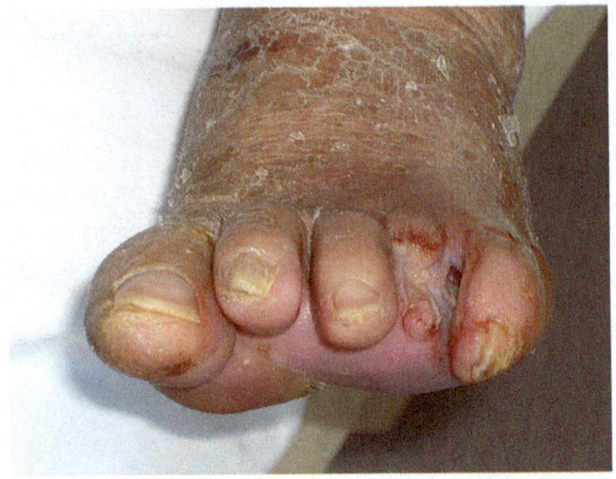

Figure 11.33 Infection of the head of the fourth metatarsal (after an amputation of the fourth toe), which spread into the central plantar space. This foot is also shown in Figure 11.34. PEDIS 4.

- the *interosseous compartment* – bounded by the interosseous fascia of the metatarsals.

Infection may enter any of these compartments after web space infections, or from an infection anywhere in the toes (Figure 11.33) by means of suppurative tenosynovitis of the flexor tendon sheath.

Draining of the abscess, together with aggressive antibiotic treatment, is the treatment of choice (Figures 11.34 and 11.35).

11.9 Gas Gangrene

Exotoxin-producing clostridia (most often *Clostridium perfringens* A strain) and other anaerobic microorganisms (anaerobic streptococci and *Bacteroides*) may cause gas gangrene (Figure 11.36). Treatment is usually debridement and excision; amputation is often necessary. Penicillin is given as an auxiliary therapy, and hyperbaric oxygen may also help.

11.10 Septic Arthritis

Septic arthritis of the metatarsophalangeal joint is often a complication of a neuropathic ulcer under the metatarsal head. The fibers of the plantar aponeurosis split and pass between the metatarsal heads; therefore, the base of an ulcer under the metatarsal head is formed by the flexor tendon, which becomes fixed to its sheath and to the underlying metatarsophalangeal joint capsule and periosteum. Infection spreads through the eroded tendon to the joint, causing septic arthritis (Figures 11.37–11.39), and to the bone, causing osteomyelitis (Figures 11.40–11.43, and see Figure 11.44).

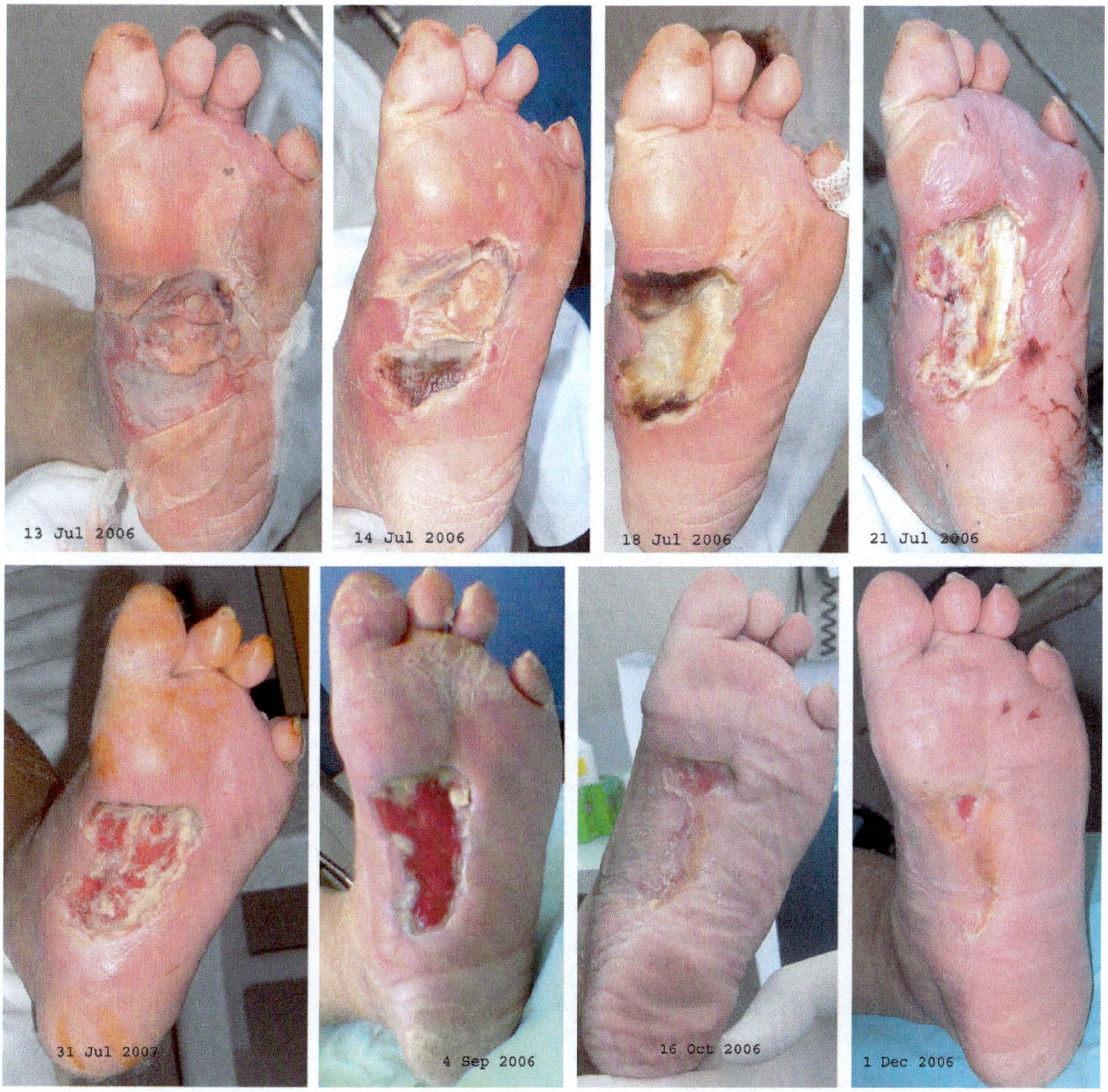

Figure 11.34 A central plantar compartment abscess. A staphylococcal infection entered the deep plantar space through an infection of the base of the amputated fourth toe (see Figure 11.33). Draining of the abscess, together with long-term antibiotic treatment and bed rest, allowed healthy granulation of the bed of the ulcer and healing (see Figure 11.35). PEDIS 4.

After osteomyelitis of the forefoot is healed a disfigurement of the member often persists, even when no amputation is performed. As mentioned in Chapter 3, this renders the forefoot prone to a new ulceration, and a custom shoe must be used (Figures 11.45–11.49).

11.11 Osteomyelitis

All patients with foot wounds, especially long-standing ulcers, should be evaluated for osteomyelitis, since this complication increases the likelihood of hospitalization, the risk for long antibiotic treatment and infection with multi-resistant microorganisms, and also the possibility of surgery and amputation.

The possibility of an ulcer being complicated by osteomyelitis increases when the diameter of the ulcer exceeds 2 cm and the depth is greater than 3 mm; the possibility of complications becomes even higher when the white blood cell count, erythrocyte sedimentation rate and C-reactive protein level are high. Osteomyelitis thwarts the healing of an ulcer that is properly treated with antibiotics, debridement and off-loading (Figures 11.44 and 11.49). Clinically, osteomyelitis should be suspected when a sterile probe penetrates to bone through an ulcer.

The treatment of acute osteomyelitis includes the parenteral administration of antibiotics for two weeks initially, and the continuation of oral treatment for a prolonged period (at least six weeks) (Figure 11.50).

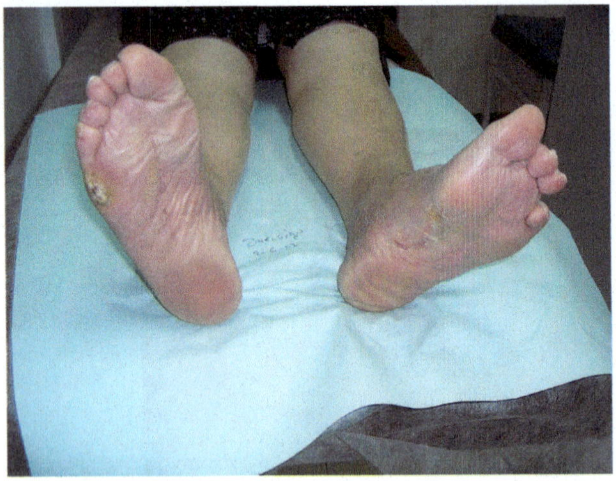

Figure 11.35 A healed abscess of the left foot, 10 months after presentation (see Figure 11.34). PEDIS 1. Callus has formed under the fifth metatarsal head of the opposite foot due to some guarding and improper footwear.

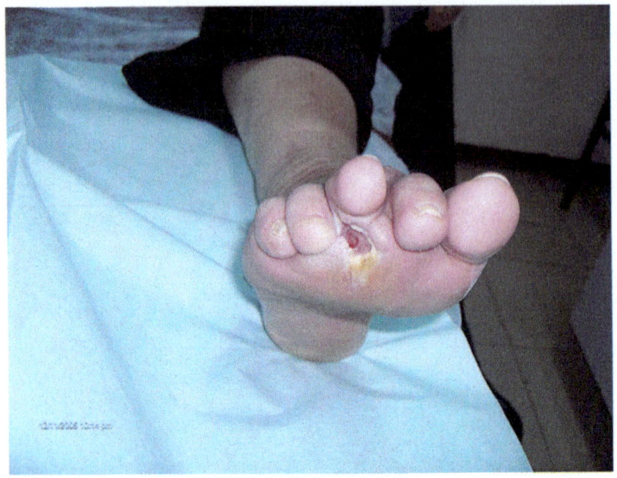

Figure 11.37 A neuropathic ulcer exposing the metatarsophalangeal joint (causing septic arthritis) is seen under the third toe. PEDIS 3.

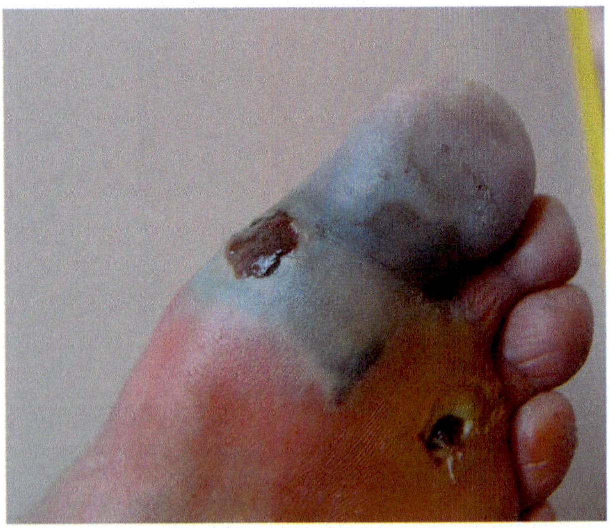

Figure 11.36 A neuro-ischemic ulcer on the medial aspect of the hallux showed a rapid change in its base from healthy pink to blue. PEDIS 4. Malodorous slime was present, and wet gangrene developed. Bluish discoloration is caused by an inadequate supply of oxygen, due to septic vasculitis of the circulation of the skin. Gas gangrene was diagnosed by a simple radiogram, and crepitus was felt through palpation. *Klebsiella pneumoniae* was isolated; this is not a common pathogen of foot infections, but is often reported as the cause of gas gangrene in the context of diabetes. A deep neuro-ischemic ulcer is present under the third metatarsal head. *Source:* Courtesy of Dr. C. Loupa.

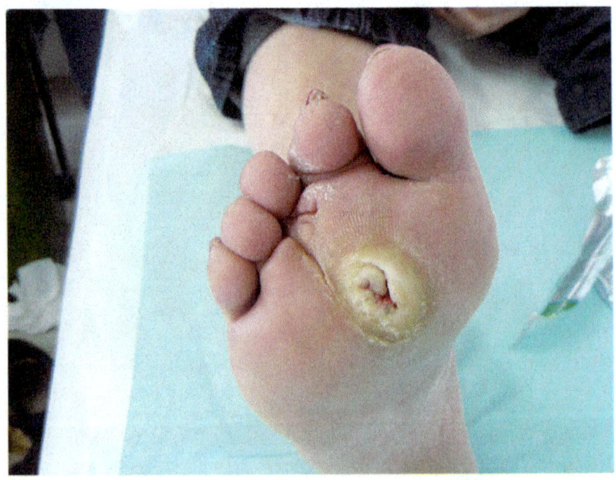

Figure 11.38 A neuropathic ulcer with extensive callosity is shown under the second metatarsal head. A scar between the third and fourth toes is due to a healed ulcer. PEDIS 3. This is the foot of the patient shown in Figure 11.39, four years after first presentation (see Figure 11.37). The damaged protruding third metatarsophalangeal joint and improper footwear caused the new ulcer.

Several methods are used for the diagnosis of osteomyelitis:

- *Probe-to-bone tests* (contacting the bone with a sterile metal probe) have a sensitivity of more than 90% and can be carried out at the bedside.
- *Plain radiographs* have a sensitivity of 55% but when repeated – usually two weeks later – the sensitivity is higher, making this the most cost-effective diagnostic procedure. Osteomyelitic lesions may cause cortical bone destruction, permeative radiolucency, focal osteopenia or osteolysis, periosteal new bone formation and/or soft tissue swelling (see Figures 11.26, 11.39, 11.52, 11.43, 11.49, 11.50 [middle panel] and 11.45).
- *Computed tomography* may reveal areas with subtle abnormalities such as periosteal reactions, small cortical erosions and soft tissue abnormalities.

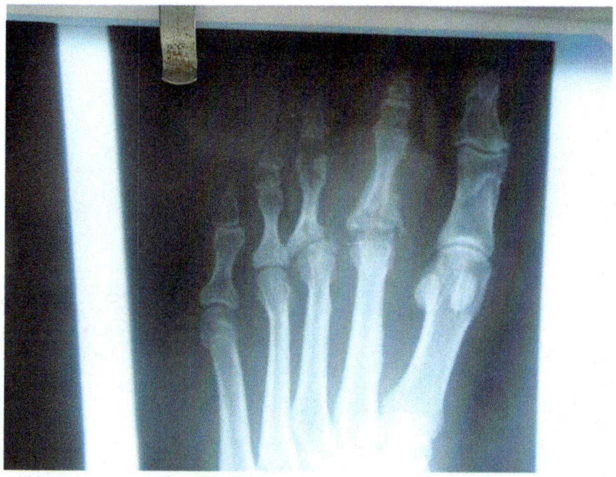

Figure 11.39 A plain radiograph of septic arthritis and osteomyelitis of the second toe of the foot shown in Figure 11.37. Note the distortion of the cortical bone and the destruction of the metatarsophalangeal joint. A damaged third metatarsophalangeal joint is due to a healed episode of septic arthritis, four years before this radiograph was taken (see Figure 11.29).

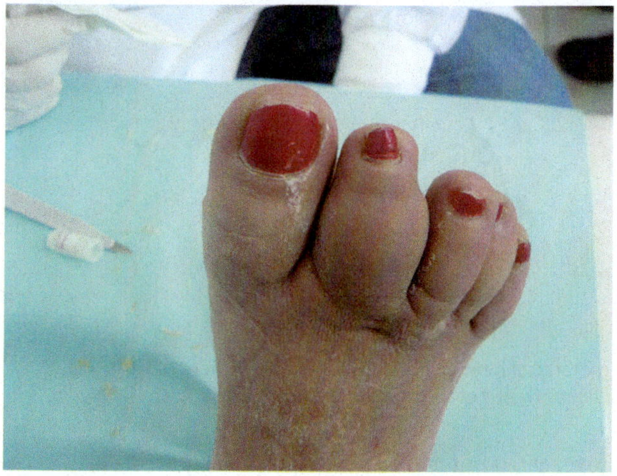

Figure 11.40 A sausage-toe disfigurement caused by bone edema and osteomyelitis of the first phalanx of the second toe. This is the foot of the patient shown in Figure 11.37. See Figure 11.39 for the radiograph of this foot.

- *MRI* has a sensitivity of almost 100% and a specificity of over 80%, and has the potential to reveal abscesses. Therefore, this is the preferred method for the diagnosis of osteomyelitis in many centers in cases where plain radiographs do not provide sufficient information to make a conclusive diagnosis. However, the specificity of MRI decreases in the presence of neuro-osteoarthropathy, prior bone biopsy, recent bone fracture or recent surgery.
- *Magnification radiography* is also a very useful method for the detection of early osteomyelitis and is used to follow up the disease.

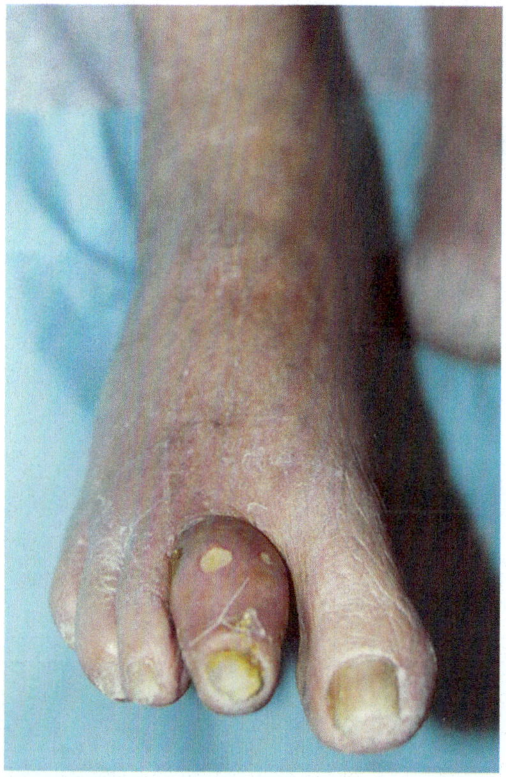

Figure 11.41 A sausage-like toe indicates osteomyelitis. PEDIS 3.

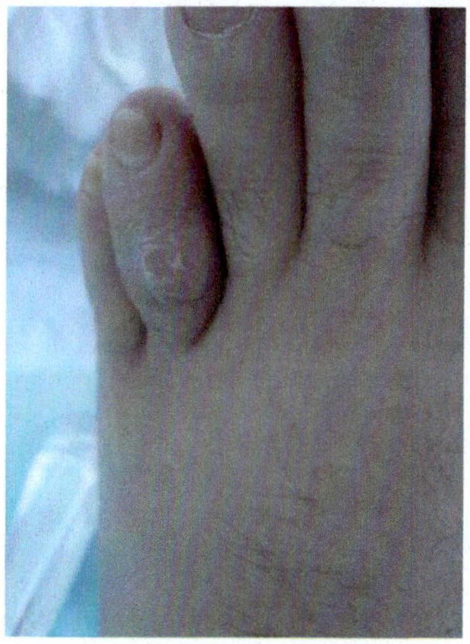

Figure 11.42 A sausage-like toe due to osteomyelitis of the first phalanx of the fourth toe. PEDIS 3.

Chronic osteomyelitis needs surgical removal of the infected bone. However, some authors suggest that prolonged treatment with antibiotics (for one or two years) may eradicate chronic osteomyelitis, although there is no consensus on this issue at present.

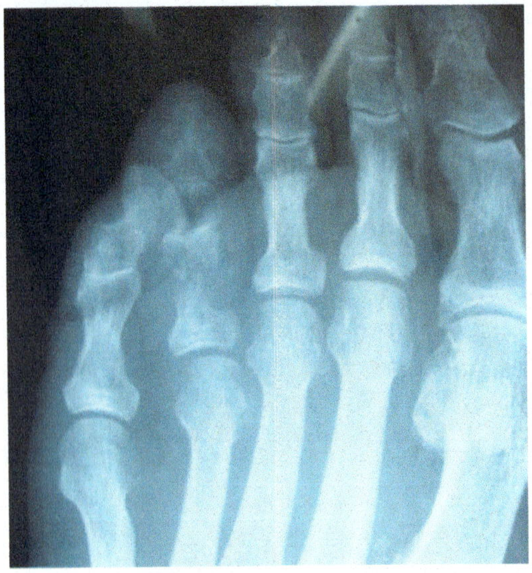

Figure 11.43 Osteomyelitis of the first phalanx of the fourth toe (radiography of the foot shown in Figure 11.42).

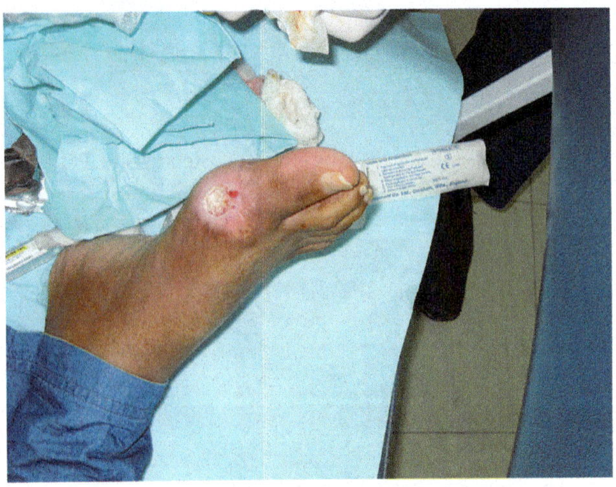

Figure 11.44 A chronic neuro-ischemic ulcer on the medial aspect of the first metatarsal head resists healing due to osteomyelitis (evident in the plain radiograph shown in Figure 11.49), despite proper footwear. PEDIS 3.

11.12 Bone Scintigraphy Imaging

Bone scintigraphy scanning with technetium-99 m (^{99m}Tc) phosphonate produces images in three different phases. During the *flow phase* (Figures 11.51 and 11.52), a series of three second image acquisitions of the site in question is obtained. A static blood pool image (the *blood pool phase*; Figures 11.51b and 11.52b) is obtained five minutes later, and a static delayed image (the *delayed phase*; Figures 11.51c and 11.52c) is obtained three hours later.

^{99m}Tc scintigraphy is useful in cases of questionable osteomyelitis (Figure 11.53). It has a high sensitivity (over 90%) but a low specificity (33%), particularly in the presence of neuro-osteoarthropathy. Although increased radionuclide uptake during the flow and pool phases is not specific to the diagnosis of osteomyelitis (as it may mean soft tissue infection, bone infection or both), delayed ^{99m}Tc scintigraphy images show increased blood flow to the bones only, thus increasing the specificity of the method in the diagnosis of bone infection. Patients with neuro-osteoarthropathy have increased bone blood flow in the absence of osteomyelitis.

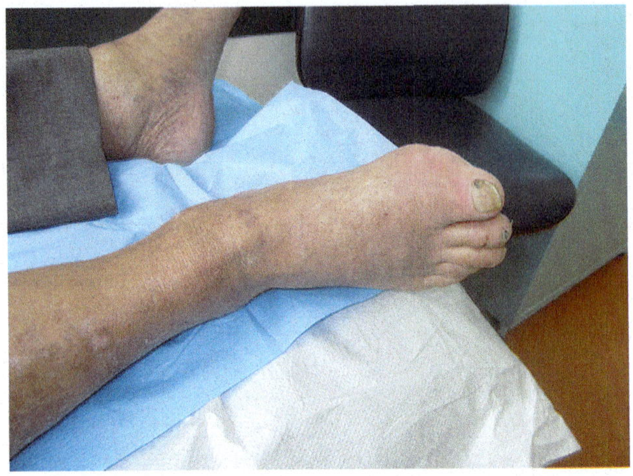

Figure 11.45 Healed osteomyelitis of the first toe. Surgical debridement of the infected bone was performed. The toe remained abnormal, yet free of infection. PEDIS 1.

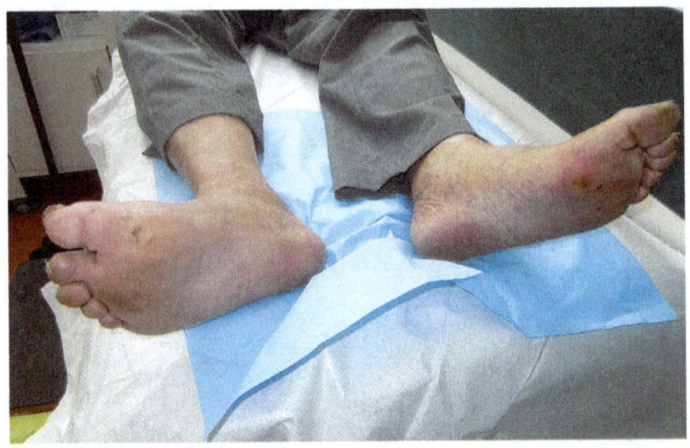

Figure 11.46 A small neuropathic ulcer is present under the first metatarsal head of the right foot of the patient of Figure 11.45. Osteomyelitis of the first toe is healed. PEDIS 1.

Gallium-67 citrate scans exclude osteomyelitis when they are normal, but since gallium accumulates at sites of both osteomyelitis and increased bone remodeling, the specificity of this scan is limited. When positive, gallium scans need a supplementary bone scan to improve their specificity.

Indium-111 (^{111}In) white blood cell imaging is expensive and time-consuming, has poor spatial resolution

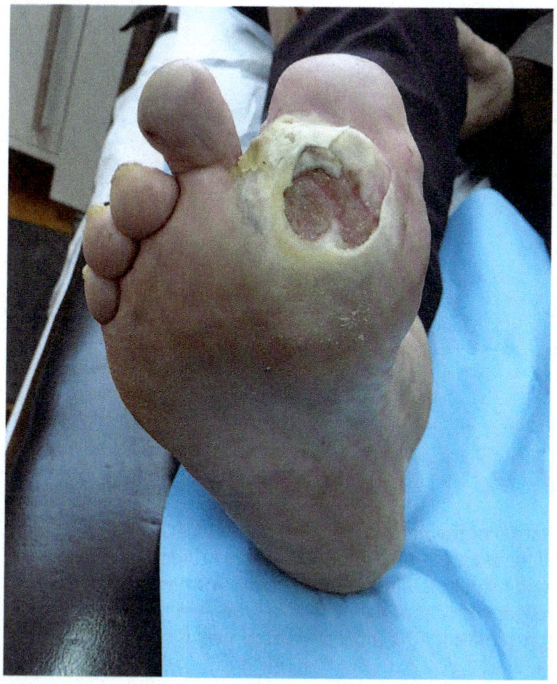

Figure 11.47 A neuropathic ulcer is seen under the first metatarsal head of the foot of the patient presented in Figures 11.45 and 11.46, three years after osteomyelitis was healed. PEDIS 2. The disfigured first toe is a risk factor for a new ulcer. This is a depressive patient, who is very reluctant to visit any doctor, and he is not following doctor's advice to use special shoes.

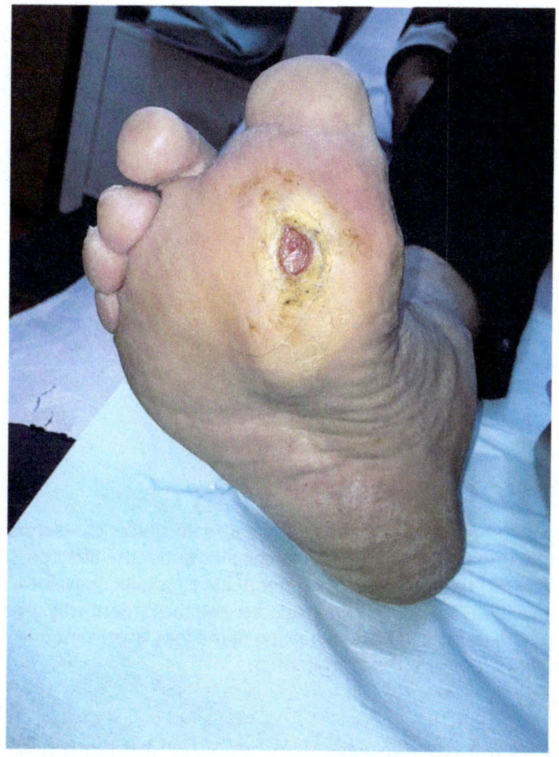

Figure 11.48 A neuropathic ulcer (PEDIS 1) is seen under the first metatarsal head of the foot of the patient presented in Figures 11.45–11.47, eight months after Figure 11.47 was taken. The disfigured first toe is a life-long risk factor for a new ulcer.

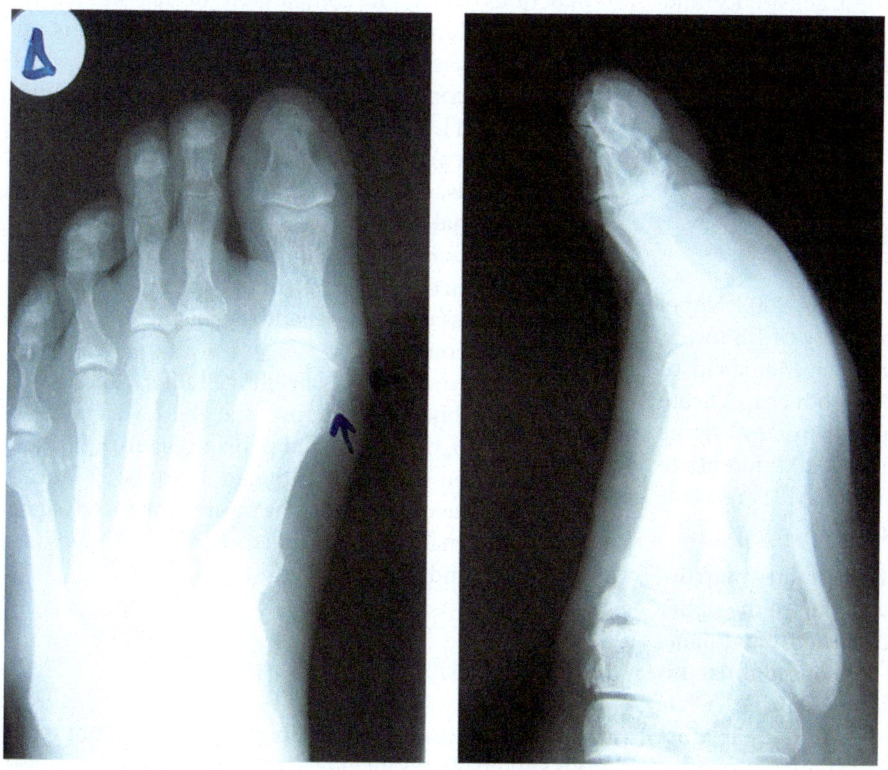

Figure 11.49 Osteomyelitis of the first metatarsal head thwarts healing of the ulcer shown in Figure 11.44.

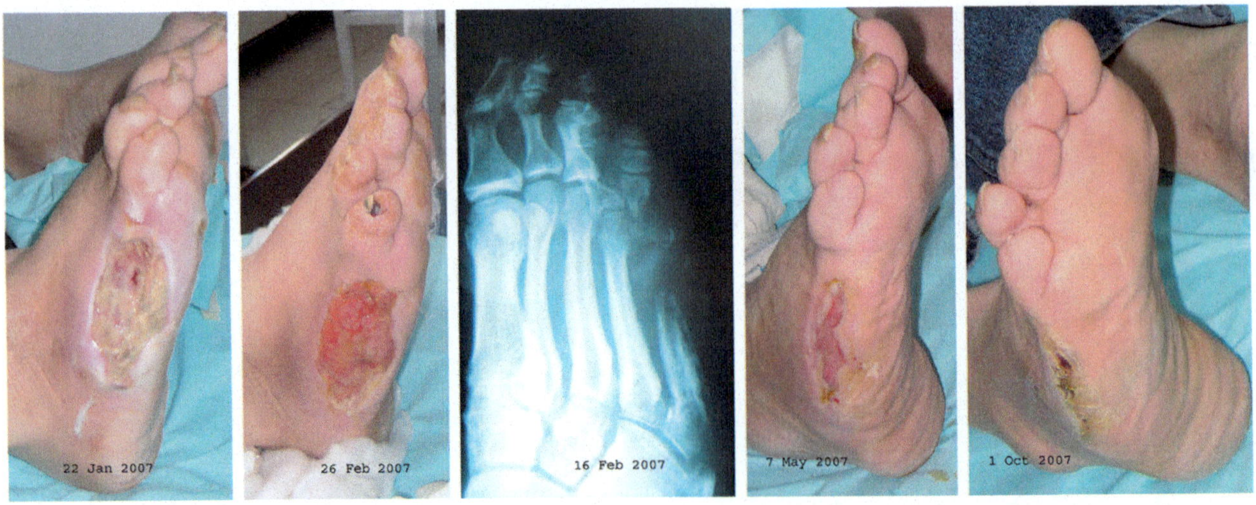

Figure 11.50 An acute infection of a neuropathic ulcer characterized by maceration of the bed and borders of the ulcer, a purulent discharge under the fibrin layer, and cellulitis under the fifth toe is seen on the lateral aspect of this foot. In a plain radiograph, bone destruction of the fifth metatarsal, permeative radiolucency, focal osteopenia and osteolysis, and periosteal bone formation are signs of osteomyelitis. No pathogen was isolated, and the patient was given antibiotic cover with ciprofloxacin and clindamicin. Granulating tissue, characteristic of healthy healing of the foot, is present one month after presentation. The ulcer and osteomyelitis were successfully treated after four months of antibiotics.

and does not distinguish soft tissue infection from bone infection.

Scintigraphy using white blood cells labeled with ^{99m}Tc hexamethyl-propylamineoxime (a gamma-emitting radionuclide imaging agent; ^{99m}Tc HMPAO-WBC), and ^{111}In-labeled leukocytes offer the best sensitivity and specificity both in diagnosing osteomyelitis and in differentiating it from neuropathic osteoarthropathy (Figures 11.52, 11.54 and 11.55).

11.13 Magnetic Resonance Imaging

The technique of MRI (which earned the 2003 Nobel Prize for Paul Lauterbur of the University of Illinois at Urbana-Champaign, USA, and Sir Peter Mansfield of the University of Nottingham, UK) produces delicate anatomic definition and offers a high intrinsic soft tissue contrast; MRI can outline an infection and differentiate tissue lesions. The following sequences of MRI are available for bone and soft tissue abnormalities:

- The *T1 sequence* shows a bright normal fatty marrow, while abnormal marrow is seen as dark (see the upper panels of Figures 11.59 and 11.60, the left-hand panel of Figure 11.61 and 11.67). In the case of cellulitis, this low signal may be diffuse and non-specific, while abscesses and osteomyelitic lesions produce a more focal low-T1 signal. The T1 sequence offers the most detailed anatomy.
- The *short tau inversion recovery (STIR) sequence* shows a dark normal marrow and bright fluid collections.
- *T1 with fat saturation* ("fat sat"; see Figure 11.70) is produced after gadolinium infusion, which reveals the bright inflammation tissue of an infectious or non-infectious cause. A comparison of fat sat against pre-gadolinium T1 (or STIR) sequence images is utilized to bypass inhomogeneous fat suppression, which may cause confusion in the case of the foot imaging (see Figure 11.69). Abscesses may produce an enhancing rim after gadolinium administration; in the case of osteomyelitis, gadolinium enhances the abnormal low marrow signal on T1 images. Interruption or destruction of the bone cortex, subperiosteal abscesses, periosteal enhancement and a contiguous sinus tract or a full-thickness ulcer are secondary magnetic resonance signs of osteomyelitis.
- The *T2 sequence* depicts bright cellulitis, fluid collections and abnormal marrow (see the lower panel of Figure 11.46, the right-hand panel of Figure 11.61 and 11.68). When combined with gadolinium (T2 fat sat), the T2 sequence produces a more enhanced signal from abnormalities of the marrow and soft tissues (see the right-hand panel of Figure 11.60).

11.14 Antibiotic Treatment

Empirical treatment with antibiotics in severe foot infections should always include agents against staphylococci, enterobacteriaceae, and anaerobes. In the case of

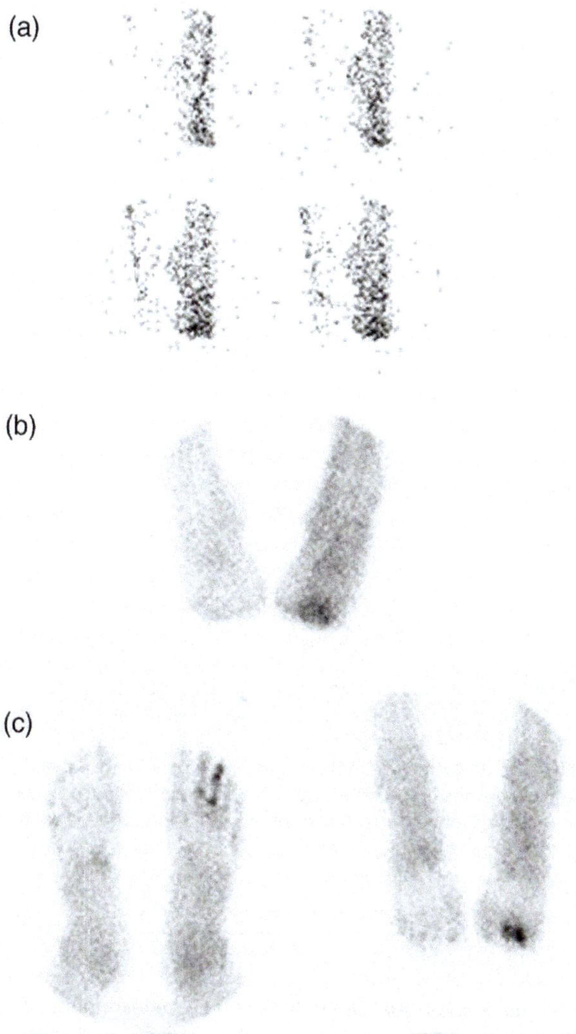

Figure 11.51 A three-phase bone scan (^{99m}Tc-MDP TPBS) of the feet of the patient shown in Figure 11.38. (a) "Flow phase," plantar aspect. There are areas of increased blood flow. (b) "Blood pool phase," plantar and dorsal aspects. Areas of increased soft tissue inflammation can be seen. (c) "Bone phase," plantar, dorsal, and lateral aspects. Areas of increased bone turn-over have incorporated the radionuclide tracer. Osteomyelitis of the third toe is evident. *Source:* Courtesy of Dr. Stamatia Georga, Papageorgiou Hospital, Thessaloniki.

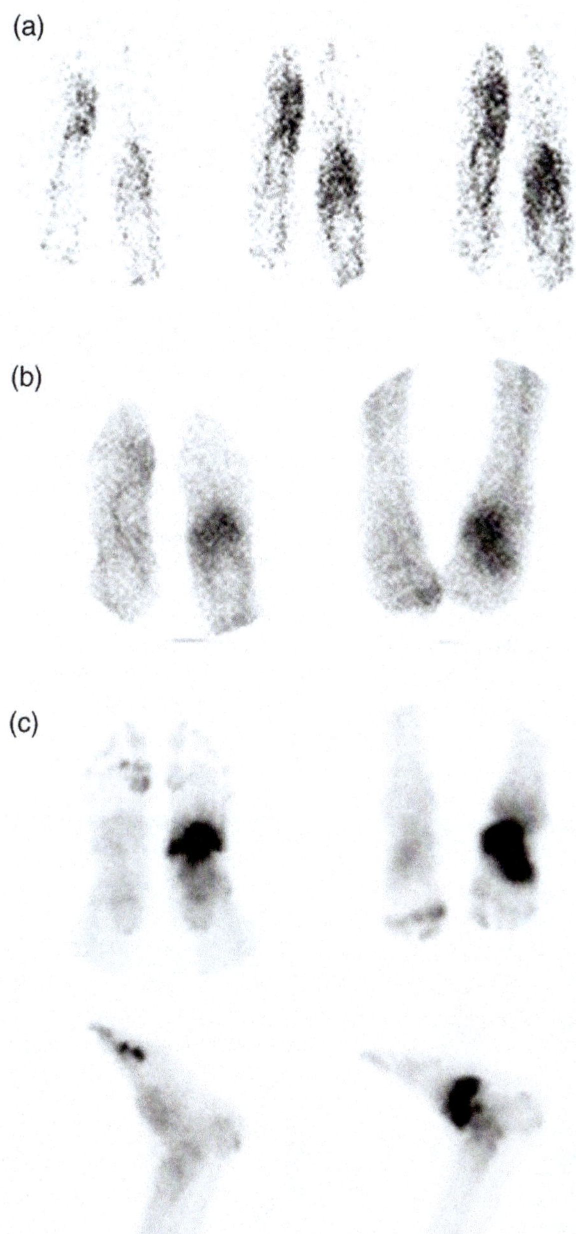

Figure 11.52 A three-phase bone scan (^{99m}Tc-MDP TPBS) of the feet of the patient shown in Figure 11.40. (a) "Flow phase," plantar aspect. (b) "Blood pool phase," plantar and dorsal aspects. (c) "Bone phase," plantar, dorsal, and lateral aspects. This scan indicates osteomyelitis of the first right metatarsal head, and a lesion of the tarsal bones that has a differential diagnosis between osteomyelitis, recent bone fracture, recent surgery and neuro-osteoarthropathy. A positive delay is seen when there is an underlying process that promotes bone remodeling. *Source:* Courtesy of Dr. Stamatia Georga, Papageorgiou Hospital, Thessaloniki.

osteomyelitis, two agents with good bone bioavailability are chosen. Therapeutic options in patients with severe foot infections include the following:

- Fluoroquinolone plus metronidazole or clindamycin. This combination is effective against *S. aureus* (meticillin-susceptible strains only), enterobacteriaceae, and anaerobes.
- β-Lactam and β-lactamase inhibitor combinations (ticarcillin–clavulanic acid, piperacillin–tazobactam). Ampicillin–sulbactam is particularly active against *Enterococcus* species. For patients who have received extensive antibiotic therapy, ticarcillin–clavulanic acid or piperacillin–tazobactam may be preferred because of the increased activity against nosocomial Gram-negative bacilli. Such regimens are also

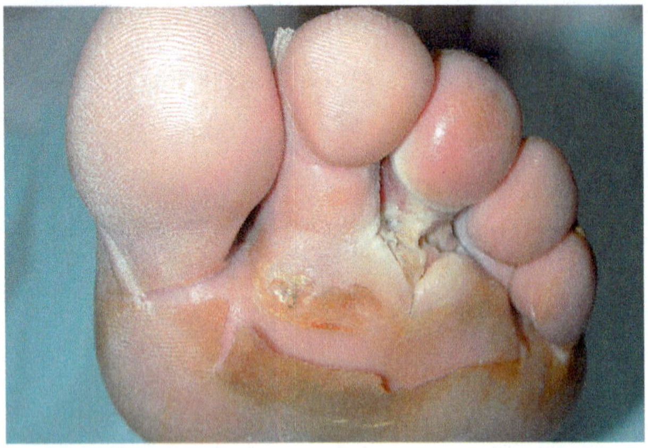

Figure 11.53 An infected neuropathic ulcer at the base of the third toe (after the removal of a corn on the lateral aspect of this toe), four days after proper antibiotic treatment. The first phalanx is exposed. Osteomyelitis of the third toe was verified by the three-phase bone scan (^{99m}Tc-MDP TPBS) shown in Figure 11.39. Note the scaling on the sole after the edema had diminished. *Source:* Courtesy of Dr. Stamatia Georga, Papageorgiou Hospital, Thessaloniki.

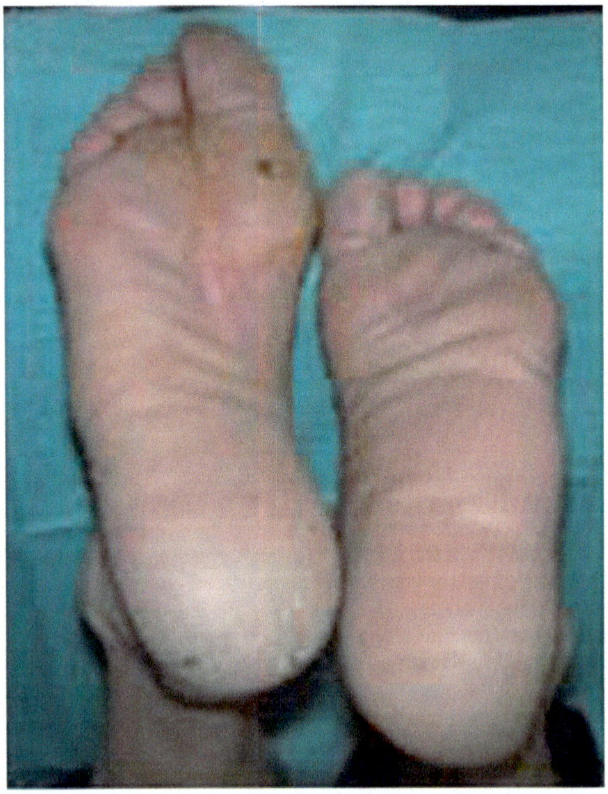

Figure 11.54 A neuropathic ulcer under the first right metatarsal head (after a recent ray amputation of the second right toe) and swelling of the left midfoot. Osteomyelitis was diagnosed under the ulcer on the right foot by means of a labeled leukocyte scan, while the lesion of the left foot is a neuro-arthropathic one. *Source:* Courtesy of Dr. Stamatia Georga, Papageorgiou Hospital, Thessaloniki.

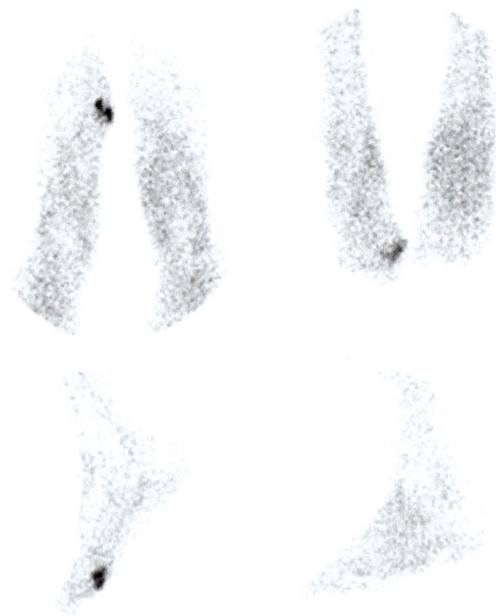

Figure 11.55 A technetium-hexamethylpropylene amine oxime (^{99m}Tc-HMPAO) labeled leukocyte scan of the feet of the patient shown in Figures 11.40 and 11.41. The labeled leukocyte scan is performed by labeling the patient's own white cells with ^{99m}Tc-HMPAO or ^{111}In-oxime and reinjecting them into the same patient (autologous white blood cells). Labeled white blood cells accumulate at sites of infection (as in the first right metatarsal head of this patient) and not at sites of increased osteoblastic activity. *Source:* Courtesy of Dr. Stamatia Georga, Papageorgiou Hospital, Thessaloniki.

Case 11.2 MRI Investigation of Osteomyelitis

A 46-year-old gentleman with type 1 diabetes mellitus of 18 years' duration with a healing neuropathic ulcer under his second metatarsal head noticed some discomfort and swelling of his forefoot (Figures 11.56 and 11.57), as well as low fever. Proper footwear was not being used.

A plain radiogram revealed destruction of his first metatarsophalangeal joint and osteolysis of the second metatarsal head (Figure 11.58). MRI of his forefoot was performed in order to diagnose soft tissue damage and abscess formation. T1-, T2-weighted and T2-weighted fat sat sequences revealed septic arthritis of the first metatarsophalangeal joint and osteomyelitis of the first metatarsal (Figures 11.59–11.61).

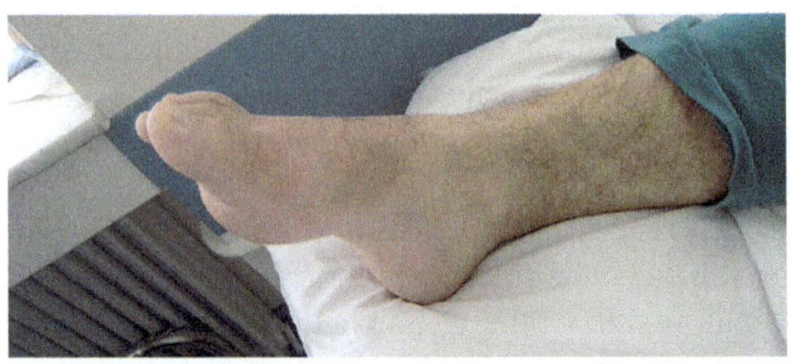

Figure 11.56 Case 11.2: swelling of the right forefoot due to osteomyelitis of the first two metatarsal heads. *Source:* Courtesy of Dr. Stamatia Georga, Papageorgiou Hospital, Thessaloniki.

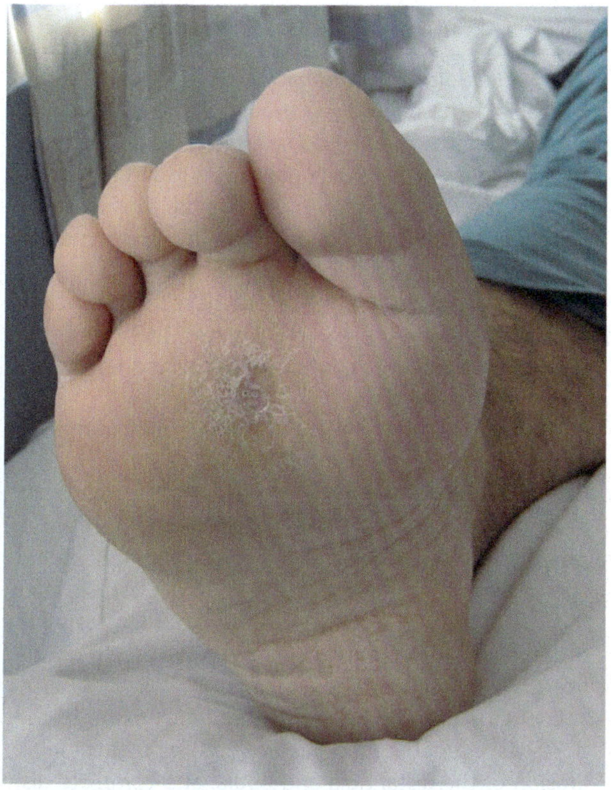

Figure 11.57 Case 11.2: swelling of the forefoot due to osteomyelitis of the first two metatarsal heads. A healing neuropathic ulcer is seen under the second metatarsal head.

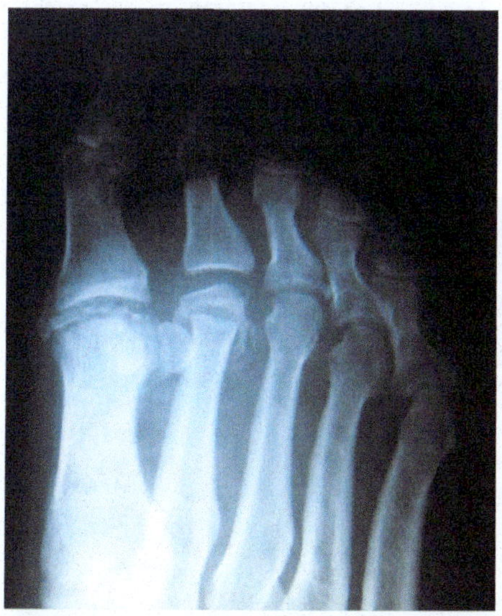

Figure 11.58 Case 11.2: A radiograph of septic arthritis and osteomyelitis of the first metatarsophalangeal joint and osteolysis of the second metatarsal head.

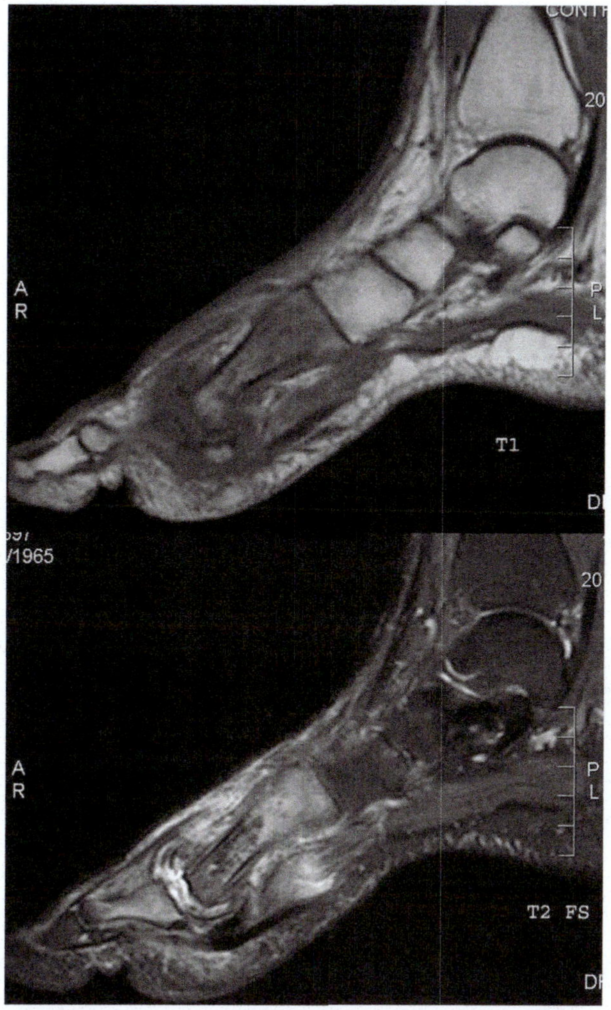

Figure 11.59 Case 11.2: Sagittal magnetic resonance imaging T1- (upper panel) and T2 fat sat (lower panel) weighted images. The first metatarsal produces a low signal in the T1 image and an enhanced signal in the T2 fat sat image, compatible with osteomyelitis. The metatarsophalangeal joint is also bright in the T2 fat sat image, due to septic arthritis.

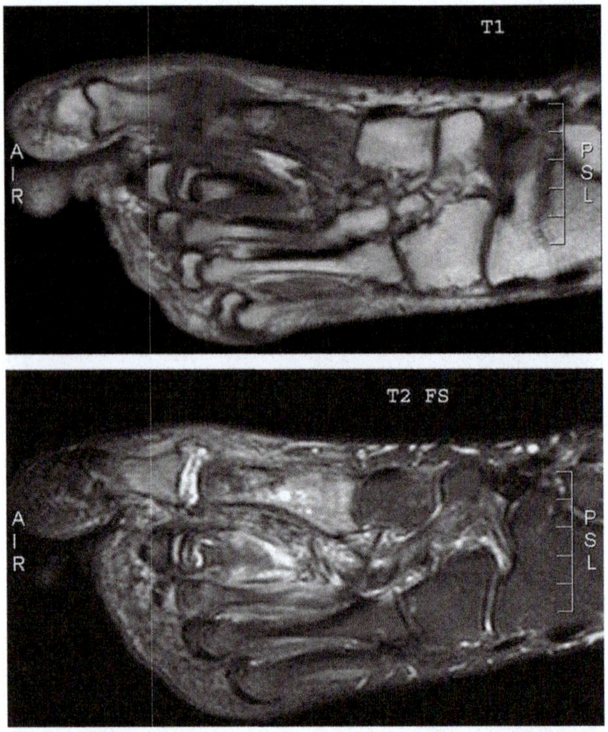

Figure 11.60 Case 11.2: T1- (upper panel) and T2 fat sat (lower panel) weighted coronary magnetic resonance images. The proximal phalanx of the hallux produces an enhanced signal in the T2 image, compatible with reactive bone edema. Edema is also evident in the soft tissue around the first metatarsal, denoting inflammation. The metatarsophalangeal joint is thickened and bright, due to septic arthritis. The whole first metatarsal gives a low signal in the T1 image and an enhanced signal in the T2 image, compatible with osteomyelitis.

Case 11.3 MRI Investigation of an Ambiguous Case

This 70-year-old lady who had had type 2 diabetes for 28 years had suffered a strain of her left ankle. Compression and some bed rest had been advised, but no off-loading. A plain radiograph was found to be normal (Figure 11.62). Three months later, however, the patient complained of left ankle swelling and some discomfort. A new radiograph was diagnosed as a healing fracture (which was supposed to have been undiagnosed three months earlier; Figure 11.63), and the patient was advised to continue with her chores without any other intervention.

Five months later, the patient noticed inflammation on the front aspect of her left swollen ankle. An eschar developed after a superficial ulcer that formed and healed automatically (Figure 11.64). Her C-reactive protein level was normal. A new radiograph of her left ankle was diagnosed as chronic Charcot joint (Figures 11.65 and 11.66), and an MRI was requested in order to exclude osteomyelitis, given the eschar on the frontolateral aspect of her ankle.

Edema is present in the subcutaneous tissue of the dorsal aspect of the foot and around the tibiotalar joint. Erosion of the distal tibia and fibula, and complete disruption of the architecture of the talus are seen, as well as partial erosion of the dorsal and lateral aspects of the calcaneus. The anterior cuboid produces an abnormal signal. The erosion produces an intermediate signal in T1 and T2 (Figure 11.67 and 11.68) and STIR (Figure 11.69)

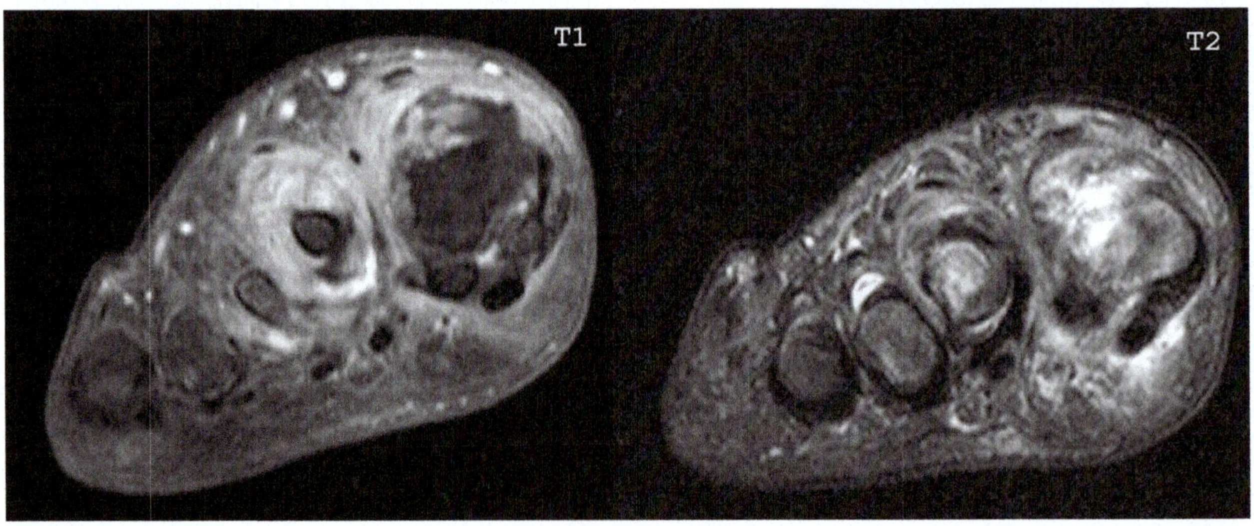

Figure 11.61 Case 11.2: T1- (upper panel) and T2- (lower panel) weighted coronal magnetic resonance images of the right forefoot. The dark marrow in the first metatarsal in the T1 image and bright marrow in the T2 image indicate osteomyelitis. A periosteal reaction and subperiosteal abscess of the first two metatarsals are secondary signs of osteomyelitis.

sequences, which is enhanced after gadolinium infusion (Figure 11.70).

Bone edema is seen as an enhanced signal in the lateral and medium cuneiforms, and at the proximal heads of the fourth and fifth metatarsals. These lesions are present only in T1 fat sat sequences (Figure 11.70) (and not in the T1 sequences), so they are attributed not to osteomyelitis or bone necrosis, but to neuropathic osteoarthropathy.

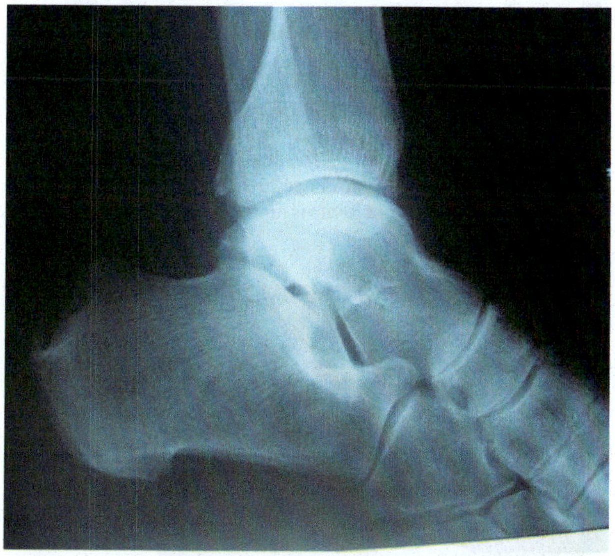

Figure 11.62 Case 11.3: A plain radiograph of a left ankle after an ankle strain.

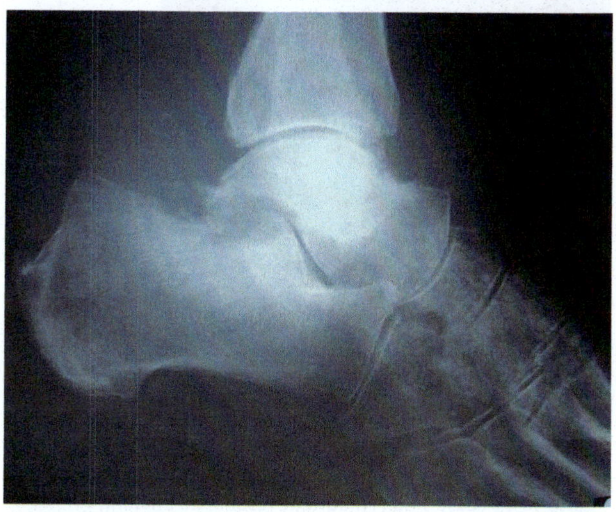

Figure 11.63 Case 11.3: A plain radiograph of an acute neuro-osteoarthropathic ankle.

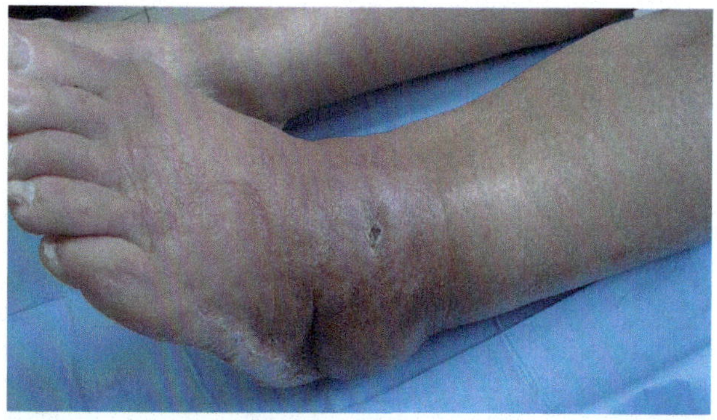

Figure 11.64 Case 11.3: Cellulitis of the front aspect of the swollen neuro-osteoarthropathic ankle (Charcot joint).

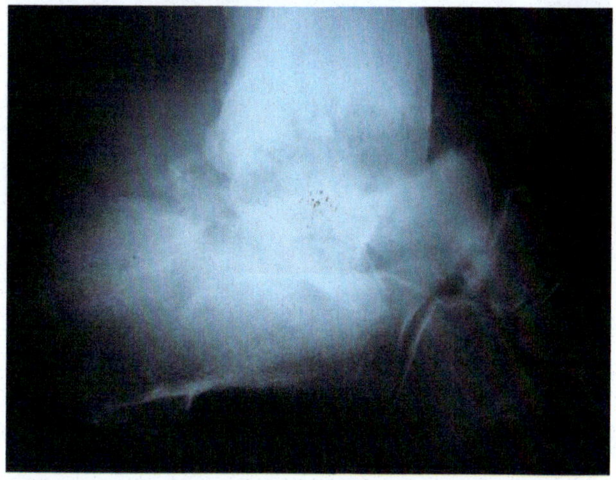

Figure 11.65 Case 11.3: Chronic neuropathic osteoarthropathy (Charcot joint) of the ankle in a lateral plain radiograph.

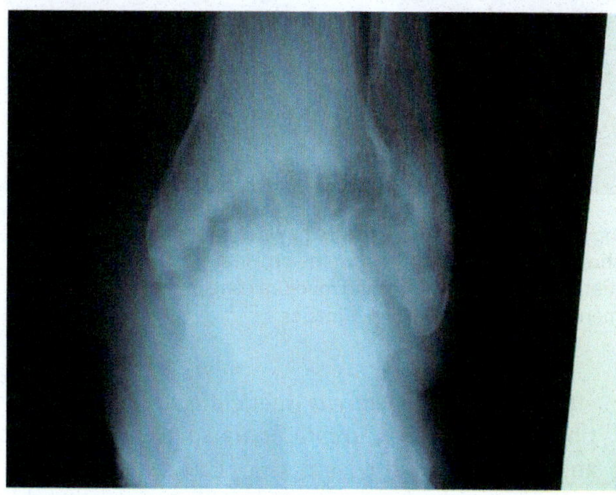

Figure 11.66 Case 11.3: A hindfoot radiograph showing chronic neuropathic osteoarthropathy (Charcot joint) of the ankle.

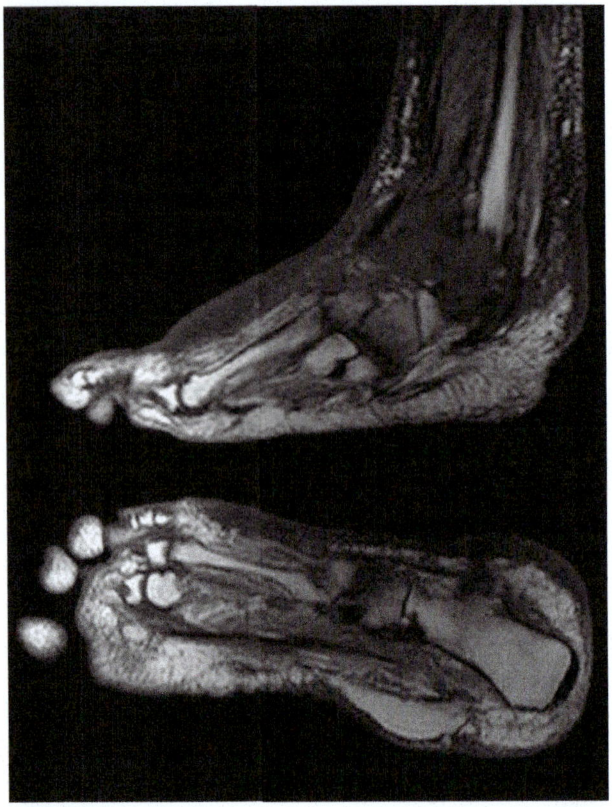

Figure 11.67 Case 11.3: A magnetic resonance imaging T1-weighted image showing erosion of the distal fibula, distraction of the talus, and an abnormal signal from the cuboid and lateral cuneiform bones and the proximal head of the fourth metatarsal. Normal fatty marrow is bright on T1 imaging.

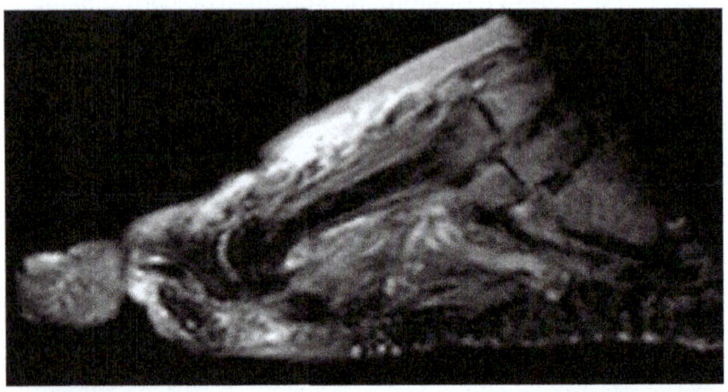

Figure 11.68 Case 11.3: A magnetic resonance imaging T2 image showing enhanced signal from the proximal head of the fourth metatarsal and the lateral and medium cuneiforms. Normal marrow is seen as dark on T2 images.

effective against *S. aureus* (meticillin sodium-susceptible strains only), *Streptococcus* species, and most anaerobes.

- In patients who have severe penicillin allergy, combination therapy with aztreonam and clindamycin, or a fluoroquinolone and clindamycin, is effective.

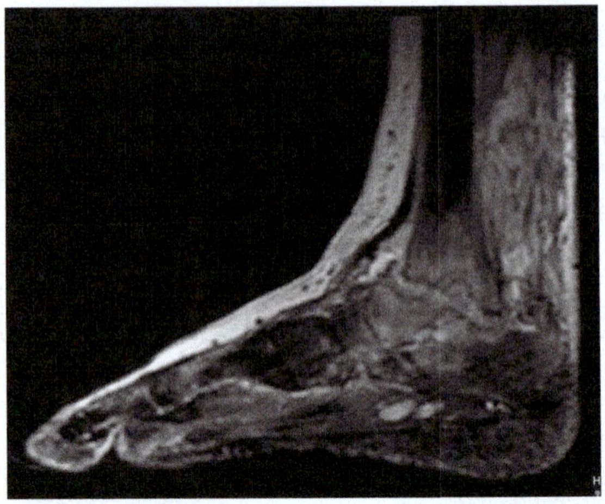

Figure 11.69 Case 11.3: A magnetic resonance imaging STIR image. Pathology is indicated by the relatively high signal from the peripheral tibia. This is a highly sensitive sequence to screen for lesions and fluid collections, yet the anatomic detail on STIR imaging is inferior to that from T1 sequences. Differentiating osteomyelitis from Charcot joints is not possible with this sequence.

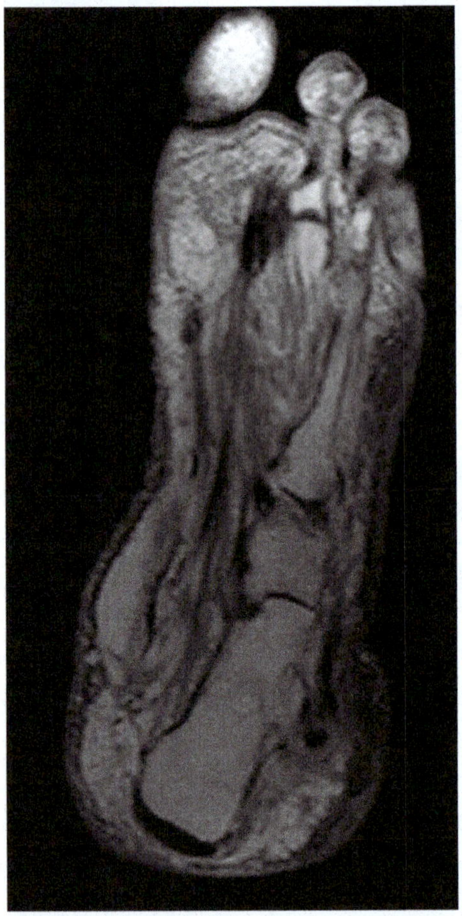

Figure 11.70 Case 11.3: A magnetic resonance imaging T1-weighted image post gadolinium with fat suppression. The fifth metatarsal and the cuboid look bright, therefore excluding osteomyelitis.

- Imipenem–cilastin or meropenem as monotherapy has broad-spectrum activity against Gram-positive and Gram-negative microorganisms, including *Pseudomonas*.

Doctors should always consider the following:

- Modification of treatment may be necessary according to the results of cultures and the level of the patient's kidney function.
- Vancomycin, teicoplanin, linezolide, daptomycin, quinupristin/dalfopristin and tigecycline are active against meticillin-resistant staphylococcal strains. Teicoplanin can be given intramuscularly. Fucidin may also be useful in combination therapy with another anti-staphylococcal agent, but not alone since resistance to it develops quickly.
- Ertapenem is active against Gram-positive and Gram-negative bacteria, and anaerobes, and can be given intramuscularly (1g once daily). It is not active against *Pseudomonas* or *Acinetobacter*.
- Third-generation cephalosporins should be used only in combination with other agents, as they have moderate anti-staphylococcal activity and lack significant activity against anaerobes. Ceftriaxone can be given in the community (1g intramuscularly) on a once-daily basis, but is not active against meticillin-resistant *S. aureus* or *Pseudomonas*.
- Aminoglycosides are nephrotoxic, are inactivated in the acidic environment of the soft tissue infection and have poor penetration into bone.

Further Reading

Aragón-Sánchez, J. (2011). Seminar review: a review of the basis of surgical treatment of diabetic foot infections. *Int. J. Low. Extrem. Wounds* 10 (1): 33–65.

Stang D, Dancer SJ, Seaton A, Leese GP; Scottish Diabetes Foot Action Group. 2017. "Diabetic foot infection: antibiotic therapy and good practice recommendations." *Int. J. Clin. Pract.*. Oct; 71(10): doi: https://doi.org/10.1111/ijcp.13006

Berendt, A.R., Peters, E.J.G., Bakker, K. et al. (2008). Specific guidelines for treatment of diabetic foot osteomyelitis. *Diabetes Metab. Res. Rev.* 24 (Suppl 1): S190–S191.

Boc, S.F., Brazzo, K., Lavian, D., and Landino, T. (2001). Acute Charcot foot changes versus osteomyelitis: does Tc-99 m HMPAO labeled leukocytes scan differentiate? *J. Am. Podiatr. Med. Assoc.* 91: 365–368.

Cheung, Y., Hochman, M., and Brophy, D. (2002). Radiographic changes of the diabetic foot. In: *The Diabetic Foot: Medical and Surgical Management* (ed. A. Veves, J.M. Giurini and F.W. LoGerfo), 179–206. New York: Humana Press.

De Berker, D. (2009). Fungal nail disease. *N. Engl. J. Med.* 360: 2108–2116.

Dumont, I.J. (2009). Diagnosis and prevalence of onychomycosis in diabetic neuropathic patients: an observational study. *J. Am. Podiatr. Med. Assoc.* 99: 135–139.

Edmonds, M.E., Foster, A.V.M., and Sanders, L.J. (2008.). *A Practical Manual of Diabetic Foot Care. Stage 4: The Infected Foot*, 130–180. Oxford: Blackwell.

Fridman R, Bar-David T, Kamen S, Staron RB, Leung DK, Rasiej MJ. 2014. "Imaging of diabetic foot infections." *Clin. Podiatr. Med. Surg.*. Jan 31(1): 43–56.

Gratz, S., Rennen, H.J.J.M., Boerman, O.C. et al. (2002). 99 mTc-HMPAO-labeled autologous versus heterologous leukocytes for imaging infection. *J. Nucl. Med.* 43: 918–924.

Heald, A.H., O'Halloran, D.J., Richards, K. et al. (2001). Fungal infection of the diabetic foot: two distinct syndromes. *Diabet. Med.* 18: 567–572.

Internal Clinical Guidelines team. National Institute for Health and Care Excellence (UK); 2015 Aug. Clinical Guidelines. Diabetic Foot Problems: Prevention and Management. NICE Clinical Guideline19 Methods, evidence and recommendations. Published [August] 2015, updated [January] 2016. Assessed January 2018.

International Working Group on the Diabetic Foot. Available at: www.iwgdf.org (accessed January 2018).

Lavery, L.A., Peters, E.J.G., Armstrong, D.G. et al. (2009). Risk factors for developing osteomyelitis in patients with diabetic foot wounds. *Diabetes Res. Clin. Pract.* 83: 347–352.

Lipsky, B.A., Aragón-Sánchez, J., Diggle, M. et al. (2016 Jan). IWGDF guidance on the diagnosis and management of foot infections in persons with diabetes. *Diabetes Metab. Res. Rev.* 32 (Suppl 1): 45–74.

Makrantonaki, E., Jiang, D., Hossini, A.M. et al. (2016 Sep). Diabetes mellitus and the skin. *Rev. Endocr. Metab. Disord.* 17 (3): 269–282.

Morales Lozano, R., González Fernández, M.L., Beneit Montesinos, J.V. et al. (2010 Oct). Validating the probe-to-bone test and other tests for diagnosing chronic osteomyelitis in the diabetic foot. *Diabetes Care* 33 (10): 2140–2145.

Nelson, E.A., O'Meara, S., Golder, S. et al. (2006). Systematic review of antimicrobial treatments for diabetic foot ulcers. *Diabet. Med.* 23: 348–359.

O'Meara, S., Nelson, E.A., Golder, S. et al. (2006). Systematic review of methods to diagnose infection in foot ulcers in diabetes. *Diabet. Med.* 23: 341–347.

O'Neal, L.W. (2001). Surgical pathology of the foot and clinicopathological correlations. In: *Levin and O'Neal's the Diabetic Foot* (ed. J.H. Bowker and M.A. Pfeifer), 483–512. St Louis: Mosby.

Peter-Riesch, B. (2016). The diabetic foot: the never-ending challenge. *Endocr. Dev.* 31: 108–134.

Peters, E.J. and Lipsky, B.A. (2013 Sep). Diagnosis and management of infection in the diabetic foot. *Med. Clin. North Am.* 97 (5): 911–946.

Rigopoulos, D., Larios, G., Gregoriou, S., and Alevizos, A. (2008). Acute and chronic paronychia. *Am. Fam. Physician* 77: 339–348.

Schaper, N.C., Van Netten, J.J., Apelqvist, J. et al. (2017 Feb). Prevention and management of foot problems in diabetes: a summary guidance for daily practice 2015, based on the IWGDF guidance documents. *Diabetes Res. Clin. Pract.* 124: 84–92.

Swartz, M.N. (2004). Cellulitis. *N. Engl. J. Med.* 350: 904–912.

Treece, K.A., Macfarlane, R.M., Pound, N. et al. (2004). Validation of a system of foot ulcer classification in diabetes mellitus. *Diabet. Med.* 21: 987–991.

Uçkay I, Gariani K, Pataky Z, Lipsky BA. 2014 Apr. "Diabetic foot infections: state-of-the-art." *Diabetes Obes. Metab.* 16(4): 305–316.

12

Methods of Prevention

K. Makrilakis and A. Kokkinos

First Department of Propaedeutic Internal Medicine, National and Kapodistrian University of Athens, Medical School, Laiko General Hospital, Athens, Greece

The causal pathways leading to foot ulceration include several component causes, the most important of which is peripheral neuropathy, leading to a loss of protective sensation; the consequent vulnerability to physical and thermal trauma increases the risk for foot ulceration sevenfold. A second causative factor is excessive plantar pressures. This is related to both limited joint mobility (at the ankle, subtalar and first metatarsophalangeal joints) and foot deformities.

A third component cause is trauma, especially when repetitive (e.g. friction from ill-fitting shoes, injuries from falls, self-inflicted from cutting toenails, cellulitis from tinea pedis, etc.). Trauma frequently results from callus formation and hematoma manifestation in the underlying tissues. Sudomotor dysfunction which leads to hyperkeratosis formation, along with increased plantar pressures, both play a crucial role. Once a foot ulcer develops in a diabetic person, several factors may contribute to an adverse outcome, including peripheral vascular disease, hyperglycemia leading to immunologic perturbations (especially in polymorphonuclear leukocyte function), and a high rate of onychomycosis and tinea infections of the toe web, leading to skin disruptions. The obesity and poor vision that are associated with diabetes may also impair self-care.

Preventing foot complications begins with identifying those at risk, that is, those with previous foot ulcers, prior lower extremity amputations, a long duration (over 10 years) of diabetes, poor glycemic control, impaired vision, structural abnormalities of the lower extremities (calluses, hammer or claw toes, flat feet, bunions, etc.), reduced joint mobility, dry or fissured skin, tinea or onychomycosis and also improperly fitting footwear. Unfortunately, the literature lacks good quality controlled studies on the prevention of a first foot ulcer. Callus must be removed regularly, because several studies have consistently shown that it is associated with high plantar pressures and ulcer formation. A demonstration of callus removal is shown in video 12.1.

When it comes to foot care, the patient is a vital member of the medical team. It is important that prophylactic advice on foot care be given to any patient whose feet are at high risk, if not to all diabetic persons. There are a series of recommendations that can markedly diminish ulcer formation; these are particularly important in patients with existing neuropathy. Patient education has been found to be effective especially on prevention of ulcer recurrence. However, one session is not enough; healthcare providers should use every opportunity to remind the patient of prevention methods.

First, the patient should be informed about the possible symptoms and signs of foot problems, so that he or she can identify them at their onset, notify the healthcare provider about their existence and seek ways of management. For example, some simple clues can point to circulatory problems: poor pulses, cold feet, thin or blue skin, and lack of hair signal that the feet are not getting enough blood.

Nerve damage may lead to unusual sensations in the feet and legs, including pain, burning, numbness, tingling and fatigue. Patients should describe these symptoms if they occur, including the timing, whether the feet, ankles or calves are affected, and what measures relieve the symptoms. Nerve damage may cause no symptoms as the foot and leg slowly lose sensation and become numb. This can be very dangerous because the person may be unaware that they have improperly fitting shoes, a stone or other irritant in a shoe, or other problems that could cause damage.

A method for evaluating the presence of peripheral neuropathy (PN) in diabetic patients has been developed, with satisfactory sensitivity and specificity (the

Atlas of the Diabetic Foot, Third Edition. Ioanna Eleftheriadou, Alexandros Kokkinos, Stavros Liatis, Konstantinos Makrilakis, Nicholas Tentolouris, Anastasios Tentolouris, and Panagiotis Tsapogas.

Companion website: www.wiley.com/go/tentolouris/atlas_diabetic_foot

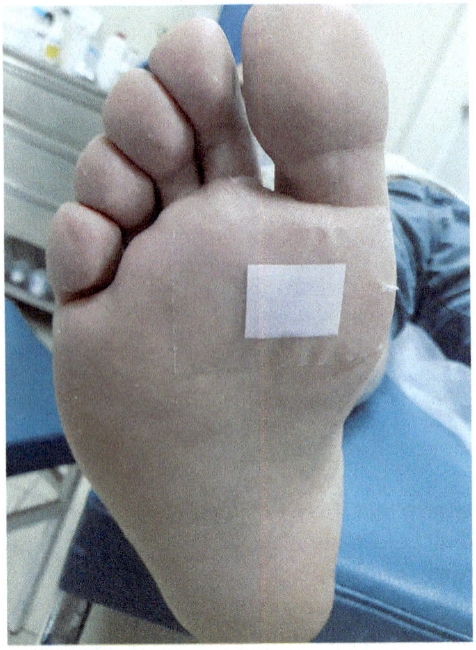

Figure 12.1 The indicator plaster Neuropad is applied to the patient's foot. After 10 minutes, a pink discoloration signifies adequate sudomotor function and indicates no peripheral neuropathy.

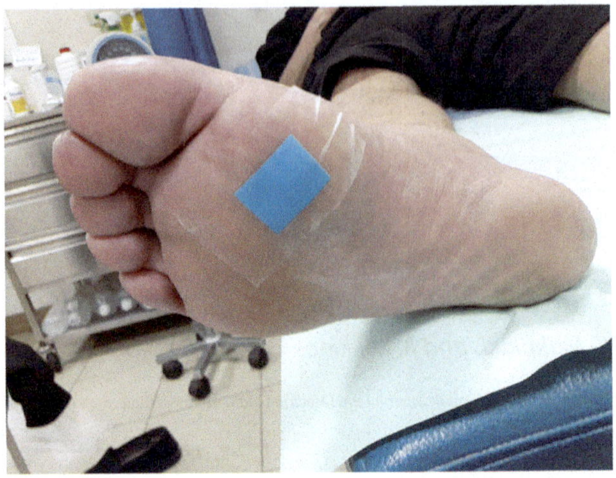

Figure 12.2 The indicator plaster Neuropad is applied to the foot of the patient. After 10 minutes, a blue discoloration signifies sudomotor dysfunction and is a sign of peripheral neuropathy.

indicator plaster Neuropad®; miro Verbandstoffe, Wiehl-Drabenderhöhe, Germany). This can be applied by patients themselves, even at home, and is based on the production of sweat by the feet (sudomotor function). It can help in the diagnosis of peripheral neuropathy (Figures 12.1 and 12.2).

Advantages of the Neuropad are its simplicity, wide availability, high performance for the diagnosis of peripheral neuropathy (PN), high reproducibility and correlation with nerve conduction velocities and neuropathy scores. In addition, recent data suggest that an abnormal Neuropad result is associated with foot ulceration.

Other recommendations to consider are:

- Controlling blood sugar levels can reduce the blood vessel and nerve damage that often leads to diabetic foot complications, and is a vital part of patient care.
- The patients should avoid smoking.
- The use of heating pads or hot water bottles, and stepping into a bath without checking the temperature, should be avoided.
- The toenails should be trimmed to the shape of the toe and filed to remove sharp edges. The patient should be advised never to cut (or allow a manicurist to cut) the cuticles. Patients should never open blisters, try to free ingrown toenails or otherwise break the skin of the feet. A healthcare provider or podiatrist should be consulted for even minor procedures.
- The feet should be inspected daily, looking between and underneath the toes and at pressure areas for skin breaks, blisters, swelling or redness. The patient may need to use a mirror or, if his or her vision is impaired, have someone else perform the examination. Foot inspection may be the single most important precaution against ulceration that a patient can take.
- The feet should be washed daily in tepid water. Mild soap should be used, and the feet should be dried by gentle patting. A moisturizing cream or lotion should then be applied. This is even more important in the case of dry or cracked skin.
- The patient should avoid walking barefoot at any time, both indoors and outdoors, even for short periods of time. Shoes should not be worn without socks, even for a short period. New shoes should not be worn for more than one hour a day, and the feet should be inspected after taking off new shoes; if there is any foot irritation, the patient should inform the healthcare provider. Patients should change their shoes at noon and, if possible, again in the evening; this prevents high pressures remaining on the same area of the foot for a prolonged time. Inspect and palpate the inside of the shoes before wearing them.
- Inappropriate footwear is a major cause of ulceration (see cases 12.1 and 12.2). The aim of providing special shoes and insoles (preventive footwear) to diabetic patients at risk for foot ulceration is to reduce peak plantar pressures over areas "at risk," and to protect the feet against injuries from friction.

Although there is limited scientific information about shoe selection, recommendations can be made in this regard based on risk stratification studies. Shoes for the patient at risk for ulceration should have certain

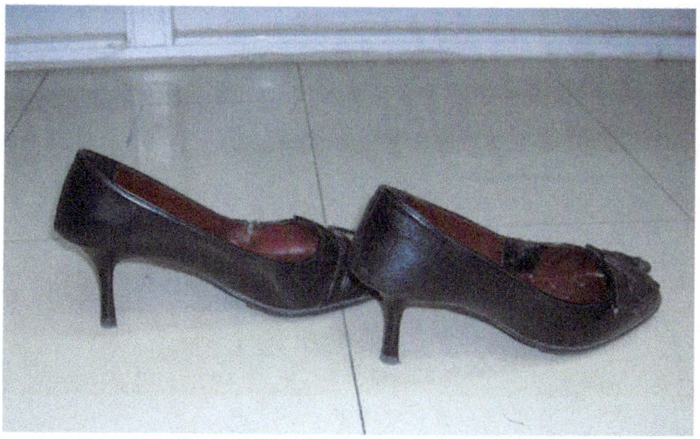

Figure 12.3 High-heel shoes worn by a female patient in the diabetic foot clinic. These shoes are completely inappropriate because they shift the body weight toward the forefoot, and increase pressure under the metatarsal heads.

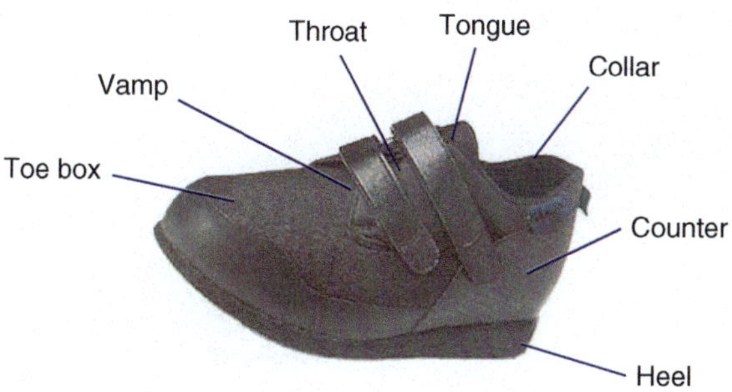

Figure 12.4 Shoe terms.

characteristics. High-heel shoes are completely inappropriate, as they shift the body weight toward the forefoot and increase the pressure under the metatarsal heads (Figure 12.3).

Patients with toe deformities need shoes with enough room at the toe box to prevent friction and pressure on the dorsum of the toes (Figures 12.4 and 12.5). Foot deformity is defined according to the International Consensus on the Diabetic Foot as "the presence of structural abnormalities of the foot such as presence of hammer toes, claw toes, hallux valgus, prominent metatarsal heads, status post neuro-osteoarthropathy, amputations or other foot surgery."

The patient's shoes should be snug, not tight, and the socks should be cotton, loose fitting and changed every day. Patients who have misshapen feet or have had a previous foot ulcer may benefit from the use of special customized shoes (Figure 12.6).

Particular care should be taken when these patients buy new shoes. Patients with a loss of protective sensation tend to select shoes that are too small because they can feel a tight shoe better. Shoes should also be neither too loose. The inside of the shoe should be 1–2cm longer than the foot itself. The internal width should be equal to the width of the foot at the metatarsophalangeal joints. The fitting must be evaluated with the patient in a standing position and preferably at the end of the day.

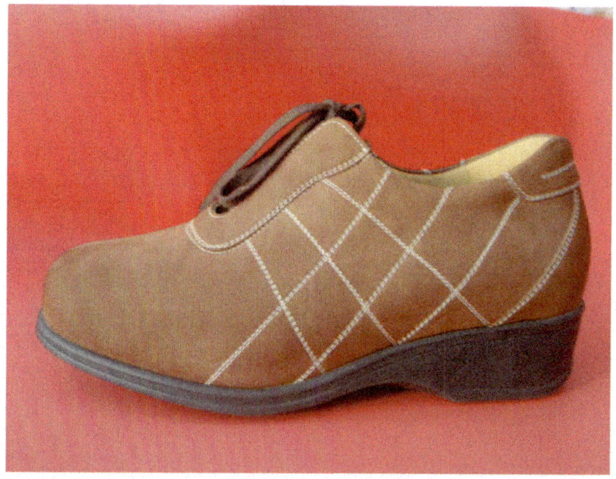

Figure 12.5 A shoe with enough room at the toe box to prevent friction and pressure on the dorsum of the toes, appropriate for feet with toe deformities. Notice the rocker bottom, which reduces pressure at the metatarsal heads.

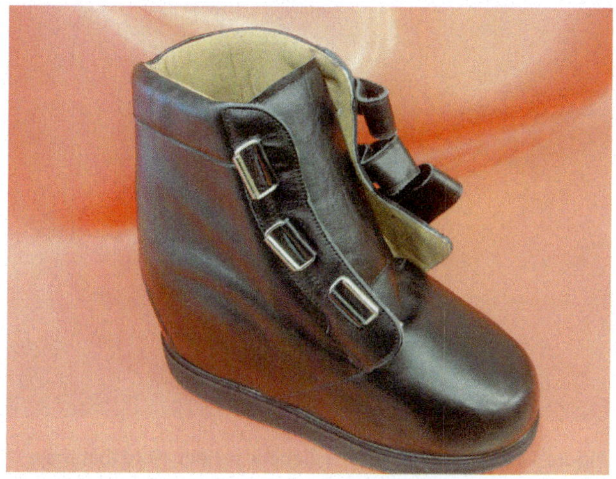

Figure 12.6 A ready-made shoe for a patient with Charcot neuro-osteoarthropathy. Note the wide base to accommodate the deformed foot.

All patients with loss of protective sensation should have soft, shock-absorbing stock insoles in all the shoes they wear (Figure 12.7). Such insoles are usually made of open-cell urethane foam, microcellular rubber or polyethylene foam (Plastazote). According to the design of the insole and the material used, peak plantar pressure reduction during walking may range from 5 to 40%. As insoles may take up considerable space in the shoe, care should be taken to allow sufficient room for the dorsum of the foot (by the use of extra-depth commercially available shoes), otherwise ulceration may develop in this area.

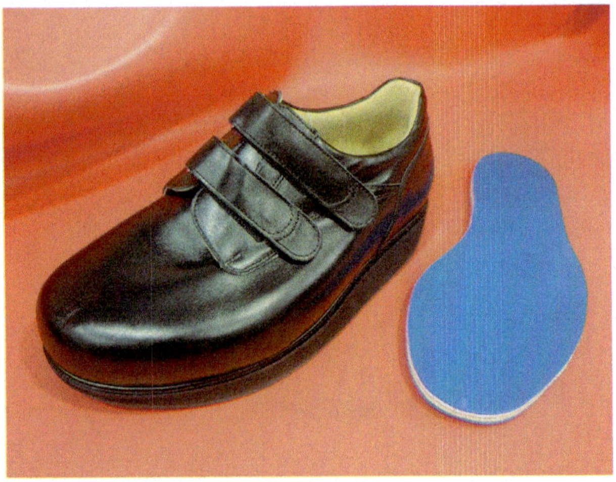

Figure 12.7 A ready-made insole for a diabetic patient's custom-made shoe.

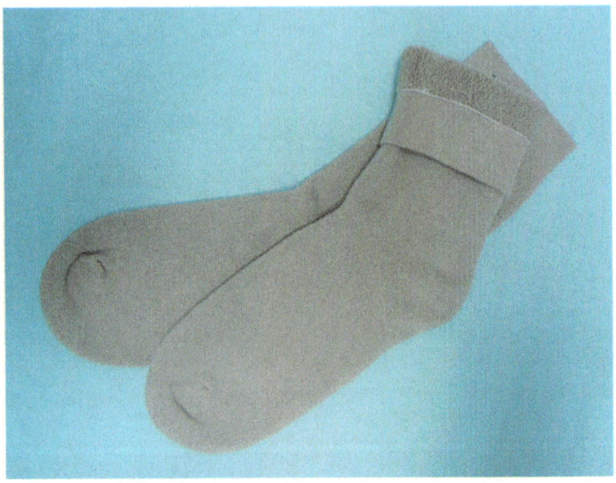

Figure 12.8 Special socks for a diabetic patient. Note that they have no seams and that there is extra padding in the soles.

Many materials used in footwear lose their effectiveness in a relatively short time, depending on the patient's activity. Therefore, regular replacement of the insoles at least three times a year is necessary. Shoes should be changed at least once a year too. Some specifically designed socks (padded socks) may also be used, since they reduce peak plantar pressures during walking by up to 30% (Figure 12.8).

The use of proper insoles, which reduce peak plantar pressures under specific areas, is also necessary for patients with increased plantar pressures (see Figure 12.9); these are inserted in commercially available extra-depth shoes. Insoles must be custom-molded and shock-absorbing. The idea is to redistribute plantar pressures by the use of such insoles, that is, to decrease the load from "at-risk" regions to "safe" regions. In addition,

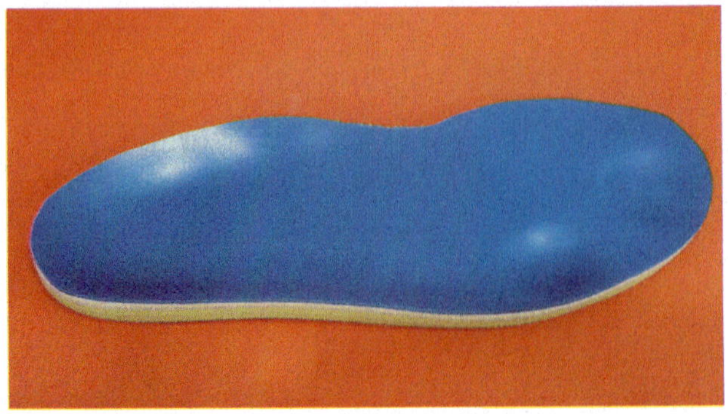

Figure 12.9 A custom-made insole for a diabetic patient's shoe. Notice the special indentations at the fifth metatarsal head and the second to third toes to decrease pressures at these areas.

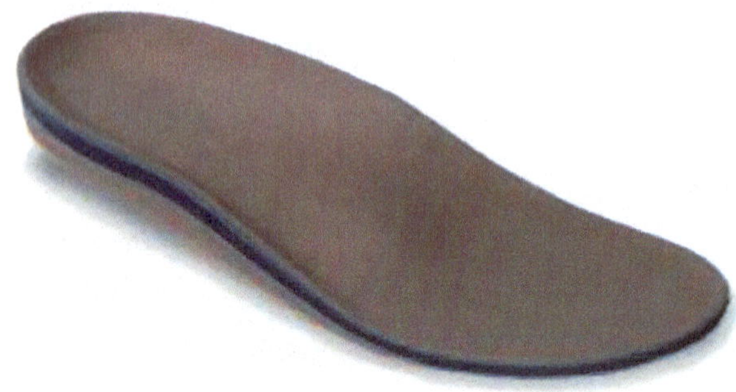

Figure 12.10 The upper side of a three-layer custom-made insole, used to off-load the forefoot. The upper layer is made of cross-linked polyethylene foam, the middle layer of polyurethane, and the lower layer of cork.

insoles reduce shear stress, since the total contact minimizes horizontal and vertical foot movement.

These insoles have two or three layers and are made of materials of different densities. A thin layer of the material with the lowest density (the most potent shock-absorbing material, usually made from cross-linked polyethylene foams) is placed at the foot–insole interface; the firmest material (acrylic plastics, thermoplastic polymers, cork) is placed at the shoe–insole interface. A soft, shock-absorbing, durable material (closed cell neoprene, rubber or urethane polymer) is placed between them (Figure 12.10 and 12.11). Proper insoles for the patient at risk for ulceration should have a minimum thickness of 6.25mm. Patients at high risk need thicker (12.5mm) insoles (Figure 12.12).

Patients with recurrent foot ulcerations or an active lifestyle often need modifications of the outsole. A **rocker**-style rigid outsole rotates over a ridge (fulcrum) in the outsole as the patient walks; this ridge is located 1cm behind the metatarsal heads (Figure 12.13). The rocker outsole allows the shoe to "rock" forward during

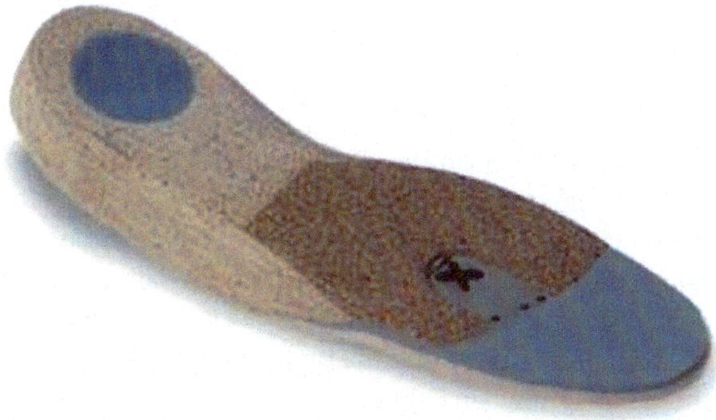

Figure 12.11 The lower side of the insole shown in Figure 12.10.

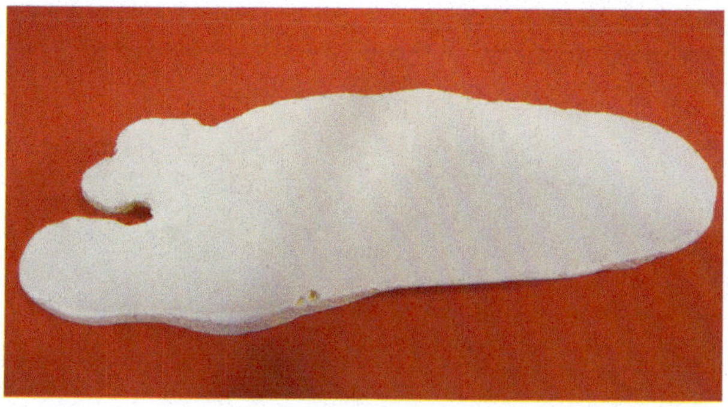

Figure 12.12 A custom-made insole for a patient with amputation of two toes.

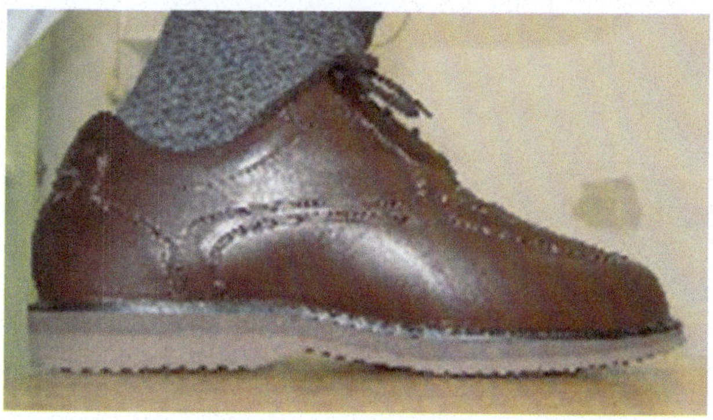

Figure 12.13 A ready-made shoe with a hard, rocker-bottom outsole. Note that the apex (ridge) of the rocker sole is located behind the metatarsal heads.

propulsion, before the metatarsophalangeal joints are allowed to flex, thereby reducing the pressure applied to the forefoot (Figure 12.14).

In a **roller**-style shoe, the contour of the outsole is a continuous curve without a ridge like the rocker style. During walking, as the person lifts the heel, the shoe rolls forward on the curved outsole. This prevents the pressures from remaining in one region. Rocker-style shoes

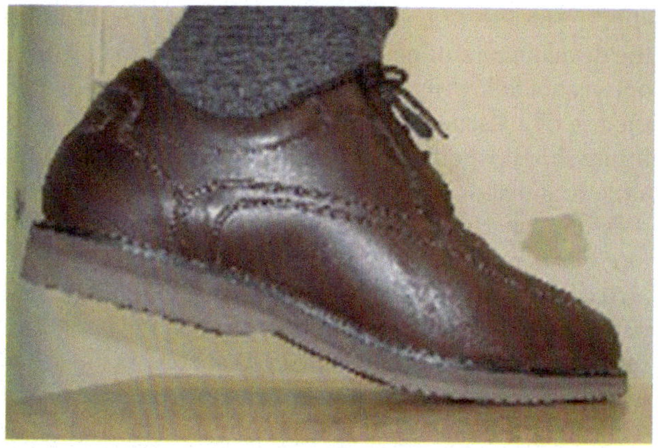

Figure 12.14 The shoe depicted in Figure 12.13, shown during walking. Note the rocking movement of the whole outsole, thus reducing the pressures applied to the forefoot.

Table 12.1 Risk classification based on a comprehensive foot examination.

Risk category	Definition	Treatment recommendations	Suggested follow-up
0	No LOPS, no PAD, no deformity	Patient education including advice on appropriate footwear	Annually (by generalist and/or specialist)
1	LOPS ± deformity	Consider prescriptive or accommodative footwear. Consider prophylactic surgery if deformity is not able to be safely accommodated in shoes. Continue patient education	Every 3–6 months (by generalist or specialist)
2	PAD ± LOPS	Consider prescriptive or accommodative footwear. Consider vascular consultation for combined follow-up	Every 2–3 months (by specialist)
3	History of ulcer or amputation	Same as category 1. Consider vascular consultation for combined follow-up if PAD present	Every 1–2 months (by specialist)

Source: Reproduced from Boulton et al. (2008).
LOPS, loss of protective sensation; PAD, peripheral arterial disease.

are more effective in reducing forefoot plantar pressures compared with roller-style shoes.

A prospective study found that shoe variables other than the recommendation for customized shoes (e.g. style, width, length or type of shoe) had no preventive effect. The use of customized shoes, however, reduced the development of new foot ulcers from 58 to 28% over one year of follow-up in a second report. In a third review, the use of a viscoelastic insole in conjunction with well-fitting shoes (whether customized, standard "comfort" or athletic shoes) was associated with a decrease in plantar pressure; whether this results in a reduced incidence of foot ulcers remains to be determined.

According to the comprehensive foot examination and risk assessment report of the Task Force of the Foot Care Interest Group of the American Diabetes Association, with endorsement by the American Association of Clinical Endocrinologists, the patient should, once he or she has been thoroughly assessed with a comprehensive physical examination, be assigned to a foot risk category (Table 12.1). These categories are designed to direct referral and subsequent therapy by the specialty clinician or team, and the frequency of follow-up by the generalist or specialist.

For patients with diabetes, foot complications are an ever-present risk. However, it is possible to design a plan for keeping the feet as healthy as possible. It is important for the patient to learn as much as possible about diabetic foot care and to take an active role in medical decisions and care. While routine medical examinations are important, everyday foot care plays the major role in stopping foot complications before they start.

12.1 Patient Cases Highlighting the Importance of Avoiding Improper Footwear

Case 12.1

A 44 year old man with Down's syndrome and type 1 diabetes since the age of 14, presented with hematomas and skin exfoliation on the tips of the first and second toes of his left foot (Figure 12.15). He had recently acquired new shoes (shiny loafers made of very hard leather), of which he was very proud, and which he wore all the time. These were found to be very tight; in fact, they were half a size smaller than his usual shoes. Due to severe sensory neuropathy, he felt no pain and allowed the lesions to develop over the space of two weeks, before his caretaker finally noticed.

Case 12.2

A 40 year old man with type 2 diabetes diagnosed two years ago, presented with ulcers on the tips of both first toes, and an ulcer on the dorsal surface of his left foot, after wearing tight sneakers for seven days in a row, during which he performed very intense manual labor. He said he noticed bullae on the tips of his toes after the first day, but did not pay any attention until he removed his shoes on the last day, and the bullae had burst, exposing the lesions shown in Figures 12.16 and 12.17. The ulceration on the foot's dorsum produced a small amount of malodorous seropurulent exudate. The patient was given instructions on local care for the ulcers, as well as a short course of antibiotics. The lesions had improved very much after 10 days.

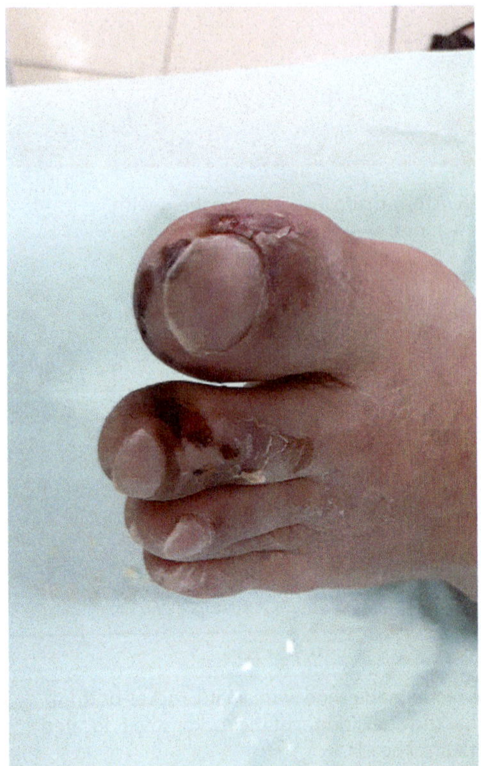

Figure 12.15 Skin exfoliation and hematomas on the toes due to the use of improperly tight shoes.

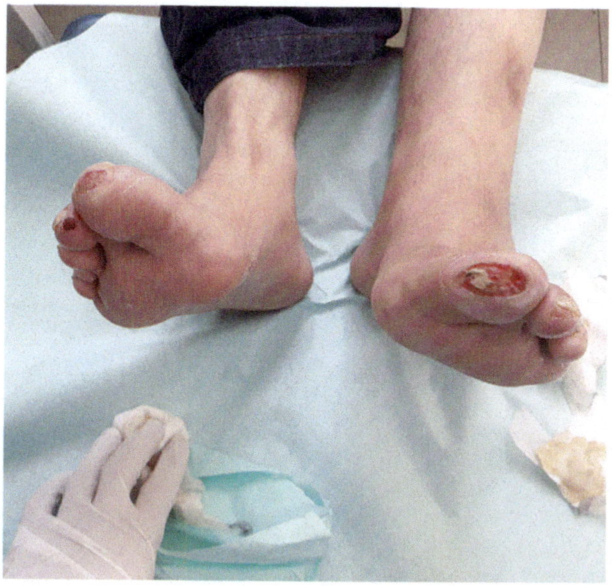

Figure 12.16 Ulcers on the tips of both first toes, as a result of constant friction inside very tight sneakers.

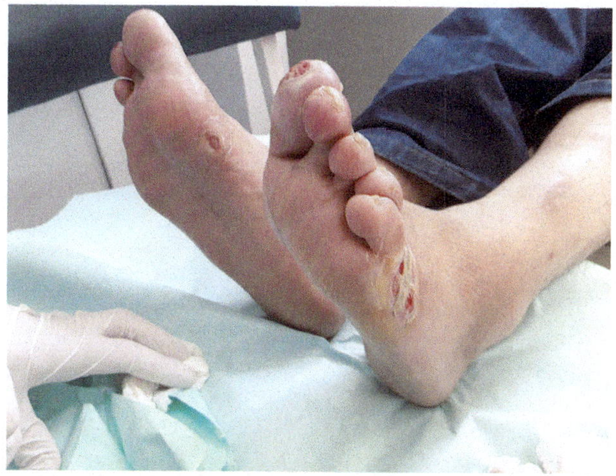

Figure 12.17 A further ulceration on the dorsal surface on the left foot of patient shown in Figure 12.16.

Reference

Boulton, A.J.M., Armstrong, D.G., Albert, S.F. et al. (2008). Comprehensive foot examination and risk assessment. A report of the Task Force of the Foot Care Interest Group of the American Diabetes Association, with endorsement by the American Association of Clinical Endocrinologists. *Diabetes Care* 31: 1679–1685.

Further Reading

Crawford, F., Inkster, M., Kleijnen, J., and Fahey, T. (2007). Predicting foot ulcers in patients with diabetes: a systematic review and meta-analysis. *QJM* 100: 65–86.

Lavery, L.A., Vela, S.A., Fleischli, J.G. et al. (1997). Reducing plantar pressure in the neuropathic foot. A comparison of footwear. *Diabetes Care.* 20: 1706–1710.

Litzelman, D.K., Marriott, D.J., and Vinicor, F. (1997). The role of footwear in the prevention of foot lesions in patients with NIDDM. Conventional wisdom or evidence-based practice? *Diabetes Care* 20: 156–162.

Tentolouris, N., Achtsidis, V., Marinou, K., and Katsilambros, N. (2008). Evaluation of the self-administered indicator plaster neuropad for the diagnosis of neuropathy in diabetes. *Diabetes Care* 31: 236–237.

Uccioli, L., Faglia, E., Monticone, G. et al. (1995). Manufactured shoes in the prevention of diabetic foot ulcers. *Diabetes Care* 18: 1376–1378.

van Netten, J.J., Price, P.E., Lavery, L.A. et al. (2016). International Working Group on the Diabetic Foot. Prevention of foot ulcers in the at-risk patient with diabetes: a systematic review. *Diabetes Metab. Res. Rev.* 32 (Suppl 1): 84–98.

13

Methods of Ulcer Healing

A. Tentolouris and N. Tentolouris

First Department of Propaedeutic Internal Medicine, National and Kapodistrian University of Athens, Medical School, Laiko General Hospital, Athens, Greece

In this chapter, we present the available methods for wound healing. Topics such as microenvironment of chronic diabetic wounds, wound preparation, the use of proper dressings and methods for off-loading the ulcer area are covered. Additionally, methods of augmenting ulcer healing, such as the topical or systemic use of growth factors, bioengineered skin substitutes, extracellular matrix proteins and regenerating agents, are discussed. Moreover, we provide information on the indications and use of negative-pressure therapy and hyperbaric oxygen.

13.1 Chronic Diabetic Wounds

A wound's exudate is rich in cytokines, platelets, white blood cells, growth factors, matrix metalloproteinases (MMPs), and other enzymes. Most of these factors facilitate healing by promoting fibroblast and keratinocyte proliferation and angiogenesis, while others, including leukocytes and toxins produced by bacteria, retard healing. Recent data described that local concentrations of growth factors such platelet-derived growth factor, vascular endothelial growth factor, epidermal and fibroblast growth factor and transforming growth factor-β are not necessarily low in patients with chronic diabetic wounds; however, in the environment of chronic wounds there is an imbalanced tuning between local neuropeptides, proinflammatory cytokines, and the down-stream proliferative response as well as fragmentation of heparan sulfate, which is a major component of the extracellular matrix in the dermis, as a result of the imbalanced production of serine proteases and matrix metalloproteinases, leading eventually to retardation in wound healing. Experimental data has shown that mast cells participate in wound healing process. Wound microbiota seems to play an important role in wound healing and may serve as prognostic biomarker. Additionally, chronic wounds exudate and biofilm has proved to degrade many of natural and synthetic substrates and derive from inflammatory cells, lytic cells, and local bacteria. Thus, diabetic chronic wounds microenvironment is hostile for local growth factors stability, chemical integrity, bioavailability, and ultimately to their physiological role as major drivers for the healing process.

In the last years many efforts have been made to find markers predictive of wound healing. Thus, patients with diabetic foot ulcers who fail to heal by 53% over a 4-week period or if the reduction in ulcers' size is less than 0.7mm per week have limited chances to achieve complete wound healing over a 12-week period. During the last decades there has been considerable research, both basic and clinical, that has resulted in the development of new treatments and requires the collaboration of a large team that includes medical doctors, nurses and other health care providers. Thus, management of chronic wounds that traditionally was part of nurses has changed, because of the availability of new treatments, mainly growth factors, bioengineered skin, and even stem cell therapy. These developments have increased the ability of the treating team to achieve complete wound healing in patients who would other fail to heal their wounds.

13.2 Wound Bed Preparation

The term "wound bed preparation" applies to facilitation of the healing process by optimizing the base and edges of the wound. Management of the infection by the

Atlas of the Diabetic Foot, Third Edition. Ioanna Eleftheriadou, Alexandros Kokkinos, Stavros Liatis, Konstantinos Makrilakis, Nicholas Tentolouris, Anastasios Tentolouris, and Panagiotis Tsapogas.

Companion website: www.wiley.com/go/tentolouris/atlas_diabetic_foot

systematic or local use of antibiotics, revascularization when indicated, debridement and reduction of edema are prerequisites for wound healing.

13.3 Debridement

Debridement should be employed to all chronic wounds to remove surface debris and necrotic tissues. Debridement can be achieved by different means, namely surgically, enzymatically, biologically and by autolysis.

13.3.1 Surgical Debridement

Surgical (sharp) debridement is rapid and effective, and can remove large volumes of hyperkeratosis and dead tissue (Figures 13.1–13.8). Wide excision of the wound has been proposed as a method of changing the biology of the chronic ulcer for that of an acute one. Care should be taken during repeated surgical debridement to protect healthy tissue, which has a red or deep pink (granulation tissue) or pink appearance at the wound borders, or isolated pink islets on the surface (epithelial tissue). Video demonstrates sharp debridement in a patient with neuropathic ulcer.

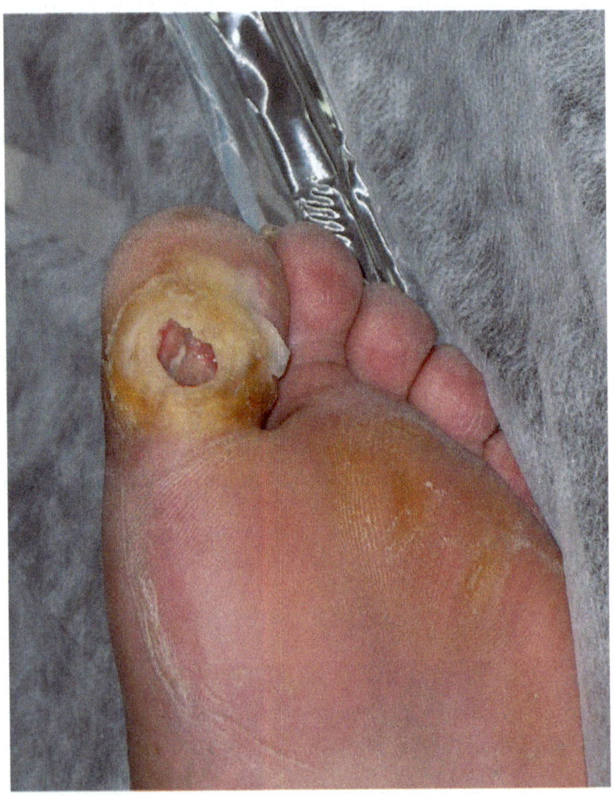

Figure 13.1 A neuropathic ulcer under the hallux before debridement.

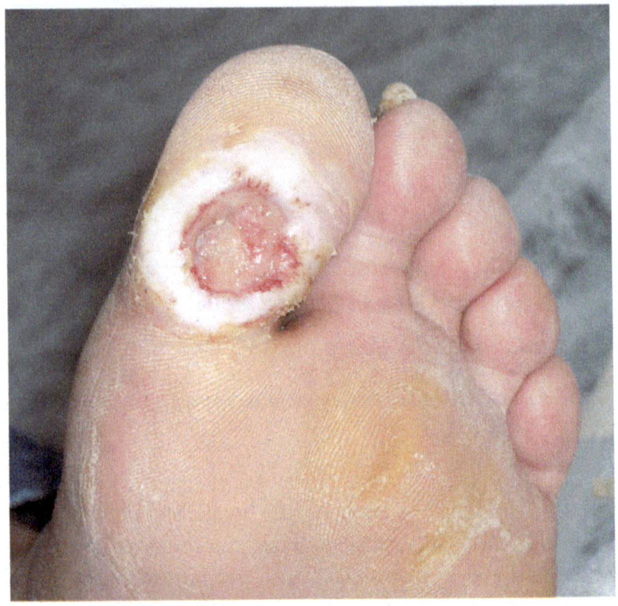

Figure 13.2 The ulcer of the patient in Figure 13.1 after sharp (surgical) debridement.

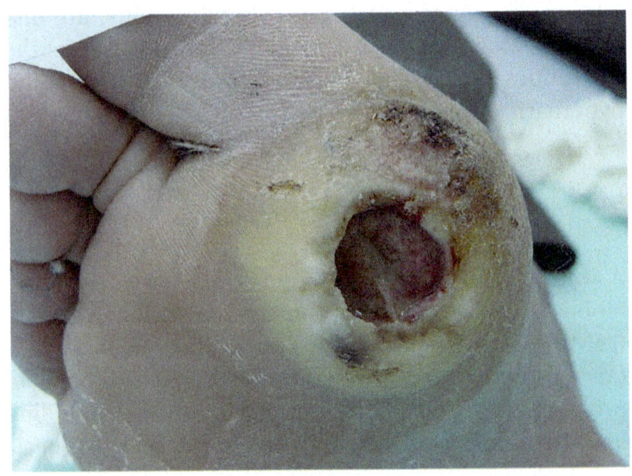

Figure 13.3 A deep neuropathic ulcer under the first metatarsal head covered by callus before debridement.

Sharp debridement can be performed using, instead of scalpels, modern technology based on ultrasound (Figures 13.9–13.11) or hydrosurgery such as Versajet (Smith & Nephew, Hull, UK). These devices are expensive and are indicated for the debridement of necrotic areas or when debridement with other methods is not possible.

13.3.2 Enzymatic Debridement

Enzymatic debridement can be achieved using of a variety of enzymatic agents including crab-derived collagenase, collagen from krill, papain, a combination of

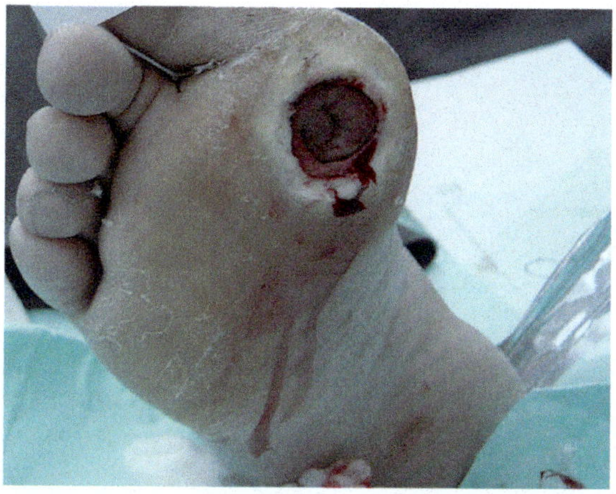

Figure 13.4 The ulcer of the patient in Figure 13.3 after surgical debridement. A hydrocolloid is indicated for dressing this ulcer after debridement.

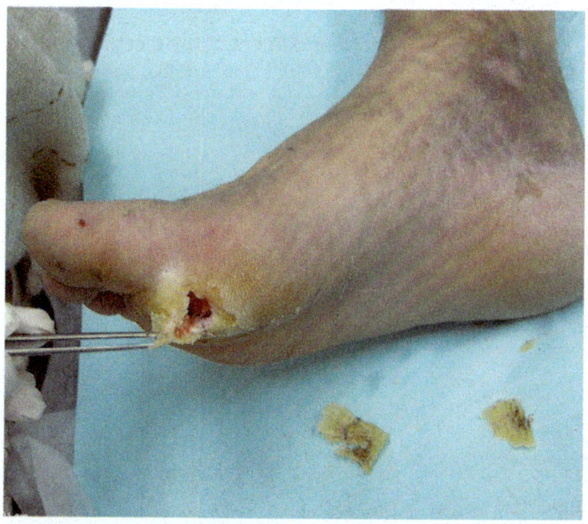

Figure 13.5 A neuropathic ulcer under the first metatarsal head covered by gross callus before debridement.

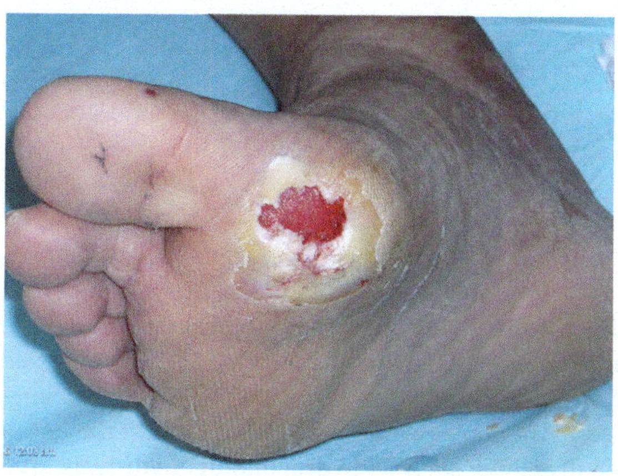

Figure 13.6 The ulcer of the patient in Figure 13.5 after surgical debridement.

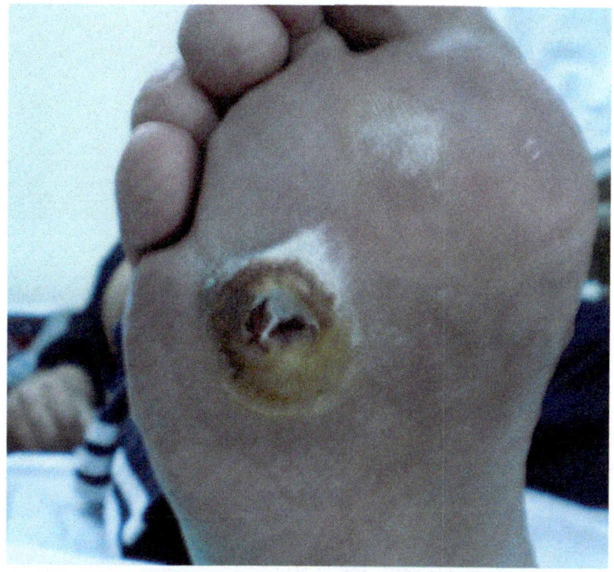

Figure 13.7 A neuropathic ulcer under the fifth metatarsal head before debridement.

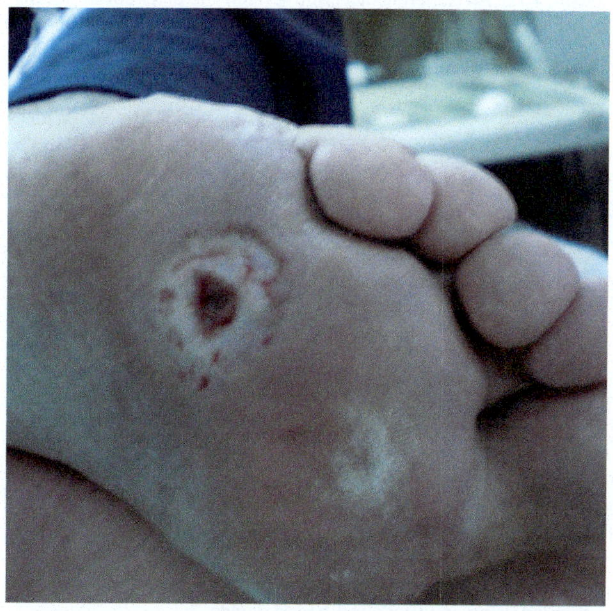

Figure 13.8 The ulcer of the patient in Figure 13.7 after surgical debridement.

streptokinase and streptodornase, and dextrans. These can remove necrotic and sloughy material without damaging healthy tissue. Enzymatic debridement is expensive and requires skill for its application. It is indicated specifically for neuro-ischemic and ischemic ulcers because surgical debridement may be extremely painful (Figures 13.12 and 13.13).

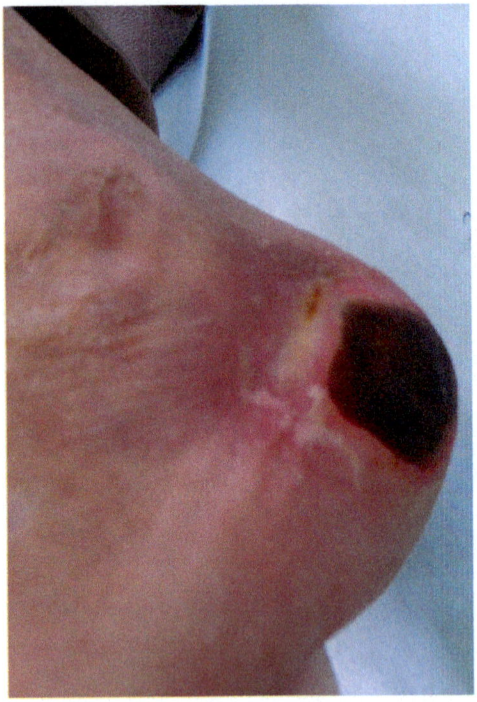

Figure 13.9 An ischemic ulcer at the heel. The ulcer could not be debrided with a scalpel because of the severe pain.

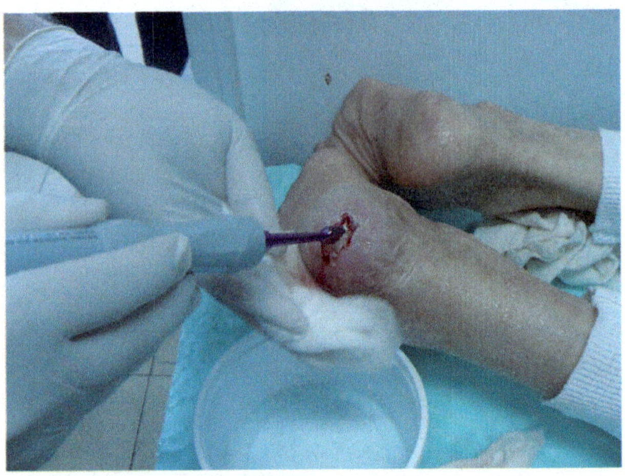

Figure 13.10 Sharp debridement of the ulcer in Figure 13.9 was achieved using an ultrasound-based device.

13.3.3 Biologic Debridement

This type of debridement has been developed in recent years using sterile maggots. Maggots, when applied to the wound, can digest surface debris, bacteria and necrotic tissues, while respecting healthy tissue. Recent reports suggest that they are particularly effective in the eradication of drug-resistant pathogens such as methicillin-resistant *Staphylococcus aureus* from wound surfaces. Larval therapy is suitable for the debridement of infected ulcers, ulcers with heavy exudate and dry gangrenous areas.

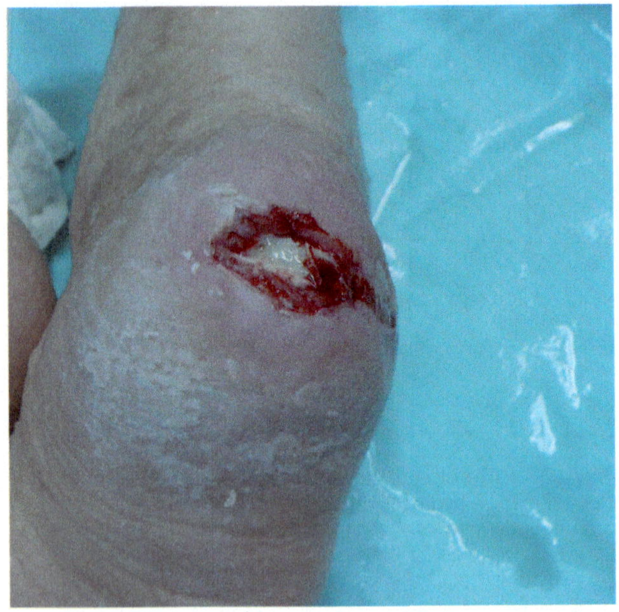

Figure 13.11 The result after debridement of the ulcer in Figure 13.9.

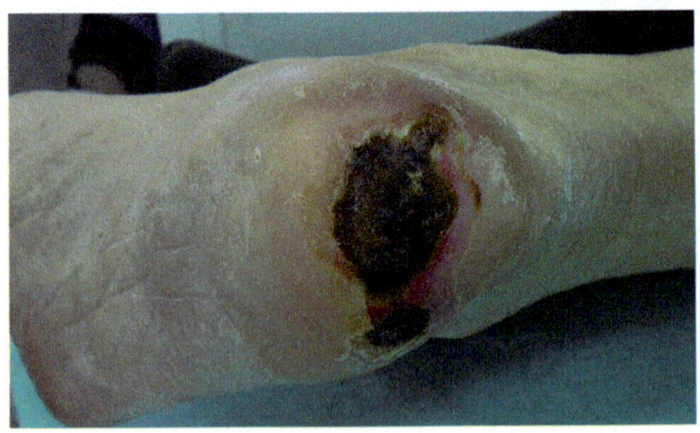

Figure 13.12 A neuro-ischemic ulcer of the heel. Enzymatic debridement is indicated for this ulcer.

13.3.4 Autolytic Debridement

This technique involves the use of dressings that permit a moist wound environment, so that host defense mechanisms (neutrophils, macrophages) will clear devitalized tissue using the body's own enzymes. Autolysis is augmented in the moist wound environment with the use of proper dressings such as hydrocolloids, hydrogels, and films. Autolysis is highly selective, with no damage to the surrounding skin.

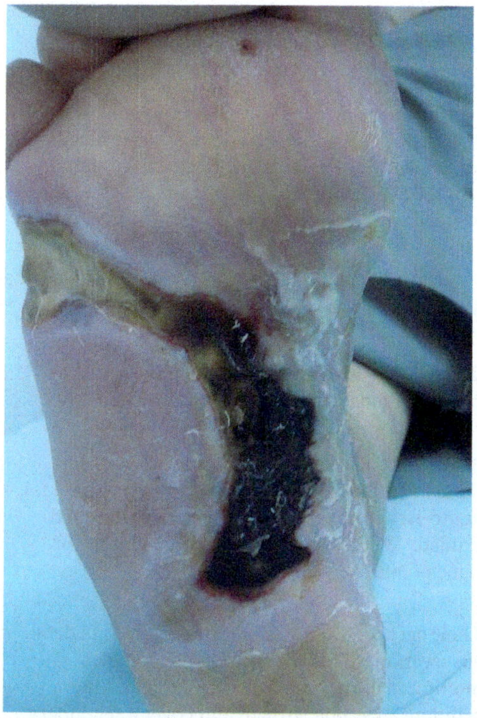

Figure 13.13 A large neuro-ischemic ulcer on the plantar area of the foot. This ulcer was painful on surgical debridement, so enzymatic debridement was used instead.

13.4 Dressings

Ulcers heal more quickly and are complicated less often by infections in the moist environment of the wound. The only exception to this rule is dry gangrene, where the necrotic area should be kept dry to avoid infection and wet gangrene.

Management of the wound environment by proper dressings, in addition to off-loading, can augment healing and prevent infections.

The characteristics for optimal wound dressings have been described as follows. Dressings should:

- be free from particulate or toxic contaminants;
- remove excess exudates and toxic components;
- maintain a moist environment at the wound–dressing interface;
- be impermeable to microorganisms, thus protecting against secondary infection;
- allow gaseous exchange;
- be easily removal without trauma;
- be transparent or changed frequently, thus allowing monitoring of the wound;
- be acceptable to the patient, be conformable and not take up too much space in the shoe;
- be cost-effective;
- be available in hospital and in the community.

A broad spectrum of materials for wound dressings is currently available. Their properties and indications are described in Table 13.1, and their advantages and disadvantages in Table 13.2. A proposal for the selection of a proper dressing according to the appearance of the wound is depicted in Table 13.3. Some types of dressing have combined properties offering a high absorbing capacity (foam or alginates) together with bactericidal activity (silver, active charcoal).

Table 13.1 Properties of and indications for available dressings.

Type of dressing	Necrotic/ gangrenous	Infection	No exudate	Low exudate	Moderate exudate	High exudate	Cavity without sinus	Cavity with sinus tract
Gauzes	+	+	+	+	+			
Dry enzymatic debriders	+							
Films			+	+				
Foams		+		+	+	+		
Hydrogels	+		+	+			+	+
Hydrocolloids				+	+		+	
Alginates		+		+	+	+	Alginate rope or gel	Alginate rope or gel
Dressings with active charcoal		+		+	+	+		
Hydrofibers		+			+	+		
Dressings with honey		+		+	+	+	+ (ointment)	+ (ointment)
Sucrose octasulfate dressing	+			+	+			
Dressings with antimicrobial properties (Sorbact)		+			+	+	+	+ (rope)

Table 13.2 Advantages and disadvantages of available types of dressing.

Type of dressing	Advantages	Disadvantages
Gauzes	Cheap and widely available. Appropriate for gangrenous lesions	Adhere to the wound bed and may cause bleeding on removal. Do not create a moist environment. Limited absorbing capacity. Provide little protection against bacterial contamination. Fibers can be incorporated into the wound tissue
Films	Semi-permeable. Allow inspection of the wound. Form a bacterial barrier. Durable. Require changing every 4–five days	Useful on flat or superficial wounds only. Some patients are allergic to the adhesive in the dressing
Foams	Appropriate for ulcers with low-to-high volumes of exudate. Provide thermal insulation. Easily conformable. May be used to fill cavities without sinus tracts	Variability of absorbency of different foams. Limited published data
Hydrogels	Effective, versatile and easy to use. Very selective, with no damage to the surrounding skin. Safe process, using the body's own defense mechanisms. Promote autolysis and healing. Decrease risk of infection. Useful in removing slough and necrosis from wounds. May be used to fill cavities with sinus tracts	Effect difficult to quantify. Not as effective and rapid as surgical debridement. Not appropriate for neuro-ischemic ulcers, which produce minimal exudate. Wound must be monitored closely for signs of infection
Hydrocolloids	Safe and selective process, using the body's own defense mechanisms. Good for necrotic lesions with low-to-moderate exudate. May be used to fill cavities without sinus tracts. Can be easily used with a shoe. Adhesive surface prevents slippage. Do not require daily dressing changes. Cost-effective	Their occlusive and opaque nature prevents daily observation of the wound. Wounds must be monitored closely for signs of infection. May promote anaerobic growth and cover a secondary infection
Alginates	Useful as absorbents of exudates. Good for infected ulcers. Some products have hemostatic properties, and some reduce bacterial load	Not appropriate for neuro-ischemic ulcers, which produce minimal exudate. Some researchers think they may traumatize the wound bed and predispose to infections. May dry out and form a plug within the wound bed. Require painstaking removal using large amounts of saline
Enzymatic debriders	Good for any wound with a large amount of necrotic debris, and for eschar formation. Promote autolysis and fast healing. Decrease maceration of the skin and risk of infection	Costly. Application must be performed carefully and only to the necrotic tissue. May require a specific secondary dressing. Irritation and discomfort may occur
Sucrose octasulfate dressing	Efficacy proven for neuro-ischemic ulcers in a large randomized-double blind, placebo controlled clinical trial	Costly. No proven efficacy in neuropathic and no indication for infected ulcers. Proper for ulcers with low-to-moderate exudate
Dressings with antimicrobial properties (Sorbact)	Bind wound bacteria rapidly and effectively. Reduce the bacterial load and support the natural wound healing process. Wide range of formats. No development of bacterial resistance. Indication for infected or heavily contaminated ulcers with a sloughy base	Costly. Limited published data
Dressings with honey	Anti-inflammatory and bactericidal properties. Reduce the formation of reactive oxygen species. Enzymatic debridement; accelerate all phases of healing. Indicated for all types of ulcer except gangrenous	Dressings proper for superficial ulcers only. For deep ulcers, ointment and additional dressing are required. Limited published data
Dressings with active charcoal	Bactericidal activity. Reduce odor. Indicated for infected/heavily contaminated ulcers	Costly. Secondary dressing may be required when the volume of exudate is large. For ulcers with little exudate, a paraffin dressing on the wound surface is recommended to prevent dryness
Microfibers	High absorption capacity. Assure a moist environment. Absorb and retain microorganisms	Costly. Limited published data

Table 13.3 Selection of dressings according to the characteristics of the ulcers.

Appearance of the wound	Type of dressing
Healthy granulous tissue	Film, hydrocolloid, foam if exudate is present
Sloughy base, exudate	Alginate, foam, microfibers, Sorbact
Sloughy base, necrosis	Hydrogels, enzymatic debriders
Sloughy base, infection	Alginates, Sorbact, dressings with active charcoal, honey, or silver. Consider dressings with active charcoal if odor is present
Dry gangrene	Keep the gangrenous area dry. Use alcohol solution or local povidone-iodine
Neuroischemic ulcers	Sucrose octasulfate dressing

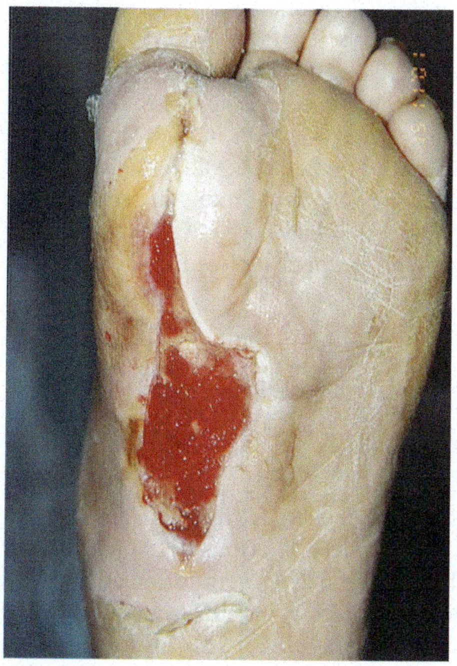

Figure 13.14 A hydrocolloid dressing is indicated for this ulcer, which has mild exudate and a surface covered by healthy granulation tissue.

In the next few paragraphs, we present cases with various types of foot ulcer, and the dressing being indicated in each case.

The patients in Figures 13.2 and 13.4 (above) and 13.14, with uncomplicated neuropathic ulcers that have mild exudate and surfaces covered by healthy granulation tissue, are best managed by the application of a hydrocolloid dressing after surgical debridement. An indication for a hydrocolloid dressing exists also for the patient in Figure 13.15 with a dry neuropathic ulcer.

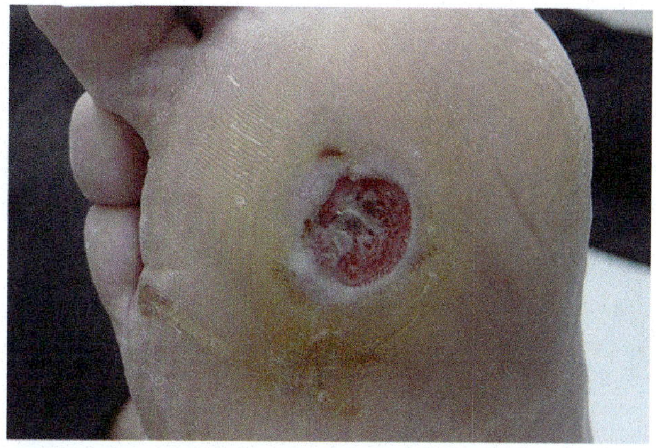

Figure 13.15 A hydrocolloid dressing can be used in this patient with a dry neuropathic ulcer.

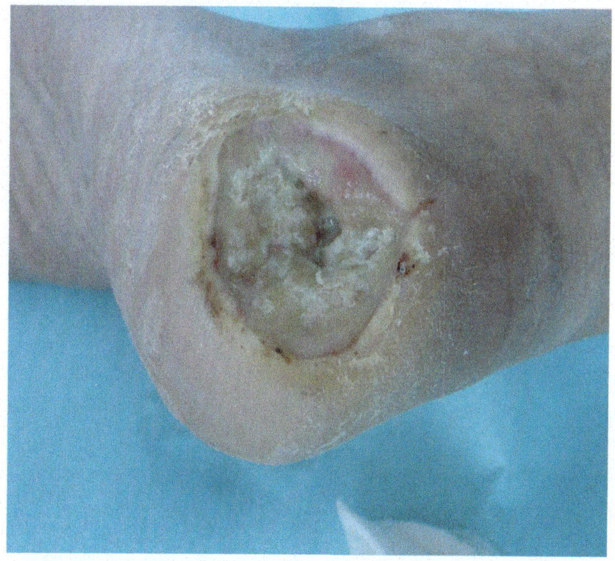

Figure 13.16 A sloughy infected ulcer of the heel. This ulcer could be dressed using an alginate, foam, microfiber or active charcoal-containing dressing or Sorbact.

The sloughy infected ulcer on the heel of the patient in Figure 13.16 should be dressed using an alginate, foam, microfiber or active charcoal-containing dressing or Sorbact®. The patient in Figure 13.17, with an infected sloughy ulcer on his great toe, which showed a large volume of exudate, is best managed by the application of an alginate or foam dressing or with Sorbact.

The patient in Figure 13.12 above with a black necrotic area at the heel is best managed by enzymatic debridement. Larval therapy is an alternative option. The ulcers of the patients in Figures 13.12 and 13.13, with necrotic areas, can be managed with larval therapy, sharp or enzymatic debridement and the application of an alginate, foam or microfiber dressing.

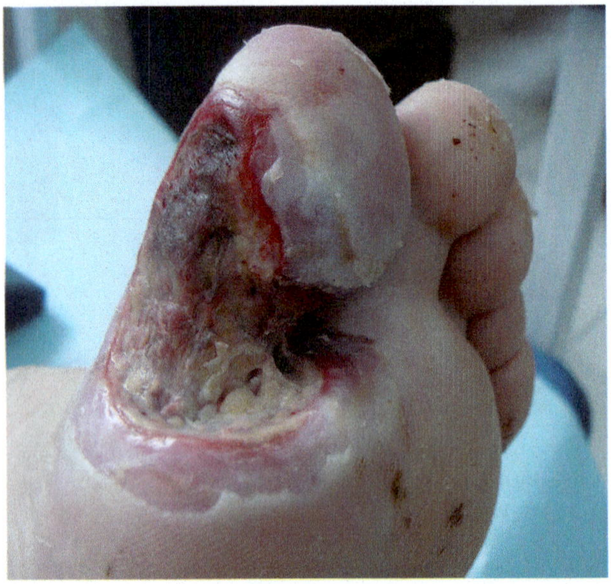

Figure 13.17 An infected sloughy ulcer of the great toe with bone exposure and a large exudate. This ulcer is best managed by the application of an alginate or foam dressing or with Sorbact.

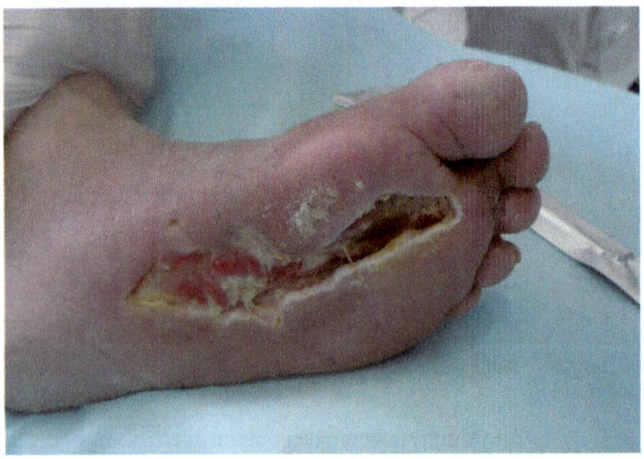

Figure 13.18 An extensive plantar infected ulcer. After debridement, this ulcer can be dressed using an alginate, foam or microfiber dressing or Sorbact.

The extensive plantar infected ulcer shown in Figure 13.18 can, after debridement, be dressed using an alginate, foam or microfiber dressing or Sorbact.

It should be remembered that the type of the dressing needs to be changed when the characteristics of the ulcer also change. For example, an alginate dressing used for a wound with a heavy exudate and sloughy base should be replaced by a hydrocolloid dressing when healthy granulation tissue covers the base of the ulcer.

The use of topical antiseptics (chlorhexidine, potassium permanganate, povidone-iodine, weak acids, and silver- as well as copper-containing preparations), alone or together with various dressings, is indicated only for infected ulcers. Alcohol and povidone-iodine solutions are indicated in dry gangrene. Hydrogen peroxide and povidone-iodine are toxic to the fibroblasts and keratinocytes, and retard healing.

Wound care products are generally expensive and add substantially to the financial burden of healthcare systems. Today, there is little scientific evidence to justify the general use of any dressing, and most of the data come from small trials and case report studies. Recently, a randomized, double-blind clinical trial (Explorer) in 43 hospitals with specialized diabetic foot clinics in four European countries (France, Spain, Italy, Germany, and the UK) was published. Eligible participants were adult inpatients or outpatients with diabetes and a non-infected neuroischaemic diabetic foot ulcer greater than $1 cm^2$ and of grade IC or IIC (as defined by the University of Texas Diabetic Wound Classification system). Participants ($n = 240$) were randomized to treatment with either a sucrose octasulfate wound dressing or a control dressing for 20 weeks. Both groups received the same standard of care throughout the trial. After 20 weeks, wound closure occurred in 48% in the sucrose octasulfate dressing group and 30% in the control dressing group (18% points difference, 95% CI 5–30, $p = 0.002$), with no difference between two groups in safety. These findings support the use of sucrose octasulfate dressing as a local treatment for neuroischaemic diabetic foot ulcers.

13.5 Off-loading

13.5.1 Total-Contact Cast

Off-loading of the ulcer area is the sine qua non for the healing of plantar ulcers. Various methods exist for off-loading. The most effective method for off-loading, which is the gold standard, is the non-removable total-contact cast (TCC; Figure 13.19). This is custom made from plaster or fast-setting fiberglass cast materials, has a relatively low cost and permits restricted activity.

Although casting is a technique prone to variation, plantar pressure measurements within TCCs have been shown to have high repeatability when the casts are applied by experienced technicians. They are indicated for the effective off-loading of the ulcers located at the forefoot or midfoot.

TCCs are contraindicated for ulcers located on the hindfoot. Severe foot ischemia (an ankle–brachial index less than 0.5 or a toe pressure below 30mmHg), a deep abscess, osteomyelitis and poor skin quality are absolute contraindications to the use of a TCC. Blindness, ataxia, obesity and fluctuating edema, usually in patients with end-stage renal disease, are relative contraindications to

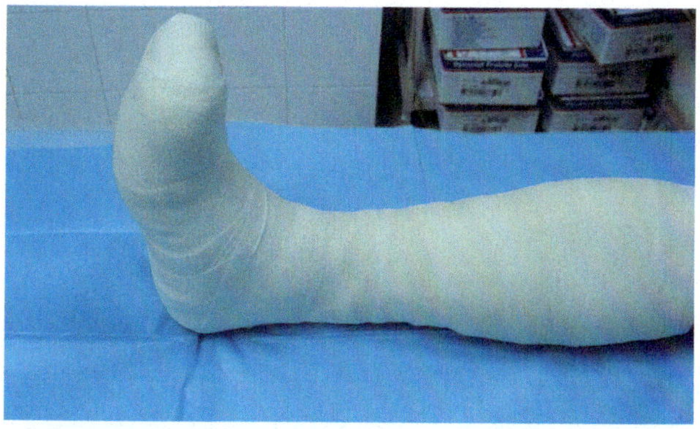

Figure 13.19 Total-contact cast.

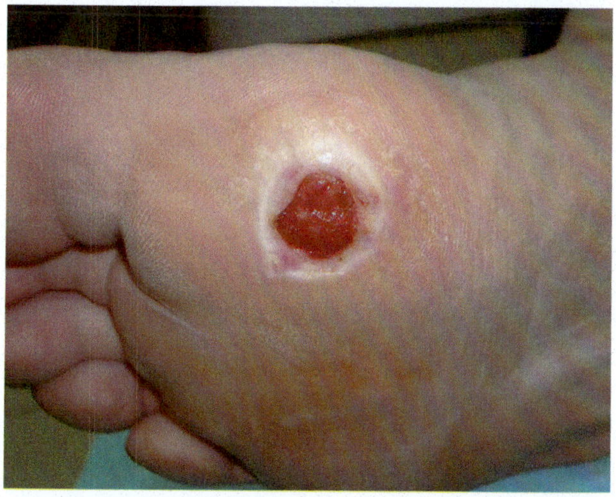

Figure 13.20 Ulcer debridement.

the use of TCCs. Infected ulcers or ulcers with a heavy exudate that need frequent changes of dressing should not be managed with a TCC unless a window is made under the ulcer area to allow inspection and regular change of the dressing.

Problems related to the use of a TCC are not uncommon, include skin abrasions, usually to the tibia or toes, and are related to a poorly fitting TCC.

Standards in the fitting of the TCC should be followed carefully. First, the ulcer should be debrided (Figure 13.20) and covered with an absorbent adhesive dressing (Figure 13.21). Toenails should be debrided, and the skin should be well hydrated using an emollient of choice. The moisture and pressure between toes should be reduced using gauze, cotton or felt (Figure 13.22).

An adherent foam is recommended for toe protection, followed by the application of a seamless stocking to the foot and leg (Figure 13.23). The stockinette should be folded over the toes dorsally and taped in place (Figure 13.24); a cut should be made on the anterior

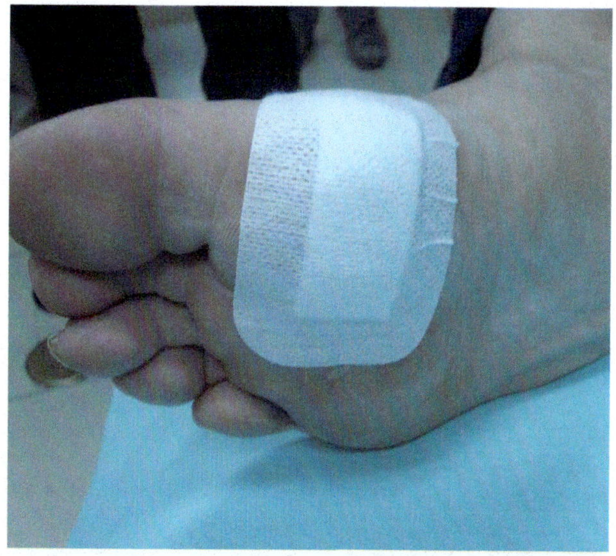

Figure 13.21 An ulcer covering using an absorbent adhesive dressing.

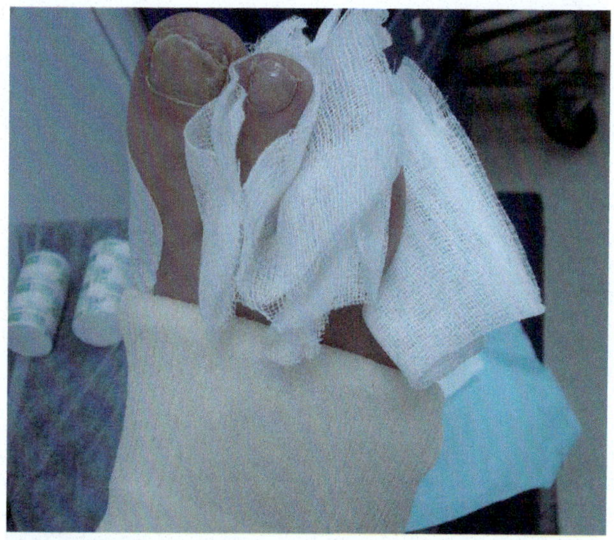

Figure 13.22 Moisture and pressure between the toes should be reduced using gauze, cotton, or felt.

aspect of the ankle (Figure 13.25) and taped in place (Figure 13.26) to reduce wrinkling.

Felt padding is then applied over bony prominences and pressure areas (Figure 13.27). The ulcer area is protected using an adherent foam (Figure 13.28), after which minimal padding consisting of an orthopedic synthetic protective material should be applied (Figure 13.29). Well-molded plaster cast material is then massaged and molded to conform to the contour of the foot and leg (Figure 13.30).

Finally, the outer layer will consist of fiberglass for strength when weight-bearing so that the patient can

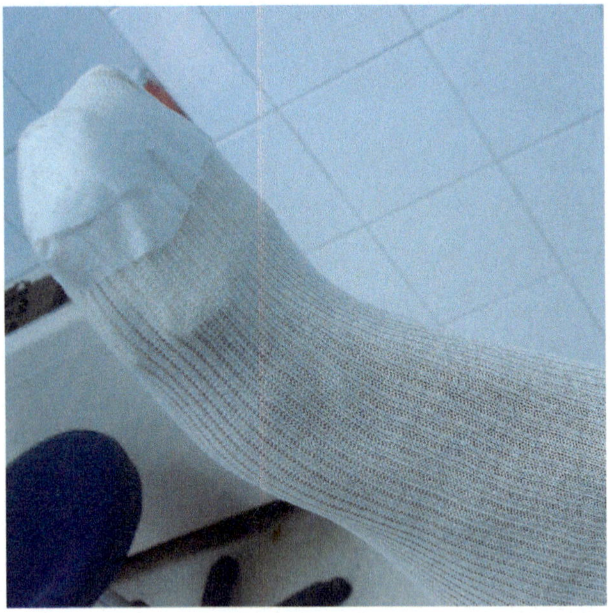

Figure 13.23 Adherent foam is placed around the toes for their protection, and a seamless stocking is applied to the feet and leg.

walk on the cast within 30 minutes (see Figure 13.19 above). A double rubber heel can be placed at the plantar aspect of the cast boot opposite the site of fore- or hind-foot ulcers or on either side of midfoot ulcers (Figure 13.31).

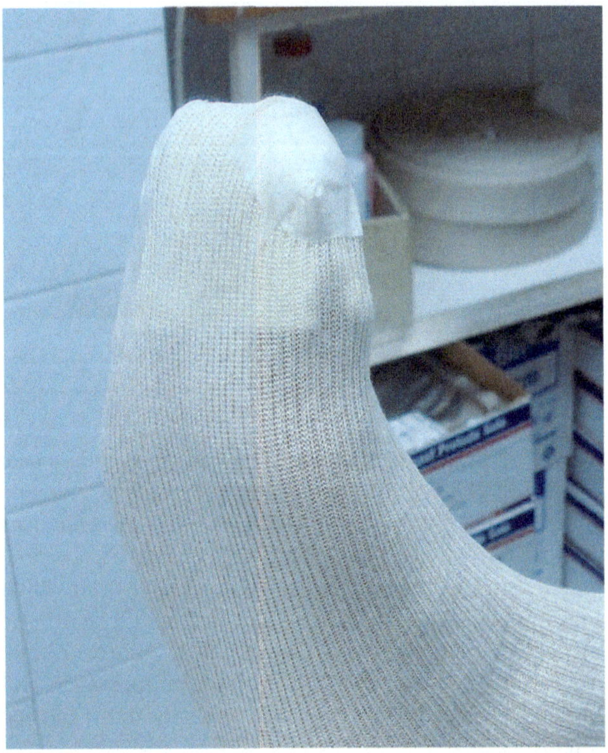

Figure 13.24 The stockinette should be fold over the toes dorsally and taped in place.

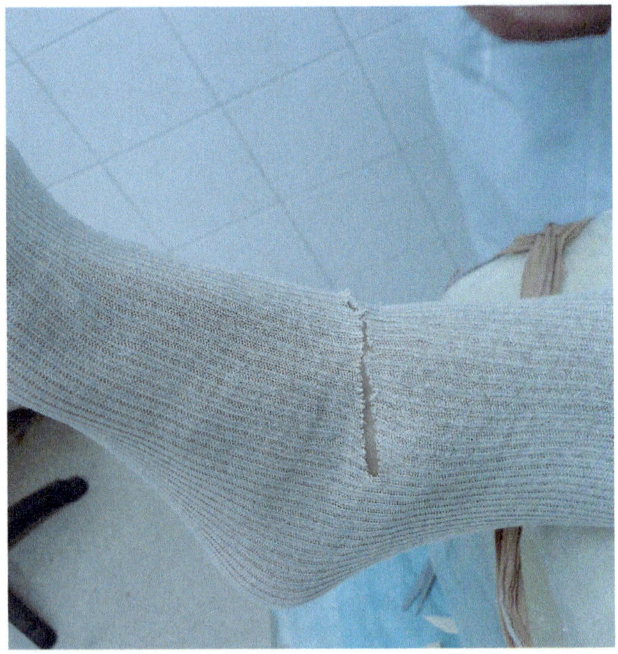

Figure 13.25 A cut on the anterior aspect of the ankle should be made in order to reduce wrinkling.

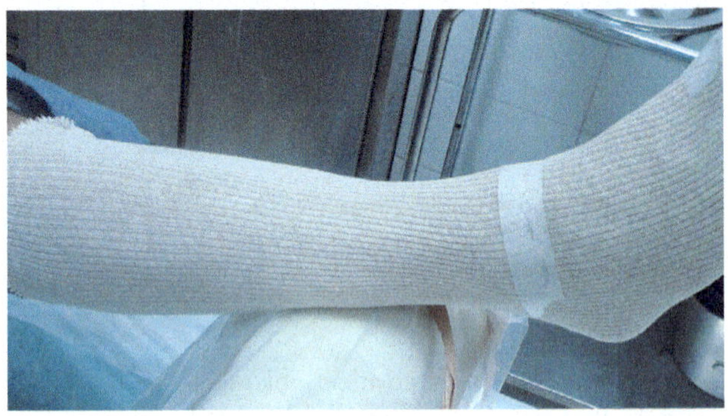

Figure 13.26 The cut is taped in place on the anterior aspect of the ankle.

TCCs allow complete rest of the foot while at the same time allowing restricted activity; they also reduce edema, and compliance with treatment is necessarily high. It is recommended that the cast be replaced after five to seven days, because a rapid reduction in edema may make the cast loose, and every two weeks thereafter.

TCCs work by redistributing the plantar pressures from the forefoot and midfoot (with reductions in peak plantar pressure of up to 80 and 30%, respectively) to the heel (increases in peak plantar pressure of up to 20%) and the calf, while up to 30% of the load is distributed to the cast.

An open-toe TCC (Figures 13.32 and 13.33) is an alternative method of casting. It is as effective as a TCC, but trauma to the top of the toes may ensue. Video 13.2 demonstrates the way a TCC is constructed (kind offer

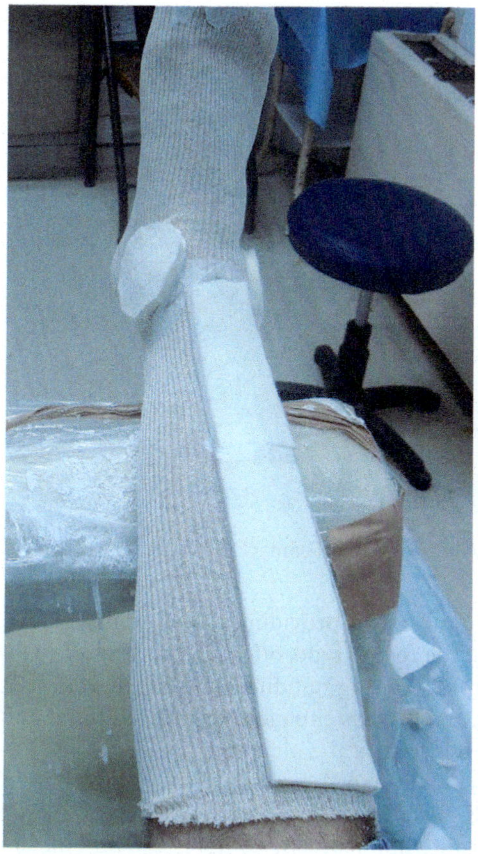

Figure 13.27 Felt padding for the protection of bony prominences.

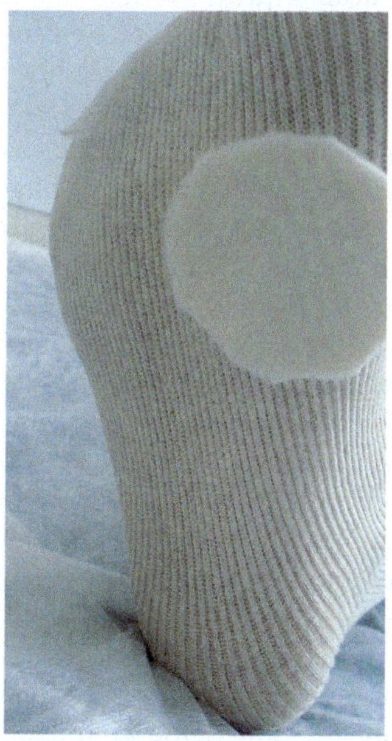

Figure 13.28 The application of adherent felt for protection of the ulcer area.

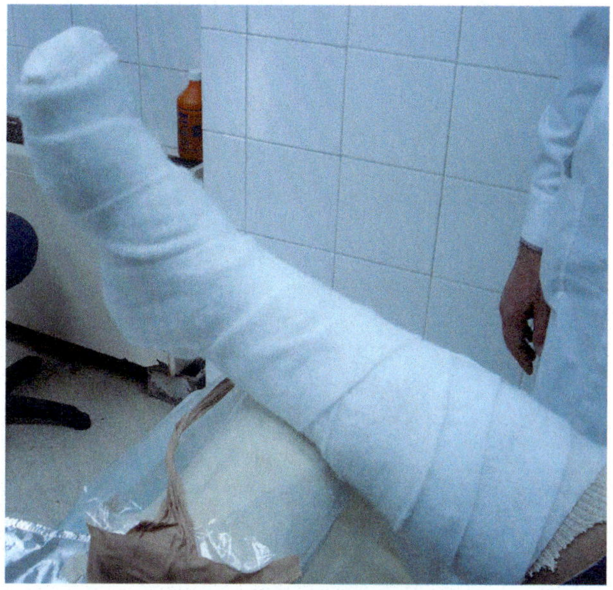

Figure 13.29 Minimal padding using orthopedic protective padding.

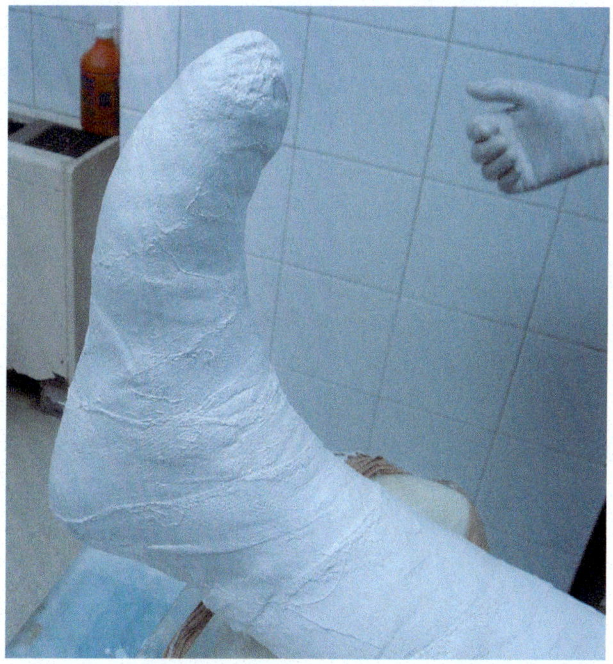

Figure 13.30 Plaster cast material to conform to the contour of the foot and ankle.

of Maureen Bates, podiatrist at the King's College Hospital, UK).

13.5.2 Removable Cast Walkers

There are many removable cast walkers (RCWs) designed specifically for individuals with diabetes. These usually have a lightweight, durable semi-rigid shell that helps

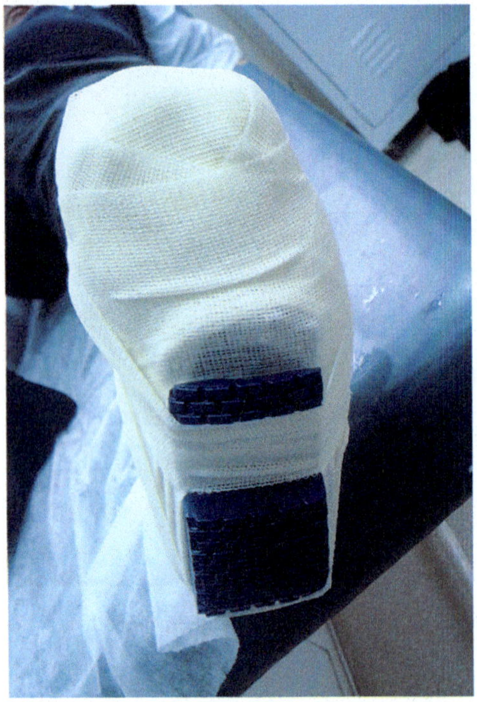

Figure 13.31 A double rubber heel can be placed on the plantar aspect of the cast opposite the site of forefoot or hindfoot ulcers, or on either side of midfoot ulcers.

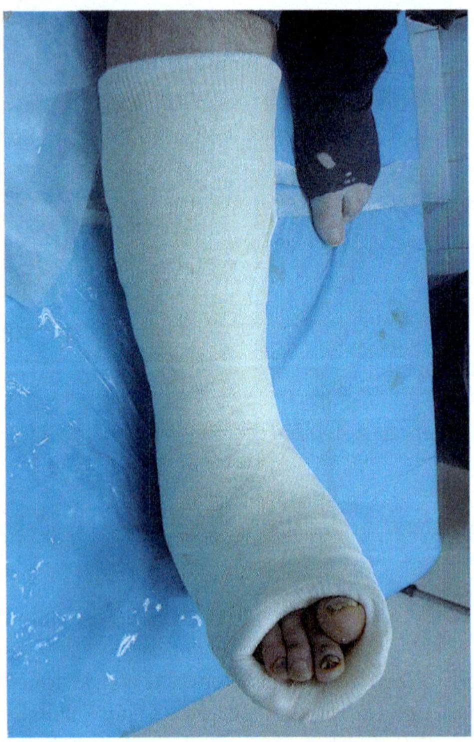

Figure 13.32 An open-toe total-contact cast.

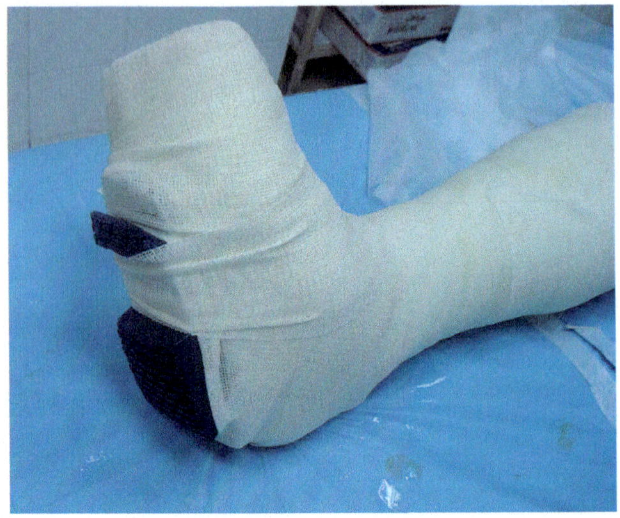

Figure 13.33 An open-toe total-contact cast.

support the limb while providing full-shell protection. The sole is of the rocker type, offering effective off-loading of the forefoot during standing and walking. The foot base is wide, and there is enough room for dressings and for windowed insoles at the ulcer area for additional off-loading of the ulcer area.

In some RCWs, overlapping air cells line the shell and provide intermittent pneumatic compression for efficient edema reduction; these can be custom-inflated using a hand bulb for a "total-contact" fit. In other RCWs, there are additional layers of foam or other soft material instead of air cells offering total contact. This adjustability allows the removable casts to accommodate changes in limb dimension throughout the healing process while maintaining stability and immobilization. Walking brace extension straps are available to increase contact and stability.

Commonly used RCWs are shown in Figures 13.34–13.36. An advantage of some walkers is that the insole is constructed of numerous independent shock-absorbing hexagons that can be removed, so various sizes, shapes and numbers of ulcers can be accommodated.

RCWs are as effective in off-loading ulcer areas as TCCs. The cost of the RCW depends on the manufacturer and currently varies between US$100 and US$300 in different countries. However, compliance with this treatment is poor, and this translates to low healing rates. An elegant study has demonstrated that patients usually underestimate their activity and removed their cast walkers or therapeutic shoes for, on average, 72% of their daily activity.

Advantages of RCWs are that no special training is required for their application, and that they can be removed for debridement and dressing of the wound, for bathing and during sleep. In addition, they can be used by patients with severe peripheral arterial disease and/or infections.

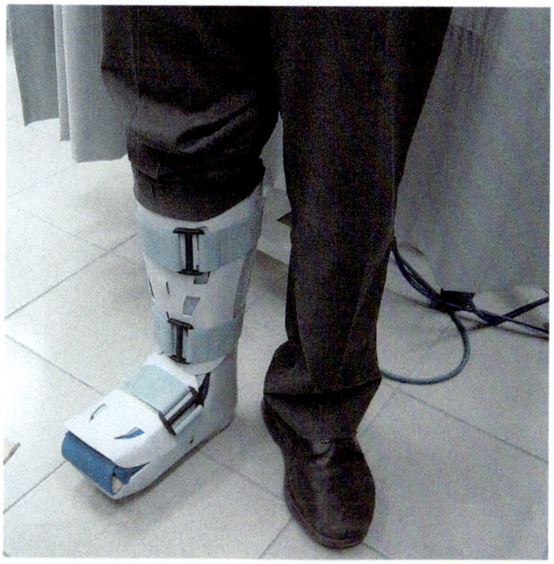

Figure 13.34 A removable cast walker – 1.

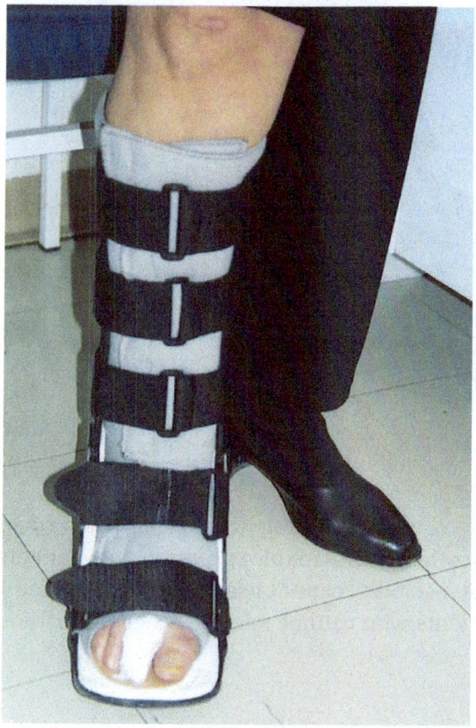

Figure 13.35 A removable cast walker – 2.

13.5.3 Instant TCC

Armstrong and Katz modified RCWs by wrapping them with a layer of cohesive tape or plaster bandage. This technique has been termed the "instant total-contact cast" (ITCC). Their aim was to take the clinical efficacy of the TCC and combine it with the ease of application of the RCW (Figure 13.37).

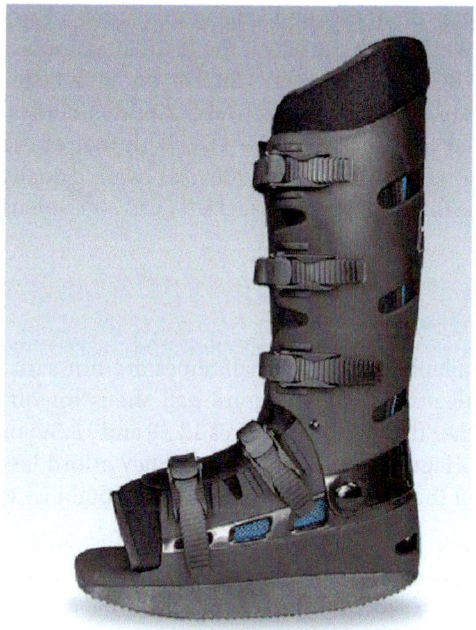

Figure 13.36 A removable cast walker – 3.

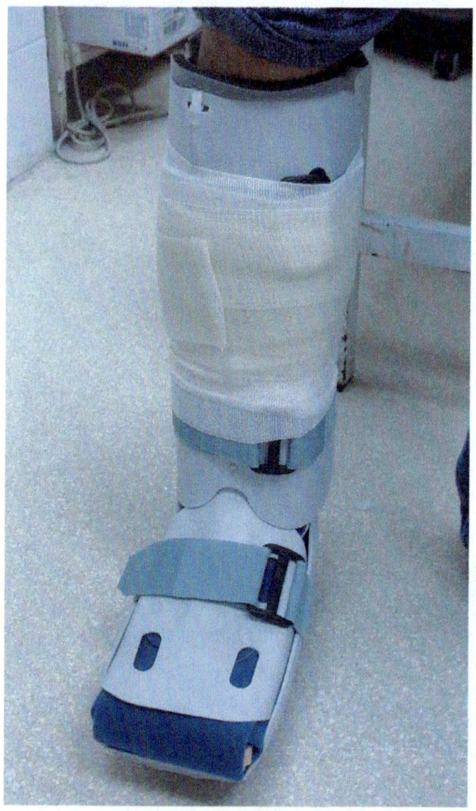

Figure 13.37 An instant total-contact cast.

Clinical data demonstrated that more foot ulcers healed at 12 weeks with the use of the ITCC in comparison with the RCW (86.4% versus 58.3%), and at a faster rate (41.6 versus 58.0 days, respectively). Another clinical trial compared the efficacy of the TCC with that of the ITCC and concluded that both devices were equally effective in healing ulcers at 12 weeks (ITCC 80% versus TCC 74%).

13.5.4 Half-shoes

Currently available off-loading half-shoes are not satisfactory for ulcer healing. There are half-shoes for off-loading of either the forefoot (Figures 13.38 and 13.39) or the hindfoot (Figures 13.40 and 13.41). They afford less pressure relief than a cast boot, and their acceptability is poor because they are difficult to walk in, they often cause pain to the contralateral extremity, and patients with postural instability cannot use them. They are indicated for patients who cannot tolerate other off-loading devices.

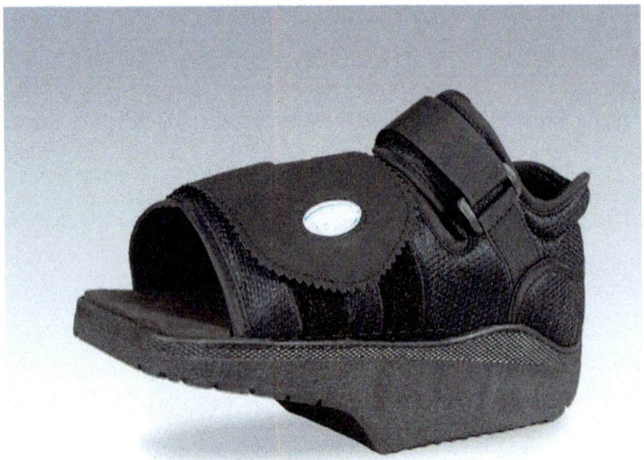

Figure 13.38 A half-shoe for off-loading the forefoot – 1.

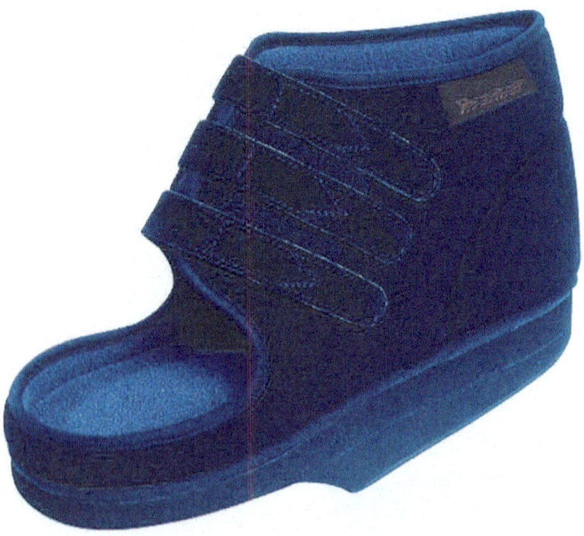

Figure 13.39 A half-shoe for off-loading the forefoot – 2.

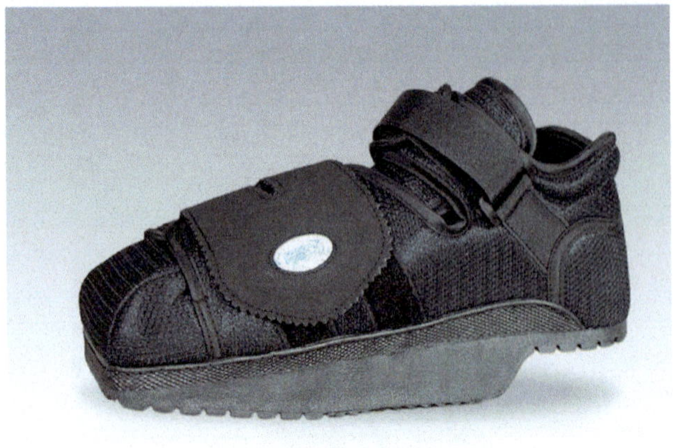

Figure 13.40 A half-shoe for off-loading the rearfoot – 1.

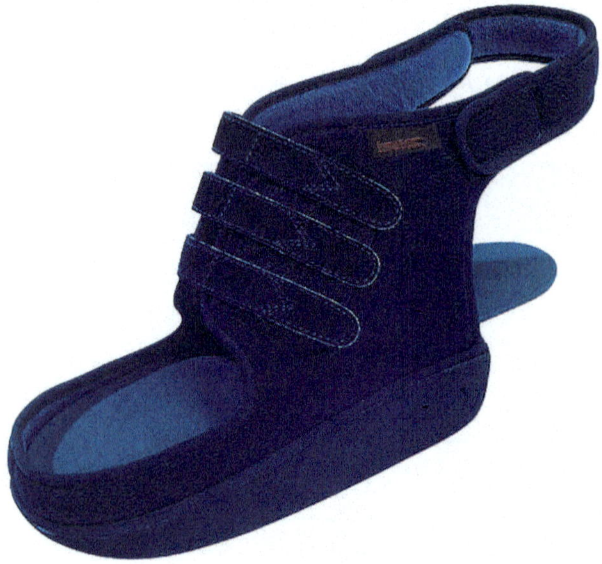

Figure 13.41 A half-shoe for off-loading the rearfoot – 2.

13.5.5 Therapeutic Shoes

Therapeutic shoes and insoles are alternative methods to off-load wounds located at the forefoot (Figure 13.42). However, they are not as effective as TCCs, ITCCs or RCWs in terms of pressure reduction. Therapeutic shoes and insoles, particularly custom-made insoles, can reduce pressure at the site of ulceration by 4–50%. They are indicated for patients who cannot tolerate other off-loading devices. Other types of shoe can be used for ulcers on the dorsal aspect of the feet (Figure 13.43).

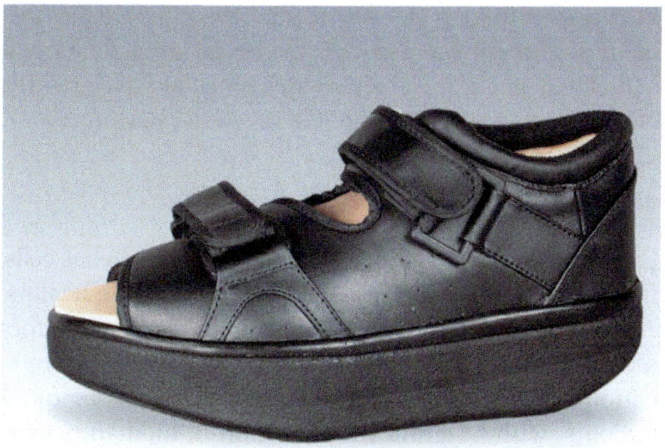

Figure 13.42 Therapeutic shoes. Note the "rocker-bottom" shape of the sole for off-loading the forefoot.

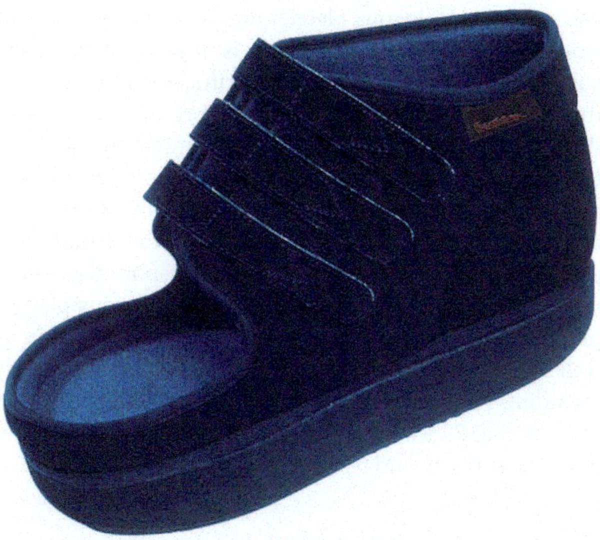

Figure 13.43 Therapeutic shoes. These are indicated to protect the dorsal aspect of the forefoot.

13.5.6 Other Methods for Off-loading

The continuous use of crutches may help in off-loading wounds located at the forefoot or midfoot. The use of a wheelchair is a very effective method for off-loading, particularly if there are large wounds or wounds of the heel and the other methods of off-loading are not indicated. Many patients with active or recurrent ulcers have had their ulcers healed completely after obligatory long-term bed rest for other medical reasons (e.g. after surgery for a hip fracture).

13.6 Growth Factors

13.6.1 Platelet-Derived Growth Factor-β

Platelet-derived growth factor-β (PDGF-β, becaplermin, Regranex; Janssen-Cilag, High Wycombe, UK) has been developed as a safe and effective topical therapy for the treatment of non-infected diabetic foot ulcers. It is applied by the patient as a gel to the ulcer surface once daily, while the ulcer is debrided on a weekly basis. A dose of 100 $\mu g\, g^{-1}$ has been demonstrated to be the most effective.

Compared with standard treatment, more ulcers treated with becaplermin healed completely and in a shorter time. The maximum time of application in the studies performed was 20 weeks. Another study failed to recruit enough patients, and no differences from the control group were found. There may be some evidence for an increased risk of death from cancers in patients who have had repeated treatments with Regranex, and the use of Regranex should be weighed against the benefit for each individual patient.

13.6.2 Platelet-Rich Plasma

Platelet-rich plasma (PRP) is an autologous product that concentrates a high number of platelets in a small volume of plasma. It mimics the last step of the coagulation cascade, leading to the formation of a fibrin clot, which consolidates and adheres to the application site in a short period of time. Absorption of the fibrin clot is achieved during wound healing within days to weeks following application. Factors secreted from platelets are serotonin, fibronectin, adenosine diphosphate, thromboxane A, platelet factor-4, PDGF-β, and platelet activating factor.

Case studies suggest clinical efficacy, but results for the complete healing process of chronic skin ulcers are inconclusive. One open-label study reported completed wound healing after seven to eight weeks of PRP application irrespectively of the wound size. In addition, there are few data about the safety of PRP. A patient with a refractory ulcer (Figure 13.44) despite off-loading with a TCC and local care was treated with PRP once weekly for four weeks; the result at that time was satisfactory (Figure 13.45).

13.6.3 Granulocyte-Colony Stimulating Factor

The effect of the subcutaneous administration of granulocyte-colony stimulating factor (GCSF) in patients with infected foot ulcers was assessed in five randomized controlled trials. The results indicated a faster resolution of

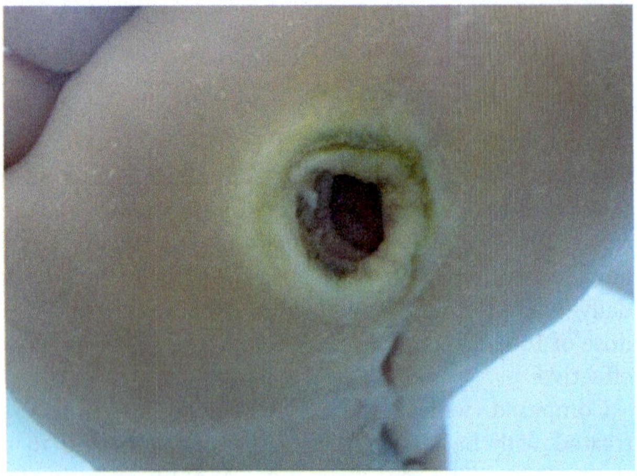

Figure 13.44 A patient with a refractory ulcer despite proper off-loading and local care.

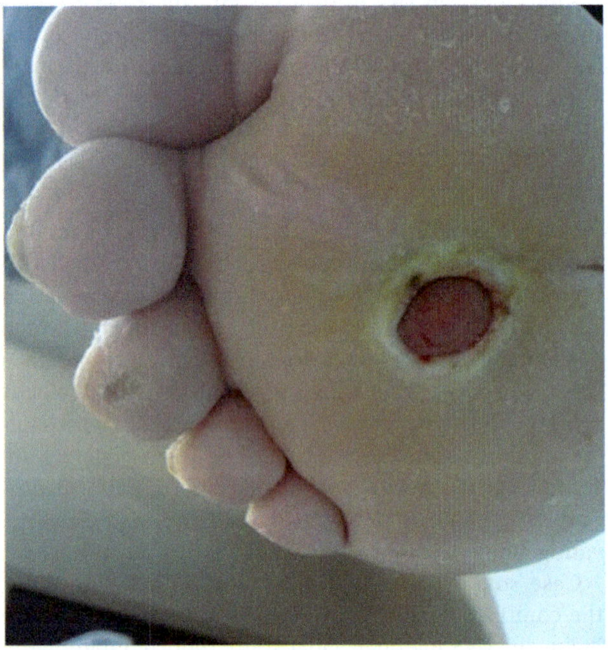

Figure 13.45 The result after four weekly applications of platelet-rich plasma.

the infection and faster healing in four of the trials. Larger controlled studies are needed to evaluate the efficacy and safety of GCSF in the treatment of infected foot ulcers.

13.6.4 Basic Fibroblast Growth Factor

Basic fibroblast growth factor (bFGF) is known to be beneficial to the formation of granulation tissue and normal healing. A randomized placebo-controlled trial of diabetic foot ulcers reported no benefit in healing rates with bFGF compared with placebo (33% versus 63%, respectively). Another study on 28 patients with chronic ulcers of diverse etiology (four with diabetes) concluded that bFGF treatment was associated with faster healing rates. More evidence from larger studies is needed to clarify the effectiveness and safety of bFGF in wound healing.

13.6.5 Epidermal Growth Factor

Epidermal growth factor (EGF) acts on epithelial cells, fibroblasts and smooth muscle cells to promote healing. A randomized trial in 61 diabetic patients with foot ulcers of moderate severity showed that the topical application of 0.04% EGF enabled healing in 20 out of 21 patients, with a significant reduction in median healing time. Recent data suggest that EGF may enhance wound healing when it is injected locally at the borders of the wound than after local application.

13.6.6 The LeukoPatch® System

The LeukoPatch® is a single-use medical device used to generate an autologous platelet and leucocyte-rich fibrin wound dressing. A LeukoPatch is produced from the patient's own venous blood by centrifugation, but without the addition of any reagents. The final product comprises a thin, circular patch composed predominantly of fibrin together with living platelets and leucocytes. The yield of platelets is close to 100% and varies minimally from patient to patient. The content and release of growth factors of this product is equal to, or higher, than other reported preparations. The product differs from other autologous platelet products by containing a high concentration of fibrin as well as both platelets and leucocytes. An open label study including 41 patients with hard-to-heal diabetic foot ulcers showed that 32% of them healed within 12 weeks of once-weekly treatment and 54% healed within 20 weeks.

13.6.7 Other Growth Factors

In a case study of the topical application of nerve growth factor (NGF) to chronic leg or foot ulcers that had failed to respond to standard treatment, healing was achieved after 5–14 weeks' treatment. This effect was ascribed to a stimulation of keratinocyte growth and new vessel formation by NGF. Accelerated cutaneous healing by means of topically administered vascular endothelial growth factor has been described in mice.

13.7 Bioengineered Skin Substitutes

Tissue-engineered skin substitutes are classified into allogenic cell-containing (Apligraf, Dermagraft, OrCel), autologous cell-containing (Hyalograft 3D, Laserskin Autograf,

TranCell) and acellular (OASIS, GRAFTJACKET) matrices. The former contains living cells such as keratinocytes or fibroblasts within a matrix, whereas the latter are free from cells and act by releasing growth factors to stimulate neovascularization and wound healing. Both represent promising therapeutic adjuncts in the management of foot ulceration. All products are indicated for ulcers free of infection.

13.7.1 Graftskin (Apligraf)

Graftskin (Apligraf; Organogenesis Inc., MA, USA) consists of an epidermal layer formed by human keratinocytes, and a dermal layer composed of human fibroblasts derived from neonatal foreskin in a bovine collagen matrix. Its efficacy has been assessed in a large randomized controlled trial. Treatment with Apligraf resulted in higher rates of complete healing of diabetic foot ulcers and shorter healing times (56% of the ulcers healing in 65 days) compared with placebo (39% of the ulcers healing in 90 days). The application of Apligraf was safe and, in addition, was followed by lower incidence of osteomyelitis and a lower amputation rate.

13.7.2 Dermagraft

Dermagraft (Smith & Nephew UK Limited, London, UK) is manufactured by obtaining human fibroblast cells from neonatal foreskin and cultivating them on a three-dimensional polyglactin scaffold; they are designed to replace the patient's own destroyed dermis. Dermagraft is stored at −70 °C, and needs to be thawed, rinsed and cut to the size of the ulcer prior to implantation. It is applied on the ulcer area on a weekly basis.

The efficacy of Dermagraft in improving wound closure was tested in two randomized placebo-controlled studies which showed that healing rates were higher than with the standard treatment. In France, the average cost per healed ulcer was lower with Dermagraft compared with standard treatment only. Nevertheless, this cost-effectiveness analysis needs to be repeated in other countries.

13.7.3 OrCel

OrCel (Ortec International, New York, USA) is a two-layered cellular matrix that contains allogenic fibroblasts and keratinocytes harvested from human neonatal skin. A randomized placebo-controlled trial of long-standing neuropathic ulcers has shown faster wound healing with OrCel in comparison with the standard treatment.

13.7.4 Hyalograft 3D and Laserskin Autograft

Grafts formed from autologous fibroblasts and keratinocytes have been developed (Fidia Advanced Biopolymers, Abano Terme, Italy). Autologous fibroblasts and keratinocytes are cultivated and grown on a scaffold made from the benzyl ester of hyaluronic acid (Hyalograft 3D and Laserskin Autograft, respectively).

Hyalograft 3D and Laserskin Autograft have been evaluated in one randomized controlled trial of diabetic foot ulcers. The healing time was shorter, and the product was more effective in healing ulcers located on the dorsal aspect of the feet. No treatment-related side-effects were observed.

A patient successfully treated first with Hyalograft 3D and one week later with Laserskin Autograft is shown in Figures 13.46–13.50. Another patient (Figures 9.18–9.22 and Figures 13.51 and 13.52) with a difficult to heal ulcer on the heel was treated successfully with Hyalograft 3D and Laserskin Autograft.

13.7.5 TranCell

TranCell (CellTran Limited, Sheffield, UK) represents a novel carrier surface for the delivery of autologous keratinocytes aiming to promote wound healing in patients with chronic neuropathic foot ulcers. A small

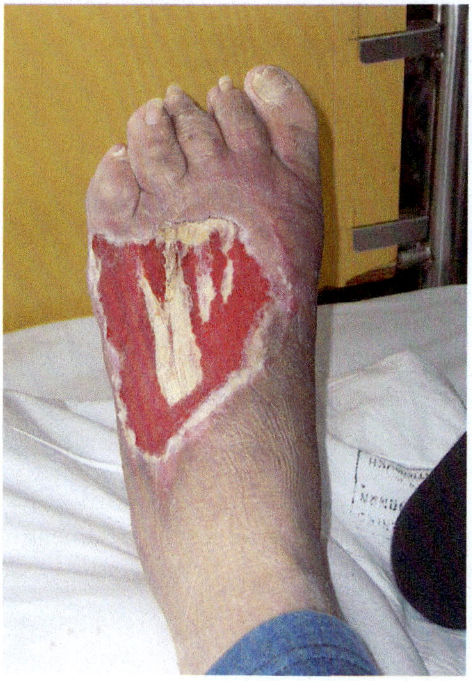

Figure 13.46 A patient newly diagnosed with type 2 diabetes with an extensive skin deficit caused by a severe foot infection. The patient was treated with the systemic use of antibiotics and vacuum-assisted closure. At this stage, Hyalograft 3D was applied.

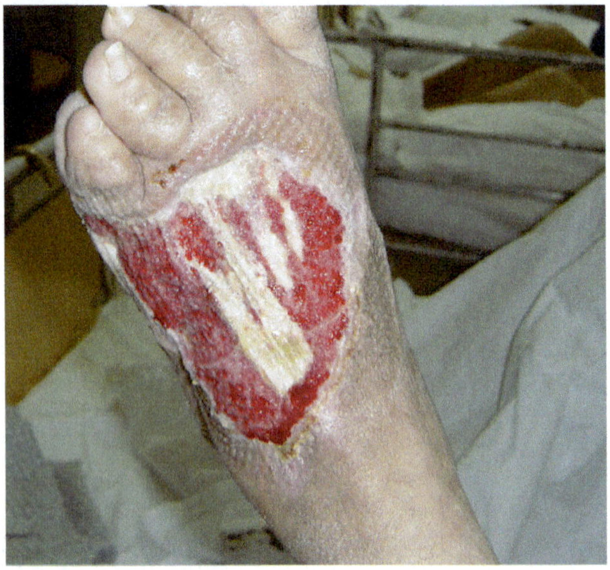

Figure 13.47 The results in the patient from Figure 13.46, one week after Hyalograft 3D application.

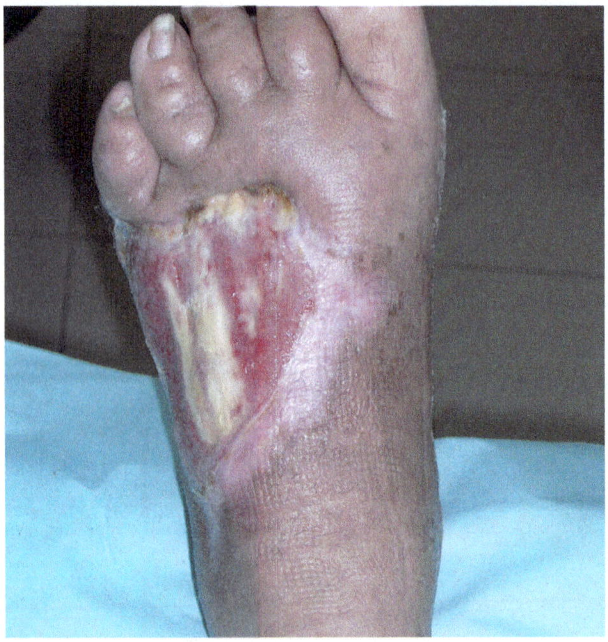

Figure 13.48 The Laserskin Autograft was next applied to the patient in Figure 13.46.

trial has shown that it is effective for the treatment of refractory neuropathic ulcers.

13.7.6 OASIS

OASIS (Healthpoint Ltd., TX, USA) is derived from porcine small intestine submucosa. It consists of a three-dimensional natural collagenous matrix, free from cells that might induce a rejection reaction. OASIS has shown

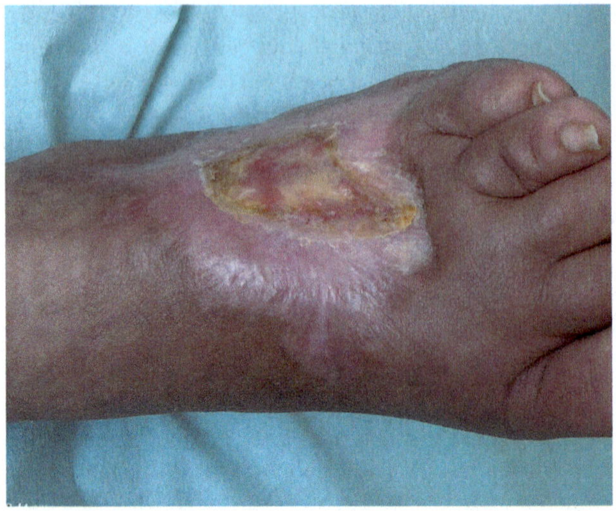

Figure 13.49 Excellent results for the patient in Figure 13.46 after treatment with Hyalograft 3D and Laserskin Autograft.

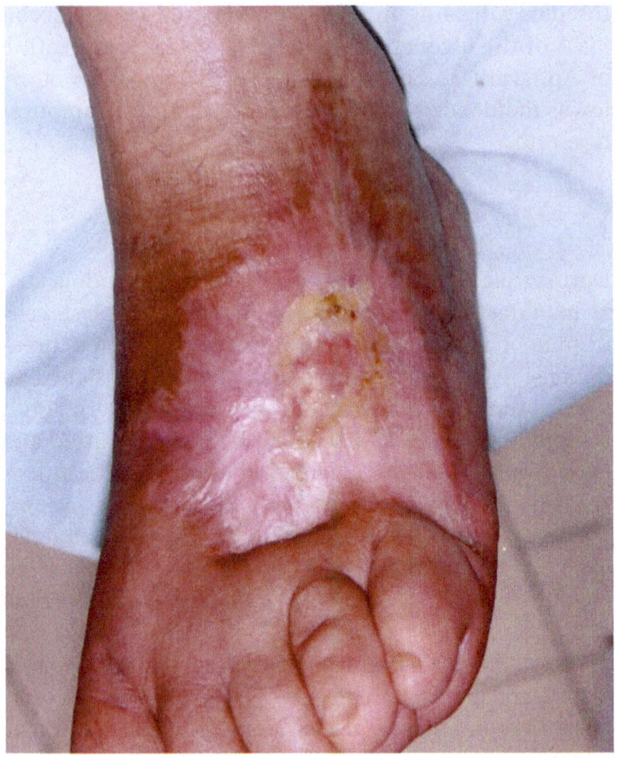

Figure 13.50 The patient in Figure 13.49, two months later: the ulcer has almost completely healed.

similar efficacy to Regranex gel in a randomized placebo-controlled trial.

13.7.7 GRAFTJACKET

GRAFTJACKET (Wright Medical Technologies, Arlington, TN, USA) is an allogeneic acellular matrix derived from donated human skin. To avoid an immune

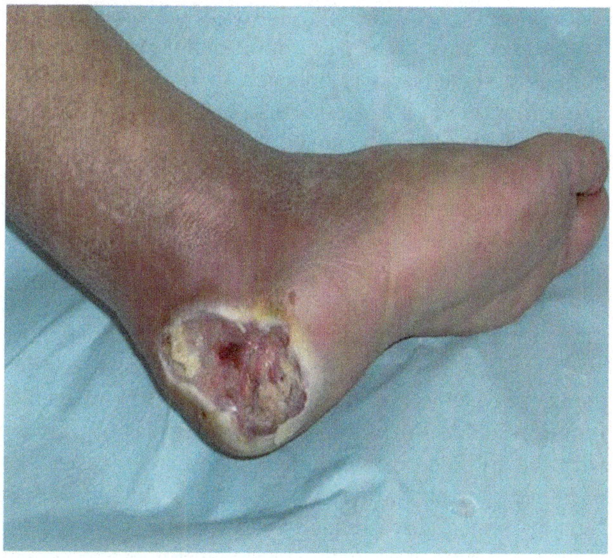

Figure 13.51 A non-healing ulcer of the heel.

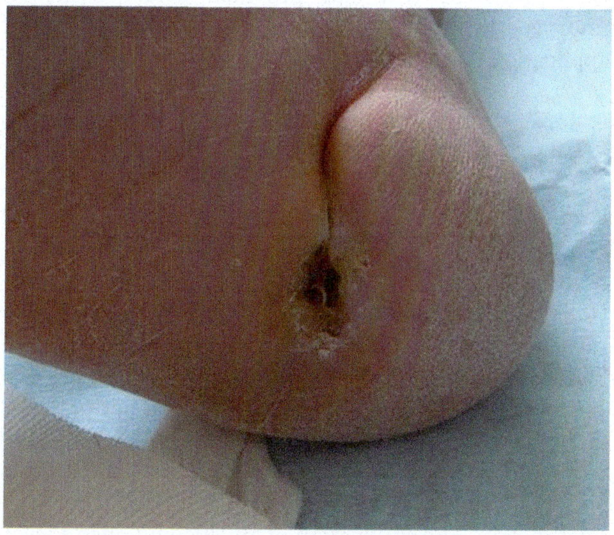

Figure 13.52 The result two months after the application of Hyalograft 3D and Laserskin Autograft (see Figure 13.51).

response, the epidermal and dermal cells are removed. It has been evaluated in two small trials and has shown superior efficacy to standard treatment in patients with foot ulcers.

13.7.8 AlloDerm

AlloDerm (LifeCell, Branchburg, NJ, USA) is an acellular dermal matrix derived from donated human skin tissue. It has been used extensively in the surgery, but there is limited experience in the treatment of diabetic foot ulcers. We have used AlloDerm successfully in a patient with a refractory ulcer of the heel (Figures 13.53–13.55).

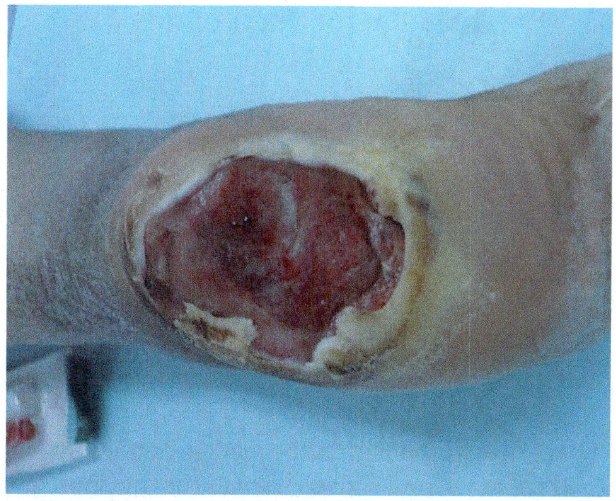

Figure 13.53 A patient with renal failure on hemodialysis developed this ulcer after rupture of a bulla. The ulcer was refractory to standard treatment.

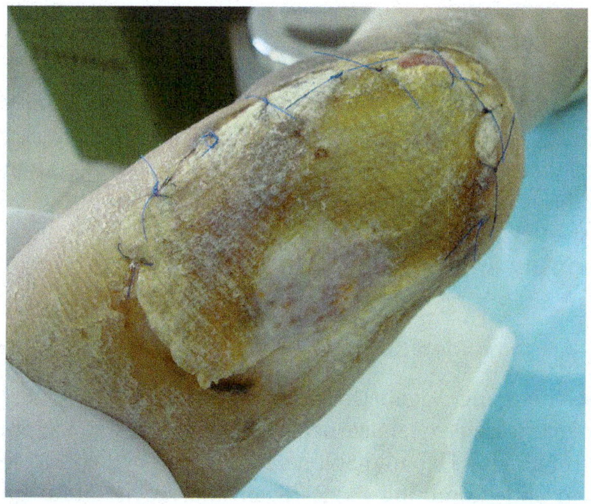

Figure 13.54 The ulcer in Figure 13.53 was covered with AlloDerm.

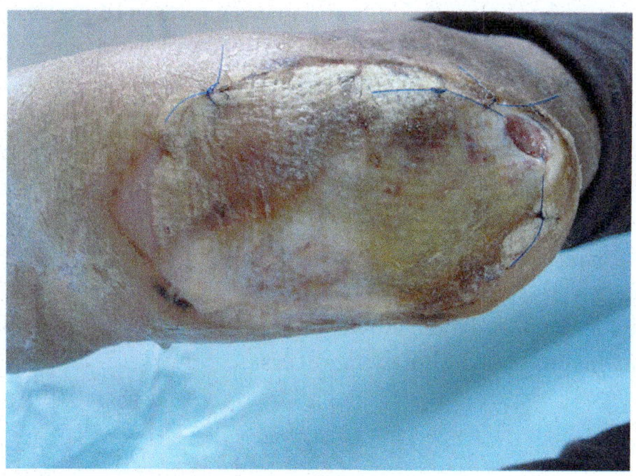

Figure 13.55 One month later, the result for the ulcer in Figure 13.54 was satisfactory.

13.8 Extracellular matrix proteins

13.8.1 Hyaff

Hyaff (Convatec, Bristol-Myers Squibb, New York, USA) is a semi-synthetic ester of hyaluronic acid. As an essential component of the wound matrix, hyaluronic acid facilitates the growth and movement of fibroblasts and controls hydration. So far, it has been used in the treatment of neuropathic ulcers with promising results.

13.8.2 Collagen

There are many products on the market containing lyophilized collagen from various sources (bovine, porcine) alone or in combination with alginates, cellulose or antibiotics. Collagen seems to induce the production of endogenous collagen and to promote platelet adhesion and aggregation; is also acts as a chemotactic factor for macrophages.

Promogran (Johnson & Johnson, Langhorne, PA, USA) consists of collagen and oxidized regenerated cellulose. A large randomized controlled trial has shown a similar efficacy of Promogran and moistened gauze for diabetic foot ulcers, and a higher efficacy for ulcers of less than six months' duration. Promogran has been shown to be cost-effective across four European countries (France, Germany, Switzerland, UK).

13.8.3 Regenerating Agends

ReGeneraTing Agents (RGTAs) are a family of polymers bioengineered to stabilize heparin-binding growth factors by mimicking Heparan Sulphate (HS) thereby protecting them and promoting tissue repair and regeneration. In inflammation, destruction of HS exposes the ExtraCellular Matrix – ECM (structural and cellular proteins within) to the actions of proteases and glycanases which break them down and act on cytokines and growth factors to prevent adequate repair. In injured tissue, RGTAs would replace destroyed HS by binding to the structural proteins and reconstruct the ECM scaffold. Growth factors will also bind to RGTA and resume position and organization resembling that of non-injured tissue. Experimental data have shown that RGTAs induce a regeneration process by restoring -the proper cellular micro-environment. More recently a RGTA named CACIPLIQ20® was adapted to skin lesions and has shown efficacy in various trials of non-healing leg and diabetic ulcers.

13.8.4 MMP Modulators

MMPs have an active role in the regulation of extracellular matrix components. During normal wound healing, there is a balance between the "construction" and "destruction" of extracellular matrix. In chronic wounds, a high expression of MMP-2 in fibroblasts and endothelium is detected and is believed to favor destruction. Experimental data suggest that a downregulation of MMP-2 expression may augment the healing process.

DerMax (Dermagenics Inc, Memphis, TN, USA) is a dressing containing metal ions and citric acid. The topical application of DerMax is associated with a lower expression of MMP-2 by fibroblasts and endothelial cells. In addition, metal ions inhibit the production of reactive oxygen species by polymorphonuclear cells, whereas citric acid acts as a scavenger of superoxide anions. A product containing DerMax with honey (MelMax; Dermagenics Inc) is available and combines the properties of DerMax with the antimicrobial and anti-inflammatory properties of honey. Currently, there are no data on the efficacy of DerMax or MelMax from large-scale trials.

The antibiotic doxycycline has been shown to have relevant inhibitory properties, mitigating inflammation in a variety of tissues. In the diabetic foot, a randomized placebo-controlled trial has provided evidence for an improved healing of diabetic foot ulcers by the topical application of doxycycline gel.

13.9 Other Agents

Lamin gel (ProCyte Corporation, Redmond, WA, USA) is a granulating agent containing a glycyl-L-histidyl-L-lysine–copper complex. A randomized placebo-controlled clinical study showed very high efficacy and lower rates of infection with the lamin gel in patients with diabetic foot ulcers.

Amelogenin (Xelma; Mölnlycke Health Care, Göteborg, Sweden) contains amelogenin protein, and manufacturers support the finding that amelogenin applied to the wound bed acts as a temporary extracellular matrix. The application of amelogenin once a week restores damaged extracellular matrix, providing adhesion sites for cells and thus promoting wound healing. Currently, no clinical data on the efficacy of Xelma for diabetic foot ulcers are available.

13.9.1 Stem Cell Therapy

There is great interest in delivery of stem or progenitor cells, either applied topically or recruited from the circulation. Some preliminary work suggests that topically applied autologous bone-marrow cultured cells can heal human chronic wounds that are recalcitrant to other treatments, including growth factors and bioengineered skin. Transplantation of stem cells derived from bone marrow, peripheral blood, umbilical cord blood, or adipose tissue have been examined in various studies. One meta-analysis reported that stem cell transplantation was favorable for wound ulcers healing irrespective of the ulcer size. Limitations of this meta-analysis is that stem cell sources, the number of delivered cells, and the routes of cell administration differed among the studies. Moreover, there are safety concerns and more research is necessary in this field.

13.9.2 Alternative Treatments

A recent multicenter open-label study found that the use of a BioPhotonic gel for two weeks resulted in healing of 52% of ulcers of various etiology including diabetic foot ulcers. The fluorescence technology of the BioPhotonic gel is based on the ability of special light-capturing molecules (chromophores) to convert light emissions from a multi-light emitting diode (LED) lamp into a different photons emission spectrum with broader and longer range of wavelengths with lower energy (fluorescence). Because of this technology, when skin is exposed to fluorescence it induces modulation of biological processes (PBM). The beneficial effects of PBM on wound healing might be attributed to anti-inflammatory signaling, cell proliferation, protein synthesis, and decreased bacterial infection.

13.9.3 Negative-Pressure Wound Therapy

Negative-pressure wound therapy (NPWT) has emerged as a new treatment for diabetic foot ulcers. This therapy involves the use of intermittent or continuous subatmospheric pressure through a special pump (vacuum-assisted closure; e.g. V.A.C. [Kinetic Concepts Inc., San Antonio, TX, USA], other such devices also being on the market) connected to a resilient open-celled foam surface dressing covered with an adhesive drape to maintain a closed environment. The pump is connected to a canister to collect wound discharge and exudate. The optimal subatmospheric pressure for wound healing appears to be approximately 125 mmHg, utilizing an alternative pressure cycle of five minutes of suction followed by two minutes off suction.

Experimental data suggest that NPWT optimizes blood flow, decreases tissue edema and removes exudate, proinflammatory cytokines and bacteria from the wound area. These physiologic changes promote the development of a moist wound environment, and may increase the rate of cell division and the formation of granulation tissue.

NPWT should be delivered after debridement and should be continued until there is the formation of healthy granulation tissue at the surface of the ulcer. Two randomized controlled trials have demonstrated that the rate of ulcer healing and the time to granulation tissue formation were in favor of V.A.C. Moreover, treatment with V.A.C. resulted in lower amputation rates in comparison to the standard therapy. NPWT is well tolerated, and the device can be portable.

This therapy is contraindicated for patients with an active bleeding ulcer. Care should also be taken in patients on anticoagulant therapy as there is a risk for bleeding. Currently, NPWT is indicated for complex diabetic foot wounds.

In Figures 13.56–13.61, we present a patient with an extensive ulcer on the dorsal aspect of the foot with gross odor and exudate caused by a severe foot infection. The plastic and orthopedic surgeons suggested a below-knee amputation. However, this patient was successfully treated with an intravenous administration of antibiotics

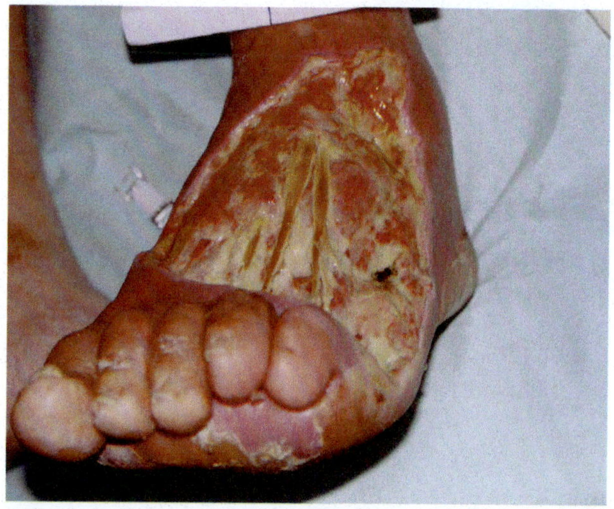

Figure 13.56 The patient from Figure 13.46 at presentation. He had a severe foot infection caused by a small, unnoticed ulcer on the plantar aspect of his foot.

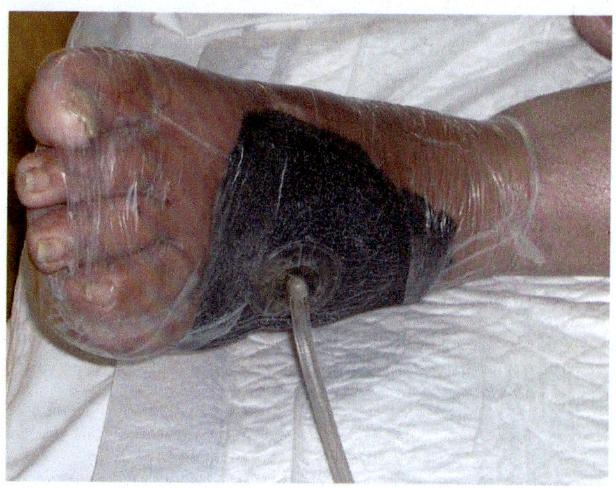

Figure 13.57 Application of negative-pressure wound therapy to the patient shown in Figure 13.56 using the vacuum-assisted closure (V.A.C.) system. The ulcer is covered with a resilient open-celled foam surface dressing covered with an adhesive drape to maintain a closed environment.

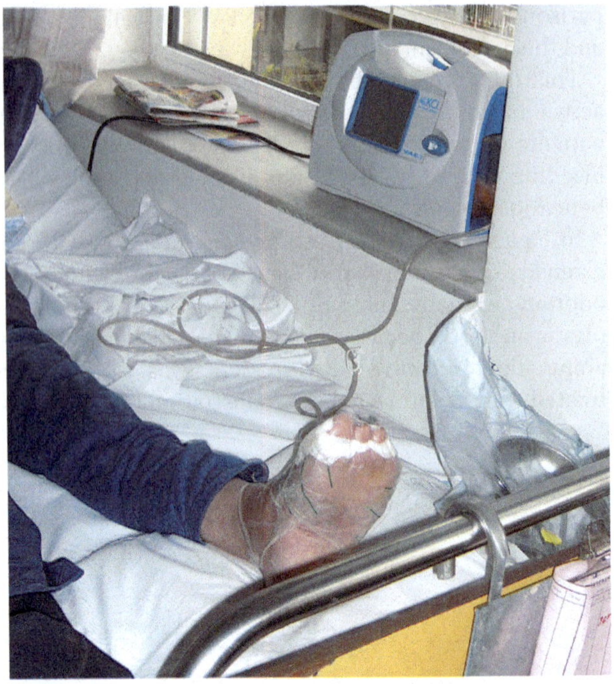

Figure 13.58 The foam dressing is connected to the V.A.C device.

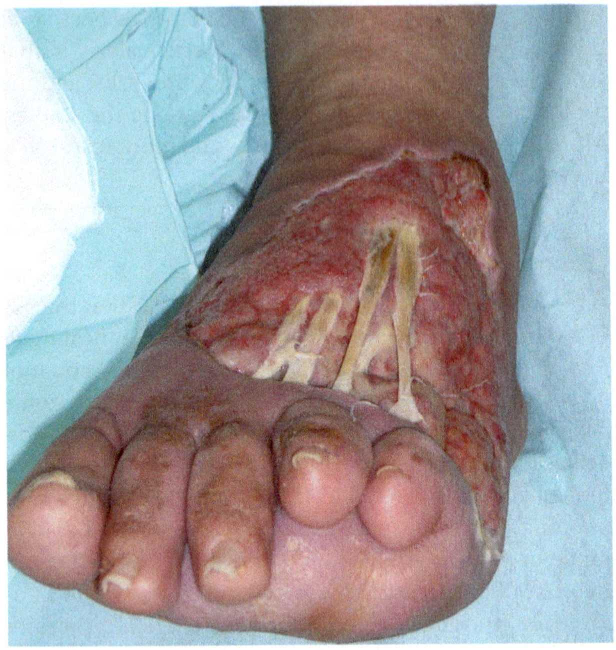

Figure 13.60 The result of V.A.C. therapy after three weeks.

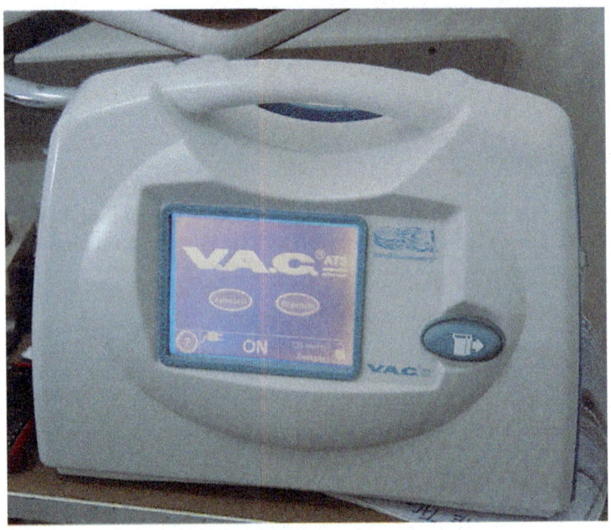

Figure 13.59 The V.A.C. in operation.

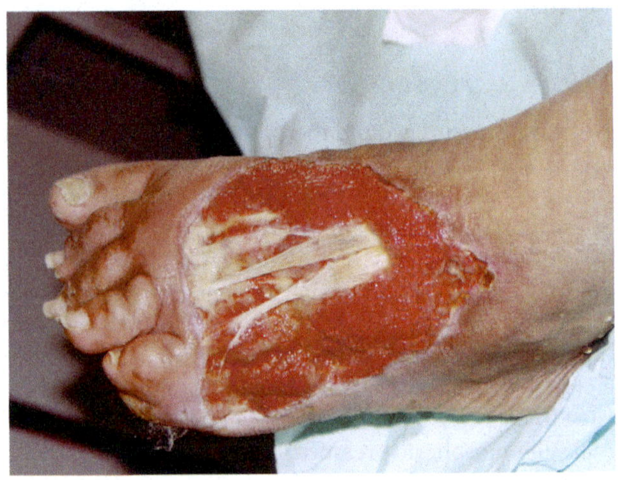

Figure 13.61 Healthy granulation tissue covers the wound area. At this time, V.A.C. therapy was discontinued.

and V.A.C. until the ulcer was covered by healthy granulation tissue. He was then (see Figures 13.46–13.50 above) treated with bioengineered skin substitutes, with complete ulcer healing.

13.9.4 Hyperbaric Oxygen

There is strong evidence suggesting that fibroblasts, endothelial cells and keratinocytes are replicated at higher rates in an oxygen-rich environment. Moreover, leukocytes kill bacteria most effectively when supplied with oxygen. It is also known that fibroblasts from individuals with diabetes show diminished cell turn-over in comparison with those from non-diabetic controls. Based on these data, the idea was that the administration of oxygen at high concentrations might accelerate wound healing in diabetes.

Treatment with hyperbaric oxygen therapy is the intermittent administration of 100% oxygen at a pressure greater than that at sea level. It is delivered in a chamber with the patient breathing 100% oxygen intermittently while the atmospheric pressure is increased to 2–3 atm

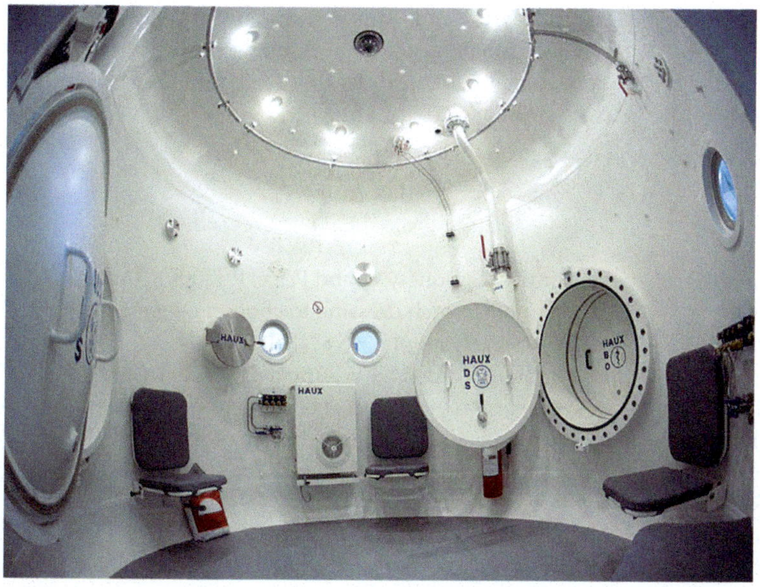

Figure 13.62 A multiplace chamber to treat multiple individuals with hyperbaric oxygen.

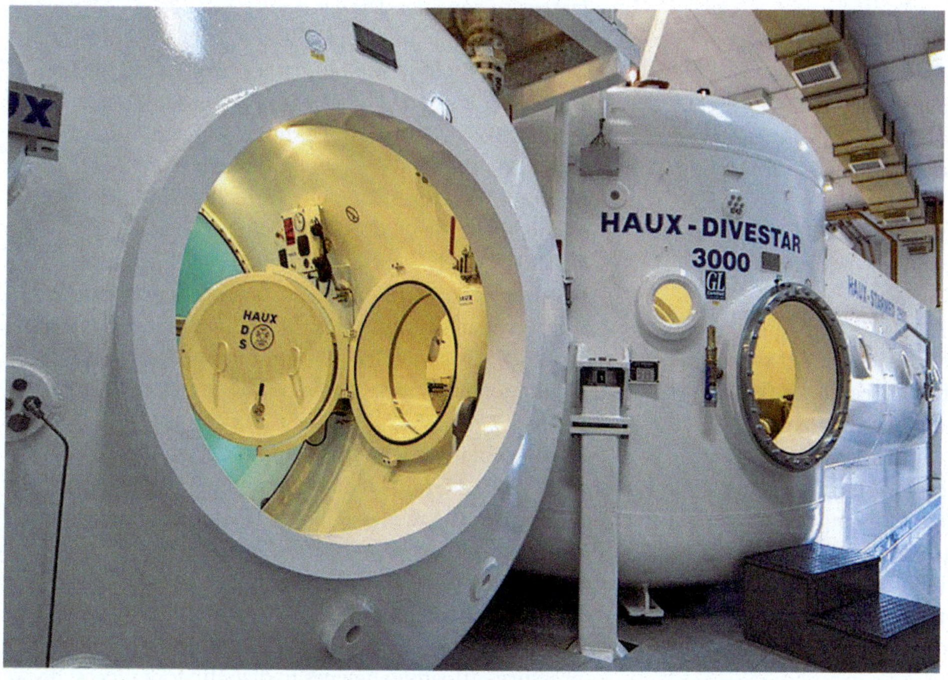

Figure 13.63 The outer aspect of the multiplace chamber.

absolute. This lasts for one to two hours. A full course typically involves 30–40 of these sessions. The technique can usually be implemented in multiplace chambers (Figures 13.62 and 13.63) compressed to depth with air while the patient breaths 100% oxygen via a face mask or head tent.

There are no controlled trials comparing the effectiveness of systemic hyperbaric oxygen therapy in the treatment of neuropathic ulcers. Small studies and a systematic review suggested that this treatment reduced amputations and accelerated healing in patients with neuropathic ulcers. A recent meta-analysis of randomized clinical trials showed no difference between hyperbaric oxygen therapy and standard therapy in the healed ulcer rate, risk of major and minor amputations, and adverse events. However, hyperbaric oxygen therapy was associated with a greater reduction in the ulcer wound area than standard treatment.

Hyperbaric oxygen therapy can be tried also as an adjunctive therapy for patients with severe soft foot infections and osteomyelitis that has not responded to other treatments. Adverse effects include barotrauma to the ears and sinuses, pneumothorax, transient changes in visual acuity and seizures. The topical use of hyperbaric oxygen does not seem to offer advantages over standard treatment.

Further Reading

Armstrong, D.G., Lavery, L.A., Wu, S., and Boulton, A.J. (2005.). Evaluation of removable and irremovable cast walkers in the healing of diabetic foot wounds: a randomized controlled trial. *Diabetes Care* 28: 551–514.

Armstrong, D.G., Nguyen, H.C., Lavery, L.A. et al. (2001). Off-loading the diabetic foot wound: a randomized clinical trial. *Diabetes Care* 24: 1019–1022.

Babaei, V., Afradi, H., Gohardani, H.Z. et al. (2017). Management of chronic diabetic foot ulcers using platelet-rich plasma. *J. Wound Care* 26: 784–787.

Bowler, P.G., Jones, S.A., Davies, B.J., and Coyle, E. (1999). Infection control properties of some wound dressing. *J. Wound Care* 8: 499–502.

Brett, D.W. (2005). Bacterial resistance to silver in wound care. *J. Hosp. Infect.* 60: 1–7.

Clark, R.A.F. (1996). Wound repair: overview and general considerations. In: *The Molecular and Cellular Basis of Wound Repair* (ed. R.A.F. Clark), 3–50. New York: Plenum Press.

Cutting, K., White, R., and Edmonds, M. (2007). The safety and efficacy of dressings with silver – addressing clinical concerns. *Int. Wound J.* 4: 177–184.

Dinh, T., Pham, H., and Veves, A. (2002). Emerging treatments in diabetic wound care. *Wounds* 14: 2–10.

Edmonts, M.E., Bates, M., Doxford, M. et al. (2000). New treatments in ulcer healing and wound infection. *Diabetes Metab. Res. Rev.* 16 (Suppl. 1): S51–S54.

Edmonds, M., Lázaro-Martínez, J.L., Alfayate-García, J.M. et al. (2018). Sucrose octasulfate dressing versus control dressing in patients with neuroischaemic diabetic foot ulcers (explorer): an international, multicentre, double-blind, randomized, controlled trial. *Lancet Diabetes Endocrinol.* 6 (3): 186–196. https://doi.org/10.1016/S2213-8587(17)30438-2.

Eneroth, M. and van Houtum, W.H. (2008). The value of debridement and vacuum-assisted closure (V.A.C.) therapy in diabetic foot ulcers. *Diabetes Metab. Res. Rev.* 24 (Suppl. 1): S76–S80.

Falanga, V. (2005). Wound healing and its impairment in the diabetic foot. *Lancet* 366: 1736–1743.

Guo, J., Dardik, A., Fang, K. et al. (2017). Meta-analysis on the treatment of diabetic foot ulcers with autologous stem cells. *Stem Cell Res. Ther.* 8 (1): 228.

Harding, K.G., Jones, V., and Price, P. (2000). Topical treatment: which dressing to choose. *Diabetes Metab. Res. Rev.* 16 (Suppl. 1): S47–S50.

Hinchliffe, R.J., Valk, G.D., Apelqvist, J. et al. (2008). A systematic review of the effectiveness of interventions to enhance the healing of chronic ulcers of the foot in diabetes. *Diabetes Metab. Res. Rev.* 24 (Suppl. 1): S119–S144.

Hinchliffe, R.J., Valk, G.D., Apelqvist, J. et al. (2008). Specific guidelines on wound and wound-bed management. *Diabetes Metab. Res. Rev.* 24 (Suppl. 1): S188–S189.

Jones, V. (1998). Selecting a dressing for the diabetic foot: factors to consider. *Diabet. Foot* 1: 48–52.

Lindley, L.E., Stojadinovic, O., Pastar, I., and Tomic-Canic, M. (2016). Biology and biomarkers for wound healing. *Plast. Reconstr. Surg.* 138 (3 Suppl): 18S–28S.

Petre, M., Tokar, P., Kostar, D., and Cavanagh, P.R. (2005). Revisiting the total contact cast: maximizing off-loading by wound isolation. *Diabetes Care* 28: 929–930.

Romanelli, M., Piaggesi, A., Scapagnini, G. et al. (2017). EUREKA study – the evaluation of real-life use of a biophotonic system in chronic wound management: an interim analysis. *Drug Des. Devel. Ther.* 11: 3551–3558.

Singer, A.J., Tassiopoulos, A., and Kirsner, R.S. (2017). Evaluation and management of lower-extremity ulcers. *N. Engl. J. Med.* 377: 1559–1567.

Veves, A., Falanga, V., Armstrong, D.G., and Sabolinski, M.L. (2001). Graftskin, a human skin equivalent, is effective in the management of noninfected neuropathic diabetic foot ulcers. *Diabetes Care* 24: 290–295.

Weiss, S.J. (1989). Tissue destruction by neutrophils. *N. Engl. J. Med.* 320: 365–376.

Wu, S.C., Jensen, J.L., Weber, A.K. et al. (2008). Use of pressure offloading devices in diabetic foot ulcers: do we practice what we preach? *Diabetes Care* 31: 2118–2119.

Wu, L., Norman, G., Dumville, J.C. et al. (2015). Dressings for treating foot ulcers in people with diabetes: an overview of systematic reviews. *Cochrane Database Syst. Rev.* 14 (7): CD010471.

Zhao, D., Luo, S., Xu, W. et al. (2017). Efficacy and safety of hyperbaric oxygen therapy used in patients with diabetic foot: a meta-analysis of randomized clinical trials. *Clin. Ther.* 39 (10): 2088–2094.

14

Amputations

K. Makrilakis and I. Eleftheriadou

First Department of Propaedeutic Internal Medicine, National and Kapodistrian University of Athens, Medical School, Laiko General Hospital, Athens, Greece

Amputation surgery on the diabetic foot is a real challenge for the surgeon since it should be regarded as a reconstructive procedure in order for the remaining foot to be functioning as before, with or without a prosthesis. The timing of the procedure, the surgical technique, the level of amputation, and the rehabilitation program are equally important.

The main reasons for a foot or leg amputation in patients with diabetes are ischemia (about 70%) and/or infection (approximately 30%). A less common reason is the presence of severe foot deformity as a consequence of the Charcot foot of the ankle, resulting in a distortion of foot function.

Amputations in patients with diabetes are performed at a younger age in comparison with the non-diabetic population. Many patients are candidates for multiple amputations. Overall, about 40% of the patients with diabetes have a second amputation on the same or the contralateral foot within a period of 1.5–2 years after the first amputation. An unnecessary amputation for a chronic non-healing neuropathic ulcer may solve the problem only temporarily; even minor amputations distort the architecture of the foot, and patients are prone to reamputation in the future. Additionally, mortality following amputation is high: approximately 40–50% of patients with diabetes die during a period of five years after the first amputation.

Until the last part of the twentieth century, partial foot amputations and disarticulations were rarely carried out on patients with diabetes, and major, usually transtibial or transfemoral, amputations were performed, aiming at safe primary healing. Currently, the trend is toward a clear reduction in the rates of major amputation in diabetes, while the rates of minor amputation have increased.

However, determination of the level of the amputation is still controversial. Currently, the level of amputation is determined preoperatively by clinical examination and the results of non-invasive arterial blood flow studies. The level of adequate circulation in the leg, determined by palpation of the pulses, an ankle–brachial index of over 0.5, a transcutaneous partial pressure of oxygen of 30–40 mmHg or more, and popliteal systolic pressures over 70 mmHg obtained on ultrasound Doppler imaging are used by many surgeons as criteria for the level of amputation because such values guarantee wound healing. Other more sophisticated techniques, including fluorescein angiography, laser techniques and radioisotope clearance, also exist. Generally, more distal levels of limb amputation reduce the need for extensive prostheses and reduce the amount of energy required for ambulation.

A careful program of medical and surgical intervention can prevent most limb amputations. However, amputation may represent an acceptable option for patients facing a prolonged course of treatment and a poor prognosis in order to obtain a successful outcome. The decision to undertake an amputation should be obtained by a team of a diabetologist with knowledge and experience in foot problems, a vascular surgeon, a specialist in infectious diseases in the presence of infection, and a general or orthopedic surgeon, and should not be left to one single healthcare professional to determine.

Currently, no consensus exists on the indications for amputation. However, the following situations are indications for a foot or leg amputation:

- the presence of severe chronic ischemic pain at rest attributable to objectively proven arterial occlusive disease that is not amenable to vascular reconstructive surgery and that cannot be controlled;
- an overwhelming foot infection that threatens the patient's life (Figure 14.1);

Atlas of the Diabetic Foot, Third Edition. Ioanna Eleftheriadou, Alexandros Kokkinos, Stavros Liatis, Konstantinos Makrilakis, Nicholas Tentolouris, Anastasios Tentolouris, and Panagiotis Tsapogas.

Companion website: www.wiley.com/go/tentolouris/atlas_diabetic_foot

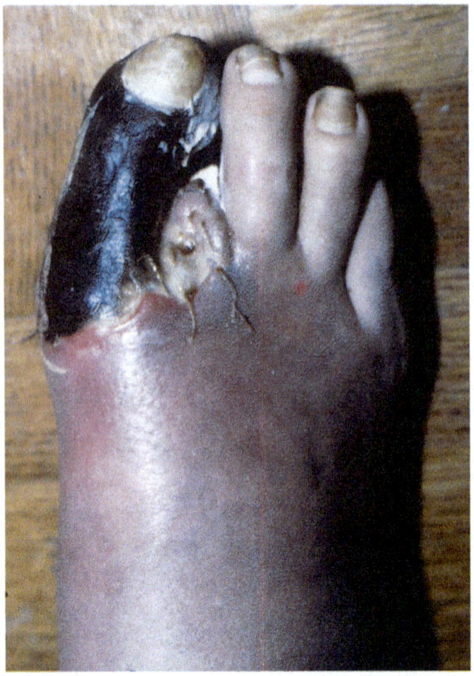

Figure 14.1 Wet gangrene, an indication for a wider amputation.

- the presence of necrosis secondary to an arterial occlusion that has destroyed the foot;
- a non-functional foot due to severe foot infection or deformity caused by neuro-osteoarthropathy that has destroyed the ankle joint, and when efforts at internal fixation or external stabilization are not possible or have failed.

Regarding revascularization, not all patients should be considered for such procedures, and primary amputation may sometimes be the best option. The degree on the mobility grading system (Box 14.1) can help with the decision between revascularization and primary amputation.

Box 14.1 Degrees of Mobility

1) Free mobility indoors and outdoors
2) Free mobility outdoors with support
3) Free mobility indoors with support
4) Wheelchair dependency
5) Bedridden: not able to move around.

Patients in categories 4 and 5 who are referred with a septic foot are a special group because extensive debridement and revascularization may be successful; however, because they are not ambulatory, the benefit from extensive procedures for limb salvage is not impressive. An exception is patients belonging to category 4 (partly independent) who have already had a leg amputation; in this particular case, it is extremely important to make every effort to preserve the remaining leg in order to avoid complete dependency (category 5).

Many orthopedic surgeons perform amputations of toes affected by osteomyelitis. Amputation of the distal phalanx of a small toe does not result in severe deformity or changes in foot biomechanics. However, many such cases can be managed successfully with long-term antibiotic administration providing there is adequate blood supply to the feet.

Foot amputations are classified as longitudinal, transverse, intercalary, through joints and through bone (Box 14.2). The level of foot amputation is depicted in Box 14.3.

It is important to create a functional stump after an amputation. As a rule, the longer the length of the stump, the better the functionality of the remaining limb. The length of the stump at foot level defines the boundary of the supporting area, which is important for the neuropathic patient. The stump must be covered with a healthy fat pad and skin, particularly in the weight-bearing area,

Box 14.2 Foot Amputations

- **Longitudinal** (+ ray amputations)
- **Transverse** (+semi transverse)
  - **close**
    - one stage
    - two stages (Syme's)
  - **open**
    - two stages (guillotine)
- **Intercalary** (i.e., scaphoidectomy)
- **Through joints** (disarticulation)
- **Through bones**

Box 14.3 Levels of foot amputation

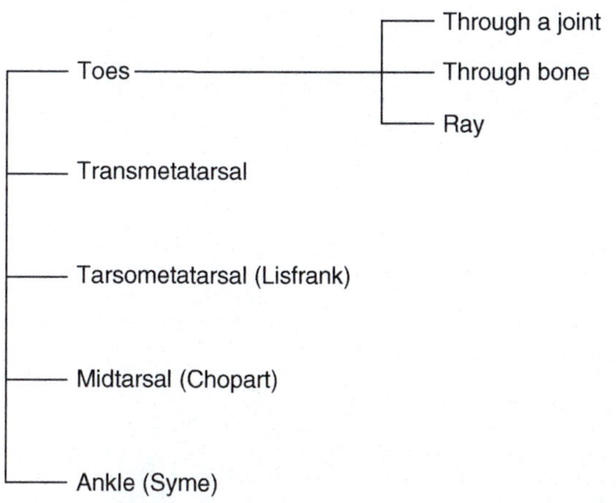

to function as a shock absorber and support the function of the prosthesis.

Prosthetic management is demanding because the prosthesis has to be weight-bearing, functional, and cosmetically acceptable. Thus, it has to:

- complete the space of the stump in the shoe;
- provide a shock-absorbing mechanism;
- distribute the loading forces to a wider area;
- be light enough;
- be easy to put on and take off;
- be stable with rotating forces, particularly in foot push-off;
- be suitable for any fashion shoes;
- be constructed with material that is friendly to the skin.

14.1 Amputation of the Toes

Removal of the great toe results in dysfunction of the foot during both stance and propulsion. This disability is related to the length of the removed metatarsal shaft. Most surgeons preserve the longest metatarsal shaft possible.

In addition, the base of the proximal phalanx must be preserved because the tendon of flexor hallucis brevis is attached with the sesamoid bones integrated in it, keeping the sesamoids in place and maintaining the windlass mechanism (Figures 14.2–14.4). This mechanism protects the first metatarsal head from overloading during the propulsion phase of gait.

In the case of an obligatory removal of the hallux, the surgeon should preserve all uninvolved portions of the metatarsal, except the avascular sesamoids and their fibrocartilagenous plate. A hallux disarticulation at the metatarsophalangeal joint exposes the head of the third metatarsal to abnormally high pressure during stance and may displace the second toe medially (Figure 14.5).

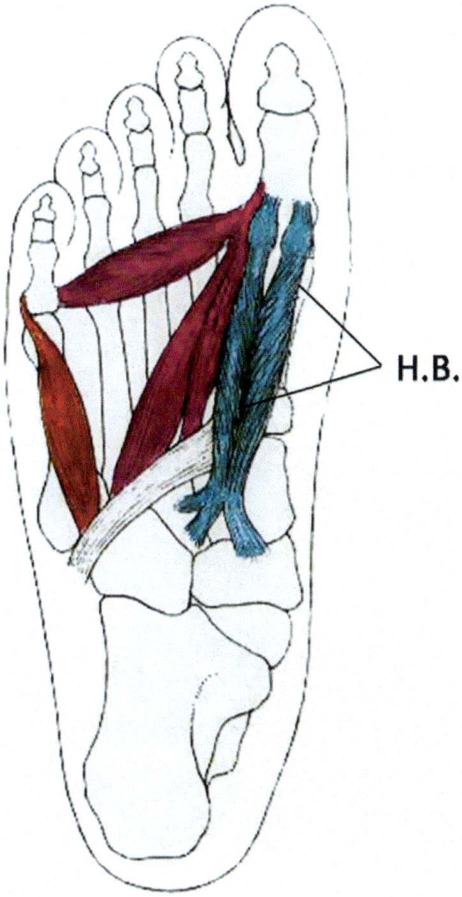

Figure 14.2 The flexor hallucis brevis (HB) attaches to the tendon of the proximal phalanx. The sesamoids are integrated into each part of the tendon.

Ablation of the second toe is not allowed because the big toe loses its lateral support, and this results in a hallux valgus deformity (Figures 14.6–14.8). Instead of second toe ablation, a second ray resection should be performed (Figure 14.9 and 14.10), so that the first ray remains intact and provides a wider supporting area during standing and in the propulsion phase of gait.

Amputations of the other toes or ray resections can be performed without major functional disturbance. The preservation of one single lesser toe is unacceptable because of lack of functionality and problems with wearing shoes. Ablation of all five toes (poblectomy) is an acceptable and functional amputation. Toe prostheses are shoe-fillers that provide stability for the remaining toes and better shoe-holding in combination with a proper insole.

In the case of a wider forefoot amputation, the prosthesis has to provide filling of the space in the shoe and a better holding and distribution of the pressures and forces in the remaining forefoot. Thus, it has to include

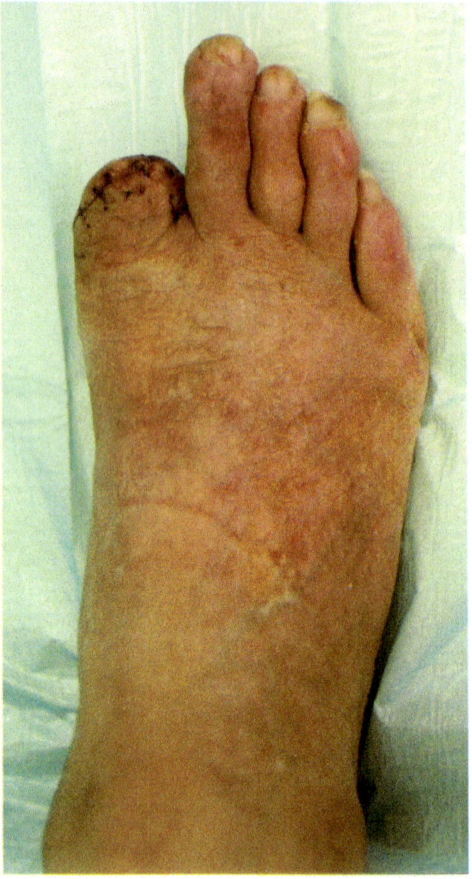

Figure 14.3 The base of the proximal phalanx has to be retained because the tendon of flexor hallucis brevis is attached with the sesamoids integrated in it, keeping the sesamoids in place and maintaining the windlass mechanism.

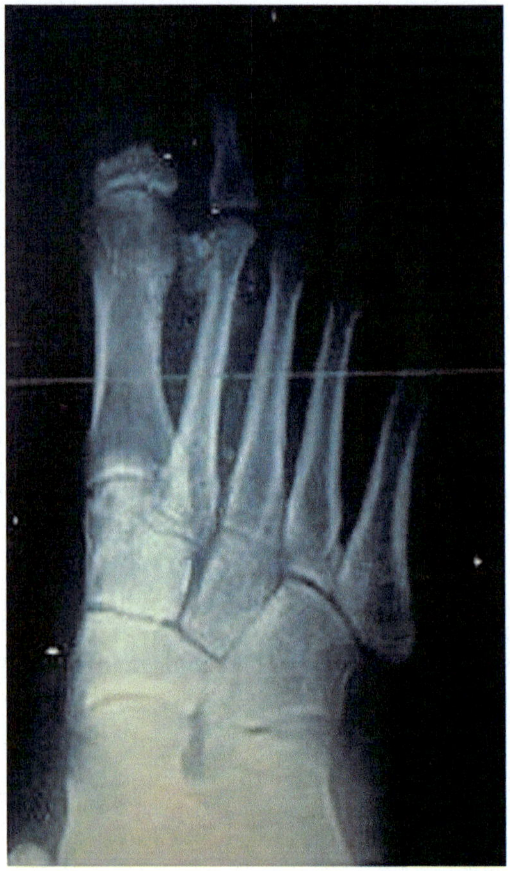

Figure 14.4 X-ray showing amputation of the distal and preservation of the proximal phalanx.

the whole foot under the ankle. In minor toe amputations, patients often require esthetic toe replacements and custom-made silicone toes.

14.2 Midfoot (Lisfranc and Chopart) Amputations

In Lisfranc (at the junction of the tarsus and metatarsus) amputations, the balance of the foot is not disturbed, and both provide an excellent weight-bearing platform for walking. In a Chopart amputation, the stump is unbalanced in an equinous position, because of detachment of the tibialis anterior, but the Achilles tendon continues functioning. The equinous deformity can be avoided by either reattachment of the tibialis anterior to the neck of talus, or performing percutaneous Achilles tendon lengthening at the time of surgery.

In midfoot amputations, the prosthesis, apart from filling the space in the shoe, has to provide stability up to the height of the metatarsal heads compatible with the

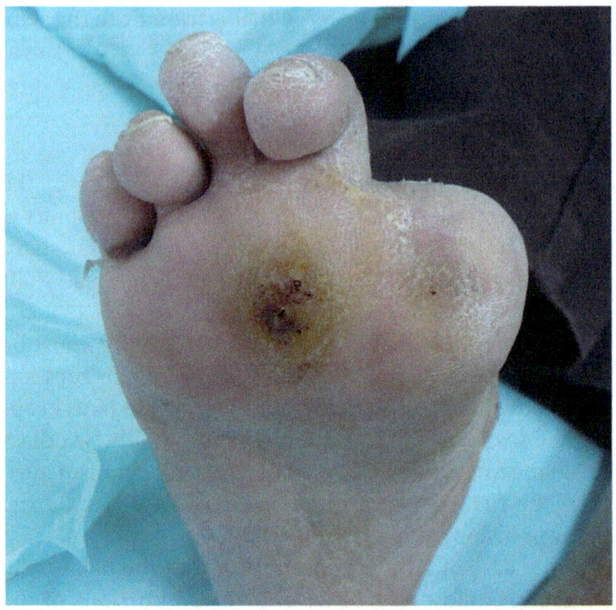

Figure 14.5 Callus formation over the third metatarsal head due to great toe disarticulation and subsequent high pressure on this area.

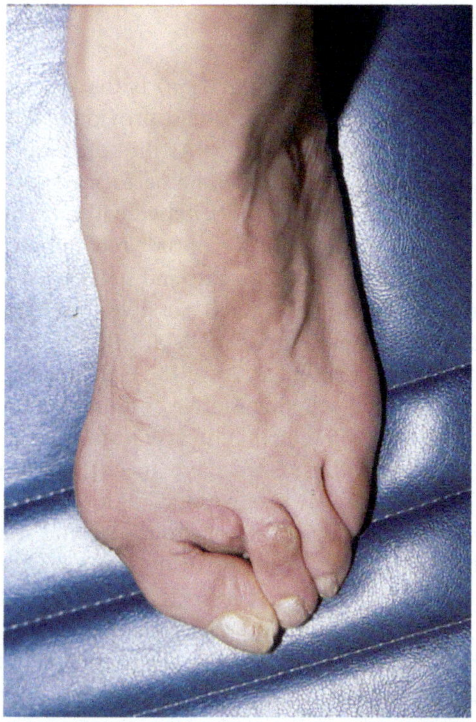

Figure 14.6 Hallux valgus deformity after second toe amputation.

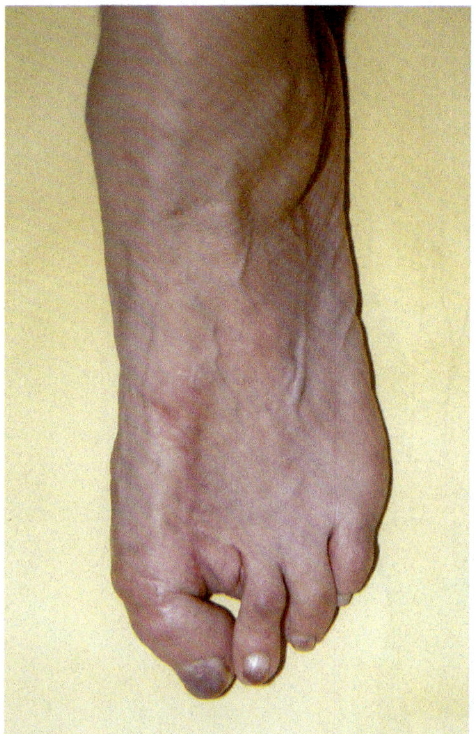

Figure 14.8 A hallux valgus deformity after second toe removal.

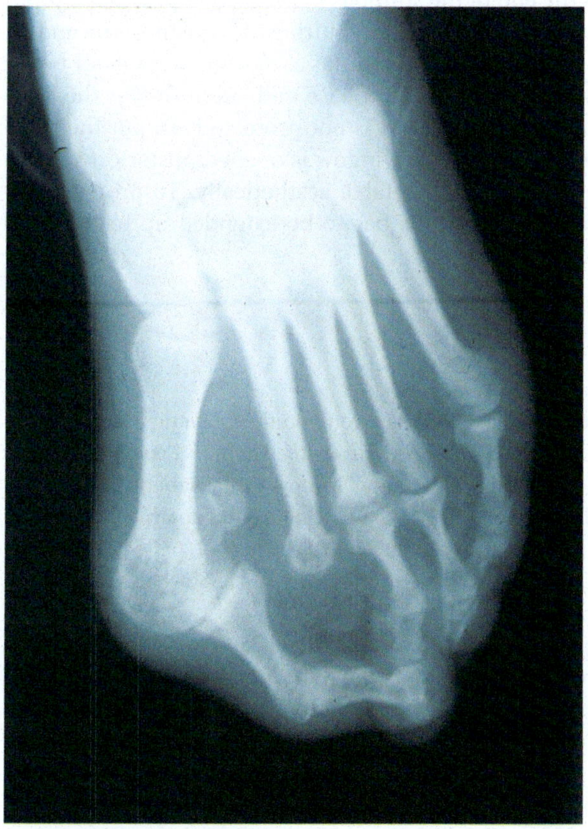

Figure 14.7 X-ray showing amputation of the second toe and severe hallux valgus deformity.

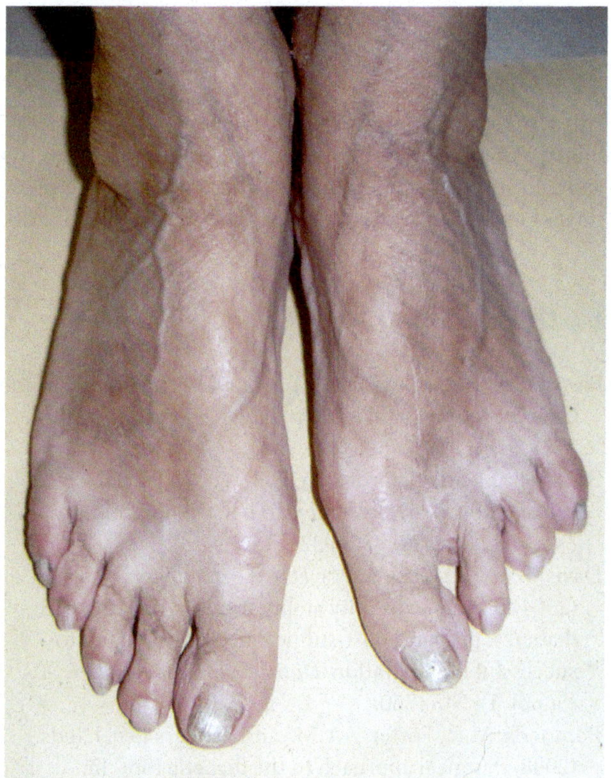

Figure 14.9 Correction of hallux valgus after completion of the second ray amputation of the patient shown in Figure 14.8.

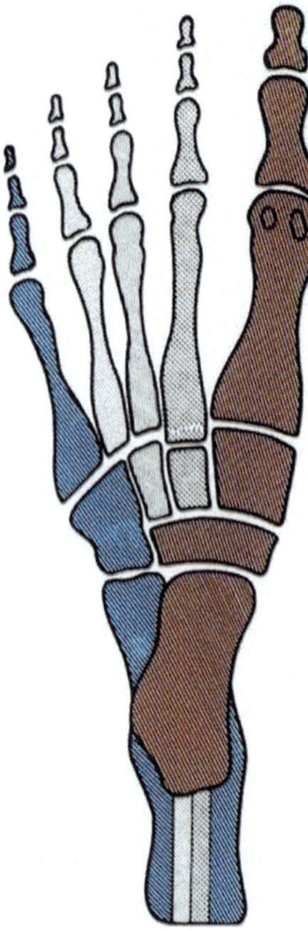

Figure 14.10 Rays of foot amputation: the lateral or calcaneal ray (in blue), and the inner or talar ray (in brown).

stiffness required in push-off. It also has to provide flexibility so that it can permit pronation and supination as the subtalar joint is functioning. For these reasons, the prosthesis can be below or above the ankle, if the ankle is stiff.

14.3 Hindfoot Amputations

Ankle disarticulation (Syme amputation) is the highest foot amputation and can be performed providing that the heel fat pad and skin are healthy. As the soft tissues are not secure, the procedure has to be performed with the minimum possible damage and stitched without any tension. For the above reasons, we do not recommend removing the malleoli in the first stage, and suggest leaving the dog ears of the skin as long as possible. After the wound has healed, we remove the malleoli with the skin of the dog ears in a second stage. After the envelope has been closed, the fat pad remains mobile and may sometimes become displaced, requiring intervention.

With the Syme prosthesis, we have to correct the limb length discrepancy and reproduce ankle motion. The space between the distal end of the stump and the floor is so limited that it is not possible to fit a joint mechanism. Therefore, the prosthesis is manufactured with a non-articulated foot, but the heel of this foot, called SACH (solid ankle–cushion heel), is collapsible and is slightly modified from the tibial-as-femoral prosthesis.

The prosthetic foot is also elastic (carbon fiber) so the cushion heel and the elastic foot provide elasticity in gait. As the end of the stump is bulbous, two prosthetic problems arise. The first is in putting the prosthesis on and off as the socket has an isthmus above the malleoli for better hanging in the swing phase and, additionally, the rotation of the prosthesis is not protected. To put the prosthesis on and off, a window is opened posteriorly, which is not usually acceptable aesthetically. To protect rotation, the prosthesis has to be extended up to the tibial condyles.

Further Reading

Baravarian, B. and Van Gils, C.C. (2004). Arthrodesis of the Charcot foot and ankle. *Clin. Podiatr. Med. Surg.* 21: 271–289.

Bollinger, M. and Thordarson, D.B. (2002). Partial calcanectomy: an alternative to below knee amputation. *Foot Ankle Int.* 23: 927–932.

Davis, B.L., Kuznicki, J., Praveen, S.S., and Sferra, J.J. (2004). Lower-extremity amputations in patients with diabetes: pre- and post-surgical decisions related to successful rehabilitation. *Diabetes Metab. Res. Rev.* 20 (Suppl. 1): S45–S50.

Edmonds, M.E., Foster, A.V.M., and Sanders Lee, J. (eds.) (2008). Surgical approach to the diabetic foot. In: *Practical Manual of Diabetic Foot Care*, 229–272. Massachusetts: Blackwell.

International Working Group on the Diabetic Foot (1999). *International Consensus on the Diabetic Foot.* Amsterdam: International Working Group on the Diabetic Foot.

Johnson, J.E. (2001). Charcot neuroathropathy of the foot: surgical aspects. In: *The Diabetic Foot*, 6e (ed. M.E. Levin, M.A. Pfeifer and J. Bowker), 587–606. St Louis: Mosby.

Lipsky, B.A. (2004). International consensus group on diagnosing and treating the infected diabetic foot. A report from the international consensus on diagnosing and treating the infected diabetic foot. *Diabetes Metab. Res. Rev.* 20 (Suppl. 1): S68–S77.

Lipsky, B.A., Berendt, A.R., Embil, J., and De Lalla, F. (2004). Diagnosing and treating diabetic foot infections. *Diabetes Metab. Res. Rev.* 20 (Suppl. 1): S56–S64.

Lipsky, B.A., Armstrong, D.G., Citron, D.M. et al. (2005). Ertapenem versus piperacillin/tazobactam for diabetic foot infections (SIDESTEP): prospective, randomized, controlled, double-blinded, multicentre trial. *Lancet* 366: 1695–1703.

Peters, E.J., Childs, M.R., Wunderlich, R.P. et al. (2001). Functional status of persons with diabetes-related lower-extremity amputations. *Diabetes Care* 24: 1799–1804.

Pinzur, M.S. (2000). Amputations in the diabetic foot. In: *The Foot in Diabetes*, 4e (ed. A.J.M. Boulton and G. Rayman), 308–322. Chichester: Wiley.

Van Ross, E.R.E. and Carlsson, T. (2000). Rehabilitation of the amputee with diabetes. In: *The Foot in Diabetes*, 4e (ed. A.J.M. Boulton and G. Rayman), 323–335. Chichester: Wiley.

Appendix

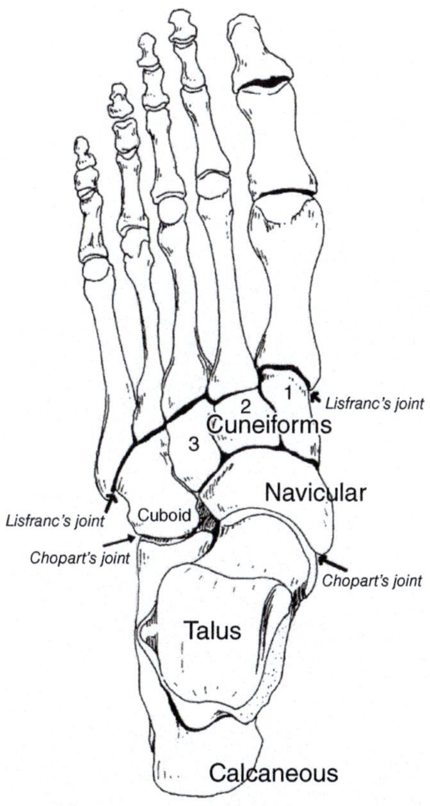

Figure A.1 Bones of the foot: dorsal aspect.

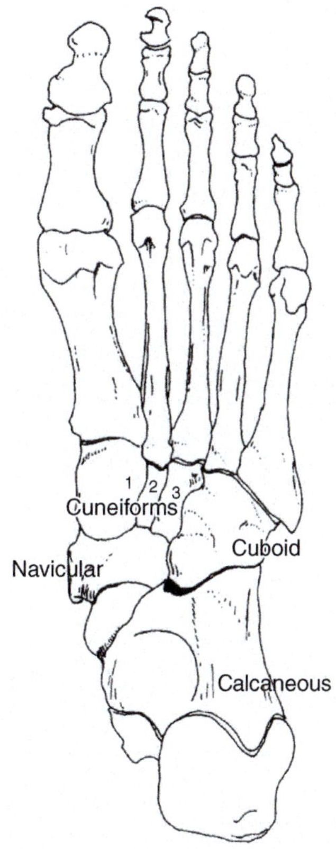

Figure A.2 Bones of the foot: plantar aspect.

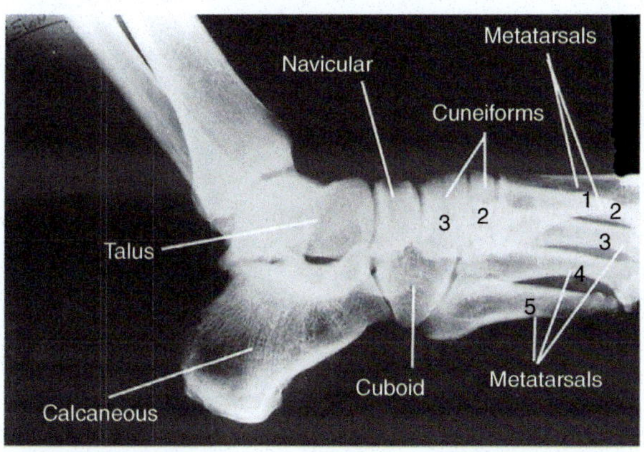

Figure A.3 Bones of the foot: plain radiograph of a lateral view.

Atlas of the Diabetic Foot, Third Edition. Ioanna Eleftheriadou, Alexandros Kokkinos, Stavros Liatis, Konstantinos Makrilakis, Nicholas Tentolouris, Anastasios Tentolouris, and Panagiotis Tsapogas.

Companion website: www.wiley.com/go/tentolouris/atlas_diabetic_foot

Index

Page locators in **bold** indicate tables. Page locators in *italics* indicate figures. This index uses letter-by-letter alphabetization.

Atlas of the Diabetic Foot, Third Edition. Ioanna Eleftheriadou, Alexandros Kokkinos, Stavros Liatis, Konstantinos Makrilakis, Nicholas Tentolouris, Anastasios Tentolouris, and Panagiotis Tsapogas.

Companion website: www.wiley.com/go/tentolouris/atlas_diabetic_foot

v

w

y

Wiley The manufacturer's authorized representative according to the EU General Product Safety Regulation is Wiley-VCH GmbH, Boschstr. 12, 69469 Weinheim, Germany, e-mail: Product_Safety@wiley.com.

Printed and bound by CPI Group (UK) Ltd, Croydon, CR0 4YY
22/09/2026
02220338-0001